Rodal

S0-CRS-767

LIBRARY OF
THE NEW YORK
STATE VET. COL. · BOOK NO.

28.00
9/81

Applied Physiology of
Respiratory Care

Applied Physiology of Respiratory Care

John Hedley-Whyte, M.D.
George E. Burgess III, M.D.
Thomas W. Feeley, M.D.
Malcolm G. Miller, M.B., Ch. B.

Harvard Medical School

Little, Brown and Company · Boston

Copyright © 1976 by Little, Brown and Company (Inc.)

First Edition

Third Printing

All rights reserved. No part of this book may be reproduced in any form or by any electronic or mechanical means, including information storage and retrieval systems, without permission in writing from the publisher, except by a reviewer who may quote brief passages in a review.

Library of Congress Catalog Card No. 75-36760

ISBN 0-316-35420-1

Printed in the United States of America

To David S. Sheridan
Upon skillful design and manufacture of equipment does respiratory care depend.

Preface

This book is intended primarily as a guide for physicians and other hospital personnel who care for critically ill patients. Emphasis is on recent advances in the understanding and management of cardiorespiratory failure. Reflecting our experience at the Harvard Medical School and particularly at Beth Israel Hospital in Boston during the last 10 years, the book describes methods that have been useful to us during this time period. Since we feel that personal experience (see Figs. 1 and 2) is highly important, a bias toward local references has been unavoidable.

In addition to our purpose of providing valuable information for medical personnel directly involved in respiratory care, another aim of this book is

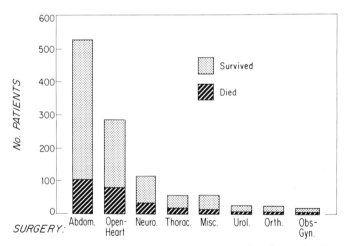

Figure 1. In seven years 1,440 patients were ventilated in the Respiratory–Surgical Intensive Care Unit of the Beth Israel Hospital for respiratory failure. Respiratory failure was defined as a vital capacity less than 10 ml per kilogram of body weight, a respiratory acidemia with an arterial pH below 7.25, or an alveolar-arterial oxygen tension gradient measured on 100% oxygen of greater than 350 mm Hg (46.6 kPa). Of these patients, 1,101 were surgical, almost half of them having had abdominal surgery, generally emergency laparotomy. Seventy-six percent of all surgical patients requiring controlled ventilation for acute respiratory failure survived. During this period there were 130 beds in the surgical wards of our hospital.

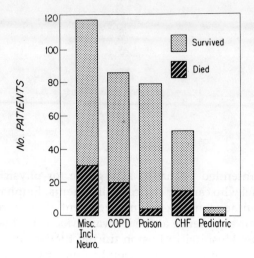

Figure 2. In our institution only 339 of 1,440 patients who required ventilation due to respiratory failure were from the medical service. Of these patients, 79 percent survived—essentially the same survival rate as after surgery. We usually do not ventilate patients with terminal chronic obstructive pulmonary disease (COPD). *CHF* = congestive heart failure.

to serve as a source of information for board examination candidates in the medical and surgical specialities, including respiratory therapy. A question ever present in our minds as we wrote and revised the manuscript was "Might a board candidate be required to give an examiner this information?"

It is our hope that this book stimulates interest in respiratory care and contributes to improved management of critically ill patients. We encourage feedback from our readers on errors or significant omissions.

J. H-W.
G. E. B. III
T. W. F.
M. G. M.

Boston

Acknowledgments

We would especially like to thank the Bushnells. Sharon Spaeth Bushnell's book *Respiratory Intensive Care Nursing* is a most useful companion to this book.[281] Her husband, Leonard S. Bushnell, is Director of Respiratory Therapy at Beth Israel Hospital.

We also thank John Joakim Skillman for his long-standing instruction of each of us in the complexities of the surgical management of critically ill patients.

We are indebted to the nursing staff of the Respiratory–Surgical Intensive Care Unit. Countless hours of work and expert care by nurses have made modern respiratory care possible. We would also like to thank Drs. Inder Malhotra, Dorothy Crawford, and L. Hans Laasberg and their colleagues for advice and criticism. While we wrote this book, they allowed us time from our more routine obligations.

We thank the respiratory therapists with whom we have worked in the last 10 years. Theirs is a difficult role and so are their examinations. Perhaps as a requisite to recertification physicians should be required to pass the respiratory therapy examination. The respiratory care team might then function with more mutual understanding.

Joan Krier, Mary Anne Becker, and Linda McAulay typed and retyped the manuscript several times; their skill and forbearance are much appreciated. Elizabeth Sheldon was of enormous help in verifying references.

Contents

I

General Management of Respiratory Failure

1

Effect of Controlled Ventilation on the Upper Airway

The presence of a tracheal tube for controlled ventilation or for airway protection is associated with some damage to the upper airway in nearly all patients.[840] The majority of these injuries are related to the pressure exerted by the tracheal tube on the air passages. Although damage can occur anywhere along the course of the tracheal tube, the most common sites are in the larynx and in the trachea. Innovations in the design of tracheal tubes have lowered the incidence of airway injury in the past few years.

PHARYNGEAL AND LARYNGEAL INJURIES

PATHOGENESIS

Damage to the oropharynx and nasopharynx during controlled ventilation is quite rare. Ulceration of the ala nasi follows prolonged nasotracheal intubation in less than 1 percent of patients.[1165] Prolonged orotracheal intubation can result in ulceration of the lips and oral mucosa, especially if the tube is taped with excessive pressure. For this reason any patient receiving prolonged orotracheal intubation should have the tube repositioned daily from one side of the mouth to the other. Ulceration of the pharynx also can occur.[525] Lacerations and contusions of the oropharynx, nasopharynx, and tongue occur most frequently when inexperienced personnel perform the intubation.

Laryngeal injury is more common. In 44 percent of patients short-term intubation (less than 24 hours) leads to gross abnormalities of the larynx. This usually consists of congestion of the vocal cords or of the membranous glottis. In a series of 100 patients receiving short-term intubation all lesions resolved completely and were associated with minor symptoms.[525]

Following prolonged (more than 24 hours) tracheal intubation, the laryngeal complications become more serious. Alterations in the mucosa can be found in areas constantly affected. The most common sites are the medial portion of the arytenoid cartilage, usually on the vocal process, the interarytenoid area, and the inner posterolateral region of the cricoid cartilage.[874,1165]

Mucosal ulcerations heal in one of two ways. Primary healing, or rapid epithelialization of the injury, occurs in 61 percent of cases. In this group there is complete resolution of the lesion within one month. In the remain-

3

der of cases a stage of granuloma formation occurs. The majority of granulomas resolve spontaneously but may take as long as 10 months to disappear completely. Some may continue to grow, leading to airway obstruction and requiring surgical removal.[1165]

Serious damage occurs most frequently when tubes are in place for more than 72 hours.[840] In such cases the majority of injuries are due to pressure necrosis. Most of the laryngeal lesions seen are posterior (Fig. 1-1), since the tracheal tube exerts the most pressure on the posterior portion of the larynx. Since the arytenoids normally move with each respiratory cycle, they are vulnerable to damage when a tube is placed through the cords.[1165]

Movement of the patient is also an important cause of laryngeal injuries. Patients who move their heads with a tracheal tube in place are more likely to develop laryngeal damage than patients who lie still. We have seen one patient who was extremely agitated during 36 hours of intubation and who went on to have a permanent loss of voice secondary to extensive vocal cord ulceration and scarring.

The size of the tube used can influence the extent of laryngeal damage. Tubes that are large in diameter in relation to laryngeal size are associated

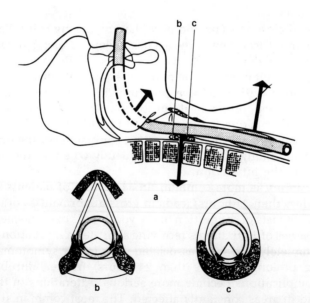

Figure 1-1.   Sites of injury during orotracheal intubation. Schematic representation of an orotracheal tube in an adult. The large arrows (*a*) demonstrate the forces that a curved tracheal tube exerts in an effort to achieve its original shape. Cross sections are drawn (*b*) through the larynx at the level of the vocal cords and (*c*) through the cricoid cartilage. The major forces are exerted on the posterolateral aspect of the larynx, in particular on the medial aspect of the arytenoid cartilages and cricoid cartilage. (From C.-E. Lindholm, *Acta Anaesthesiol. Scand.*[1165])

with a greater number of injuries. This possibly accounts for the greater incidence of laryngeal injuries seen in women. Improper aeration of tracheal tubes following ethylene oxide sterilization can lead to laryngeal damage. Plastic tubes are associated with less laryngeal injury than rubber tubes.[840]

Shock increases laryngeal injury, probably by decreasing blood flow to areas already compromised by the pressure of a tracheal tube.[840] Local infection also can lead to more serious laryngeal damage when a tracheal tube is in place.[1165] Dislocation of the arytenoid cartilage can follow prolonged tracheal intubation.[1553] In addition to damage occurring to the larynx while the tracheal tube is in place, several important complications can ensue following extubation. The first is the sudden development of laryngeal edema. This is most common after prolonged tracheal intubation, but it can follow short-term intubation. The etiology of this entity is unclear; it may result from acute ulceration, acute laryngitis, sudden heart failure, or epiglottitis. We have seen allergy to rubber cause complete airway obstruction after extubation.

Following extubation, laryngeal protection of the airway from aspiration is often inadequate.[483,840] For several hours or even days or weeks after extubation patients may experience difficulty in receiving fluids orally. A high incidence of aspiration during the first 12 hours after extubation has been demonstrated both clinically and radiographically. The reason for this functional impairment of the larynx is unclear. The constant pressure that the tracheal tube places on the submucosal neuronal plexuses may cause insensitivity of the pharynx and larynx and could explain the apparent functional incapacity of the larynx following extubation.

Dionosil dye is useful in evaluating the function of the larynx after extubation. Five ml of dionosil dye is given orally, and a portable chest x-ray is taken one hour later. The degree of aspiration is indicated by the amount of dye in the tracheobronchial tree. This test may be especially helpful in evaluating function in obtunded patients.[483]

DIAGNOSIS

Nasal and oral lesions secondary to tracheal intubation usually can be detected by simple inspection. Pharyngeal ulcerations lead to a persistent sore throat. Complaints should not be dismissed but should be followed up with a careful inspection of the oropharynx, especially in the patient who has had a prolonged period of tracheal intubation.

Lesions involving the larynx usually are detected by complaints of hoarseness, sore throat, and cough. A complaint of hoarseness for more than 48 hours should be investigated by indirect laryngoscopy.

Detection of laryngeal edema following extubation is usually straightforward. Within 3–15 minutes following extubation the patient will develop inspiratory stridor and respiratory distress. The edema is seen during laryngoscopy for reintubation of the trachea. Photographs are valuable for documenting progress.

TREATMENT

A complete discussion of the surgical management of laryngeal lesions is beyond the scope of this text; however, several points should be mentioned. Most granulomas that form will resolve without surgical intervention. Some may progress to produce complete airway obstruction. Permanent hoarseness can occur as a result of prolonged tracheal intubation, caused not by any surgically correctable lesion but by general scarring of the larynx.[840,1165]

PREVENTION

Because of the nature of the lesions that are formed and their occasional irreversible nature, every effort should be made to prevent laryngeal injuries.

The size of the tube is important. The smallest diameter tube with which ventilation can be efficiently maintained should be selected for each patient. Women need smaller diameter tubes than men. Plastic tubes should be used if prolonged orotracheal or nasotracheal intubation is necessary. Patients should not be allowed to become agitated while a tube is present in the larynx.

The exact time at which a tracheostomy should be done is controversial. Timing should vary from patient to patient. Tracheostomy is rarely needed if less than 72 hours of controlled ventilation is necessary. After 72 hours of controlled ventilation the chances of developing laryngeal complications increase, so that if it seems likely that more than 72 hours of controlled ventilation will be necessary, we prefer tracheostomy. It is often quite difficult to predict when a patient will be able to be weaned from the ventilator. One should therefore make a daily assessment of the patient's course in considering when to perform a tracheotomy.

We perform our tracheotomies in the operating room. This provides a controlled situation with sufficient lighting, instruments, and operative personnel. There are many individual variations in the surgical approach to the creation of a tracheostomy. The one constant feature is that the stoma should be made in the region of the second and third tracheal rings. If the stoma is too high, the complications of laryngotomy are severe. Placing the stoma too low results in having the tip of the cannula near the carina. This leads to selective ventilation of one lung and collapse of the other. Furthermore the presence of a foreign body near the carina can lead to bronchospasm.[594,1832,1911] A chest x-ray film should therefore be taken following every tracheostomy to ascertain the position of the tip of the tracheostomy cannula.

TRACHEAL INJURIES

The majority of the tracheal complications of tracheal intubation are related to the presence of a cuff on the tracheal tube.[301,775,953,1053,1272] The possible complications are tracheal stenosis, tracheomalacia, tracheo-esophageal fistula, and tracheoinnominate artery fistula.[841]

PATHOGENESIS

The pathogenesis of injuries produced by tracheal tube cuffs is well documented. The first change is mucosal inflammation under the cuff. This is followed by ulceration of the trachea. Infection in the area hastens the destruction of the trachea. After several days the tracheal rings become exposed[413] (Fig. 1-2) and then begin to soften and disappear. Following extubation this area of tracheomalacia may be extensive enough to collapse and cause airway obstruction. Usually it does not, and over several months

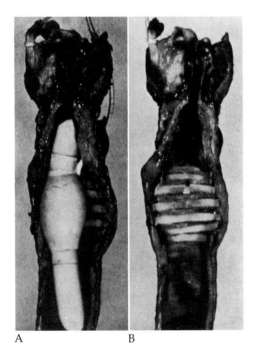

A   B

Figure 1-2. Effect of the high-pressure tracheal tube cuff on the gross anatomy of the trachea. The trachea of a dog after one week of controlled ventilation with a high-pressure cuff is shown. A. Trachea opened and tracheal tube still in place. There is marked dilatation of the trachea at the site of the cuff. B. Severe tracheal damage with exposure of the tracheal rings. This progresses to softening, fragmentation, and eventual sloughing of the affected rings of cartilage. (From J. D. Cooper and H. C. Grillo.[413] By permission of *Surgery, Gynecology & Obstetrics.*)

a band of scar tissue develops which becomes the area of tracheal stenosis.[413,414,1313,1856]

If the lesion is severely destructive, there is erosion posteriorly into the esophagus, which leads to a tracheoesophageal fistula. This lesion is usually found at the site of the tracheal tube cuff.[841] Erosion anteriorly or anterolaterally can lead to the formation of a tracheoinnominate artery fistula also at the site of the cuff.[414]

The tip of the tracheal tube can lead to tracheal damage; however, its importance has been overshadowed by the high incidence of cuff-related injuries.[1910] Perhaps when cuff design prevents injury at the site of the cuff, we will see more injuries at the site of the tip of the tracheal tube.

In order to provide a complete seal of the trachea during positive pressure ventilation, the pressure inside the cuff must be equal to or greater than the pressure needed to inflate the lung. Standard cuffs must distend the trachea until it is occluded[413] (Fig. 1-3), and pressures as high as 180–250 mm Hg (24–33 kPa) are necessary to get occlusion.[414,1272] External pressure on a capillary will stop flow when the pressure is 32–60 mm Hg (4–8 kPa). In many instances the tracheal wall pressures exerted by conventional tracheal tube cuffs far exceed this capillary occlusion pressure and lead to ischemia and ulceration.[1053]

DIAGNOSIS

Signs of tracheal stenosis or tracheomalacia may be seen while the patient is in respiratory failure. Tracheomalacia is suspected when increasing amounts of air are needed to seal the trachea; tracheal stenosis is suspected when smaller volumes of air are needed to occlude the trachea. One should

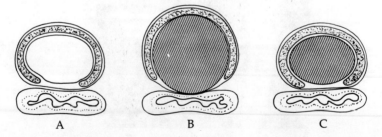

      A   B   C

Figure 1-3. Method of sealing the trachea with high- and low-pressure tracheal tube cuffs. A. The trachea and esophagus of a normal adult. The cartilage is lightly stippled. The lumen of the trachea is neither round nor oval. B. High-pressure cuffs produce a seal by expanding in all directions, thus distorting the trachea in a circular fashion. The high pressure can easily lead to erosion into the esophagus or innominate artery. C. Low-pressure cuffs seal the trachea by conforming to its configuration. The amount of pressure needed to prevent air leaks is therefore nearly equal to the peak pressure needed to inflate the lungs. (From J. D. Cooper and H. C. Grillo.[413] By permission of *Surgery, Gynecology & Obstetrics.*)

therefore keep careful records of the minimum amount of air necessary to seal the trachea.

The symptoms of tracheal stenosis and tracheomalacia are usually insidious in onset. Only minimal symptoms may be present up to the time that nearly complete airway obstruction develops with respiratory distress. Tracheal stenosis often occurs several weeks to months following an episode of acute respiratory failure.

The best diagnostic tool in the evaluation of tracheal stenosis and tracheomalacia is the x-ray. An air tracheogram with tomography can give an accurate evaluation of the location and extent of a stenotic area. Fluoroscopy with a cough or forced expiration can also document areas of tracheomalacia. Proper radiographic demonstration of stenotic areas and areas of malacia is necessary prior to any surgical correction.[953] Bronchoscopy can locate a stenotic area, but if the area is touched by the bronchoscope, edema may occlude the already compromised airway. Pressure-volume studies of the lungs may also be helpful in evaluating the course of tracheal stenosis.

The diagnosis of a tracheoesophageal fistula is often difficult. One may see pulmonary aspiration or find evidence of gastric dilatation during controlled ventilation.

A tracheoinnominate fistula is a dramatic finding and requires immediate tamponade.

TREATMENT

Tracheal stenosis that is causing airway obstruction can be treated effectively with tracheal resection. The stenotic portion of trachea can be excised, and a primary anastomosis done. Surrounding areas of tracheomalacia which frequently are present, make the operation more difficult.

Tracheoesophageal fistulas should be corrected surgically if possible. Tracheoinnominate fistulas require emergency surgery on total cardiopulmonary bypass. Bleeding may be minimized by maximum inflation of the tracheal tube cuff at the time of the acute hemorrhage.[414] Late deaths are due to paratracheal infection.

PREVENTION

A multitude of cuffs and other devices have been developed in the hope of enabling controlled ventilation to be carried out with minimal tracheal injury.[302] Techniques that have not been effective in preventing tracheal injury, or that do not give adequate alveolar ventilation, include a large-bore needle placed in the trachea,[1832] intermittent cuff deflation of high-pressure cuffs, tracheal tubes without cuffs,[302] inflation of the cuff during inspiration only,[1035,1114,1179] underinflation of the cuff so that a constant leak is present,[258] and use of double-cuffed tubes.[302]

The most effective way of preventing tracheal injury is to use large residual volume, large diameter, low-pressure cuffs.[300,1178] This type of cuff occludes the lumen of the trachea by conforming to the configuration of the tracheal wall (see Figure 1-3). According to measurements of tracheal wall pressures, this type of cuff exerts the lowest pressure of all available cuffs.[301,302] In experimental animals use of the low-pressure cuff is associated with less tracheal damage (Fig. 1-4).[413] The same is true in studies on patients requiring controlled ventilation.[414,775]

A danger of the low-pressure cuff is overinflation. Cuffs should be inflated only to the point where a seal is obtained at peak airway pressure. This is determined by auscultation of the neck while air is being injected into the cuff and the patient is being ventilated. If more air is inserted than necessary, the cuff pressure and the cuff tracheal pressure will increase markedly, defeating the purpose of the soft cuff. Overinflation also can lead to herniation of the cuff over the end of the tracheal tube, obstructing the airway.[302,414] The careful filling of the cuff with air to the no-leak point is the simplest method of preventing overinflation. A system of preventing overinflation by use of a device that limits pressure in the cuff is available.[300,1272]

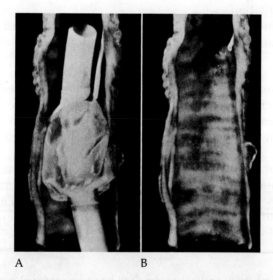

A   B

Figure 1-4.   Effect of a low-pressure tracheal tube cuff on the gross anatomy of the trachea. A dog was ventilated for 13 days via a tracheal tube with a low-pressure cuff. A. The trachea is shown open with the tracheal tube in place. There is no apparent dilatation of the trachea at the site of the cuff. The softness and large volume of the cuff allow it to conform to the anatomy of the trachea without distorting it. B. After removal of the tracheal tube the structure of the trachea remains intact. The mucosa appears unaltered. (From J. D. Cooper and H. C. Grillo.[413] By permission of *Surgery, Gynecology & Obstetrics.*)

Use of a liquid to inflate the cuff passively is also reported to be a safe method of preventing overinflation.[950]

Measurement of the intracuff pressure is best made by a simple aneroid pressure gauge. The pressure needed to occlude the airway yet permit maximal capillary blood flow is estimated to be 20–25 cm H_2O (1.9–2.4 kPa) at exhalation in cuffs that do not have any circumferential tension.[302]

Other types of low-pressure cuffs have also been designed.[65,709] Cuffs composed of polyurethane foam provide minimal tracheal wall pressures, but this type of cuff has the potential for uneven pressure distribution if the tube lies asymmetrically in the trachea.[302,990] Prestretching high-pressure polyvinyl chloride cuffs to produce a low-pressure system was common practice prior to the commercial availability of soft cuff tubes.[694] This practice is associated with several serious complications, especially tracheal ring necrosis, cuff herniation and bronchial occlusion, and inability to deflate the cuff.[1123,1245] With the commercial availability of soft cuffs the practice of prestretching is unnecessary and should be abandoned. Progress in tube and cuff design is lowering morbidity. Persons looking after intubated patients must keep abreast of the interdisciplinary problems of long-term intubation of the airway.

2

Effect of Controlled Ventilation on the Lungs and Cardiovascular System

In the past ten years considerable advances have been made in the understanding of the physiologic effects that both intermittent positive pressure ventilation and continuous positive pressure ventilation have on the lung and the cardiovascular system.

INTERMITTENT POSITIVE PRESSURE VENTILATION

During intermittent positive pressure ventilation (IPPV) the lungs are ventilated with a device that provides positive pressure on the airway during inspiration and allows the airway pressure to return to atmospheric pressure during expiration. In the Respiratory–Surgical Intensive Care Unit of the Beth Israel Hospital we use volume-constant ventilators to administer IPPV to patients in acute respiratory failure. Because this type of patient undergoes frequent changes in total respiratory compliance, we try to avoid using pressure-controlled ventilators. Numerous changes in alveolar ventilation result from pressure-controlled ventilators.

EFFECT ON GAS EXCHANGE IN PATIENTS WITH CARDIORESPIRATORY DISEASE

Numerous factors can influence the arterial oxygen tension in patients who require controlled ventilation. The most common reason for alterations in the arterial oxygen tension is changes in the percent of cardiac output that is shunted through the lungs during acute respiratory failure. In most patients this can be attributed to atelectasis, pulmonary edema, or pneumonia. Occasionally pulmonary hemorrhage or pulmonary embolus can lead to an increased degree of intrapulmonary right-to-left shunt.

The role that controlled ventilation with IPPV plays in affecting this shunt is controversial. When patients receive IPPV during anesthesia, there is sometimes a fall in arterial oxygen tension, which has been attributed to ventilation of the lungs with constant low tidal volumes.[851,1894] It has been postulated that at constant low tidal volumes of ventilation atelectasis progressively develops, leading to a fall in arterial oxygen tension.[153] This concept is supported by the fact that patients who breathe spontaneously at low tidal volumes show a fall in total lung compliance, which can be reversed by the taking of a deep breath or sigh.[630] The use of intermittent hyperinflation of the lung has been suggested as a possible solution to the

13

problem of progressive atelectasis.[153] Other studies have not substantiated this suggestion.[1120] Nunn found that hyperinflation was effective only in a few patients in whom a pressure of 40 cm H_2O (3.9 kPa) was produced for 40 seconds.[1447] With lower pressures for hyperinflation there was no improvement in the degree of shunt. Consequently we do not use sighing mechanisms on our ventilators.

The tidal volume at which a patient is ventilated probably affects the degree of shunting. In anesthetized patients the degree of atelectasis that occurs can be minimized by ventilation with large tidal volumes.[1894,1995] In patients in acute respiratory failure, ventilation with tidal volumes of 15 ml per kilogram or above is frequently associated with a fall in the intrapulmonary shunt.[854] This effect depends upon the underlying pulmonary disease. In an evaluation of patients in acute respiratory failure who received controlled ventilation with tidal volumes increasing up to 30 ml per kilogram patients with emphysema showed a progressive fall in cardiac index with increasing tidal volumes associated with a decrease in the physiologic shunt. In those patients who had significant cardiopulmonary disease but did not have emphysema there was no effect of increasing tidal volumes on either the cardiac index or the degree of right-to-left shunt. In all patients there was an increase in alveolar ventilation associated with increases in tidal volume. The degree of increase in alveolar ventilation depended upon the deadspace-to-tidal-volume ratio (Fig. 2-1).[855]

A number of other factors can affect gas exchange during controlled

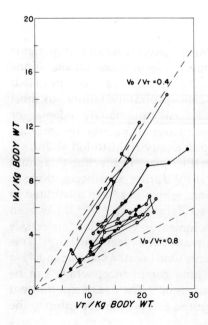

Figure 2-1. Relationship between tidal volume and alveolar ventilation. In 12 patients with acute respiratory failure alveolar ventilation (V_A) was increased by increasing the tidal volume (V_T) (respiratory rate constant at 20 breaths per minute). With large increases in tidal volume there is little change in deadspace-to-tidal-volume ratio (V_D/V_T). Alveolar ventilation increases in proportion to tidal volume, with the plot falling along the isopleth of each patient's V_D/V_T. *Solid circles* = patients with emphysema. *Open circles* = patients with respiratory failure without emphysema. (From J. Hedley-Whyte, H. Pontoppidan, and M. J. Morris, *J. Clin. Invest.*[855])

ventilation with IPPV. Increases in the inspiratory flow rate above 25 liters per minute produce a marked increase in the deadspace-to-tidal-volume ratio, which can lead to alveolar hypoventilation if no changes in the rate or tidal volume of the ventilator are made. High flow rates do not affect the degree of right-to-left shunt.[607]

The relationship between closing volume and functional residual capacity is an important determinant of the degree of shunting that will develop during IPPV. In normal patients undergoing general anesthesia with IPPV, if the functional residual capacity exceeds the closing volume preoperatively, there is no increase in physiologic shunt during IPPV at tidal volumes of 5 or 10 ml per kilogram. In patients whose closing volume exceeds the inspiratory lung volume (functional residual capacity plus tidal volume) there is a significant increase in physiologic shunt during IPPV. When there is an increase from low to high tidal volume, there is a decrease in physiologic shunt only if the increase in tidal volume produces an increase in inspiratory lung volume from below to above the closing volume. The relationship between closing volume and functional residual capacity is therefore an important determinant of the development of an increased physiologic shunt during IPPV.[2040]

The pattern of controlled ventilation has a small effect on the surface tension properties of the lungs. Hyperventilation ($V_T - 50$ ml/kg) with the elimination of pulmonary blood flow is associated with a fall in the surface activity of the lung secondary to changes in the rate of production of surfactant.[1261,2107] Extreme overinflation of the lungs results in a fall in the lung surface activity secondary to a depletion or alteration in surfactant, which does not occur with ventilation at normal pressures and volumes.[764] Additional studies in open-chest dogs showed the development of pulmonary edema after eight hours of overinflation with a tidal volume of 50 ml per kilogram. These changes are associated with a fall in the surface activity of the lungs of the hyperinflated dogs. Closed-chest dogs showed no such changes.[2108] A later study confirmed that closed-chest dogs who are hyperinflated with a tidal volume of 50 ml per kilogram for 24 hours show no alterations in the surfactant system.[1920] In summary it is likely that the pattern of ventilation does not affect the surfactant system of normal lungs when arterial carbon dioxide tension and cardiac output are kept within normal ranges, but extremes of lung volume can lead to insufficient production of surfactant.[1920]

Changes in the tidal volume can lead to changes in the deadspace-to-tidal-volume ratio. Patients in respiratory failure due to cardiopulmonary disease, if given increasing tidal volumes while in a sitting position, show a significant fall in this ratio. There is no change in the deadspace-to-tidal-volume ratio if the tidal volume is changed while the patients are supine (Fig. 2-2).[847] Expiratory pulmonary flow resistance not surprisingly increases significantly when tidal volume increases (Fig. 2-3).

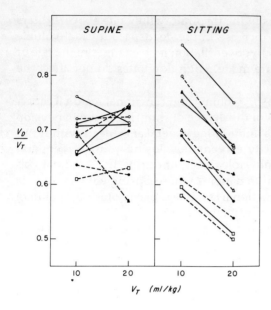

Figure 2-2. Effect of posture on the relationship between the deadspace-to-tidal-volume ratio (V_D/V_T) and tidal volume (V_T). Twenty patients with respiratory failure secondary to bronchopneumonia had measurements of V_D/V_T made at two levels of V_T (rate constant at 24 breaths per minute) in either the supine or the sitting position. Doubling the tidal volume in sitting patients resulted in a uniform decrease in V_D/V_T. No such fall occurred in the patients who were supine when the V_T was doubled. (From J. Hedley-Whyte, P. Berry, L. S. Bushnell, H. K. Darrah, and M. J. Morris, *Progress in Anaesthesiology*.[847])

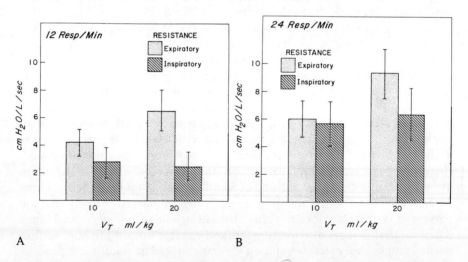

A   B

Figure 2-3. Effect of tidal volume and respiratory rate on airway resistances. Ten patients in respiratory failure from bronchopneumonia had inspiratory and expiratory resistance measured at different tidal volumes and at (A) 12 and (B) 24 breaths per minute. Measurements represent flow in the lungs below the tracheostomy tube. Inspiratory pulmonary flow resistance is always less than expiratory resistance. At 24 breaths per minute there is less of a difference. Values shown are means (± 1 SE). (From J. Hedley-Whyte, P. Berry, L. S. Bushnell, H. K. Darrah, and M. J. Morris, *Progress in Anesthesiology*.[847])

When a patient is in the lateral position, there are significant alterations in ventilation-perfusion relations. In the lateral position during IPPV the nondependent lung receives a greater part of the tidal volume than does the dependent lung.[1236,1605] The dependent lung receives the greater part of the perfusion.[292,524,1579,1606] With emphysema, controlled ventilation with 100% oxygen generally leads to a marked reduction in pulmonary artery pressure and pulmonary vascular resistance with only a small fall in cardiac index. IPPV with 100% oxygen may therefore decrease pulmonary vasoconstriction in emphysematous patients.[916]

EFFECT ON METABOLISM IN PATIENTS WITH CARDIORESPIRATORY DISEASE

Patients with significant cardiopulmonary disease who are treated with controlled ventilation usually show a fall in oxygen consumption. The greatest fall occurs in patients in respiratory distress with a high oxygen cost of breathing during spontaneous respiration.[770] This lessened oxygen consumption probably is related to a decrease in the work of the respiratory muscles. The metabolic cost of ventilation is not merely a function of the respiratory muscles, however. Studies of excised dog lungs show that mechanical ventilation is associated with a higher oxygen consumption and uptake of glycogen and phospholipids than static inflation. Mechanical deformation of the lung during ventilation therefore contributes to the metabolic cost of breathing.[614,615]

EFFECT ON THE CARDIOVASCULAR SYSTEM IN PATIENTS WITHOUT SIGNIFICANT CARDIORESPIRATORY DISEASE

The initiation of intermittent positive pressure ventilation is associated with a fall in the cardiac index in patients without significant lung consolidation.[430,770,1354] This decrease is often associated with a small fall in arterial blood pressure.[1570] Cardiac output and stroke volume fall as the peak airway pressure increases. There is also a fall in cardiac output with increasing inspiratory-to-expiratory ratios (Fig. 2-4).[1354] With increasing intrathoracic pressure there is a progressive fall in venous return, reflected by a fall in vena caval blood flow. The majority of the circulatory effects of IPPV are therefore a result of the effect of increased intrathoracic pressure on venous return.[1353,1354] Patients with normal lungs behave differently from patients with significant cardiopulmonary disease.

In addition to causing a decrease in stroke volume and cardiac output, IPPV results in a fall in pulmonary artery pressure and arterial blood pressure. Left atrial pressure does not change. There is no change in pulmonary vascular resistance. The systemic vascular resistance increases slightly when IPPV is begun.[770]

The fall in cardiac output that occurs during IPPV is rarely of any clinical significance, since it is compensated for by an increase in peripheral vascu-

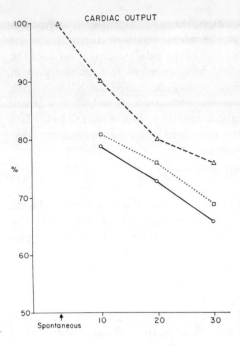

Figure 2-4. Effect of airway pressure and inspiratory-to-expiratory ratio (I/E) on cardiac output. *Dashed line* = I/E of 1:2; *dotted line* = I/E of 1:1; *solid line* = I/E of 2:1. The ordinate expresses cardiac output as a percent of control value. The abscissa represents the peak positive airway pressure in cm H_2O starting with spontaneous respiration. Cardiac output progressively declined with increasing airway pressure and increased I/E ratio in six lightly anesthetized dogs. (From B. C. Morgan, W. E. Martin, T. F. Hornbein, E. W. Crawford, and W. G. Guntheroth, *Anesthesiology*.[1354])

lar resistance, so that hypotension secondary to the institution of IPPV is rare. Furthermore the fall in oxygen consumption with IPPV makes the fall in cardiac output less harmful.

CONTINUOUS POSITIVE PRESSURE VENTILATION

During continuous positive pressure ventilation (CPPV), the lungs are inflated with a ventilator that provides positive pressure to the airway during both inspiration and expiration. This form of ventilation differs from IPPV only in the expiration phase, during which positive pressure is applied, usually by placing the expiratory hose under a column of water. For this reason CPPV is often referred to as *positive end-expiratory pressure* (PEEP).

EFFECT ON GAS EXCHANGE

The major use of CPPV is to increase the arterial oxygen tension without increasing the inspired oxygen concentration. Considerable evidence has accumulated regarding the harmful effects of high inspired oxygen concentrations (Chap. 31). The mechanism of the increase in arterial oxygenation that occurs with CPPV (Fig. 2-5) is related to an increase in the functional residual capacity. The functional residual capacity expands linearly with increases in the end-expiratory pressure (Fig. 2-6)[393,608,2115], usually at a rate of 400 ml or more for each 5 cm H_2O (0.5 kPa) end-expiratory pres-

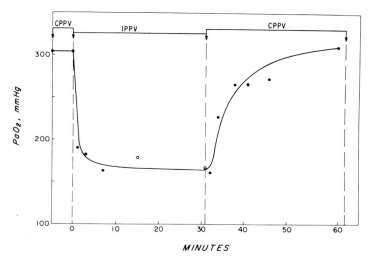

Figure 2-5. Change in arterial oxygen tension (Pa_{O_2}) with continuous positive pressure ventilation (CPPV) and intermittent positive pressure ventilation (IPPV). Eight patients who required CPPV had frequent measurements of Pa_{O_2} following conversion from CPPV to IPPV for 30 minutes and then back to CPPV. *Open circles* represent the mean values of six of the patients. Within one minute of discontinuation of CPPV the mean Pa_{O_2} fell 129 mm Hg (17.1 kPa). Over the next 30 minutes the mean Pa_{O_2} continued to fall gradually. Following reapplication of CPPV the Pa_{O_2} gradually returned to control values within 30 minutes. (From A. Kumar, K. J. Falke, B. Geffin, C. F. Aldredge, M. B. Laver, E. Lowenstein, and H. Pontoppidan.[1074] Reprinted by permission from the *New England Journal of Medicine* 283:1430–1436, 1970.)

sure.[276,324,393,1074,1139,1200,1236,1552,1965] This increase in functional residual capacity represents alveoli that remain open and available for gas exchange during all phases of the ventilatory cycle. The increase in functional residual capacity with CPPV improves the relationship between functional residual capacity and closing volume and therefore also improves gas exchange, as was discussed in the section on IPPV.[435]

EFFECT ON PULMONARY FUNCTION

In addition to the increase in functional residual capacity with CPPV, static total respiratory and lung compliance is increased. Dynamic lung compliance decreases with increasing levels of positive end-expiratory pressure above 10 cm H_2O (1.0 kPa).[608]

The deadspace-to-tidal-volume ratio falls progressively with increasing amounts of positive end-expiratory pressure to the point where the highest static lung compliance is reached. As positive end-expiratory pressure is increased beyond this point, cardiac output decreases and there is an increase in the deadspace-to-tidal-volume ratio.

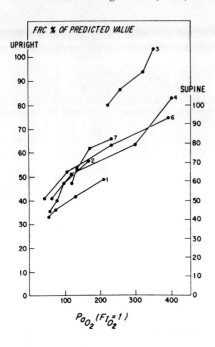

Figure 2-6. Relationship between the functional residual capacity (FRC) and arterial oxygen tension (Pa_{O_2}) at four different levels of end-expiratory pressure (EEP). Seven patients in respiratory failure had measurements of FRC and Pa_{O_2} at EEP of 0 cm, 5 cm H_2O (0.05 kPa), 10 cm (0.1 kPa), and 15 cm (0.15 kPa). The lowest FRC in each patient corresponds to 0 cm EEP. FRC is expressed as a percent of its predicted value for each patient. Increasing levels of EEP resulted in increasing both FRC and Pa_{O_2} in each patient. (From K. J. Falke, H. Pontoppidan, A. Kumar, D. E. Leith, B. Geffin, and M. B. Laver, *J. Clin. Invest.*[608])

EFFECT ON VENTILATION-PERFUSION RELATIONS

During CPPV the distribution of ventilation changes, a large amount of the ventilation going to areas where the ventilation-perfusion ratios are high (Fig. 2-7).[2054] Changes in airway pressure result in greater changes in alveolar pressure than in pulmonary arterial pressure, leading to improvement in ventilation-perfusion ratios.[1607,1608]

EFFECT ON THE CARDIOVASCULAR SYSTEM

The use of CPPV is often reported to be associated with a significant reduction in cardiac output (Fig. 2-8).[393,584,1074,1214,1938] Other reports, however, suggest varying effects or none at all on cardiac output.[394,608]

The reason for this discrepancy in findings is that the effects of CPPV on the cardiovascular system depend upon the intravascular volume, the contractility of the heart, and the pulmonary vasculature. When cardiac output falls with the institution of CPPV, it does so as a result of a fall in ventricular filling pressure. If allowed to continue, the new low level of cardiac output then persists without compensation. Increase in the blood volume by transfusion will result in a return of cardiac output to normal. Once the positive end-expiratory pressure is discontinued, however, the full effects of hypervolemia will be seen. Filling pressures will rise, and the ultimate effect on cardiac output will depend upon the individual patient's ventricular contractility.[1574]

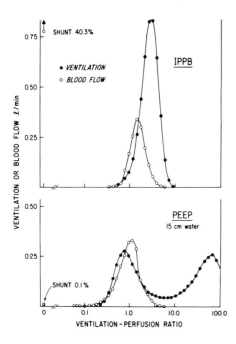

Figure 2-7. Effect of positive end-expiratory pressure (PEEP) on the ventilation-perfusion relationship. Acute respiratory failure was induced in a dog by the injection of oleic acid, which produced an acute hemorrhagic pulmonary edema. During intermittent positive pressure breathing (IPPB) the intrapulmonary shunt is 40.3 percent. With the start of PEEP the shunt falls to 0.1 percent and the majority of the ventilation goes to areas with high ventilation-perfusion ratios. Due to problems with experimental methods and analyses, these results should be regarded as descriptive rather than strictly quantitative. (From J. B. West, *Anesthesiology.*[2054])

The cardiovascular effects of CPPV cannot be considered separately from the pulmonary effects. Oxygen transport is a function of the oxygen content of blood and the cardiac output. In patients receiving CPPV oxygen transport rises progressively to a certain level of positive end-expiratory pressure and then declines. This level of best positive end-expiratory pressure falls between 0 and 15 cm H_2O (0–1.5 kPa) (Fig. 2-9). The increase in oxygen transport occurs because of increases in the arterial oxygen tension, while the fall in oxygen transport at excessive levels of positive end-expiratory pressure occurs because of falls in the cardiac output. The level of best positive end-expiratory pressure in patients in respiratory failure corresponds to the level at which the cardiac output and the total respiratory compliance are maximal while the deadspace-to-tidal-volume ratio is minimal (Fig. 2-10). The precise level of best positive end-expiratory pressure will depend upon the functional residual capacity of the patient before CPPV is begun (Fig. 2-11).[1880]

When using CPPV one must aim at maximizing the oxygen transport. The arterial oxygen tension and the intrapulmonary shunt are not good indicators of the optimal level of positive end-expiratory pressure, since they continue to improve even after this level has been reached (Fig. 2-12). Measurements of cardiac output and total respiratory compliance are good indicators of best positive end-expiratory pressure. Since total respiratory compliance is simple to measure in patients receiving controlled ventilation, it should be monitored during the application of positive end-

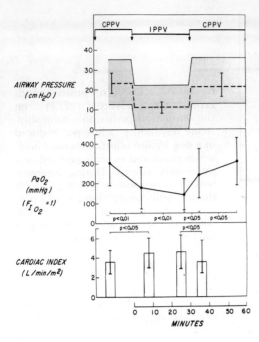

AIRWAY PRESSURE
(cm H₂O)

PaO₂
(mmHg)
(F_{I_{O_2}} = 1)

CARDIAC INDEX
(L/min/m²)

MINUTES

Figure 2-8. Effect of continuous positive pressure ventilation (CPPV) on arterial oxygen tension and cardiac index. Eight patients in acute respiratory failure who were receiving CPPV had a 30-minute period of intermittent positive pressure ventilation (IPPV), following which they were returned to CPPV. Mean, peak, and expiratory pressures are shown (*upper panel*). During IPPV there is a significant fall in arterial oxygen tension (Pa_{O_2}) (*middle panel*), and there is a significant rise when CPPV is restarted. During CPPV the mean cardiac index is 3.6 l/min/m² (*lower panel*), which rises significantly to 4.5 l/min/m² after only seven minutes of IPPV. When CPPV is restarted, the cardiac index is again reduced to 3.6 l/min/m². *Vertical bars* represent 1 ± SD. Statistically significant values are noted by *P* values. (From A. Kumar, K. J. Falke, B. Geffin, C. F. Aldredge, M. B. Laver, E. Lowenstein, and H. Pontoppidan.[1074] Reprinted by permission from the *New England Journal of Medicine* 283:1430–1436, 1970.)

expiratory pressure to determine the optimal level of cardiopulmonary function during CPPV.[1880]

Preexisting pulmonary vascular disease can modify the cardiovascular response to CPPV. The response to CPPV following aortic is different from the response following mitral valve replacement. The administration of CPPV following aortic valve replacement in patients without pulmonary vascular disease results in a fall in the alveolar-arterial oxygen tension gradient breathing 100% oxygen, a decrease in right-to-left shunt, and a decrease in cardiac index. In patients with pulmonary vascular disease who are given CPPV following mitral valve replacement there is a decrease in cardiac index, an increase in the deadspace-to-tidal-volume ratio, and no change in the calculated right-to-left shunt. One hour after discontinuation of CPPV patients with normal pulmonary vasculature have a return of all intravascular pressures and flows to normal. Patients with pulmonary vascular disease have persistent depression of the cardiac index after CPPV is discontinued. In patients with preexisting pulmonary vascular disease the hemodynamic response to CPPV is not predictable and varies according to myocardial competence.[1938]

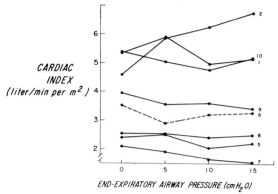

Figure 2-9. Relationship between cardiac index and level of end-expiratory pressure (EEP). Ten patients in respiratory failure had measurements of cardiac index at four levels of EEP. Patient 6 (*dashed line*) required infusions of metaraminol, 8 μg per minute, and isoproterenol, 8 μg per minute, during IPPV. Metaraminol infusion was increased to 75 μg per minute at 5 cm (0.05 kPa) PEEP, 150 μg per minute at 10 cm (0.10 kPa) PEEP, and 204 μg per minute at 15 cm (0.15 kPa) PEEP. One patient (7) demonstrated a progressive fall in cardiac index with increasing levels of EEP. (From K. J. Falke, H. Pontoppidan, A. Kumar, D. E. Leith, B. Geffin, and M. B. Laver, *J. Clin. Invest.*[608])

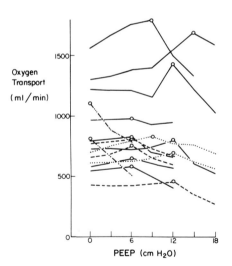

Figure 2-10. Effect of different levels of positive end-expiratory pressure (PEEP) on oxygen transport. Fifteen patients in acute respiratory failure had measurements of oxygen transport made with increasing levels of PEEP during controlled ventilation. Different lines represent different patients. *Circles* represent the level of PEEP at which maximum oxygen transport occurred (best PEEP). Increases in PEEP beyond the level of best PEEP result in a fall in oxygen transport. In all patients the level of best PEEP is between 0 and 15 cm H_2O (0.15 kPa). (From P. M. Suter, H. B. Fairley, and M. D. Isenberg.[1880] Reprinted by permission from the *New England Journal of Medicine* 292:284–289, 1975.)

COMPLICATIONS OF CONTROLLED VENTILATION

PNEUMOTHORAX

Pneumothorax is a common complication of controlled ventilation in the presence of acute lung disease. The diagnosis is sometimes unnecessarily delayed. Pneumothorax occurs with increasing frequency at high mean airway pressures. When unnecessarily high levels of PEEP are used (25–44 cm H_2O) (2.4–4.3 kPa), the incidence of pneumothorax is 14 percent.[1033] The

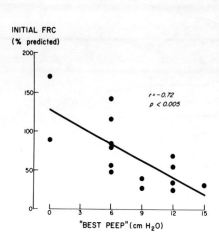

INITIAL FRC
(% predicted)

"BEST PEEP"(cm H₂O)

$r = -0.72$
$p < 0.005$

Figure 2-11. Relationship between functional residual capacity (FRC) before positive end-expiratory pressure (PEEP) and the level of PEEP at which optimum oxygen transport occurs (best PEEP). Fifteen patients receiving controlled ventilation for acute respiratory failure had measurements of FRC before institution of constant positive pressure ventilation (CPPV). PEEP was then added in 3 cm H_2O (0.03 kPa) increments to determine the level of PEEP at which oxygen transport was maximal (best PEEP). There is an inverse relationship between the initial FRC and the level of best PEEP. (From P. M. Suter, H. B. Fairley, and M. D. Isenberg.[1880] Reprinted by permission from the *New England Journal of Medicine* 292:284–289, 1975.)

site of rupture is often in an emphysematous bleb or an area of acute lung disease.

Pneumothorax should be suspected when there is a sudden rise in right-to-left shunt or in peak inflation pressures. Other signs include decreased or absent breath sounds, hyperresonance to percussion, and tracheal deviation. Shock can occur when there is a tension pneumothorax.

Immediacy of treatment depends on the clinical appearance of the patient. In most cases in which there is a suspicion of a pneumothorax the patient is stable enough to await a chest x-ray for confirmation before treatment is begun. Occasionally a patient will develop a tension pneumothorax and go into shock or have a cardiac arrest. Resuscitation is not possible until the pneumothorax is treated. In such a case the placement of a 14-gauge needle in the anterior second or third intercostal space of the affected side can be lifesaving. Following that, and in patients receiving controlled ventilation who have a documented pneumothorax, closed-chest drainage is mandatory. Even a 10 percent pneumothorax can rapidly become a tension pneumothorax in a patient receiving positive pressure ventilation.[2137]

SUBCUTANEOUS EMPHYSEMA

Patients receiving CPPV via a tracheostomy may develop subcutaneous emphysema in the neck. Serious consequences from it are rare, but subcutaneous emphysema may be so severe that the distance from the skin of the neck to the trachea increases to the point that a standard tracheostomy tube cannot reach the trachea. In such cases an orotracheal tube has to be placed into the trachea via the tracheostomy.

Subcutaneous emphysema can go into the mediastinum, or mediastinal

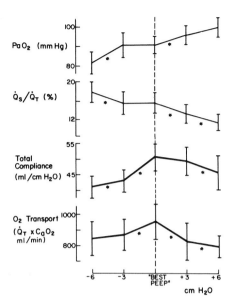

Figure 2-12. Effect of increasing levels of positive end-expiratory pressure (PEEP) on arterial oxygen tensions (Pa_{O_2}), intrapulmonary shunt ($\dot{Q}s/\dot{Q}T$), total compliance, and oxygen transport ($\dot{Q}T \times Ca_{O_2}$). Fifteen patients in acute respiratory failure requiring controlled ventilation had measurements of Pa_{O_2}, $\dot{Q}s/\dot{Q}T$, total compliance, and oxygen transport made with increasing levels of PEEP. In each patient there was a level of PEEP associated with optimal oxygen transport (best PEEP). The level of best PEEP corresponds to a point where total respiratory compliance is maximal. With increase in PEEP in excess of the best PEEP there is continued increase in the Pa_{O_2} and continued fall in the $\dot{Q}s/\dot{Q}T$. Significant changes ($P < 0.05$) brought about by 3 cm H_2O (0.03 kPa) increments of PEEP are indicated by *. (From P. M. Suter, H. B. Fairley, and M. D. Isenberg.[1880] Reprinted by permission from the *New England Journal of Medicine* 292:284–289, 1975.)

emphysema can develop without subcutaneous emphysema. No matter how it develops, one should be aware that air in the pericardium can produce cardiac tamponade, which requires immediate needle aspiration. Subcutaneous emphysema can also be a sign of pneumothorax.

HYPOTENSION ASSOCIATED WITH CONTINUOUS POSITIVE PRESSURE VENTILATION

In those situations in which a fall in cardiac output occurs with CPPV despite a normal intravascular volume, expansion of the blood volume will return the cardiac index to normal as described previously. This form of therapy can be dangerous, especially when there is some degree of cardiac failure. Hepatic and renal function can be compromised (see Chapter 3). Therefore we prefer to use dopamine to manage hypotension in normovolemic patients on CPPV.

OTHER COMPLICATIONS

Fluid retention frequently occurs in association with controlled ventilation.[1801] The many aspects of this problem are discussed in Chapter 6.

Acquired pulmonary infection also is frequently seen in patients who require controlled ventilation. This is discussed in Chapter 4.

3

Effect of Pattern of Ventilation on
Hepatic, Renal, and Splanchnic Function.

The vast majority of deaths of patients in respiratory failure are caused chiefly by failure of organ systems other than the lungs. Increases in upper airway pressure cause deterioration of hepatic, renal, and splanchnic function. Thus patients with liver, kidney, or gastrointestinal insufficiency often sustain serious complications from controlled ventilation.

HEPATIC FUNCTION

Mean serum bilirubin values rise to more than 3.5 mg per 100 ml (59.8 μmol/l) in 32 percent of patients in our intensive care unit who have no preexisting liver disease and who receive intermittent positive pressure ventilation for acute respiratory failure. Seventy-seven percent of patients in our hospital who receive continuous positive pressure ventilation (CPPV) show evidence of hepatic dysfunction (serum total bilirubin > 2.5 mg per 100 ml [42.8 μmol/l] plasma). While the etiology of this dysfunction in patients in respiratory failure obviously is extremely diverse, we have been concerned that the splanchnic effects of high airway pressure may contribute to hepatic dysfunction.

Downward motion of the diaphragm, if exaggerated or prolonged, may result in splanchnic hemodynamic disturbances. Portal vein pressure is increased by increased intraabdominal pressure, either directly by external pressure on the surface of the compressible liver or indirectly by interference with venous outflow.[1408] During intermittent positive pressure ventilation, portal venous flow can be reduced by 27–62 percent more than with spontaneous ventilation. If tidal volumes approximately twice normal are used, a 45 percent reduction in splanchnic blood flow and a 118 percent increase in splanchnic resistance can occur.[418] The splanchnic hemodynamic response to passive hyperventilation with tidal volumes of 40 ml per kilogram of body weight in dogs is the same during normocapnia and hypocapnia (Fig. 3-1). Hepatic venous pressure is doubled by this level of controlled passive hyperventilation from 3 to 6 mm Hg (0.4–0.8 kPa) in normocapnia and in hypocapnia. Mesenteric vascular resistance is increased from 360 to 480 mm Hg per liter per minute (48–64 kPa/l/min). Splanchnic venous outflow, taken as the difference between suprahepatic and infrahepatic flows, is decreased during ventilation with a tidal volume

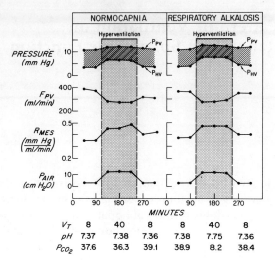

Figure 3-1. Effect of hyperventilation on hepatic and mesenteric hemodynamics. Two groups of seven dogs each were subjected to hyperventilation. One group had normocapnia maintained during hyperventilation, and the others became hypocapnic. V_T = tidal volume (ml/kg body weight). During hyperventilation there is an increase in hepatic venous pressure (Phv), portal venous pressure (Ppv), and mesenteric vascular resistance (Rmes) as well as a decrease in blood flow in the portal vein (Fpv). These changes do not seem to be related to changes in pH or arterial carbon dioxide tension. P_{AIR} = mean airway pressure. (From E. E. Johnson, *J. Appl. Physiol.*[968])

of 40 ml per kilogram. Portal blood flow is decreased due to this level of hyperventilation by 27 percent during normocapnia and 22 percent during hypocapnia (Fig. 3-2). Oxygen transport to the mesenteric bed decreases by 22 percent and to the liver by 20 percent. As blood flow to the liver decreases, the oxygen extraction ratio increases to maintain normal oxygen consumption. In the mesenteric bed, however, the extraction ratio fails to increase (Fig. 3-3).[968]

The application of 5–7 cm H_2O (0.5–0.7 kPa) positive end-expiratory pressure causes a 42–75 percent reduction in portal flow with a significant elevation in portal pressure (Fig. 3-4). This elevation in portal pressure, which accompanies a reduction in portal flow, indicates that this reduction in flow is not solely a reflection of a reduced blood supply to the viscera drained by the portal vein. Reduction in portal flow renders the liver more susceptible to ischemia should the arterial supply be compromised.[970]

When comparisons are made between the effects of IPPV and CPPV, resistance to flow through the choledochoduodenal junction is consistently elevated by the application of CPPV and always reversed by the release of expiratory resistance (Fig. 3-5). CPPV does not appear to affect the rate of bile flow. Local application of vasoconstrictor drugs to the chole-

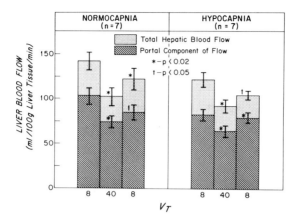

Figure 3-2. Effect of ventilation with large tidal volumes on hepatic blood flow. Fourteen anesthetized dogs were subjected to hyperventilation with large tidal volumes (V_T 40 ml/kg body weight). Half the dogs had normocapnia maintained, and the others became hypocapnic. Hyperventilation results in a significant reduction in total liver blood flow which is unrelated to pH and arterial carbon dioxide tensions. *Vertical bars* signify SE of mean. (From E. E. Johnson, *J. Appl. Physiol.*[968])

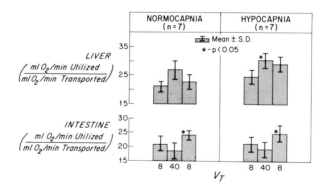

Figure 3-3. Effect of decreased O_2 transport during hyperventilation on the O_2 extraction ratio in the hepatic and mesenteric portion of the splanchnic vasculature. Hyperventilation was achieved in fourteen dogs using large tidal volumes ($V_T = 40$ ml/kg body weight) while keeping half the dogs normocapnic and the remainder hypocapnic. During decreased blood flow to the liver with hyperventilation the oxygen extraction ratio increases to allow near normal oxygen consumption. The mesenteric vasculature responds differently with the oxygen extraction ratio decreasing with decreasing blood flow. *P* values reflect comparisons with the preceding variables. (From E. E. Johnson, *J. Appl. Physiol.*[968])

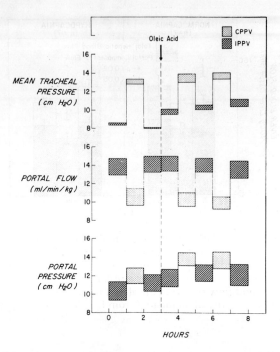

Figure 3-4.   Effect of continuous positive pressure ventilation (CPPV) and intermittent positive pressure ventilation (IPPV) on portal blood flow and pressure in eight dogs who had pulmonary edema induced by intravenous injection of oleic acid. CPPV produces a significant reduction in portal blood flow as well as a rise in portal blood pressure both before and after oleic acid–induced pulmonary edema. The combination of the pressure and flow changes suggests that CPPV increases the resistance to portal venous flow. (From E. E. Johnson and J. Hedley-Whyte, *J. Appl. Physiol.*[969])

dochoduodenal junction abolishes the increased resistance to flow caused by CPPV, suggesting that passive vascular engorgement causes the increased resistance to flow.[970]

RENAL FUNCTION

In contrast to conventional IPPV continuous positive pressure ventilation is associated with a reduction in urine output and salt and water retention (Fig. 3-6). Release of antidiuretic hormone and changes in renal perfusion are two mechanisms responsible for these changes.[95,546] Total renal blood flow generally remains almost unchanged during continuous positive pressure ventilation, but a redistribution of intrarenal blood flow occurs (Figs. 3-7 and 3-8). Fractional perfusion of the outer cortex decreases, while perfusion of the inner cortex and outer medullary tissue increases.[795] Consequently with positive end-expiratory pressure of 10 cm H_2O (1.0 kPa)

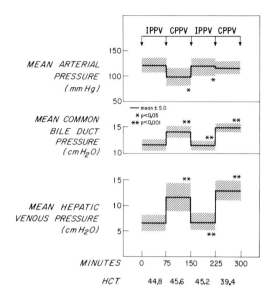

Figure 3-5. Effect of continuous positive pressure ventilation (CPPV) on mean common bile duct (CBD) pressure. Measurements are made during a continuous infusion of 0.8 ml per minute of saline into the CBD. Dogs were ventilated with either intermittent positive pressure ventilation (IPPV) or with CPPV. During CPPV there is a significant rise in common bile duct pressure, which reverses when IPPV is reinstituted. The increases in CBD pressures are associated with an increase in mean hepatic venous pressure. Values shown are mean ± SD. *P* values refer to significant changes in comparison to the preceding ventilatory period. (From E. E. Johnson and J. Hedley-Whyte, *J. Appl. Physiol.*[970])

urine output falls by 40 percent, creatinine clearance by 23 percent, and sodium excretion by 63 percent. Fractional reabsorption of sodium increases with increased perfusion of the juxtamedullary zone. Juxtamedullary nephrons are more efficient in conserving sodium than are outer cortical nephrons.[925] The redistribution of intrarenal blood flow is not related consistently to changes in total renal vascular resistance. Increased perfusion of the juxtamedullary zone with sodium retention is also present in congestive heart failure,[1826] hemorrhage,[299,1844] stimulation of the renal sympathetic nerves, partial occlusion of the thoracic inferior vena cava,[1025] and low-sodium diets.[912]

Renal function is not adversely affected by portal venous hypertension, unless systemic hypotension is also present. No change in systemic hemodynamics occurs until portal venous pressure exceeds 30 cm H_2O (3.0 kPa). An acute increase in portal venous pressure results in worsening of renal function after systemic arterial hypotension has already occurred; thus the deleterious effects of portal venous hypertension and systemic arterial hypotension on renal function cannot be dissociated.[1153,1154]

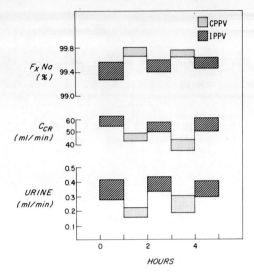

Figure 3-6. The effect of continuous positive pressure ventilation (CPPV) and intermittent positive pressure ventilation (IPPV) on renal function. During CPPV there is a significant increase in the fractional reabsorption of sodium by the kidney (Fx_{Na}), a decrease in creatinine clearance (C_{CR}), and a decrease in urine output during CPPV. All changes related to changing pattern of ventilation are significant ($P <$ 0.05). Each shaded area represents the mean ± SE. (N = 10). (From S. V. Hall, E. E. Johnson, and J. Hedley-Whyte, *Anesthesiology*.[795])

SPLANCHNIC FUNCTION

Massive gastrointestinal bleeding from multiple gastric ulcers used to occur in 5 percent of patients in our Respiratory–Surgical Intensive Care Unit. Gastric mucosal changes can be demonstrated photographically in all critically ill patients.[1194] Etiologic factors include respiratory failure, hypotension, sepsis, and jaundice.[816,1778,1779]

Positive end-expiratory pressure increases splanchnic resistance and may contribute to gastric mucosal ischemia (Fig. 3-1). Gastric acid hypersecretion and disruption of the gastric mucosal barrier are important factors in the pathogenesis of these acute gastric ulcers (Figs. 3-9, 3-10, and 3-11).[742,1792,1797] Hypercapnia has no demonstrable effect on gastric secretion.[903] Agents that increase gastric mucosal permeability include aspirin, indomethacin, alcohol, and bile salts.[374,1448,1807] The list of compounds containing aspirin is extensive.[1143] Direct intraarterial infusion of vasopressin in the treatment of gastric mucosal hemorrhage does not disrupt the gastric mucosal barrier initially; after three hours back-diffusion of hydrogen ions begins to occur.[529]

Aggressive antacid therapy reduces the occurrence of massive gastrointestinal bleeding from acute stress ulceration. We administer antacids

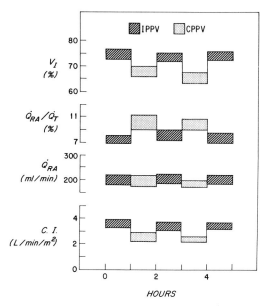

Figure 3-7. Effect of continuous positive pressure ventilation (CPPV) and intermittent positive pressure ventilation (IPPV) on renal blood flow. During CPPV in ten
dogs the proportion of the cardiac output going to the kidneys ($\dot{Q}_{RA}/\dot{Q}_T$) increases,
while the total renal blood flow ($\dot{Q}_{RA}$) does not change. The percent volume of
kidney perfused at outer cortical flow rates (V_I) decreases during CPPV. All changes
are significant ($P < 0.05$). Shaded areas indicate the mean ± SE. (From S. V. Hall, E.
E. Johnson, and J. Hedley-Whyte, *Anesthesiology*.[795])

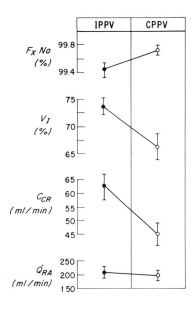

Figure 3-8. Effect of continuous positive
pressure ventilation (CPPV) and intermittent
positive pressure ventilation (IPPV) on renal
blood flow and function. During CPPV the
creatinine clearance (C_{CR}) and the percent
volume of kidney perfused at outer cortical
flow rates (V_I) decrease while the total renal
blood flow ($\dot{Q}_{RA}$) is unchanged. This intrarenal redistribution of blood flow results in an
increase in the fractional reabsorption of
sodium. Mean values ± SE are recorded.
(From S. V. Hall, E. E. Johnson, and J.
Hedley-Whyte, *Anesthesiology*.[795])

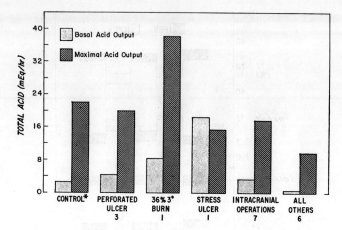

Figure 3-9. Basal and maximal gastric acid output in critically ill patients. Basal acid output (BAO) and maximal acid output (MAO) after histamine stimulation were studied in eighteen critically ill patients. The one patient who developed a lethal stress ulceration of the stomach had a BAO which was equal to the MAO of seven patients following intracranial operations and three patients with perforated duodenal ulcers. Control values (*) are the normal BAO and MAO of males. (From J. J. Skillman, L. S. Bushnell, H. Goldman, and W. Silen, *Am. J. Surg.*[1790])

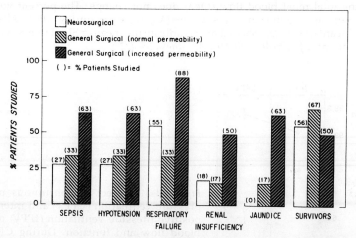

Figure 3-10. Incidence of sepsis, hypotension, respiratory failure, renal insufficiency, and jaundice and the survival rate with reference to the permeability of the gastric mucosal barrier (GMB) in neurosurgical and general surgical patients. Data on gastrointestinal bleeding in these patients are also shown in the succeeding figure. The greatest incidence of complications and the lowest survival rate occur in general surgical patients with increased permeability of the GMB. General surgical patients with normal permeability of the GMB and neurosurgical patients have approximately the same incidence of complications. (From M. J. Gordon, J. J. Skillman, N. T. Zervas, and W. Silen, *Ann. Surg.*[742])

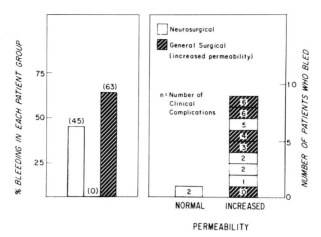

Figure 3-11. Incidence of gastrointestinal bleeding and other complications in postoperative patients. (*Left*) Percent bleeding in each patient group. No general surgical patients with normal gastric mucosal permeability had gastrointestinal bleeding. (*Right*) Gastric mucosal permeability and the number of other clinical complications in each patient who developed gastrointestinal bleeding. Only one patient with normal gastrointestinal permeability developed gastrointestinal bleeding. Five of the nine patients with increases in the gastric mucosal permeability and who bled had multiple other complications such as respiratory failure, shock, jaundice, renal failure, or septicemia. (From M. J. Gordon, J. J. Skillman, N. T. Zervas, and W. Silen, *Ann. Surg.*[742])

hourly to maintain a gastric luminal pH greater than 5. We have used as much as 4 liters of antacid daily in some patients to achieve this goal. After the adoption of this regimen of antacid prophylaxis the occurrence of major gastrointestinal bleeding (4 units of blood or more) was reduced from 5 percent to the point where out of more than 1,000 admissions to our Respiratory–Surgical Intensive Care Unit only two patients required surgery for uncontrollable bleeding. Maintenance of intravascular volume with crystalloid or colloid replacement to correct or prevent mucosal ischemia plays an important role in the prevention of stress ulceration.[1345,1798]

If surgical intervention for uncontrollable hemorrhage becomes necessary for patients with gastrointestinal bleeding, partial gastrectomy combined with vagotomy is more effective operative treatment than vagotomy and pyloroplasty.[737,1790]

In summary abnormal patterns of ventilation adversely alter hepatic and renal function and probably splanchnic function as well. Aggressive antacid therapy has greatly lessened gastrointestinal bleeding in patients in respiratory failure. Increased understanding of the interrelationships between airway pressure and hepatic and renal function should further improve the management of acute respiratory failure.

4

Problems of Nosocomial Pulmonary Infection

In the past fifteen years the problem of nosocomial infections has reached epidemic proportions. Nosocomial infection occurs in 4 to 15 percent of patients.[625] Respiratory tract infections account for about 15 percent of all acquired infections (Fig. 4-1).[582,1958]

The emergence of gram-negative organisms in hospital-acquired infections is of great importance. The rate of infection and the organisms responsible for infection vary from hospital to hospital. In one series prevalence rates for infections with *Pseudomonas, Serratia*, and *Klebsiella* were as high as 46 percent of all infected hospitalized patients. In the same series, 71 percent of patients who had gram-negative bacteremias had acquired their organisms in the hospital. The longer a patient is hospitalized, the greater the risk for acquiring a gram-negative infection (Fig. 4-2).[1402]

In a respiratory–intensive care unit the majority of acquired infections are found in the respiratory tract. In the Respiratory–Surgical Intensive Care Unit at the Beth Israel Hospital in Boston the overall mortality in a two and one-half year period was 13 percent. Patients who had no evidence of pneumonia had a mortality of 3.8 percent. Patients with gram-positive pneumonias had a mortality of 5 percent. Patients with gram-negative pneumonia not caused by *Pseudomonas aeruginosa* had a mortality of 33 percent. Patients who had pneumonia caused by *Pseudomonas aeruginosa* had a mortality of 70 percent (Fig. 4-3).[1852]

The 70 percent mortality for *Pseudomonas* pneumonia can be explained at least in part by the organism's resistance to all but a few antibiotics.[762] Gentamicin, carbenicillin, and polymyxin are frequently effective against *Pseudomonas* in vitro;[10] however, when they are given systemically to treat pneumonia, their effectiveness is questionable.[1852] The problem of nosocomial pulmonary infections in a respiratory intensive care unit is therefore great.

TRANSMISSION OF GRAM-NEGATIVE BACTERIA

Investigation of the reservoirs, routes of transmission, and routes of infection is of prime importance in eradicating nosocomial infections. The respiratory–intensive care unit poses many problems for prevention of infection in terms of its relatively small size, the critical nature of the

37

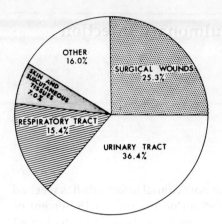

Figure 4-1. Types of nosocomial infections. Six community hospitals in various parts of the United States were surveyed for nosocomial infection over an 18-month period. Urinary tract infections were the most frequent hospital-acquired infections. A quarter of all acquired infections involved surgical wounds. Acquired respiratory tract infections were the third most common type of infection. (From T. C. Eickhoff, P. S. Brachman, J. V. Bennett, and J. F. Brown, *J. Infect. Dis.*[582] By permission from The University of Chicago Press, Copyright, 1969.)

patient's illness, and the multitude of personnel who must come into frequent contact with the patient.

Potential reservoirs of gram-negative organisms are many. Patients obviously harbor many potentially pathogenic organisms in their digestive tracts. These include the usual enteric gram-negative organisms as well as other gram-negative organisms, such as *Pseudomonas* and *Klebsiella*, which can colonize the digestive tract.[1725] Pathogenic organisms also may infect patients' surgical wounds or urinary tracts and eventually reach their lungs.

In the Respiratory–Surgical Intensive Care Unit we found that the most common reservoir of *Pseudomonas* was the hand-washing sinks used by the intensive care unit personnel. Organisms found in the drains of the hand-washing sinks were of similar pyocine types to those causing respiratory tract infection (Fig. 4-4).[714,1399] Back-splashing of organisms from the drain contaminated the hands of the user, and organisms were then transmitted to patients. [1188,1914]

Other sources of organisms were in the water traps of the ventilators. *Pseudomonas* was isolated from several of these traps and subsequently found on the hands of the respiratory therapist emptying the trap.[1914]

Following an outbreak of respiratory tract colonization with *Flavobacterium meningosepticum* we encountered a case of pneumonia caused by the same species.[1912] This prompted a search for the environmental source, and it was discovered that *Flavobacterium meningosepticum* could be cultured from a sink in the medication room of the Respiratory–Surgical Intensive Care Unit. This organism was also cultured from the tube feedings that were being administered to another patient as well as from the basement kitchen in close proximity to where the tube feedings are prepared.

Gram-negative organisms, especially *Pseudomonas*, have also been found on floors and in wash basins, suction apparatus, nail brushes, mops, ice machines, flower vases, medications, food, distilled water, and hospital disinfectants containing chlorhexidine.[270,618,1059,1346,1765,1766,1899]

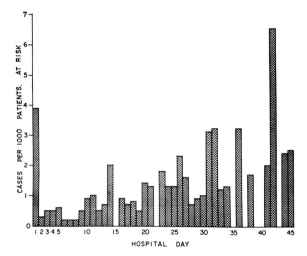

Figure 4-2. Relationship of incidence of gram-negative bacillemia to duration of hospitalization. For the period of this study the number of bacillemic episodes that began on each hospital day is divided by the total number of patients still in the hospital on that day, yielding a rate of attack for the population at risk..There is an increase in the risk of gram-negative bacteremia with increasing duration of hospital stay. (From R. L. Myerowitz, A. A. Medeiros, and T. F. O'Brien, *J. Infect. Dis.*[1402] By permission from The University of Chicago Press, Copyright, 1971.)

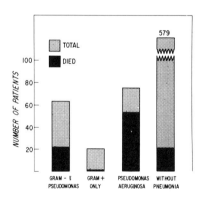

Figure 4-3. Effect of the bacterial organism on the mortality for pneumonia in 732 admissions to the Respiratory–Surgical Intensive Care Unit (R-SICU) of the Beth Israel Hospital, Boston. Pneumonia caused by gram-positive organisms had a mortality of 5 percent. Pneumonias caused by gram-negative organisms excluding *Pseudomonas aeruginosa* had a mortality of 33 percent. The mortality for patients with pneumonia where *Pseudomonas aeruginosa* was one of several organisms isolated was 68 percent. The patients who had pneumonia with *Pseudomonas aeruginosa* as the only organism isolated had a mortality of 73 percent. (Drawn from data in R. M. Stevens, D. Teres, J. J. Skillman, and D. S. Feingold, *Arch. Intern. Med.* 134:106–111, 1974.[1852] Copyright, 1971–74, American Medical Association.)

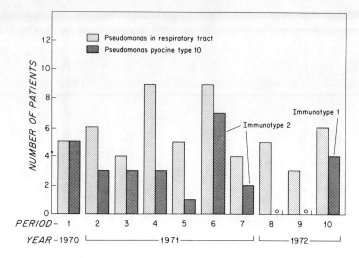

Figure 4-4. Incidence of *Pseudomonas aeruginosa* respiratory tract colonization in the R-SICU from December 1970 to June 1972. The overall incidence of airway colonization with *Pseudomonas aeruginosa* was 8.7 percent over the entire 19-month period. Many of the isolates were of pyocine type 10, which was the "resident strain" often found in the unsterilized hand-washing sinks. (From D. Teres, P. Schweers, L. S. Bushnell, J. Hedley-Whyte, and D. S. Feingold, *Lancet.*[1914])

Inhalation therapy equipment has often been implicated as a main source of gram-negative organisms.[15,279,686,772,1527,1528] The piece of equipment most frequently associated with transmission of gram-negative organisms is the nebulizer. *Pseudomonas, Flavobacterium,* and *Acinetobacter* have been found in reservoir nebulizer jets,[1612] from which they are aerosolized into particles small enough to reach small airways and alveoli. Large-volume nebulizers such as the Venturi, spinning disc, and ultrasonic types all have been implicated. Respiratory infections occur due to contaminated nebulization equipment (Fig. 4-5).[772] Hypersensitivity pneumonitis secondary to contaminated vaporizers also can be a problem.[904] Humidifiers also can be a source of microbial organisms.

Ventilators without nebulizers are probably not significant reservoirs of gram-negative organisms.[1527,1914] Experimental evidence suggests, however, that bacteria can spread in a retrograde fashion from the expiratory port of the ventilator, through the expiratory limb, to the patient.[78,488] The trap bottles that collect condensed water from the ventilator tubing can harbor organisms, which may be transmitted to other patients when the bottles are emptied.

Although there have been reports that hospital personnel may carry gram-negative organisms in their respiratory tracts, by far the most common means of transmission is through contamination of the hands of intensive care unit workers from some environmental source.[1188,1577,1914]

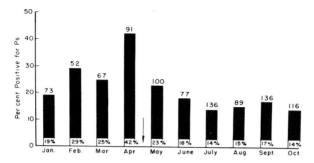

Figure 4-5.   Fine-particle humidifiers as sources of *Pseudomonas aeruginosa* (Ps). In a respiratory disease ward, fine-particle humidifiers were found to emit *Pseudomonas aeruginosa*. From January through April *Pseudomonas aeruginosa* was isolated in 19–42 percent of all sputum cultures that grew pathogenic bacteria. All humidifiers were removed at the end of April (*arrow*), and in May through October the incidence of *Pseudomonas aeruginosa* airway colonization decreased to 14–23 percent of positive respiratory tract cultures. The numbers on the top of each bar represent the number of pathogens isolated each month. The figures on the bottom of each bar give the percent positive for *Pseudomonas aeruginosa*. (From H. G. Grieble, F. R. Colton, T. J. Bird, A. Toigo, and L. G. Griffith.[772] Reprinted by permission from the *New England Journal of Medicine* 282:531–535, 1970.)

COLONIZATION OF UPPER RESPIRATORY TRACT

In the majority of cases the mode of entry of gram-negative organisms into the lung is by aspiration of organisms from the upper respiratory tract.[966] Aspiration of organisms is a normal occurrence during sleep or unconsciousness.[965]

Colonization of the upper respiratory tract with gram-negative organisms is therefore a predisposing factor to the development of a gram-negative pneumonia.[766,1048] In one study 23 percent of patients whose upper airways were colonized with gram-negative bacteria developed gram-negative pneumonias with the same organisms, while only 3.3 percent of patients who showed no evidence of colonization developed gram-negative pneumonias.[966]

ROLE OF HOST DEFENSES

The normal mechanisms of defense against bacterial infection are frequently diminished or absent in the patient in the intensive care unit. Bacteria usually are removed from the lungs by one of several mechanisms. Alveolar macrophages and other phagocytes clear the alveoli of bacteria. Mucus has an inherent bactericidal activity and also provides a mechanical mode of removal of organisms. Organisms also may be eliminated via blood or lymph.[1682] Impairment of any of these mechanisms can lead to the development of respiratory infection.

Alterations in normal immune mechanisms can predispose a patient to nosocomial respiratory infections. Patients receiving immunosuppressive treatment for organ transplantation have been reported to have a greatly increased incidence of hospital-acquired respiratory infection.[887] Patients with agammaglobulinemia or cancer of the lymphatic system also have increased susceptibility to nosocomial infections because of alterations in the immune system.[625] Alterations in either white blood cell numbers or function increase the risk of developing nosocomial infection. Conditions causing these alterations include granulocytopenia during chemotherapy of tumors, chronic granulomatous disease, acidemia, and corticosteroid therapy.[844]

Diminution in alveolar macrophage effectiveness increases the risk of nosocomial infection. Experimentally it has been shown that the use of positive end-expiratory pressure reduces alveolar macrophage function. Whether or not this is clinically significant has yet to be determined.

Whether or not the presence of a tracheal tube for controlled ventilation increases the risk of nosocomial infection is a controversial question. A tracheal tube bypasses the normal defenses of the upper airway. In our experience with patients who "acquired" pneumonia, the large majority had pneumonia prior to tracheal intubation.[1852] It was later found that all patients who received controlled ventilation for more than 72 hours developed colonies of gram-negative bacteria in the respiratory tract.[766] We therefore feel that tracheal intubation and controlled ventilation do play a part in the development of nosocomial pulmonary infections.

Prior treatment with antibiotics can alter the patient's own flora and affect the development of nosocomial pulmonary infections. This has been shown most clearly in patients receiving antibiotic therapy for pneumonia. In a series of 149 patients with pneumonia 59 percent became colonized with other organisms during treatment with antibiotics; 24 patients developed superinfections, of which 16 were fatal.[1924]

ORGANISMS CAUSING NOSOCOMIAL PNEUMONIA

In our Respiratory–Surgical Intensive Care Unit patients with acquired pneumonia were studied over a 20-month period. During that time 48 patients acquired pneumonia while in the unit. The organisms responsible were: *Pseudomonas aeruginosa*, 20 cases; *Serratia* or *Proteus* species, 14 cases; *Staphylococcus aureus*, 7 cases; *Enterobacter* species, *Klebsiella pneumoniae*, or *Escherichia coli*, 4 cases; *Flavobacterium meningosepticum*, *Pseudomonas maltophilia*, and *Candida albicans*, 1 case each.[1048]

DIAGNOSIS

The diagnosis of an acquired pneumonia frequently is difficult to make because the patient's sputum is often colonized with potentially pathogenic organisms, and because his chest x-ray film often shows infiltrates of atelectasis or pulmonary edema. One must therefore take all the data into consideration and make a clinical decision based on one's own experience.

The patient may complain of increasing cough or sputum production. Most patients in intensive care units are unable to complain; therefore it is necessary to rely on clinical examination and laboratory findings. On physical examination the patient usually is found to be febrile, often with a tachycardia. If the patient is breathing spontaneously, he is often tachypneic. Examination of the chest frequently reveals rales or rhonchi over the affected area. There may be signs of pulmonary consolidation.

Laboratory evaluation sometimes reveals an elevated white blood count and a shift to the left in the differential count. This, however, can be very misleading, as many patients with gram-negative pneumonias have normal leukocyte counts. Furthermore patients may have elevated leukocyte counts secondary to a recent operative procedure. The leukocyte count, therefore, may be indicative when it is extremely high or extremely low; otherwise it is of little help in making the diagnosis of nosocomial pneumonia.

The sputum gram stain is of great help in diagnosing a nosocomial infection. The gram stain of a patient with a tracheal tube typically shows many polymorphonuclear leukocytes and often a mixture of various gram-negative rods and gram-positive cocci. Through daily monitoring of the sputum gram stain in patients who are developing a gram-negative pneumonia, one often sees a dramatic change in the flora of the sputum. Polymorphonuclear leukocytes continue to be numerous; however, one type of gram-negative rod will appear to predominate. Often it is possible to find intracellular gram-negative rods that are quite characteristic of gram-negative pneumonia.

The sputum culture is helpful only when there are other signs of gram-negative pneumonia, however, as many patients develop colonies of one or more potentially pathogenic organisms. A positive culture per se is not diagnostic. When there are signs of pneumonia, the culture helps to determine the organism primarily responsible for the pneumonia and antibiotic sensitivities.

Arterial blood gases are helpful as indicators of pneumonia. In the presence of pulmonary consolidation there is an increase in right-to-left shunt, which is reflected either by hypoxemia or by an elevation of the alveolar-arterial oxygen tension gradient. In the Respiratory–Surgical Intensive Care Unit we measure this gradient on 100% oxygen in most patients every morning following chest physical therapy. We therefore have a method of comparing the degree of shunting on a day-to-day basis in nearly every patient. An elevation of the alveolar-arterial oxygen tension gradient is of course not in itself diagnostic of pneumonia, but it is very helpful in following the course of patients with pneumonia. Hypocapnia and later carbon dioxide retention and respiratory acidemia frequently complicate the course of acquired pneumonia in a patient who is not already receiving controlled ventilation.

Radiographic findings are most helpful in evaluation of the patient with acquired pneumonia. Chest x-ray film should be obtained if evidence of pneumonia is shown by physical examination, sputum gram stain, or elevation of the alveolar-arterial oxygen tension gradient. Since most patients are too ill to travel to the x-ray department and stand up for posteroanterior and lateral chest x-ray, one must usually rely on a portable anteroposterior x-ray film. This method has some limitations in evaluation of the heart size; however, evaluation of lung fields usually is adequate especially if an airway pressure of 20 cm H_2O (2.0 kPa) is applied.

In summary the diagnosis of nosocomial pneumonia is based on a number of clinical observations and tests. The most useful are findings of fever and tachypnea, findings of consolidation on chest physical examination, radiographic evidence of consolidation, predominance of one organism on sputum gram stain and culture, and elevation of the alveolar-arterial oxygen tension gradient.

TREATMENT

The treatment of nosocomial gram-negative pneumonia is based on three principles: removal of secretions from the tracheobronchial tree, support of oxygenation and ventilation, and proper use of antibiotics. During acute lung disease, chest physical therapy is essential. When a patient is diagnosed as having pneumonia, he should receive percussion and vibration to the entire chest, with special concentration on the affected lobe, every four hours. This helps to mobilize secretions to the larger bronchi and trachea, from which they can be removed either by the patient's coughing or by tracheal suction. Every one to two hours the patient is turned from side to side or placed prone to prevent secretions from collecting in one particular area. Patients are also encouraged to cough and take deep breaths at least every hour.

Fever is controlled with antipyretics to prevent excessive oxygen consumption and carbon dioxide production. If this is ineffective, an external cooling blanket is used (Chap. 30).

The role of antibiotics in the treatment of nosocomial pneumonia varies, depending upon the organism responsible for the pneumonia. There is evidence that the use of appropriate antibiotics in patients with gram-negative bacteremia reduces the mortality rate.[1402] There is no evidence to suggest that antibiotic treatment of nonbacteremic *Pseudomonas* pneumonia alters its course.[1150,1852]

In summary the treatment of nosocomial gram-negative pneumonia by our present methods is unsatisfactory, with mortality rates of 70 percent for *Pseudomonas* pneumonia and 33 percent for other gram-negative pneumonias. Thus, we make every effort to prevent the development of nosocomial pneumonias in these high-risk patients. Methods of doing this will be discussed fully in the next section.

PREVENTION

Since it has been clearly shown that nosocomial gram-negative infections are preceded by colonization of the upper respiratory tract, the most obvious means of attack is to focus on prevention of colonization by the most dangerous pathogens.[766]

BACTERIOLOGIC SURVEILLANCE

The numerous reservoirs of gram-negative organisms have been discussed earlier in this chapter. In our Respiratory–Surgical Intensive Care Unit there is regular bacteriologic surveillance of the environment. Handwashing sinks are cultured monthly, and ventilator traps are cultured weekly. Three times a year the unit is closed and the patients moved to another location. The unit then is cleaned extensively. During that time, swab cultures are taken from beds, floors, sinks, mops, dispensers, vents, and windows. Settling plates are placed around the unit at various stages during cleaning. Air sampling devices are also used. These precautions help ensure early detection of any reservoir of pathogenic bacteria.[1914] In addition, in the event of an epidemic with a single strain of gram-negative bacteria, all areas are again cultured as are the hands of all personnel. If necessary the unit is closed again and recleaned. Such surveillance methods have been shown to be effective in reducing the incidence of nosocomial infection.[582]

SINK STERILIZATION

As mentioned previously in this chapter, during the course of surveillance it was noted that the hand-washing sinks were frequently contaminated with *Pseudomonas aeruginosa*. In an effort to eliminate this source of bacteria a method of sink sterilization was developed. In each sink a valve is inserted in the S-trap, so that drainage can be stopped. The sink is then filled with a solution containing 5% phenol. A 500-watt immersion heating element, 1 inch in diameter, is inserted into the drain and heats the sink and drain pipe to 70°C. This is done to each sink daily for 90 minutes. This method has dramatically reduced the number of organisms in the sink drains and reduced the airway colonization rate of patients in the unit.[1048,1914]

EQUIPMENT

Respiratory therapy equipment, especially nebulization devices, can harbor potentially pathogenic gram-negative organisms, as was discussed previously in this chapter. In order to prevent this all ventilator hoses, Mörch swivels, tracheal tubes, ventilator traps, and nebulizers are sterilized with ethylene oxide after use by each patient. Ventilator hoses are changed every two days. Corrugated tubing and face masks used with heated nebulizers, as well as some tracheal tubes, are made of sterile disposable plastic and are not reused. With these methods it has been our experience, and the experience of others, that respiratory therapy equipment is not an important source of gram-negative organisms.[1188,1914]

PERSONNEL

Personnel in an intensive care unit are the usual vectors of transmission of gram-negative organisms from patient to patient and from environmental source to patient, as was discussed earlier in this chapter. The simplest way to control this is by strict hand washing when going from one patient to another. This concept is easy to understand, but often difficult to enforce, especially among physicians, who for some reason feel they are immune to being carriers of gram-negative organisms. In addition to washing hands meticulously it is extremely important to obey strict sterile technique during tracheal suctioning and during care of the tracheostomy site.

ANTIBIOTICS

There is no place for systemic antibiotics in the prevention of nosocomial pneumonia.[1147,1561] It has been known since the 1950's that systemic antibiotics are inefficient in preventing pneumonia.[2045] Patients with poliomyelitis and respiratory insufficiency were three times more likely to develop nosocomial pulmonary infection if given prophylactic systemic antibiotics than if given no antibiotics.[2045] Patients on antibiotics for other infections are at greater risk of developing nosocomial pulmonary infections with organisms resistant to those antibiotics.[1924] Therefore systemic antibiotics offer no protection against gram-negative pneumonia and actually place the patient at an increased risk.[259,976]

The use of topical antibiotics applied to the upper airway does appear to be promising in the prevention of nosocomial pulmonary infection.[766,1041,1042,1048,1234] The successful use of aerosol antibiotics for gram-negative infections was first reported in 1970, when sodium colistimethate in aerosol form proved effective in reducing the number of sensitive gram-negative organisms in the sputum of 20 patients with chronic lung disease.[1655] Later that year endobronchial polymyxin B was reported to be effective in the reduction of infections with *Pseudomonas aeruginosa* in patients with chronic lung disease.[1583]

Polymyxin B Aerosol

In 1971, in an attempt to reduce colonization of patients in respiratory failure we studied the effectiveness of polymyxin B aerosol. Polymyxin was chosen because of its very high tissue-binding capacity, its broad spectrum against gram-negative bacilli, especially *Pseudomonas*, and its lack of systemic absorption when applied topically.[766,1076]

During 21 months 58 patients were studied. They were divided into a polymyxin group and a placebo group. Patients receiving polymyxin were given a total dosage of 2.5 mg per kilogram per day divided into six doses. At each dose a solution of 0.5% polymyxin was atomized into the pharynx.

If a tracheal tube was present, half the dose was injected into the tracheal tube. The results of this study showed a significant decrease in colonization by gram-negative bacteria in those patients treated with polymyxin. Of the 25 control patients 17 became colonized with gram-negative bacilli. Of the 33 polymyxin-treated patients only 7 became colonized with gram-negative bacilli ($P < 0.01$) (Fig. 4-6). During the study no polymyxin-treated patients became colonized with *Pseudomonas aeruginosa*. Polymyxin treatment successfully reduced colonization in patients who remained in the unit for more than one week (Fig. 4-7). Polymyxin also prevented colonization in two-thirds of the patients who required controlled ventilation for more than three days, whereas control patients all became colonized after three days of controlled ventilation (Fig. 4-8).[766]

From late 1972 until mid-1974 a double-blind prospective study of 744 patients admitted to our unit demonstrated that polymyxin aerosol significantly reduced the incidence of acquired *Pseudomonas* pneumonia. For two months polymyxin B aerosol was administered to all patients as just described. During the next two months a placebo of physiologic saline was administered to all patients. Therapy was alternated in this manner for eleven two-month cycles. It was again demonstrated that upper airway colonization with *Pseudomonas aeruginosa* was significantly reduced (Figs. 4-9 and 4-10). During placebo cycles 17 patients acquired *Pseudomonas* pneumonia, whereas during polymyxin cycles only 3 patients developed *Pseudomonas* pneumonia ($X^2 = 10.2$, $P < 0.01$) (Figs. 4-11 and 4-12). There

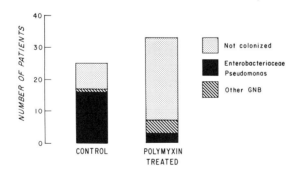

Figure 4-6.   Types of organisms causing colonization of the upper respiratory tract of patients in the R-SICU. Of 25 randomly selected control patients (who received no therapy) 17 became colonized with gram-negative bacteria (GNB); 16 of these 17 had species of Enterobacteriaceae or *Pseudomonas aeruginosa*. Of 33 patients treated with 2.5 mg per kilogram of body weight of polymyxin aerosol daily, only 7 became colonized with GNB ($P < 0.01$); only three of seven predominating organisms were species of Enterobacteriaceae. Polymyxin aerosol markedly reduces airway colonization with sensitive GNB. (From S. Greenfield, D. Teres, L. S. Bushnell, J. Hedley-Whyte, and D. S. Feingold, *J. Clin. Invest.*[766])

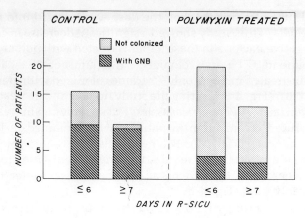

Figure 4-7. Effect of time on respiratory tract colonization with gram-negative bacteria (GNB). In 25 control patients the longer the stay in the R-SICU the greater the incidence of colonization of the upper airway by GNB. Polymyxin aerosol given to 33 patients prevented this colonization in 75 percent of treated patients, even after a week in the R-SICU. (From S. Greenfield, D. Teres, L. S. Bushnell, J. Hedley-Whyte, and D. S. Feingold, *J. Clin. Invest.*[766])

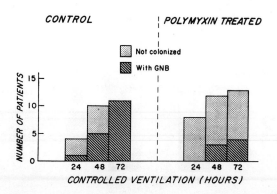

Figure 4-8. Bacterial airway colonization related to duration of controlled ventilation. Patients without a tracheal tube or those who received controlled ventilation for less than 24 hours rarely become colonized with gram-negative bacteria (GNB); 50 percent of control patients who required 24–72 hours of controlled ventilation became colonized with GNB. All 11 control patients became colonized after 72 hours of controlled ventilation ($P < 0.02$). By contrast, polymyxin aerosol prevented colonization of two-thirds of patients who required at least 72 hours of controlled ventilation. (From S. Greenfield, D. Teres, L. S. Bushnell, J. Hedley-Whyte, and D. S. Feingold, *J. Clin. Invest.*[766])

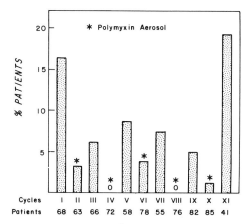

Figure 4-9. Effect of alternating cycles of polymyxin aerosol on airway colonization with *Pseudomonas aeruginosa*. Polymyxin aerosol was evaluated in a prospective double-blind study in which all patients in the Respiratory–Surgical Intensive Care Unit received polymyxin aerosol in a dose of 2.5 mg per kilogram per day for two months. During the next two months all patients received a placebo of physiologic saline. Polymyxin and placebo were alternated in this manner for 11 two-month cycles. Polymyxin aerosol (even-number cycles) reduced the incidence of airway colonization with *Pseudomonas aeruginosa*. The number of patients in each cycle is indicated. (From J. M. Klick, G. C. du Moulin, J. Hedley-Whyte, D. Teres, L. S. Bushnell, and D. S. Feingold, *J. Clin. Invest.*[1048])

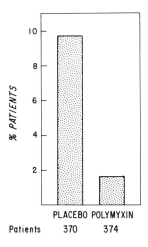

Figure 4-10. Effect of alternating cycles of polymyxin aerosol on airway colonization with *Pseudomonas aeruginosa*. Polymyxin aerosol and a placebo were given in alternating two-month cycles, as described in Figure 4-9. During placebo cycles of normal saline 36 of the 370 patients were colonized with *Pseudomonas aeruginosa* (9.7 percent). During the cycles when polymyxin aerosol was given in a dose of 2.5 mg per kilogram of body weight per day only 6 out of the 374 patients were colonized with *Pseudomonas aeruginosa* (1.6 percent). The reduction in colonization is significant ($x^2 = 23.2$, $P < 0.01$).

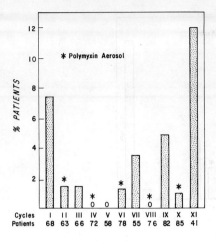

Figure 4-11. Effect of alternating cycles of polymyxin aerosol on the incidence of pneumonia caused by *Pseudomonas aeruginosa*. Polymyxin aerosol and a placebo were given in alternating two-month cycles, as described in Figure 4-9. The incidence of R-SICU–acquired pneumonia with *Pseudomonas aeruginosa* was reduced in each cycle that polymyxin was used (even-number cycles). The total number of patients in each cycle is indicated. (From J. M. Klick, G. C. du Moulin, J. Hedley-Whyte, D. Teres, L. S. Bushnell, and D. S. Feingold, *J. Clin. Invest.*[1048])

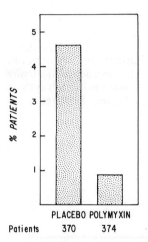

Figure 4-12. Effect of alternating cycles of polymyxin aerosol on the incidence of *Pseudomonas aeruginosa* pneumonia. Polymyxin aerosol and a placebo were given in alternating two-month cycles, as described in Figure 4-9. During placebo cycles 17 out of 370 patients (4.6 percent) acquired a pneumonia with *Pseudomonas aeruginosa*, while only 3 out of 374 patients (0.8 percent) acquired a *Pseudomonas aeruginosa* pneumonia during the polymyxin cycles. The reduction in the incidence of *Pseudomonas aeruginosa* pneumonia was significant ($x^2 = 10.2$, $P < 0.01$).

was no increase in either colonization or pneumonia caused by polymyxin-resistant organisms during polymyxin cycles. The results suggest that polymyxin aerosol prophylaxis, if given in alternating two-month cycles, may be an effective means of preventing acquired pneumonia due to *Pseudomonas*.[1048]

A subsequent study evaluated the effectiveness of polymyxin aerosol when given to all patients in our Respiratory Intensive Care Unit continuously for a seven-month period. Polymyxin was administered as described previously to all 292 patients. During that period only 1 patient acquired a pneumonia due to *Pseudomonas aeruginosa*, confirming polymyxin aerosol's ability to prevent *Pseudomonas* pneumonia (Fig. 4-13). There was an increase in the frequency of pneumonia due to polymyxin-resistant

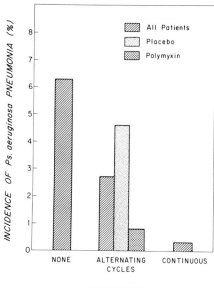

POLYMYXIN

Figure 4-13. Effect of the method of administration of aerosol polymyxin on the incidence of R-SICU–acquired *Pseudomonas aeruginosa* pneumonia. When no polymyxin was given during a period of two and one-half years *Pseudomonas* pneumonia occurred in over 6 percent of all patients. When polymyxin was alternated with a placebo of normal saline in 11 two-month alternating cycles (as described in Figure 4-9), the incidence of *Pseudomonas* pneumonia was significantly reduced during polymyxin use. Continuous use of polymyxin over a seven-month period resulted in a further reduction in the incidence of *Pseudomonas* pneumonia. Polymyxin-resistant organisms, however, posed major problems and we do not recommend long-term use of aerosol polymyxin. (From T. W. Feeley, G. C. du Moulin, J. Hedley-Whyte, L. S. Bushnell, J. P. Gilbert, and D. S. Feingold.[620] Reprinted by permission from the *New England Journal of Medicine* 293:471–475, 1975.)

organisms, however. Ten out of eleven pneumonias acquired within the intensive care unit were caused by polymyxin-resistant organisms. Although the overall incidence of acquired pneumonia fell to 3.9 percent (Fig. 4-14) the mortality associated with acquired pneumonia rose to 64 percent (Fig. 4-15). The continuous administration of polymyxin aerosol is therefore hazardous, since polymyxin-resistant organisms are selected out and appear to be as lethal as *Pseudomonas aeruginosa*. The organisms that caused pneumonia during this study and the outcome of the cases are summarized in Table 4-1.[620]

We presently use polymyxin aerosol only intermittently when patients are at increased risk to acquire *Pseudomonas aeruginosa* pneumonia. Polymyxin aerosol is given to all patients in our unit if a patient is admitted

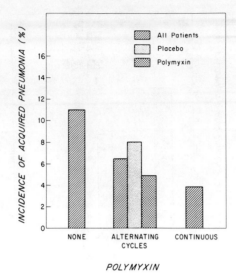

POLYMYXIN

Figure 4-14. Effect of the method of administration of polymyxin aerosol on the overall incidence of nosocomial pneumonia in our R-SICU. When no polymyxin was given for two and one-half years, 10.9 percent of patients acquired pneumonia. When polymyxin was alternated with a placebo of normal saline in 11 two-month cycles (as described in Figure 4-9), the overall incidence of acquired pneumonia fell to 6.4 percent. During the continuous use of polymyxin aerosol to all patients over seven months the incidence of acquired pneumonia fell to 3.9 percent. (From T. W. Feeley, G. C. du Moulin, J. Hedley-Whyte, L. S. Bushnell, J. P. Gilbert, and D. S. Feingold.[620] Reprinted by permission from the *New England Journal of Medicine* 291: 471–475, 1975.)

Table 4-1. Organisms Causing Pneumonia during Polymyxin Prophylaxis

Organism	Polymyxin Sensitivity*	No. Cases	No. Deaths
Pseudomonas aeruginosa	S	1	1
Proteus species	R	3	2
Pseudomonas cepacia	R	2	2
Pseudomonas maltophilia	R	2	0
Serratia species	R	1	0
Flavobacterium species	R	1	1
Streptococcus faecalis	R	1	1
Total		11	7

*S = polymyxin sensitive; R = polymyxin resistant.

SOURCE: T. W. Feeley, G. C. du Moulin, J. Hedley-Whyte, L. S. Bushnell, J. P. Gilbert, and D. S. Feingold.[620] Reprinted by permission from the *New England Journal of Medicine* 293: 471–475, 1975.

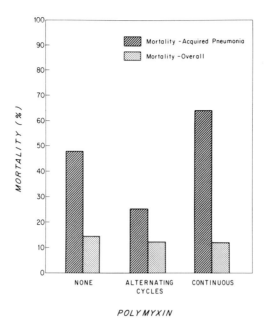

Figure 4-15. Effect of the method of administration of polymyxin aerosol on the overall mortality and the mortality for patients who acquire pneumonia. The mortality for patients who acquire pneumonia during the period of two and one-half years when no polymyxin was given was 48 percent. When polymyxin is alternated with a placebo in two-month cycles the mortality for acquired pneumonia is lowest (25 percent). When polymyxin aerosol was used in all patients over a seven-month period the mortality for acquired pneumonia rose to 64 percent due to the emergence of polymyxin-resistant organisms. (From T. W. Feeley, G. C. du Moulin, J. Hedley-Whyte, L. S. Bushnell, J. P. Gilbert, and D. S. Feingold.[620] Reprinted by permission from the *New England Journal of Medicine* 291:471–475, 1975.)

with a *Pseudomonas* infection or if a patient develops a *Pseudomonas* infection in the unit. Polymyxin aerosol is also begun if three or more of seven patients in the unit simultaneously have respiratory tracts colonized with *Pseudomonas aeruginosa*. Polymyxin aerosol is continued until cultures from all patients in the unit are free from *Pseudomonas aeruginosa*. In the last 544 patients admitted to our unit, the incidence of upper airway colonization with polymyxin-resistant organisms was reduced to 28 percent and the incidence of pneumonias acquired in the intensive care unit was reduced to 1.5 percent. The overall intensive care unit mortality rate fell to 6.4 percent with this regimen.

Gentamicin

Endotracheal gentamicin also has been suggested as an agent for the prevention of gram-negative pneumonia. Studies evaluating this treatment have been plagued by the emergence of strains of bacteria which are resistant to gentamicin. These bacteria have produced devastating infections.[1041,1042] Endotracheal gentamicin therefore is probably dangerous for the routine prophylaxis of nosocomial pneumonia in critically ill patients.

MONITORING

Of great importance in the prevention of gram-negative infections is the close monitoring of the patient.[620,1343] Environmental monitoring has been discussed previously in this chapter. Early detection of acquired pneumonia can be helpful in providing treatment as early as possible. In all patients who are at high risk for developing gram-negative pneumonia, routine monitoring should include daily cultures and gram stain of the sputum as well as a careful daily clinical examination. In our unit all patients have a daily clinical examination, and most have a daily measurement of the alveolar-arterial oxygen tension gradient. If any of these examinations suggest the development of infection, a chest x-ray will help to confirm the diagnosis. All too often there is a tendency to obtain a daily chest x-ray on all patients. This is an extremely costly way of obtaining the same information as can be gained by a careful clinical evaluation of the patient.

In summary nosocomial pulmonary infection in patients in intensive care units is a serious problem and, in spite of therapy, carries a high mortality. Since these infections are preceded by colonization of the upper respiratory tract, prevention of colonization is of prime importance in reducing the incidence of this disease. This can be accomplished by evaluation and elimination of the many environmental sources of these organisms. There is also evidence that prophylactic administration of polymyxin B aerosol to the upper airway reduces the incidence of acquired *Pseudomonas* pneumonia in critically ill patients.

5

Effect of Sepsis on Respiratory Function

The most common cause of acute respiratory failure in general surgical patients without trauma is sepsis. Respiratory insufficiency occurs in 62 percent of patients with proved gram-negative septicemia, 8–21 percent dying of respiratory failure as the primary cause.[869] In 40 percent of surgical patients respiratory failure is the first manifestation of severe gram-negative sepsis.[53,1996] Even if the lung is not seeded by the bacteria during septic shock, its defenses are devastated. Phagocytosis is inhibited by hypotension, by decreased complement,[867,1451] and by oxygen administration.[936] Electrocardiographic evidence of myocardial ischemia is found in 89 percent of patients with gram-negative septicemia.[2041]

RESPONSE OF THE RESPIRATORY SYSTEM

EFFECT OF BACTERIA

The response of the respiratory system to sepsis is brought about both by circulating microorganisms and by the products of those organisms. The bacteria themselves cause antigen-antibody reactions. The lipopolysaccharide of the gram-negative bacterial wall acts as antigen. Bacteremia or septicemia causes a temporary increase in pulmonary artery pressure with no increase in left atrial pressure and only a slight increase of pulmonary capillary wedge pressure. This elevation lasts one-half to one hour after a single intravenous infusion of either endotoxin or whole bacteria, after which pulmonary artery pressure returns to baseline values.[234,711,1073] The mechanism for this rise in pressure is not known but is in part due to precapillary vasoconstriction, which is blocked by pretreatment with acetylsalicylic acid and oxygen but not by antihistamines, antiserotonins, or adrenergic agents.[1604] The pulmonary vasoconstriction of hypoxemia is abolished by endotoxin and not modified by acetylsalicylic acid.[777]

The majority of pulmonary capillary pores are estimated to be approximately 25–58 Å. There are also pores of 125 Å.[233,234,1000,1716,1902] The infusion of whole bacteria causes an increase in pulmonary capillary permeability, resulting in a leak of fluid and protein into the pulmonary interstitium. Lymph flow from the lungs increases (Fig. 5-1).[365,1623,1839,1895,2000] Once the

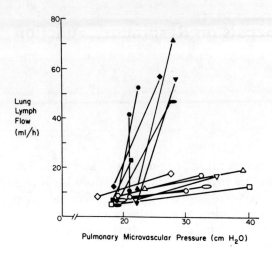

Figure 5-1. Responses of lung lymph flow to increased pulmonary microvascular pressure and to a *Pseudomonas* infusion in seven sheep. Each animal is indicated by a differently shaped symbol. *Open symbols* indicate studies in which pressure was increased mechanically by inflation of a left atrial balloon. *Closed symbols* indicate *Pseudomonas* infusion studies. Lines connect baseline and experimental observations in a single experiment. Each point is an average of at least two hours of steady state. After *Pseudomonas* bacteremia, lymph flow is much higher than would be expected on the basis of increased pressure alone. (From K. L. Brigham, W. C. Woolverton, L. H. Blake, and N. C. Staub, *J. Clin. Invest.*[234])

leak of fluid and protein exceeds the ability of the lymphatic system to drain the interstitium, fluid fills the alveoli, and pulmonary edema results.[825,942,1547,1636,1838] Surfactant activity is reduced.

Other mechanisms also have been proposed to explain the occurrence of respiratory failure in septicemia. A direct endotoxin effect on endothelial oxidative metabolism may result in inability to maintain pore structure. Endotoxin effects on the central nervous system may cause cellular hypoxia, resulting in a neurogenic increase in pulmonary venular resistance and therefore increased capillary hydrostatic pressure despite normal left atrial pressures.[1078,1296,1371] The endotoxin causes complement consumption by directly activating the properdin pathway with the release of vasoactive products.[401,895,1816,1987] This pathway consists of properdin, factor IX (C3 proactivator), C5, C6, and C9. This postulate is supported by evidence showing decreased levels of C3 in patients with gram-negative bacteremia (Fig. 5-2).[619,1259]

VASOACTIVE AGENTS

The role of vasoactive agents in the pulmonary response to septicemia is not fully understood. Vasoactive agents include amines (acetylcholine, serotonin, histamine, epinephrine, norepinephrine, dopamine, and iso-

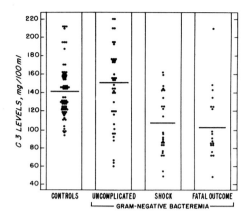

Figure 5-2. C3 (complement component) levels are significantly lower in patients with gram-negative shock and in those patients with gram-negative bacteremia who die. There is no difference in C3 levels between patients with uncomplicated sepsis and controls. *Horizontal bars* indicate mean. (From W. R. McCabe.[1259] Reprinted by permission from the *New England Journal of Medicine* 288:21–23, 1973.)

proterenol), peptides (bradykinin, angiotensin, vasopressin, fibrinopeptides A and B), and prostaglandins. Each affects pulmonary blood flow and airway size in a species-dependent fashion.[859] Leukocytes interact with endotoxin to form kinins or activate plasma kallikrein.[363] Leukocytes also release locally toxic lysosomes.[89,722]

Many vasoactive agents are stored and metabolized in the lung.[86,360,646,859,1921,1922] Serotonin, which is released by platelets, causes an increase in both pulmonary artery pressure and airway constriction.[203,1748] Acetylcholine causes airway constriction.[390] Epinephrine in high doses worsens pulmonary edema.[321] Human fibrinopeptide A increases pulmonary artery pressure and the alveolar-arterial oxygen tension difference while decreasing compliance.[115] Bradykinin causes a 10 percent decrease in pulmonary artery pressure in the dog, and in man it constricts the alveolar ducts and reduces vital capacity without changes in large or small airways.[1151,1420] Histamine, which is not significantly inactivated by the lung, raises pulmonary artery pressure in animals but reportedly not in man.[895] In man it constricts all airways, decreases vital capacity, and increases respiratory system resistance and closing volume.[1420] The ability of endotoxin to cause airway constriction is inhibited by severe thrombocytopenia, serotonin antagonism, or heparin pretreatment.[1847] In heart-lung preparations, epinephrine, norepinephrine, angiotensin, vasopressin, histamine, bradykinin, or serotonin infusions are able to cause pulmonary edema.[321] In the whole animal, infusions of epinephrine, norepinephrine, angiotensin, vasopressin, levarterenol bitartrate, serotonin, and bradykinin cause pulmonary edema in the presence of endotoxin.[321,371]

CARDIOVASCULAR EFFECTS

Eighty percent of patients who develop gram-negative bacteremia become hypotensive. However, only 20–30 percent of patients develop septic shock—a circulatory collapse in which cellular nutrition is inadequate for oxidative cellular metabolism.[869,2005,2046] Female patients account for 60 percent of gram-negative bacteremias but only 44 percent of cases of shock. Infusion of live *Escherichia coli* to conscious baboons was followed by a 2- to 4-hour period of decreased vascular resistance and increased cardiac output despite hypotension. After this period there was a progressive increase in systemic vascular resistance and a fall in cardiac output.[260,332,368,778,866]

EARLY PHASE

In patients with simple bacteremia there is an early phase of normal or elevated cardiac output compensating for a fall in peripheral resistance.[712,784,2080,2083,2089] Although the cardiac index is normal as compared to that of healthy individuals, the flow is probably inadequate for the needs of a febrile patient with peritonitis.[14,570,783,866,922,1243] The decreased peripheral vascular resistance may be due to opening of peripheral arteriovenous shunts because of circulatory vasoactive substances or locally released vasodilator substances.[14,495] This supposition is supported by studies showing increased levels of kinins in bacteremia only for the first few hours.[400,401,1027] The arteriovenous oxygen content difference is narrowed, indicating either failure of effective capillary blood flow, arteriovenous shunting, or a direct endotoxic depression of cellular oxidative metabolism.[1295] Platelets or platelet thrombi obstruct capillary flow, resulting in release of serotonin from platelets. The serotonin and other metabolic vasoactive agents cause opening of arteriovenous shunts.

LATE PHASE

In later shock, cardiac output falls. This may be due to a possible myocardial depressant factor, decreased myocardial flow, coronary vascular obstruction, or circulating toxins.[949,1136,1772,1774,2021] Endotoxin seems to have no direct myocardial depressant effect.[894] In late shock peripheral vascular resistance increases due to circulating catecholamines.[784,952] This hemodynamic picture may be the presenting one in patients with hypovolemia at the onset of bacteremia (Fig. 5-3).[712,2080] Once shock has occurred, blood volume gradually decreases due to sequestration of red cells and plasma loss.[309,893,928]

Further evidence to support the concept of two phases of septic shock is given by the effects of hemorrhage during endotoxemia in unanesthetized monkeys. After the loss of 30 percent of blood volume, endotoxin-induced hypotension with decreased vascular resistance and normal cardiac output changes to an increased vascular resistance and decreased cardiac output.[893,1322]

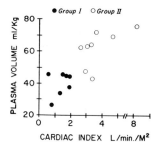

Figure 5-3. Relationship of plasma volume and cardiac index in patients in bacteremic shock. Those with plasma volumes greater than 50 ml per kilogram maintained a cardiac index greater than 3 l/min/m² *(open circles, Group II)*; those with plasma volumes less than 50 ml per kilogram had cardiac indices less than 3 l/min/m² *(closed circles, Group I)*. (From V. N. Udhoji and M. H. Weil, *Ann. Intern. Med.*[1954])

Puerperal sepsis and shock follow similar patterns to that just described.[391,1653]

METABOLISM IN SEPTICEMIA

Gram-negative septicemia is associated with multiple metabolic changes. Circulating lactate levels are increased due to anaerobic cellular metabolism.[239] An initial hyperglycemia is followed by hypoglycemia because of the increased sensitivity to epinephrine and norepinephrine of glycogenolysis in the liver. Plasma lipids increase in gram-negative septicemia but not in gram-positive septicemia.[681,819,1698]

In the presence of fever and in the absence of shock, oxygen demand and metabolic rate increase in proportion to the increase in temperature. The work done by DuBois in medical patients with fever showed a 13 percent increase in caloric expenditure or carbon dioxide production per degree Celsius increase in temperature (7.2 percent per degree Fahrenheit) (Fig. 5-4).[549,550] Tidal volume increases 9 percent per degree

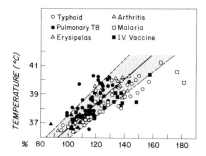

Figure 5-4. Increase in metabolic rate with increase in temperature. The abscissa shows percent of normal metabolic rate. Data are from medical patients, not in shock, with pulmonary tuberculosis, erysipelas, arthritis, malaria, intravenous vaccine, or typhoid. (From E. F. DuBois, *Basal Metabolism in Health and Disease.*[550])

Celsius in patients without cardiorespiratory disease.[1545] In patients with fever or peritonitis but without shock, however, the actual carbon dioxide production, oxygen consumption, and caloric expenditure can be 25–50 percent greater than the value predicted by DuBois (Fig. 5-5).[1031,1032,1545,1647] DuBois studied medical patients who were febrile. Larger differences from normal occur in patients who have sustained trauma, who have undergone surgery, or who have peritonitis. In such patients the increase in oxygen consumption or cardiac index is unrelated to body temperature (Fig. 5-6).[782,783] If shivering occurs, oxygen consumption and therefore carbon dioxide production can increase to five times the resting value.[114] The increased ventilatory requirements are due both to the increased metabolic rate and to an increased physiologic deadspace. In such patients without shock, the increase in oxygen consumption and carbon dioxide production stimulate an increase in cardiac output and a decrease in peripheral vascular resistance, resulting in a widening of the arteriovenous oxygen difference and a fall in blood lactate.[1031,1206]

Metabolism is affected differently if septic shock occurs. Because of arteriovenous shunting, vasoconstriction, and toxic effects on cellular oxidative metabolism, oxygen consumption falls[1875] in early and late septic shock.[1761,1762,1774] Lactate production increases (Fig. 5-7).[1280,1830] The subcellular response in shock includes a fault in ATPase activity and adenine nucleotide translocase activity at the mitochondrial level.[1295] Only in the low flow types of septic shock will an increase in cardiac output oxygenate cells and reduce cellular lactate production; in the high flow type of shock, increasing the cardiac output has no effect on lactate (Fig. 5-8). In fact, as total peripheral resistance is decreased in the high flow states, the arteriovenous oxygen difference narrows (Fig. 5-9). This is due both to ar-

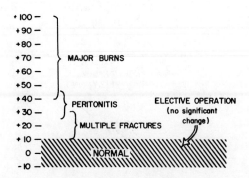

Figure 5-5. Increase in metabolic rate in patients with burns, peritonitis, and multiple fractures. These patients' metabolism often increases above that predicted by DuBois. Figures represent percentage of normal metabolic rate (0 = normal). (From J. M. Kinney. In S. G. Hershey, L. R. M. Del Guercio, and R. McConn (Eds.), *Septic Shock in Man.*[1031] Copyright, 1971, Little, Brown and Company, by permission.)

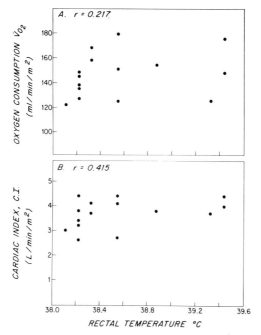

Figure 5-6. Cardiac index (CI) and oxygen consumption ($\dot{V}O_2$) in 15 patients with peritonitis with reference to the rectal temperature at the time of the measurements. Normal values for well individuals in the age group of the patients tested are CI 2.8 1/min/m² and $\dot{V}O_2$ 120 ml/min/m². Rectal temperature is not a useful predictor of CI or $\dot{V}O_2$ in patients with peritonitis. (From F. E. Gump, J. B. Price, Jr., and J. M. Kinney, *Ann. Surg.*[783])

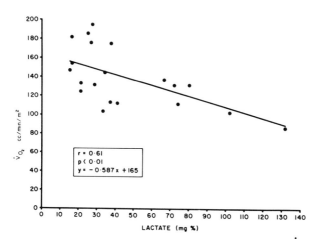

Figure 5-7. The increase in blood lactate as oxygen consumption ($\dot{V}O_2$) decreases in patients in septic shock. The raised lactate under these circumstances is indicative of cellular anoxia. (From L. D. MacLean, A. P. H. McLean, and J. H. Duff, *Postgrad. Med.*[1206])

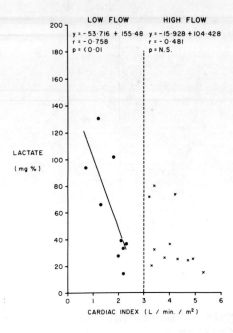

Figure 5-8. Changes in blood lactate with an increase in the cardiac index. The blood lactate level improves only in the low flow type of septic shock. In patients with normal or high flow states, further increasing the cardiac output does not decrease blood lactate. (From A. P. H. McLean, J. H. Duff, A. C. Groves, R. Lapointe, and L. D. MacLean. In S. G. Hershey, L. R. M. Del Guercio, and R. McConn (Eds.), *Septic Shock in Man.*[1280] Copyright, 1971, Little, Brown and Company, by permission.)

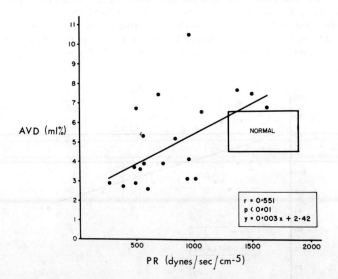

Figure 5-9. Changes in arteriovenous oxygen difference (AVD) with increasing peripheral vascular resistance (PR). In patients in septic shock the peripheral vascular resistance is usually low and is associated with a narrowed arteriovenous oxygen difference. (From A. P. H. McLean, J. H. Duff, A. C. Groves, R. Lapointe, and L. D. MacLean. In S. G. Hershey, L. R. M. Del Guercio, and R. McConn (Eds.), *Septic Shock in Man.*[1280] Copyright, 1971, Little, Brown and Company, by permission.)

teriovenous shunting and to failure of uptake of oxygen by the cell for oxidative metabolism, despite the presence of oxygen in the capillary.

COAGULATION

Both whole bacterial and endotoxin infusion can activate factor XII (Hageman factor), initiating the intrinsic clotting cascade.[145,146,427,1248,1592] Clinically septicemia is associated with disseminated intravascular coagulation, which often precipitates respiratory failure.[369,1559] Masses of platelets and fibrin can be trapped in the pulmonary bed as microthrombi.[470] These thrombi adhere to and expand on endotoxin-damaged pulmonary capillary endothelial cells.[371,500,1281,2062] Platelets and platelet membranes stimulate leukocyte procoagulant activity.[1429] Heparin administration is effective in preventing death due to endotoxic shock in the rat but not in the dog or in man, although clotting parameters are returned to normal. Heparin does not improve blood gas values.[426,1227,1560]

RENAL FUNCTION

In most human septic shock, although effective renal plasma flow does decrease, true renal plasma flow actually increases. Only when the glomerular filtration rate falls below 40 percent of the norm does blood urea nitrogen rise.[1193,1939] If the inappropriate diuresis is not compensated for by fluid administration, renal shutdown occurs.

FLORA ENCOUNTERED IN SEPTICEMIA AND SHOCK

Gram-negative organisms account for approximately 66 percent of hospital-acquired cases of bacteremia.[184,2046,2080] Gram-positive bacteria account for an additional 30 percent; the remainder are due to miscellaneous organisms such as fungi, viruses, rickettsiae, and protozoa.[1207] The organisms isolated by blood culture in patients with bacteremia with or without shock depend upon the underlying disease, the site of infection, and the prevalent organisms to which the patient is exposed. In 30 percent of cases of septicemia with shock no bacteria can be isolated.[1051] In those cases in which bacteria are isolated *Escherichia coli* is the most common and is followed by *Klebsiella, Proteus, Pseudomonas,* and *Providencia*.[2041,2046] In gram-positive bacteremias *Staphylococcus* is the most common organism and the next most common is *Streptococcus*.[2080,2089] Of the rarer miscellaneous organisms, *Candida* is the most common type and can now be diagnosed in man by gas-liquid chromatography of serum.[1314]

GRAM-POSITIVE SEPTICEMIA

Patients with gram-positive septicemia exhibit the same degree of hypotension as those with gram-negative septicemia. Cardiac output remains normal or elevated with a decreased systemic vascular resistance even in late or prolonged gram-positive septicemia.[590,780,784,1081,2089]

ANAEROBIC SEPTICEMIA

Anaerobes are isolated as the causative agent in 8–11 percent of bacteremias. Common sources are the gastrointestinal tract, the female genitourinary tract, and the lung. The lung is particularly subject to anaerobic infection, especially following aspiration. *Bacteroides* and *Fusobacteria* species are commonly encountered. The clinical picture presented by anaerobic sepsis is similar to that of gram-negative sepsis. Hypotension occurs in 40 percent of cases, and the mortality rate is approximately 30 percent.[627,741,1438,2086]

PERITONITIS

Peritonitis is associated with the majority of cases of septicemia in surgical patients.[843,2080] The effect of peritonitis on the lungs is to cause decreased diaphragmatic excursion with rapid, shallow breathing. Lung parenchyma is compressed and atelectatic. Lung water is generally increased. Mortality is elevated; 86 percent of our patients with respiratory failure without peritonitis survive, whereas only 20 percent of patients with both respiratory failure and peritonitis survive. In our study of 58 patients with and without peritonitis and with and without respiratory failure, the greatest reduction of vital capacity was found in the group with both respiratory failure and peritonitis (Fig. 5-10). Pulmonary compliance was lower in

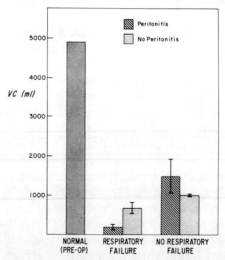

Figure 5-10.   Vital capacity (VC) in patients in respiratory failure with and without peritonitis. Vital capacities were obtained daily on 58 consecutive patients admitted to our Respiratory–Surgical Intensive Care Unit (R-SICU) following abdominal operations. Twenty-nine patients were in respiratory failure and twenty patients had peritonitis. Seventy-five percent of the patients with peritonitis were in respiratory failure. Those patients with respiratory failure and peritonitis had the lowest vital capacities compared to the other three groups ($P < 0.005$). Results were based upon the lowest vital capacity for each patient and are shown as the mean ± SE. (From J. J. Skillman, L. S. Bushnell, and J. Hedley-Whyte, *Ann. Surg.*[1791])

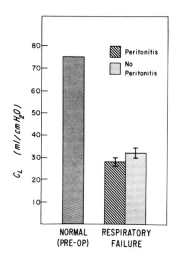

Figure 5-11. Total static compliance (CL) in respiratory failure after abdominal surgery. Values were obtained from 58 patients admitted to the R-SICU. The compliance (mean ± SE) of 15 patients with peritonitis was slightly lower than the compliance of patients without peritonitis. Results are based on the lowest compliance measurement from each patient. (From J. J. Skillman, L. S. Bushnell, and J. Hedley-Whyte, *Ann. Surg.* [1791])

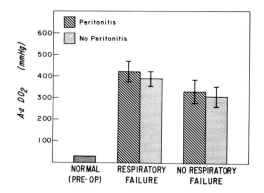

Figure 5-12. The alveolar-arterial oxygen tension difference (A-aD_{O_2}) on 100% oxygen in postoperative patients with or without peritonitis with or without associated acute respiratory failure. In patients with both peritonitis and respiratory failure the mean A-aD_{O_2} is 422 mm Hg (56.1 kPa). Results are based on the highest alveolar-arterial oxygen tension difference measured in the R-SICU on each patient. All values are mean ± SE. (From J. J. Skillman, L. S. Bushnell, and J. Hedley-Whyte, *Ann. Surg.* [1791])

those patients with peritonitis (Fig. 5-11).[1791] The effects of peritonitis and respiratory failure on the alveolar-arterial oxygen tension difference are recorded in Figure 5-12. There was no difference in deadspace-to-tidal-volume ratio (Fig. 5-13). The highest carbon dioxide production was 208 percent of the predicted value. Although metabolic rate and consequently oxygen consumption and carbon dioxide production are increased in peritonitis, contrary to previous reports these factors alone do not cause respiratory failure after major abdominal operations.[275,1545,1791]

An increased metabolic rate requires an increase in cardiac output. When the heart is no longer able to compensate or is depressed, vasoconstriction

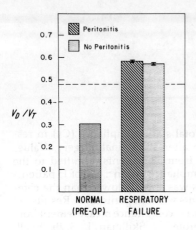

Figure 5-13. Deadspace-to-tidal-volume ratio (V_D/V_T) in patients in respiratory failure with or without peritonitis. Those patients with respiratory failure had an average V_D/V_T of 0.48 (*dashed line*), and normal individuals averaged 0.3. An increase in minute ventilation is needed to compensate for the increased deadspace. Results are based on the maximum V_D/V_T of each patient and are shown as the mean ± SE. (From J. J. Skillman, L. S. Bushnell, and J. Hedley-Whyte, *Ann. Surg.*[1791])

may occur. Survival is related to ability to maintain a normal or low peripheral vascular resistance and pulmonary vascular resistance (Fig. 5-14).[357,366] In patients with peritonitis but without hypotension or respiratory failure, oxygen consumption increases in 60 percent but is normal in 40 percent, whereas cardiac output is elevated in almost all patients.[783,1663]

MANAGEMENT

PLASMA EXPANDERS

In the case of damaged and leaking pulmonary vasculature the administration of concentrated protein plasma expanders alone will not elevate plasma oncotic pressure above pulmonary interstitial oncotic pressure, because proteins cross into the interstitium.[693,1795] As pulmonary artery pressure is increased by therapy, more fluid and protein pass into the interstitium, eventually at a rate surpassing that of lymph drainage. Fluid then rapidly accumulates in the interstitium and eventually fills the alveoli. Frank pulmonary edema results.[234] In undamaged pulmonary vasculature the elevation of plasma oncotic pressure by hemoconcentration does increase the pulmonary artery pressure at which pulmonary edema occurs.[676,717] In patients with severe peritonitis there is a large loss of plasma proteins with a lowering of plasma oncotic pressure.[503] These patients often do need plasma volume expansion with albumin to return oncotic pressures to normal. Excessive administration of albumin is to be avoided.

DOPAMINE AND OTHER VASOPRESSORS

If cardiac depression is diagnosed, dopamine 500–1500 μg per minute (1.6 mg per milliliter of solution) is administered. This is preferable to rapid digitalization or glucagon administration, since dopamine's effect is immediate and untoward consequences are relatively easily controlled. Vasoconstricting drugs such as phenylephrine, methoxamine, levarterenol, and metaraminol are usually detrimental, especially if given during the vasoconstrictive phase of shock.[779,998,1176,1177,1203,1288,1897] Vasoconstricting drugs do not increase survival rates.[921] Isoproterenol is also detrimental, if its vasodilatory effect causes further hypotension with decrease in coronary flow. The administration of vasopressors does not improve pulmonary blood gas exchange, and lactic acidemia worsens.

HEPARIN AND OTHER DRUGS

If disseminated intravascular coagulation is present, heparin is administered intravenously (Chap. 29). Metabolic acidemia is corrected by administration of sodium bicarbonate. Antibiotics are administered according to the sensitivity of the organisms. Broad-spectrum antibiotics are administered initially. When antibiotic sensitivities of the organism have been measured, antibiotic therapy is changed appropriately. Endotoxin is released from killed bacteria after antibiotic administration.[2041] Ionized calcium should be repeatedly checked.[503] Steroids have been advocated in the treatment of septic shock; however, we find the evidence for their effectiveness unconvincing, and the clinical results are equivocal in our hands.[340,868,1263,1656,2041,2077] Nitroprusside has a use in patients in endotoxic shock.[1522]

PROGNOSIS

Patients with septicemia who exhibit a sustained increase in pulmonary vascular resistance and an early fall in oxygen consumption have a poor prognosis (Fig. 5-14).[366,1762] The probable outcome is also poor for patients unable to maintain an increased cardiac output.[1954] There is a significant correlation between increasing IgG and decreasing frequency of shock and death.[1260,2138] In addition the greater the number of bacteria in the blood the higher the mortality.[1051] Survival is favored by a blood lactate level of less than 3.0 mEq per liter (3.0 mmol/1) and a normal blood volume and P_{50}.[1435] The mortality is influenced chiefly by the underlying disease: the better the prognosis for the disease, the better the prognosis if septic shock intervenes. If a patient has bacteremia, he or she should be examined frequently to exclude the possibility of pneumonia, endocarditis, meningitis, brain abscess, acute tubular necrosis, or disseminated intravascular coagulation.

Case report. A 19-year-old female, gravida O, para O, was admitted to the Beth Israel Hospital for a diagnostic laparoscopy because of continuous dull, lower abdominal pain, first noted five months prior to admission and unaffected by the removal of an intrauterine device and a 10-day course of ampicillin. Physical examination on admission revealed a 5 cm × 5 cm, soft, cystic, tender mass attached to the left ovary. The blood pressure was 116/67 mm Hg (15.4/8.9 kPa), pulse rate 82 beats per minute, respiratory rate 20 per minute, and temperature 36.7°C. The remainder of the history and physical examination was unremarkable.

A laparoscopy was performed under general anesthesia. There was difficulty in obtaining gas flow through the laparoscopy trocar prior to insertion into the abdomen, until flushing with normal saline relieved an apparent obstruction. Thereafter gas flowed freely, and the laparoscopy proceeded. An edematous left fallopian tube

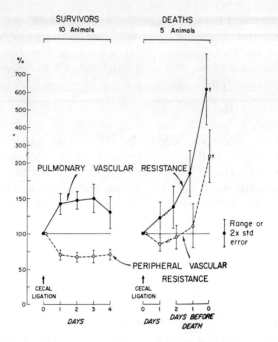

Figure 5-14.   The increase in both pulmonary and peripheral vascular resistance in dogs about to die as a result of experimental peritonitis. The average values are expressed as percent change from control values prior to onset of peritonitis. (From G. H. A. Clowes, Jr., G. H. Farrington, W. Zuschneid, G. R. Cossette, and C. Saravis, *Ann. Surg.*[366])

was noted to be adherent to the left ovary. Blood pressure during and immediately postoperatively was stable at 130/80 mm Hg (17.3/10.6 kPa), and the heart rate was 92 beats per minute.

Two hours postoperatively the patient had a shaking chill, a temperature of 39.0°C, and a blood pressure of 100/65 mm Hg (13.3/8.6 kPa). The hematocrit was unchanged from the preoperative level of 40 percent. The white blood cell count was 900 per cubic millimeter (0.9 10⁹/1) (preoperative value, 8,550 per cubic millimeter [8.5 $10^9/1$]). Cultures of blood, throat, cervix, and urine were taken, and ampicillin 1 gm every six hours was then given intravenously. The intravenous fluid bottle had been discarded and was not cultured. Four hours postoperatively the temperature was 40.8°C and the blood pressure 75/0 (10/0 kPa). The extremities were warm with full pulses. Clotting tests were drawn, the ampicillin dosage was doubled, and aggressive fluid therapy consisting of 1,500 ml Ringer's lactate and 50 gm of salt-poor albumin restored the blood pressure to 90/50 mm Hg (12/7 kPa). Urine output was 120 ml per hour and had never fallen below 40 ml per hour.

During the next sixteen hours the patient's blood pressure and urine output remained stable. One episode of bleeding at venipuncture sites was associated with a prothrombin time of 16.2/11.8, a partial thromboplastin time of 45.9/23.8, a platelet count of 70,000 per cubic millimeter (70 10⁹/1), and a fibrinogen range of 60–120 mg per 100 ml (1.8–3.5 μmol/1). Two units of fresh frozen plasma corrected the fibrinogen level and bleeding. Arterial blood gases determined while she was breathing 40 percent oxygen changed from Pa_{O_2} 234 mm Hg (31.1 kPa), Pa_{CO_2} 49 mm Hg (6.5 kPa), and pH 7.34 immediately postoperatively to Pa_{O_2} 83 mm Hg (11.1 kPa), Pa_{CO_2} 51 mm Hg (6.8 kPa), and pH 7.32 nineteen hours postoperatively.

Twenty-one hours postoperatively, due to a change in abdominal signs, an exploratory laparotomy was performed to rule out an intraabdominal abscess or contamination. No abscess or bowel perforation was found; the peritoneal fluid, which was clear, was cultured. Central venous and pulmonary artery catheters were inserted intraoperatively with initial values of 16 cm water (1.6 kPa) and 18/14 mm Hg (2.4/1.9 kPa) respectively. Arterial blood gases on 100% oxygen with controlled ventilation were Pa_{O_2} 85 mm Hg (11.3 kPa), Pa_{CO_2} 40 mm Hg (5.3 kPa), and pH 7.38. Controlled ventilation was therefore maintained postoperatively with the addition of positive end-expiratory pressure in increments of up to 15 cm water (1.5 kPa). Clindamycin 600 mg intravenously every six hours and gentamicin 60 mg intravenously every eight hours (dependent on renal function) were added to antibiotic coverage when the preliminary blood culture report was positive for gram-negative rods.

Five hours after the exploratory laparotomy the patient's blood pressure again fell to 80/0 mm Hg (10.6/0 kPa); cardiac output was 5.3 liters per minute. Administration of dopamine (400 mg in 250 ml dextrose in water) was begun; central venous pressure fell to 10 cm water (1.0 kPa) and pulmonary artery pressure to 11/6 mm Hg (1.5/0.8 kPa) with a wedge pressure of 1 mm Hg (0.13 kPa). Urine output gradually declined; a trial of levarterenol with fluid therapy in addition to dopamine increased the systolic blood pressure to 110 mm Hg (14.6 kPa), at which point urine output increased. The results of laboratory tests at this time included prolonged prothrombin and partial thromboplastin times, a thrombin time of 27/17.1, positive ethanol gelation, fibrin degradation products as high as 1,000 mg per milliliter (normal: less than 8 mg per milliliter), and decreased hematocrit and platelets. Other coagulation factor assays gave normal results. Because of continued intravascular coagulation a low dosage of heparin infusion was begun, 5–10 units per kilogram per hour, and continued for three days until fibrin degradation products disappeared and fibrinogen levels returned to normal. The chest x-ray showed poorly delineated and sometimes confluent parenchymal densities in both lung fields, of an alveolar character without vascular engorgement.

The patient required vasopressors and intermittent positive pressure ventilation with positive end-expiratory pressure for the next three days. Attempts to wean her from mechanical ventilation were not successful until the seventh postoperative day. Thereafter the patient recovered uneventfully and was discharged on the fifteenth hospital day. Final blood culture reports from the specimen taken after the first operation disclosed *Enterobacter agglomerans;* all other cultures were negative. *Enterobacter agglomerans* is occasionally found in infected intravenous solutions. Later the Food and Drug Administration ordered a general recall of intravenous solutions made at the same factory that manufactured the intravenous solution used during the laparoscopy.

6

Problems of Fluid Balance

Maintenance of a correct fluid balance in the critically ill patient is frequently difficult. There are a multitude of factors that affect fluid balance in critically ill patients, especially postoperatively, and that must be considered during the daily management of these patients. This chapter will discuss several important aspects of fluid balance that influence the management of critically ill patients.

OVERHYDRATION DURING CONTROLLED VENTILATION

During both intermittent and continuous positive pressure ventilation fluid retention occurs and can lead to pulmonary edema without evidence of cardiac failure.[701,1801] About 20 percent of patients in acute respiratory failure in the Massachusetts General Hospital demonstrated a gain in weight, positive water balance, hyponatremia, and a fall in hematocrit associated with a clinical picture of pulmonary edema but without any other signs of cardiac failure.[1801]

The mechanism for the development of this syndrome of fluid retention is not entirely clear. Alteration in circulating levels of antidiuretic hormone is postulated as one possible mechanism. Elevations in antidiuretic hormone occur in subjects receiving continuous positive pressure ventilation.[1801] During continuous negative pressure breathing a diuresis occurs which is related to an inhibition of antidiuretic hormone.[215] Left atrial stretch receptors influence levels of antidiuretic hormone via a vagal reflex arc. If the left atrium is stretched, these receptors send impulses via the vagus to the hypothalamus and reduce the output of antidiuretic hormone from the posterior pituitary, leading to a diuresis. During positive pressure ventilation the venous return is reduced, left atrial pressure falls, and increased peripheral levels of antidiuretic hormone result.[485]

Other mechanisms are also postulated, and it is likely that there are not one but many reasons for fluid retention during controlled ventilation. The effect of positive pressure breathing on the kidney has been discussed in Chapter 3. Undoubtedly intrarenal redistribution of blood flow contributes to fluid retention. Extravasation of fluid into the extravascular space when the serum oncotic pressure is low probably also contributes to fluid retention. Osmoreceptors in the hypothalamus may also play some part.[485] The humidification systems on volume-constant ventilators prevent the normal insensible loss of water from the respiratory system. A net water gain of 300–500 ml can occur daily during controlled ventilation with an adequate humidification system. If not allowed for, this water can lead to fluid overload.

Under most circumstances the fluid requirements of a patient receiving controlled ventilation are less than those of a patient breathing spontaneously. The only way to prevent fluid overload is by careful daily measurement of intake, output, and body weight and by examination of the serum electrolytes and the alveolar-arterial oxygen tension gradient.

If fluid overload with pulmonary edema does occur during mechanical ventilation, the administration of diuretics usually reverses the process. If fluid overload develops without pulmonary edema, the daily intake of fluid should be restricted so that a negative fluid balance ensues.

HYPOVOLEMIA DURING CONTROLLED VENTILATION

There are various reasons for volume depletion during controlled ventilation. During a major surgical procedure the functional extracellular space is reduced due to a loss of fluid, electrolytes, and albumin at the operative site. The longer procedures with the most retraction of organs are associated with the greatest loss.[932,1756,1758] If the losses are not replaced with salt-containing solutions at the time of surgery, the patient will arrive in the intensive care unit in a hypovolemic state. This so-called *third space* loss does not stop when the patient's incision is closed. Third space losses probably continue at a slower rate for 24–48 hours following a major surgical procedure. Therefore, to prevent hypovolemia, the patient should be given an increased amount of fluid in the first day or two following surgery.

Excessive loss of fluid can occur from nasogastric suction, ileostomy drainage, bile drainage, or diarrhea in the postoperative period. These losses must be replaced also to prevent volume depletion. Increased insensible loss of water occurs with fever and sweating. Hemorrhage in the postoperative period is a common cause of hypovolemia. Large amounts of fluid can be lost from extensive burns and can lead to severe hypovolemia if not promptly replaced. The type of solutions used to replace these various types of losses will be evaluated with specific reference to their effects on the lung.

REPLACEMENT OF FLUID LOSSES WITH
ELECTROLYTE SOLUTIONS

Replacement of the fluid losses that occur at surgery and in the immediate postoperative period can be accomplished effectively by fluids that have the electrolyte characteristics of the extracellular fluid.[1756] If physiologic saline solutions are used intraoperatively at a rate of 7.5 ml per kilogram per hour, no change in the alveolar-arterial oxygen tension gradient is seen.[964] Replacement of losses of fluid from the gastrointestinal tract should be done by replacing the lost fluid milliliter for milliliter with a solution having a similar electrolyte composition to the fluid that was lost.

Resuscitation of the patient with shock secondary to a burn injury has been associated with excessive retention of salt and water, leading to excessive weight gain and pulmonary insufficiency (see Chapter 16). When hypertonic solutions of sodium are used for resuscitation of experimental animals in burn shock, less fluid is required.[659] The use of this type of solution in burned men results in small weight gains secondary to the small volume of fluid needed for resuscitation, but in several patients significant hyperosmolality has developed.[1341]

The most controversial subject in fluid balance is the choice of fluid for the resuscitation of hemorrhagic shock. Several experimental studies on animals have suggested that the use of Ringer's lactate or similar solutions for resuscitation of hemorrhagic shock does not significantly affect the lung water. When excessive volumes of electrolyte solutions are used, however, pulmonary edema develops, but the course of pulmonary edema following resuscitation for hemorrhagic shock probably is not chiefly related to the type of fluid used for resuscitation.[1711] During hemorrhagic shock increased amounts of both sodium and water collect in the alveolar-capillary membrane.[1376,1377] Changes in skeletal muscle cell membrane function during hemorrhagic shock have suggested to Shires and co-workers a reduction in the efficiency of the sodium pump mechanism or an increased permeability to sodium.[1757] There may be a similar derangement in the alveolar-capillary membrane to account for the accumulation of water and sodium during hemorrhagic shock. This concept of the retention of salt and water may partially explain the development of respiratory insufficiency following trauma and shock.[4] We feel, however, that the mechanisms discussed in Chapter 5 are more important causes of pulmonary edema.[1637,1641,1839]

REPLACEMENT OF FLUID LOSSES WITH COLLOID SOLUTIONS

ALBUMIN LOSS

During major surgical procedures, especially abdominal, there is extensive loss of albumin from the operative site.[932,933,1083,1382] During major cancer operations 2.4–3.7 gm of albumin per kilogram of body weight are lost; that is, 158–237 gm of albumin per patient. This loss results in a significant fall in colloid oncotic pressure. Albumin loss is thought to be secondary to excessive breakdown in the postoperative period. Some feel that gastrointestinal losses are increased, but this has not been demonstrated.

The renal excretion of albumin increases during the postoperative period. Macbeth suggests that the handling of proteins by the renal tubules is compromised for several days following uncomplicated abdominal surgery, but the magnitude of this loss is only 300–500 mg daily for the first three postoperative days.[1202]

ALBUMIN THERAPY

Albumin is the major protein responsible for the maintenance of the colloid oncotic pressure.[787,1152] It is prepared from human plasma but does not carry the risks of viral hepatitis. It is extremely effective in expanding the intravascular volume. As compared to saline, considerably smaller volumes are needed to restore the intravascular volume. There is little argument concerning the importance of the use of albumin in the postoperative period in a patient who has had a major surgical procedure with excessive (> 50 gm) loss of albumin. In such a situation the maintenance of a normal intravascular volume is critical, and returning the colloid oncotic pressure to normal is necessary to achieving a normal intravascular volume.[503]

In other areas the use of albumin is more controversial. The administration of albumin in conjunction with a diuretic in patients with pulmonary edema has been shown to decrease the degree of right-to-left shunt in experimental animals and in humans. The rationale for this therapy is maintenance of the intravascular volume with a small volume of albumin at a time when there is a rapid depletion of salt and water. Some benefit may be gained by transiently increasing the colloid oncotic pressure and encouraging the movement of fluid from the interstitium of the lung to the intravascular space.[693,1795] Opponents to the use of albumin in this situation claim that in pulmonary edema there is disruption of the alveolar-capillary membrane and that protein exudes from the intravascular space into the pulmonary interstitial space and into the alveolus, thereby worsening the pulmonary edema. Investigation of the problem has so far led only to equivocal results.

Measurements of lung water following resuscitation of baboons with hemorrhagic shock with either Ringer's lactate plus blood or Plasmanate plus blood demonstrated the greatest increase in lung water in those resuscitated with Plasmanate (Fig. 6-1).[909] The results of the study have been criticized on the grounds of the possibility of an allergic pulmonary reaction in baboons treated with Plasmanate (human). The resuscitation of rats in hemorrhagic shock with various solutions has demonstrated that pulmonary edema can occur when excessive quantities of any solution are given; however, a greater degree of pulmonary edema is produced with Plasmanate than with Ringer's lactate when equal volumes of each are given.

When albumin was given to healthy human volunteers, the rate of escape of albumin from the intravascular space to the interstitium of the lung increased as the plasma volume expanded.[1489] All these studies have been used to suggest that albumin should not be given for the resuscitation of hemorrhagic shock patients because of its possible adverse effects on the lungs. Other studies do not support this conclusion.

For example, dogs that were subjected to hemorrhagic shock and received either no therapy or 25 gm of albumin during the period of shock, followed by reinfusion of the shed blood, had reversal of shock. The pulmonary

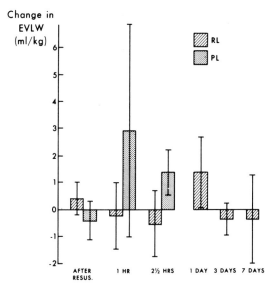

Figure 6-1. Effect of Ringer's lactate (RL) and Plasmanate (PL) on the change in extravascular lung water (EVLW) following resuscitation from hemorrhagic shock. Eight baboons had hemorrhagic shock induced to a systolic blood pressure of 60 mm Hg (8.0 kPa). Half were resuscitated with Ringer's lactate followed by their shed blood and the other half were resuscitated with Plasmanate plus their shed blood. Adequacy of fluid replacement was judged by maintaining the pulmonary capillary wedge pressure within 5 mm Hg (0.7 kPa) of the preshock levels. The animals were sacrificed and EVLW was measured. The postshock EVLW is expressed on the ordinate as the change from the preshock value, so that each animal serves as its own control. By one hour and two and one-half hours there were significant ($P < 0.05$ and $P < 0.001$) increases in the EVLW of the baboons treated with Plasmanate. These increases are consistent with the development of acute pulmonary edema since an increase in EVLW of 1–2 ml per kilogram is associated with interstitial edema. Values are represented as mean and $\pm$ 1 SD. (From J. W. Holcroft and D. D. Trunkey, *Ann. Surg.*[909])

vascular resistance of the control (no therapy) animals rose significantly following reinfusion of blood, however, while the pulmonary vascular resistance of the albumin-animals fell to baseline values (Fig. 6-2).[717] This suggests that albumin may prevent pulmonary complications of hemorrhagic shock, at least in the dog.

Resuscitation of baboons in hemorrhagic shock with either Ringer's lactate alone or with Ringer's lactate plus albumin resulted in no difference in lung water, deadspace-to-tidal-volume ratio, or lung sodium content. The amounts of fluid needed for resuscitation were significantly less when albumin was used.[1379]

When patients undergoing a major abdominal surgical procedure, such as the resection of an abdominal aortic aneurysm, received either Ringer's lactate alone intraoperatively or albumin, those patients who received Ringer's lactate had higher alveolar-arterial oxygen tension gradients when

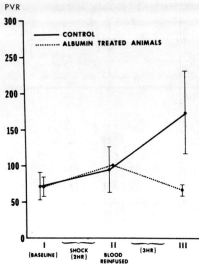

Figure 6-2.   Effect of albumin resuscitation on the pulmonary vascular resistance (PVR). The ordinate shows the PVR in resistance units (R), which are calculated based on the formula : resistance = pulmonary artery pressure − pulmonary wedge pressure (mm Hg)/cardiac index (liters per minute per kilogram of body weight). Eleven dogs were anesthetized and had hemorrhagic shock induced to a level of a mean arterial pressure of 40 mm Hg (5.3 kPa) after baseline measurements of pulmonary vascular resistance were made (*I*). After two hours of shock, shed blood was reinfused into all dogs, and measurements of PVR were repeated (*II*). Following shock there was a persistant elevation in PVR in all animals. Following this period 25 gm of albumin were given to half the dogs, and the others received nothing, to serve as controls. After three hours the PVR was measured in both groups (*III*). In the control group the PVR increased to a level 140 percent above the baseline PVR. The albumin-treated animals had a fall in PVR to baseline values. (From J. M. Giordano, D. A. Campbell, and W. L. Joseph.[717] By permission of *Surgery, Gynecology & Obstetrics.*)

breathing 100% oxygen than those who received albumin. Three patients who received an excessive amount of Ringer's lactate had florid pulmonary edema with very high gradients by the end of the procedure.[1796]

   When various solutions were used in rats in hemorrhagic shock, and the wet-to-dry-weight ratios were studied, those rats resuscitated with shed red cells had the driest, lightest lungs. In those animals not receiving red cells there was no difference between the lungs of those resuscitated with colloid and the lungs of those resuscitated with Ringer's lactate.[396]

   One final point should be made before terminating discussion of the albumin controversy. When baboons were resuscitated from hemorrhagic shock with either albumin plus red cells or Ringer's lactate plus red cells, the group receiving albumin had a marked depression of the tubular reabsorption of Na^+ and K^+ as well as a slower return of urinary output. This suggests that the use of albumin for resuscitation has a detrimental effect on the renal tubules.[1770]

7

Problems of Ionic Balance

The maintenance of a normal fluid balance in critically ill patients is closely related to the state of their intracellular and extracellular ions. In critically ill patients the severe ionic disorders most frequently measured are those involving the hydrogen ion.

RESPIRATORY DISTURBANCES

The maintenance of a normal pH is chiefly dependent upon the maintenance of a normal level of arterial carbon dioxide tension, which is in turn dependent on the correct level of alveolar ventilation. Respiratory acidemia is produced by alveolar hypoventilation and respiratory alkalemia is produced by alveolar hyperventilation.

During acute changes in the level of alveolar ventilation there are no marked alterations in the extracellular fluid volume.[708] There are changes in the electrolyte concentration of the extracellular fluid as the tissues aid in the buffering of the extracellular fluid. Chloride is transported across the erythrocyte membrane in acute hyperventilation as well as hypoventilation. During severe hyperventilation there is an increase in lactate and a fall in phosphate. The opposite occurs in hypoventilation. The magnitude of these changes is indicated in Figures 7-1 and 7-2. During controlled ventilation the level of alveolar ventilation should be adjusted so that the pH is at the desired level, somewhere between 7.30 and 7.45.

METABOLIC DISTURBANCES

Metabolic acidemia usually occurs in critically ill patients in respiratory failure as a result of a lactic acidemia secondary to anaerobic metabolism caused by poor perfusion and tissue hypoxia (see Chapter 5). Renal failure leads to a metabolic acidemia secondary to the inability of the kidney to excrete acid. Excessive loss of bicarbonate in diarrhea can produce a metabolic acidemia. Metabolic acidemia also can be produced by chronic alveolar hyperventilation with mechanical ventilation, if shivering is allowed.[581] The usual treatment of metabolic acidemia is administration of sodium bicarbonate in an amount calculated to return the bicarbonate concentration to normal. Bicarbonate has been said to distribute itself in a space equal to about 50 percent of the body weight in kilograms, and calculations of base deficit have been based on this figure. This figure is

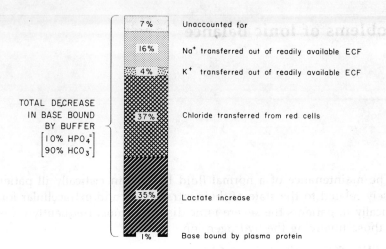

Figure 7-1.   Respiratory alkalosis leads to changes in extracellular buffers. In dogs with a marked respiratory alkalosis (Pa_{CO_2} < 10 mm Hg [1.3 kPa]) the changes in extracellular buffers are depicted. The total height of the column represents the decrease in total base bound by buffer in the extracellular fluid (ECF). Lactate increase contributes to buffer anion displacement (35 percent). Transfer of chloride into the extracellular fluid also affects buffer ion displacement (37 percent). There is also a loss of sodium (16 percent) and potassium (4 percent). The 7 percent which is unaccounted for may represent changes in other ions such as calcium or keto acids. (From G. Giebisch, L. Berger, and R. F. Pitts, *J. Clin. Invest.*[708])

unfortunately not constant and increases with the severity of the acidemia such that in severe metabolic acidemia bicarbonate may distribute itself in a space the equivalent of 200 percent of the body weight. Therefore this method of calculation of the required amount of bicarbonate underestimates the need especially in severe metabolic acidemia. Bicarbonate replacement should be closely monitored with arterial blood gases.[688]

Metabolic alkalemia is seen most often in critically ill patients in respiratory failure following diuretic therapy and chloride depletion.[1001] Nasogastric suction also produces a metabolic alkalemia. Other causes of metabolic alkalemia in respiratory failure are ingestion of alkali, hyperaldosteronism, chronic corticosteroid therapy, and very rarely, diarrhea. Elevation of the bicarbonate concentration occurs in chronic alveolar hypoventilation as a compensatory mechanism. Metabolic alkalemia can lead to a mild compensatory alveolar hypoventilation in which the arterial carbon dioxide tension rarely goes above 50 mm Hg; however, there have been several case reports of severe carbon dioxide retention with arterial carbon dioxide tensions in the 60's, and even one report of a patient with an arterial carbon dioxide tension of 88 mm Hg (11.7 kPa), who required controlled ventilation. The combination of metabolic alkalemia and narcotic administration produces respiratory depression, which is additive as demonstrated by carbon dioxide response curves.[938,1162,1746]

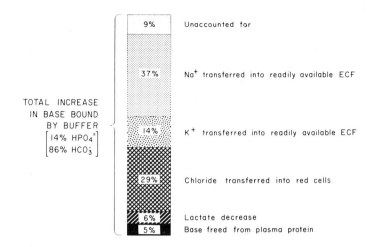

Figure 7-2. Effect of respiratory acidosis on the extracellular buffers. Dogs had respiratory acidosis induced to levels of arterial carbon dioxide tensions of 170 mm Hg (22.6 kPa) with a pH of 6.8. The height of the column represents the total increase in buffer ions in the extracellular fluid (ECF). Increase in bicarbonate accounts for the largest fraction of buffer anions. Chloride leaves the extracellular fluid and is replaced by base. The cations sodium and potassium increase (37 percent and 14 percent respectively). Lactate decrease accounts for a small portion (6 percent) of the total increase in buffer ions. (From G. Giebisch, L. Berger, and R. F. Pitts, *J. Clin. Invest.*[708])

SODIUM

Sodium exists for the most part in the extracellular fluid, kept there by means of the sodium pump mechanisms in cell walls. The concentration of sodium in the serum is determined chiefly by the amounts of total exchangeable sodium, total exchangeable potassium, and total body water.

In critically ill patients abnormalities of serum sodium are related most commonly to changes in total body water. Excessive administration of intravenous fluids to patients postoperatively is the most common reason for hyponatremia. Losses of sodium occur in the urine and from gastrointestinal drainage but are less important. Inappropriate antidiuretic hormone release is an infrequent cause of hyponatremia. Dilutional hyponatremia is treated by restriction of fluid intake. The calculation of the excess volume of fluid is based on total body water by serial measurements of body weight. Calculation of the degree of sodium deficit, in cases in which loss of sodium is the problem, is done by adding the number of milliequivalents of sodium lost daily from the various drainage sources and replacing that number over 48 hours.

Hypernatremia in critically ill patients is usually related to volume depletion (see Chapter 6). It also can be caused by administration of hypertonic saline. Patients are treated by volume replacement with isotonic fluid, the amount calculated from the total body water.

CHLORIDE

The most serious disorders of chloride in patients in respiratory failure occur in relation to excess loss of chloride during diuretic therapy or gastrointestinal drainage. The result is usually a hypokalemic, hypochloremic metabolic alkalemia. Chloride replacement is necessary to restore the normal potassium and acid-base balance.[1001] Chloride is also important as a buffer during acute changes in pH that are of respiratory origin, as discussed under Respiratory Disturbances.

POTASSIUM

Acute renal failure is the most common reason for hyperkalemia in critically ill patients in respiratory failure. Other causes include excessive administration of potassium, crush injuries, and massive hemolysis. Hypokalemia often develops secondary to diuretic therapy. Potassium must be monitored closely in patients receiving diuretics. Excess potassium also can be lost through gastrointestinal drainage, renal tubular acidosis, hyperaldosteronism, and steroid therapy.

CALCIUM

The calcium ion is extremely important to the contraction of muscle, the coagulation of blood, neuromuscular transmission, and the release of insulin. The development of a method for the rapid and reproducible measurement of the calcium ion has led to new knowledge of the importance of this ion in critically ill patients. Abnormally low levels of ionized calcium occur in critically ill patients who are in shock and require vasopressor therapy. Such patients have none of the "classic" signs of hypocalcemia and do not respond to administration of calcium chloride.[544]

The exact relation of ionized calcium to hemodynamic function is not clearly worked out. The administration of 10 ml of calcium chloride (0.72 mol) to critically ill patients is associated with a rise in ionized calcium of 0.26 mmol/l measured after 5 and after 10 minutes. After 30 minutes the increase in ionized calcium has fallen to 0.12 mmol/l. The administration of 20 ml of calcium gluconate (0.72 mol) is associated with an identical rise in ionized calcium, despite the fact that calcium in this form is chelated. With the administration of either of the above doses of calcium there is an increase in the mean arterial pressure of 4–7 mm Hg (0.5–0.9 kPa). The mechanism of the increase in arterial pressure is probably related to the effect of calcium on the peripheral vasculature, since there are no changes in cardiac output.[545]

PHOSPHATE

Changes in serum inorganic phosphate can influence the position of the oxyhemoglobin dissociation curve by changing erythrocyte 2,3-DPG concentration. During hyperphosphatemia there are increases in 2,3-DPG; however, no increase in oxygen transport or utilization can be demonstrated.[611]

The physiologic importance of alterations in erythrocyte 2,3-DPG and subsequent changes in hemoglobin oxygen affinity is unclear, because no data clearly substantiate any importance in critically ill patients. Alterations in thyroid function lead to changes in 2,3-DPG, possibly as a compensatory mechanism for changes in oxygen consumption. Total parenteral nutrition leads to hypophosphatemia, alteration in erythrocyte 2,3-DPG, and a shift of the hemoglobin-oxygen dissociation curve (see Chapter 8). Chronic renal failure leads to hyperphosphatemia and an increase in red cell 2,3-DPG. Considerable theoretic importance has been placed on these changes, but it should be remembered that as pH changes from 7.35 to 7.45 there is a lowering of the oxygen tension at which hemoglobin is 50 percent saturated, which is equivalent to a 20 percent fall in erythrocyte 2,3-DPG.[1116]

Some answers to the question of the physiologic importance of 2,3-DPG in critically ill patients may be found in investigations of organs with high arteriovenous oxygen content differences such as the heart and brain. Coronary blood flow does appear to change with alterations in hemoglobin oxygen affinity. At different levels of myocardial oxygen consumption in the dog there are changes in coronary blood flow in response to pH-induced changes in hemoglobin oxygen affinity (Fig. 12-1).[1293]

MAGNESIUM

Magnesium exists for the most part intracellularly. This ion is important for adequate neuromuscular and cardiovascular function in patients in acute respiratory failure. Hypomagnesemia occurs with diuretic therapy, diarrhea, polyuric renal failure, hyperparathyroidism, cirrhosis, and diabetic ketoacidosis. The clinical signs are similar to those of increased neuromuscular activity seen in hypocalcemia. Hypomagnesemia is best corrected by replacement with magnesium sulfate over 24–48 hours.

Hypermagnesemia occurs in chronic renal failure. Magnesium intoxication is a problem associated with the administration of large doses of magnesium for the management of eclampsia or preeclampsia. It may be manifested by cardiovascular collapse or respiratory arrest or both. In high doses magnesium acts as a potent peripheral vasodilator that produces hypotension. High doses of magnesium act as a neuromuscular blocking agent. Magnesium reduces the sensitivity of the motor endplate to acetylcholine and decreases the excitability of muscle fibers to stimulation. As the serum level of magnesium increases, there is a progressive reduction of the deep tendon reflexes, which is followed by generalized weakness and muscle paralysis. Complete heart block also has been reported to occur with magnesium intoxication at serum levels of less than 10 mEq per liter (5 mmol/l). The adverse effects of magnesium poisoning can be reversed within minutes by the administration of calcium chloride. The effect of magnesium administration on ionized calcium has not yet been clearly determined.[739]

Magnesium also potentiates the neuromuscular blockade produced by nondepolarizing muscle relaxants. We have had to ventilate three patients secondary to the therapeutic use of intravenous or intramuscular magnesium given for the treatment of eclampsia. Two patients survived without permanent sequelae; one died with irreversible cardiovascular collapse.

8

Nutrition

The nutritional status of a critically ill patient is an important factor in overall management. Postoperatively and during respiratory failure prolonged starvation increases morbidity and mortality. Ideally all of a patient's nutritional requirements should be met during all phases of an acute illness. This goal is difficult and usually impossible to achieve. Nevertheless we search for the best method of meeting the nutritional needs of each individual patient.

NUTRITIONAL REQUIREMENTS OF THE CRITICALLY ILL

Critically ill patients have higher nutritional requirements than healthy resting persons. The acutely ill surgical patient begins to lose excessive amounts of nitrogen even preoperatively. The net loss of nitrogen in an ill, fasting patient ranges from 11 gm daily in the patient with a small bowel obstruction to 31 gm daily in the burned patient. During an operation there are also significant losses of nitrogen due to losses of blood and albumin. Major abdominal surgery both intraoperatively and postoperatively is associated with a greater degree of nitrogen loss than is minor abdominal or peripheral surgery. The average degree of loss over the first ten postoperative days ranges from 1.5 gm daily for a radical mastectomy to 17.5 gm daily for a gastrectomy. The patient undergoing major abdominal surgery requires a 60–120 percent increase in nitrogen intake to maintain nitrogen balance in the postoperative period. This corresponds to a 50–60 percent increase over basal caloric requirements. In the burned patient and the severely injured patient the nitrogen and caloric requirements are probably twice that magnitude.[1617]

There is very little information concerning the vitamin requirements of acutely ill patients. The ascorbic acid requirement of burned patients is quite high, in the range of 1,000 to 2,000 mg daily.[1617] Except for patients with preexisting vitamin deficiency there is no evidence to suggest that vitamin replacement alters the morbidity or mortality of surgery or respiratory failure.

The results of starvation in critically ill patients are difficult to document, since many other factors affect their physiologic performance. Our experience is that patients in respiratory failure who for prolonged periods have received no nutritional replacement except 5% dextrose and water are often extremely difficult to wean from controlled ventilation, even when other aspects of their lung disease have resolved. Later it is possible successfully to wean these patients from controlled ventilation, after they have received a high caloric intake for one to two weeks.

There are other important sequelae of starvation in the postoperative period. There is a tendency toward wound disruption in protein-depleted animals secondary to inadequate fibroplasia. There is also decreased gastric emptying and reduced gastrointestinal motility associated with postoperative starvation. Healing of bone is delayed by poor nutrition. Lack of proper nutrition increases the risk of infection.[1617]

Weight loss and negative nitrogen balance postoperatively can be prevented by providing the critically ill patient with a normal intake of calories and nitrogen.[910] The nutritional route must be carefully evaluated for each patient.

ALIMENTATION VIA THE GASTROINTESTINAL SYSTEM

The most satisfactory method of providing adequate nutrition for the ill patient in respiratory failure is to use his own gastrointestinal tract. In the postoperative period the presence of ileus is the most frequently encountered reason that the gastrointestinal tract cannot be used. The complete absence of bowel sounds usually indicates that an ileus is present. The return of bowel sounds, however, does not necessarily indicate that the ileus is resolved. A small area of peristalsis can produce bowel sounds, but this does not necessarily mean that gastrointestinal function has returned to normal. A far more sensitive sign that an ileus has resolved is the passage of flatus or stool per rectum or via an enterostomy. Once these signs appear in conjunction with the presence of bowel sounds, it is usually safe to feed the patient via the gastrointestinal tract. Exceptions to this are patients who recently have had a gastrointestinal anastomosis, acute pancreatitis, acute peritonitis, major gastrointestinal hemorrhage, or bowel obstruction. If the patient is awake, alert, and does not have a tracheal tube in place, feeding by mouth is begun. As many patients are intubated, oral feedings often are impossible.

TUBE FEEDINGS

In most cases tube feedings can be started as soon as gastrointestinal function returns. If a nasogastric tube is already in place, we use it. If one is not in place, we prefer to insert a #8 French adult feeding tube into the stomach. The advantage of this type of tube is that its diameter is quite small, and the risks of nasal or esophageal damage therefore are minimized.

Because of its small size the feeding tube often is difficult to pass in an obtunded or uncooperative patient. Therefore the usual procedure is to pass it in conjunction with a larger, stiffer, conventional nasogastric tube.

The distal tip of the feeding tube is connected in parallel with the distal tip of a #16 French red rubber or Silastic nasogastric tube. This is done by placing the tips of both tubes into half of an empty gelatin medication capsule. The tubes then are lying parallel to each other. The joined tip is lubricated and passed through the patient's nose into the stomach. Both tubes are allowed to remain in place in the stomach for 30–60 minutes while the capsule dissolves. After that time the larger nasogastric tube is removed and the feeding tube remains in place in the stomach. Position in the stomach is confirmed by aspiration of gastric contents through the feeding tube.

Tube feedings are begun by administering 30–60 ml of skim milk every two hours. Prior to each feeding the tube is aspirated. If a significant amount of milk remains from the previous feeding, no further feeding is given until the stomach empties. If the gastric aspirates are persistently elevated, tube feedings must be discontinued. If skim milk is tolerated for 24 hours, the diet is advanced to the standard material used for tube feedings.

The preparation used for tube feedings in our intensive care unit is a mixture of beef, milk, egg, farina, applesauce, vegetable oil, and salt, which is blended at high speeds to produce a liquid. Water is added in sufficient amounts to enable the mixture to pass through a feeding tube after it is strained. Usually 2,000–3,000 ml is given daily in divided doses every hour, provided that the gastric aspirate is minimal prior to each feeding. Modified tube feedings can easily be prepared: low-sodium, low-protein, no-protein, milk-free, or clear liquid, depending upon the needs of the patient.[168]

The results of using tube feedings to provide nutrition to the acutely ill patient are excellent. A normal dietary intake can be maintained in spite of severe illness, as long as gastrointestinal function is adequate.[1481] Many of our patients in prolonged respiratory failure have normal gastrointestinal function.

The most common complication of this type of feeding is diarrhea. Diarrhea can occur secondary to a high osmolarity of the feeding, high concentration of simple sugars, rapid administration, or bacterial contamination. If a patient develops diarrhea while receiving tube feedings, his stool and the feedings should be cultured. If no contamination is found, the diarrhea usually can be controlled by adding pectin to the feeding or by administering tincture of opium or Kaopectate.

Patients with severe gastrointestinal dysfunction who cannot tolerate a conventional diet and patients in whom reduction of fecal elimination is desirable can be supplied with normal nutritional requirements by a liquid elemental diet instead of by conventional tube feedings. These elemental solutions contain a mixture of glucose, amino acids, minerals, and vitamins and can meet nutritional requirements for an indefinite period.[1850]

ORAL FEEDINGS IN TRACHEOSTOMIZED PATIENTS

The presence of a tracheostomy is not necessarily a contraindication to oral feedings. Once gastrointestinal function has returned, it may be possible to feed a patient orally with a tracheostomy.

One must first ascertain whether the patient will aspirate his feedings. We use the methylene blue test. The patient is helped to sit up and asked to swallow 2–3 ml of methylene blue. Several minutes later the tracheobronchial tube is suctioned by placing a suction catheter through the tracheostomy tube. If there is no methylene blue suctioned through the catheter, then it is safe to feed the patient. If there is any blue dye in the catheter, then it is probably unsafe to proceed with oral feedings.

Usually the patient with a tracheostomy will be able to eat only a soft diet, since the inflated tracheostomy tube cuff often produces some difficulty in swallowing. If the patient cannot eat a sufficient amount, another method of alimentation is attempted.

INTRAVENOUS ALIMENTATION

Critically ill patients whose gastrointestinal function is inadequate for prolonged periods require some form of alimentation, hence the use of intravenous solutions to provide complete nutritional requirements. The solutions available at the present time often are of questionable value to acutely ill patients, and their use is associated with many severe and sometimes fatal complications.

GLUCOSE

The administration of glucose intravenously has a definite protein-sparing effect. When 100 gm of glucose are administered, there is maximum protection from the breakdown of protein. Additional amounts of glucose have no further protein-sparing effect; however, the caloric intake is increased. The routine administration of 5% dextrose and water does have a protein-sparing effect, but it is completely ineffectual in providing the daily nutritional requirement of an acutely ill patient. In order to supply sufficient glucose to provide a normal caloric intake, hypertonic solutions of glucose must be administered. Since these solutions cause sclerosis of small veins, they can be given only via a centrally placed catheter.

AMINO ACID AND HYPERTONIC GLUCOSE SOLUTIONS

The administration of solutions of amino acids and hypertonic glucose has been reported to be associated with protein synthesis and weight gain both in infants and in chronically ill adults.[559,946,1993,1998,2073] There have also been reports of weight gain and apparent protein synthesis in postopera- and other acutely ill patients.[557,1842]

The usual constituents of these solutions are protein hydrolysates containing 4–7 gm of nitrogen per liter in the form of amino acids, 15–25% glucose, and trace elements, vitamins, and electrolytes as needed.[559,1347]

Solutions of this kind usually provide about 1,000 cal per liter (4,200 J/l). Patients are given from 2 to 5 liters of solution daily, which supplies them with 2,000–5,000 cal per day (8,400–21,000 J/day) and 8–35 gm of nitrogen per day. Since these solutions are hypertonic, they must be infused into a central vein, preferably the innominate or the vena cava, to prevent sclerosis of smaller veins.[558,2073]

Infants and puppies fed exclusively with these solutions grow and develop in a nearly normal manner.[558,559,2073] Evidence that adults can synthesize protein when fed exclusively with these solutions is less clear. Studies claiming beneficial results from these solutions rely upon caloric intake, weight gain, and positive nitrogen balance as evidence for protein synthesis.[558,1467] Although it is clear that low caloric intake, negative nitrogen balance, and weight loss indicate protein breakdown, there is little evidence to suggest that protein synthesis is demonstrated by the presence of positive nitrogen balance, high caloric intake, and weight gain.

Amino acids and hypertonic glucose solutions also can be used for long-term management of patients with irreversible gastrointestinal failure. The solutions can be administered via an arteriovenous shunt.[1723,1754] The administration of essential L-amino acids and hypertonic glucose is helpful in minimizing azotemia in postoperative patients with renal failure who cannot be fed in any other way, but we are not yet persuaded that this form of treatment is better than conventional management of surgical patients with renal failure.[557]

Complications

Weight gain. Our experiences with hyperalimentation solutions in sick adult patients in respiratory failure in the intensive care unit often have been disappointing. The major disadvantage has been unwanted weight gain secondary to fluid retention, especially in patients requiring controlled ventilation.[1240] When a solution is discontinued, we frequently have seen the patient undergo a large diuresis for several days and return to near "pre-hyperalimentation" weight. We therefore feel that, for many of our critically ill adult patients in respiratory failure, this form of nutrition is ineffectual and in some respects detrimental to their care.

Catheter complications. In addition to fluid retention there are many other potential complications that should be appreciated. Many of the complications are related to the presence of a central venous catheter. Subclavian thrombosis can occur following percutaneous placement of a subclavian catheter, especially when it is used for the administration of hypertonic solutions.[1270] Location of the catheter in a large vein is mandatory. Fatal hepatic necrosis has been reported secondary to placement of a hyperalimentation catheter in a hepatic vein. The presence of a central catheter for hyperalimentation is associated with episodes of sepsis in 11 percent of patients. *Candida* sepsis is frequently associated with this form of alimentation.[57,462] Most of the septic complications can be prevented by strict aseptic technique in placement of the catheter and daily cleansing of the insertion site.[1679] Instillation of low doses of amphotericin B may be effective in reducing the incidence of *Candida* septicemia, since *Candida* has been reported as contaminating solutions used for hyperalimentation.[231,490,732] Daily sterile cleansing of the catheter insertion site in conjunction with changing of the administration tubing reduces the infection rate to 5–6 percent. The practice of changing the catheter every several days does not significantly alter the infection rate. Air embolism also can occur during hyperalimentation and its consequences can be severe.[758]

Metabolic complications. The metabolic complications of parenteral hyperalimentation are seen frequently, since hypertonic solutions of glucose and amino acids have to be used.[312,556,860] A great danger is that hyperglycemia may go unrecognized and nonketotic hyperosmolar coma may ensue. Patients receiving hyperalimentation should have frequent determination of their urinary sugar. Some patients may not be able to mobilize enough endogenous insulin and may need supplemental insulin. Another metabolic complication related to glucose metabolism is that a rebound hypoglycemia develops when the solution is abruptly stopped.[556]

Use of hypertonic glucose and amino acid solution can result in azotemia in patients with impaired renal or hepatic function, since the protein hydrolysates used contain variable amounts of nonessential amino acids which are not utilized. This can be avoided by using essential L-amino acids. Hyperammonemia may be worsened in patients with liver failure receiving hyperalimentation.[556]

Hypophosphatemia is another serious complication associated with hyperalimentation.[1160,1674] When hyperalimentation solutions are used, serum phosphorus levels can fall to 0.5 mg per 100 ml (0.16 mmol/l) after 2–10 days of administration. Hypophosphatemia is associated with a marked reduction in the phagocytosis of bacteria by leukocytes (Fig. 8-1). In patients receiving hyperalimentation chemotaxis of leukocytes is also markedly reduced (Fig. 8-2). This is probably related to reduction of leukocyte ATP; when ATP is replenished, chemotaxis returns to normal (Figs. 8-3 and 8-4).[434,2117] During hypophosphatemia other cells become depleted of ATP. The red blood cell becomes depleted of ATP and 2,3-DPG, which results in an increased affinity of hemoglobin for oxygen. Depletion of red cell ATP is associated with a hemolytic anemia.[1935]

Most of the complications associated with hypophosphatemia can be prevented by addition of phosphate to the hyperalimentation solution in amounts of 10–15 mEq per liter (5–7.5 mmol/l). The solution used in our hospital contains 10 mEq of phosphate per liter (5 mmol/l). Since adminis-

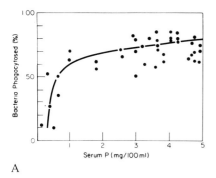

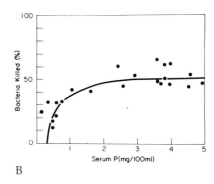

A   B

Figure 8-1. Effect of intravenous hyperalimentation–induced hypophosphatemia on phagocytosis and bacterial killing by leukocytes. Intravenous hyperalimentation was used as the only nutrition in 18 previously malnourished dogs. Blood was sampled periodically for studies of serum phosphate (P) and leukocyte phagocytosis. When the serum phosphate fell below 1 mg per 100 ml (0.32 mmol/l), there was a significant reduction in phagocyte activity ($P < 0.001$) as judged by (A) phagocytosis and (B) killing of bacteria. (From P. R. Craddock, Y. Yawata, L. VanSanten, S. Gilberstadt, S. Silvis, and H. S. Jacob.[434] Reprinted by permission from the *New England Journal of Medicine* 290:1403–1407, 1974.)

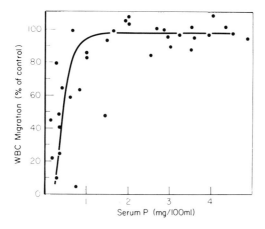

Figure 8-2. Effect of intravenous hyperalimentation–induced hypophosphatemia on white blood cell chemotaxis. Following a period of starvation 14 dogs were fed exclusively by intravenous hyperalimentation. In most animals there was a progressive fall in the serum phosphate (P). White blood cell (WBC) migration was studied in a Boyden chamber. Each point represents the mean of three assays. As the serum phosphate falls below 1 mg per 100 ml (0.32 mmol/l), there is a marked reduction in white blood cell migration. (From P. R. Craddock, Y. Yawata, L. VanSanten, S. Gilberstadt, S. Silvis, and H. S. Jacob.[434] Reprinted by permission from the *New England Journal of Medicine* 290:1403–1407, 1974.)

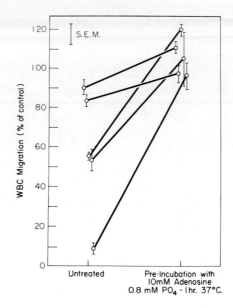

Figure 8-3. Reversal of abnormal white blood cell chemotaxis by replacement of leukocyte adenosinetriphosphate (ATP). Previously starved dogs were made hypophosphatemic by intravenous hyperalimentation. White blood cells from these animals showed marked reductions in chemotaxis in a Boyden chamber. The chemotaxic defect can be reversed by incubation of the cells in a solution of adenosine and phosphate, which restores cellular ATP. (From P. R. Craddock, Y. Yawata, L. VanSanten, S. Gilberstadt, S. Silvis, and H. S. Jacob.[434] Reprinted by permission from the *New England Journal of Medicine* 290: 1403–1407, 1974.)

tration of phosphate may lead to hypocalcemia, calcium must be administered at the same time. Both calcium and phosphate levels should be followed periodically in all patients receiving hyperalimentation.

A fatal syndrome associated with hyperalimentation has been reported to occur in humans and experimental animals. All the reports are of patients and animals who were chronically starved prior to treatment with amino acid and hypertonic glucose. After 4–7 days the development of muscle weakness, paresthesias, seizures, and coma is noted. The only metabolic abnormality detected is a marked hypophosphatemia. Whether or not a low serum phosphate is responsible for this syndrome is not clear. There is no satisfactory explanation for this syndrome at present.[1576,1781]

ISOTONIC AMINO ACIDS

Isotonic amino acid solutions without glucose may be better than amino acid solutions with hypertonic glucose as a means of sparing protein breakdown.[180,1994] In studies comparing the various methods of preventing protein catabolism, the administration of isotonic amino acids via a peripheral vein is associated with less nitrogen loss than the administration of glucose

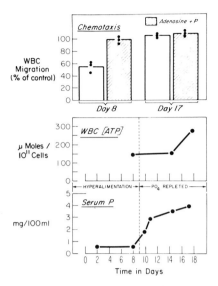

Figure 8-4. Intravenous hyperalimentation–induced hypophosphatemia, white blood cell (WBC) migration, and infection in an adult patient. A 44-year-old woman was treated with intravenous hyperalimentation because of severe cachexia thought to be secondary to an occult carcinoma. The patient developed a severe hypophosphatemia (*lower panel*). At that time a mild bronchitis progressed to pneumonia with an empyema despite appropriate antibiotic treatment of the bronchitis. Leukocyte ATP levels were about half the normal level (*middle panel*). Leukocyte migration in a Boyden chamber was also markedly reduced (*top panel*) but could be reversed with incubation of the cells in a solution of adenosine and phosphate (P). After termination of hyperalimentation and start of phosphate supplement on day 9 (*vertical dotted line*) there was an increase in serum phosphate which was associated with a return of WBC chemotaxis and return of white blood cell ATP to normal. (From P. R. Craddock, Y. Yawata, L. VanSanten, S. Gilberstadt, S. Silvis, and H. S. Jacob.[434] Reprinted by permission from the *New England Journal of Medicine* 290:1403–1407, 1974.)

and amino acids or glucose alone (Fig. 8-5). Possibly glucose-free solutions stimulate less insulin release, thereby reducing the antilipolytic activity of insulin and permitting greater utilization of fat stores.[181]

After a severe thermal injury, when protein catabolism is high, the administration of human growth hormones in addition to any form of high caloric feeding is associated with a marked protein-sparing effect. This addition of growth hormone to the management of critically ill patients may prevent nitrogen loss, but it is unclear whether it promotes protein synthesis.[2074]

FAT EMULSIONS

The use of fat emulsions to provide the nutritional requirements of critically ill patients has been gaining increasing importance, especially in

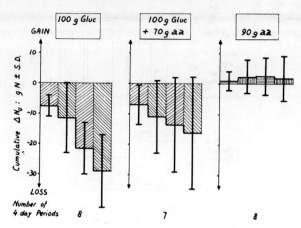

Figure 8-5. The effect of three intravenous alimentation solutions on nitrogen balance in man. Ten patients requiring intravenous alimentation received three different types of solutions rotating every four days. The ordinate represents the difference between the grams of nitrogen administered and the urinary nitrogen excretion. Administration of 100 gm of glucose in the form of 5 percent dextrose and water resulted in the largest net nitrogen loss (*left*). A solution containing 70 gm of amino acids and 100 gm of glucose given over 24 hours resulted in less of a nitrogen loss than did glucose alone (*middle*). A solution of 3 percent amino acids to give 90 gm of amino acids daily demonstrated the best protein sparing of any method (*right*). (From G. L. Blackburn, J. P. Flatt, G. H. A. Clowes, Jr., and T. F. O'Donnell, *Am. J. Surg.*[180])

Europe.[2119] Investigations suggest that this may be a better therapy than hypertonic glucose and amino acids. One of the main advantages is that the solution is isotonic.[2075]

The fat emulsions that were evaluated for use initially are associated with frequent complications of fever, dyspnea, cyanosis, nausea, vomiting, headache, jaundice, hyperlipemia, coagulopathies, and anemia. The fat emulsion now most commonly used, Intralipid, has reduced the incidence of many of these complications. Intralipid is an emulsion of soybean oil, egg yolk phosphatide, and glycerol in a 10% solution. Administration of fat emulsions to critically ill patients is associated with a positive nitrogen balance, high caloric intake, and weight gain.[118,2075] There is also an increase in oxygen consumption.[1611]

The use of Intralipid does not appear to change lung function. Arterial blood gases, lung diffusion capacity, and xenon lung scans are unaltered by use of this fat emulsion in burned patients.

Acute side effects when Intralipid is used are predominantly febrile reactions. Only 2.7 percent of infusions of fat emulsions are associated with a febrile reaction. Other common reactions are a sensation of warmth (8 percent), chills without fever, back pain, chest pain, and vomiting. With the exception of the sensation of warmth and febrile reactions these side effects are uncommon. There is no apparent adverse effect on liver function or blood count.[796]

Fluid retention as a complication of therapy with fat emulsion must be looked for. At present Intralipid is produced as an emulsion providing 1,100 cal per liter (4,620 J/l), while hypertonic glucose and amino acid solutions provide 1,000 cal per liter (4,200 J/l). Thus fat emulsions seem to offer little advantage over conventional hyperalimentation solutions in terms of the amount of fluid that must be administered.

MONITORING

No matter what form of nutrition is being provided for the critically ill patient, a daily record of the dietary intake should be kept. This should include the caloric intake as well as a breakdown into the amounts of protein, carbohydrate, and fat that the patient receives. An accurate daily account of body weight is also essential in determining the results of the fluid and nutritional management of the patient.

9

Problems of Monitoring

ARTERIAL CANNULATION

Radial arterial cannulation is useful for arterial blood gas sampling, blood pressure and pulse rate determination, pulse analysis, cardiac output determination, drawing of blood for laboratory analysis, therapeutic phlebotomy, exchange transfusion, pulse triggering of an aortic balloon, and angiography.[31,98,161,165,1173,1901]

The incidence of hematoma and ecchymosis following removal of a radial arterial cannula varies from 19 to 83 percent.[136,246,687] Bleeding usually is not troublesome if continuous pressure is applied for at least five minutes after cannula removal and if clotting abnormalities are absent.

Thrombosis occurs in up to 38 percent of arteries cannulated for longer than two hours, even with dilute heparin infusion.[136,538,687,1681,1879] Thrombosis of the radial artery forces the thenar tissues to depend on collateral circulation from the ulnar artery through the volar arches,[392] until recannulation of the radial artery occurs (Fig. 9-1).[136] If radial artery blood flow is dominant or if collateral flow is insufficient, ischemia may occur.[1003]

Ischemic complications requiring thrombectomy occur in 0.2–0.6 percent of radial artery cannulations.[106,687,1695] The result of failure may be amputation.[1003] In an attempt to avoid such tragedies we perform the modified Allen test on all patients prior to radial artery cannulation.[27] There are some patients whose need for arterial monitoring becomes evident only intraoperatively or postoperatively, when the patient is unable to tighten his fist actively for the Allen test. In such cases we have found that either passive tightening of the patient's hand for the Allen test or the use of the Brodsky test can predict ulnar artery patency. The Brodsky test uses a pulse transducer placed onto the thumb to monitor flow during compression of the radial or ulnar artery (Fig. 9-2).[240] A Doppler detector or pulsimeter may also be used to detect collateral ulnar flow. Its findings have a good correlation with results of the Allen test.[136,143,1385,1681] The Allen test is abnormal in approximately 3 percent of young healthy individuals;[135,667] this agrees with Doppler studies of the hand showing 1.6–2.0 percent of persons to have inadequate collateral circulation after radial artery compression.[1171,1385] Reports of cannulation of the radial artery in the presence of an abnormal Allen

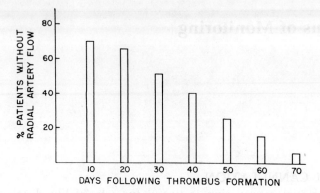

Figure 9-1.   Radial artery patency after decannulation. Every 10 days following removal of a polypropylene radial artery cannula, 20 patients were examined with a Doppler flow detector to determine radial artery patency. Fifty percent of patients who had developed thrombosis recanalized by the thirtieth day after decannulation and all patients by the seventy-fifth day. (From R. F. Bedford and H. Wollman, *Anesthesiology.*[136])

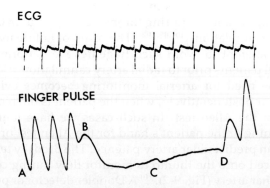

Figure 9-2.   In the Brodsky test the finger-pulse transducer is placed on the thumb of a patient with a positive Allen test (*A*). The compression of both the radial and the ulnar artery abolishes the finger pulse, as shown in the lower tracing at point *B*. Release of the ulnar artery at point *C* shows no change in the abolished finger pulse, indicating inadequate ulnar artery flow. Release of the radial artery at point *D* restores the finger pulse. Radial artery cannulation is contraindicated in this patient. (From J. B. Brodsky, *Anesthesiology.*[240])

test are few. In six patients whose response to the Allen test took from 7 to 15 seconds radial artery cannulation produced no complications.[136]

The incidence of thrombosis is directly related to the size and shape of the catheter used. In adults 20-gauge catheters produce fewer cases of thrombosis than 18-gauge catheters. Catheters with nontapered shafts produce fewer thromboses than those with tapered shafts.[538] Polypropylene catheters are reported to be associated with thrombosis more often than Teflon.[135] With 18-gauge catheters the incidence of thrombosis is proportional to the duration of cannulation (Fig. 9-3).[136] The relationship of catheter length to complication rate has not been studied, although the insertion of catheters into the aorta through the radial artery has been reported to have surprisingly few complications.[687] One reported instance of ischemia proximal to the site of catheter insertion may have been related to catheter length.[972] With intermittent heparin flush, proximal and distal emboli occur in 24 percent of cannulations studied by angiography; however, symptoms of embolization are seen in only 1.9 percent of cannulations.[136,538,1253] Emboli distal to the site of insertion produce small areas of discoloration of the thumb or hand. Proximal emboli of particulate matter or air may occur. If the bolus of flush solution injected is greater than 3 ml in the adult, then a portion may enter the carotid artery.[1189] One infusion set currently in use provides a continuous flush through an arterial cannula of a maximum of approximately 3.0 ml per hour. However, by pulling back on a rubber plunger, the flow rate can be increased to slightly greater than 1.5 ml per second. Therefore, to avoid cerebral embolization, such high flow flushes should be limited to a maximum of two seconds.[1111]

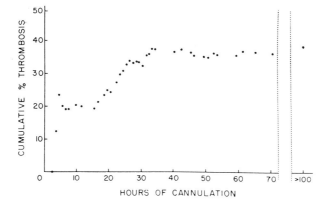

Figure 9-3. Incidence of radial artery thrombosis with duration of cannulation. The cumulative incidence of radial artery thrombosis increases to a maximum of 38 percent after 40 hours of cannulation. Polypropylene cannulas in place longer than 40 hours do not substantially increase the incidence of thrombosis. (From R. F. Bedford and H. Wollman, *Anesthesiology.*[136])

A serious complication is disconnection of the arterial cannula from its stopcock or tubing, resulting in a rapid arterial phlebotomy. This accident is preventable by careful taping, constant observation, and placing the cannula in a site which can be observed easily.

Four percent of arterial catheter tips show positive culture results. The arteriotomy site may become infected, either primarily, from the skin, or secondarily, from bacteremia.[9,598,687,836,1306,1835] Other complications include radial artery aneurysm,[1254] an Osler's node,[1306] arteriovenous fistula,[230] and arterial spasm.[472]

The ulnar artery can be cannulated in patients whose ulnar artery is not dominant and whose collateral filling by the radial is adequate. The dorsalis pedis artery may also be cannulated.[978] The technique is no more difficult than that of radial artery cannulation and is especially useful for patients with burns of the upper extremities. The pulse wave recorded from the dorsalis pedis differs from that obtained from the radial artery because of decreased compliance of the peripheral vessels. The dorsalis pedis pulse is delayed 0.1 second and is 5–20 mm Hg (0.7–2.7 kPa) greater; also the incisure is lost. If the dorsalis pedis is not available or it is undesirable to use it, the temporal artery may be cannulated. The axillary, subclavian, femoral, and brachial arteries also have been used but are not preferred, as they have a higher complication rate.[9,32,598,1363,1681,2141]

The patency of arterial cannulas is prolonged by the continuous infusion of a dilute heparin solution; we use 50 mg of heparin per 500 ml of 5% dextrose in water for this solution. Heparin itself often can be seen to cause vasoconstriction when injected into the artery, and more concentrated solutions are avoided. No other solutions are injected into the arterial line. An accurate record is kept of amount of blood drawn and flush solution used. Infants can be monitored with a 22-gauge catheter placed into the radial artery percutaneously as an alternative to an umbilical artery catheter.[1927] Blood drawn from a cannulated artery is acceptable for laboratory analysis if at least 5 ml of blood is allowed to flow prior to sample collection.

Arterial cannulation provides a method for rapid reduction of blood volume in a fluid-overloaded patient, if phlebotomy is indicated. It may be used also for blood withdrawal during exchange transfusions or during cardiac surgery. The retrograde flow of solutions administered through the radial artery cannula allows angiography to be performed in infants.[1901]

Figures that relate the number of radial artery punctures to the rate of thrombosis are not available.[1520] However, single punctures made with a 25-gauge or 22-gauge needle reduce trauma to a minimum.[246,248,1253,2025]

BLOOD PRESSURE

Blood pressure is measured continuously and directly via the arterial cannula. Transducers are of various types: variable resistance, piezoelectric, capacitance, and inductance change. Indirect methods of blood pressure determination include auscultation, palpation, plethysmography, oscillometry, flush, Doppler flow detection,[295,817,955,1233,1307,2028] and Doppler arteriokinetography.[1034,1308,1355,1548,1550,1675,1841]

The value of the majority of these indirect methods in shock states is questionable.[214,692,1268] The Doppler principle allows effective detection of peripheral pressure in hypotension (Figs. 9-4 and 9-5).[817,1006,1015,1549,2019] We use it in patients who do not require an arterial cannula, in infants, and in patients in whom an arterial line cannot be placed.

ARTERIAL BLOOD GAS TENSIONS

Blood gases are analyzed from an aliquot of arterial blood by Clark and Severinghaus electrodes.[991,1014,1731] Efforts continue to develop a reliable method of continuous arterial blood gas analysis.[1805,2084] Continuous readings of arterial oxygen tension can be obtained from a bare platinum wire electrode inserted into the arterial lumen with silver skin electrodes. Over long-term use, however, its accuracy is reduced due to protein deposition on the arterial electrode.[2084] Bare platinum and silver electrodes also can be placed in the earlobe. A silver-lead galvanic electrode inserted into the artery delivers a linear output of 0–150 mm Hg (0–20 kPa) of oxygen tension for up to 16 hours.[362,1022,1024,1482,1630] A self-powered polarographic electrode has been developed.[1427] A different method requires the arterial insertion of a gas-permeable catheter; the gas that diffuses into the lumen of the catheter is then analyzed by mass spectrometer.[220,827,2006,2099] An automated system of analysis of oxygen, carbon dioxide, and pH by microelectrodes has also been developed.[354,1988] An indwelling pH electrode has been used for continuous measurement of carbon dioxide. Its dependence on a gas-permeable membrane makes it susceptible to flow and pressure changes and to fibrin deposition.[827,1065,1086,1717] Mixed venous oxygen saturation has been monitored continuously by means of a catheter that carries separate beams of red and infrared light via fiberoptics.[385,1244] The intensities of light reflected by oxygenated and deoxygenated hemoglobin are converted to an oxygen saturation reading. Clotting on the catheter tip becomes troublesome after approximately 48 hours.[1244] We have not yet used or tested a satisfactory intraarterial system for continuous measurement of blood gases despite claims of others to have done so.

RESPIRATORY MONITORING

In addition to arterial blood gases, various respiratory parameters are measured intermittently. These include respiratory rate, tidal volume, vital capacity, peak inspiratory force, and inspired oxygen concentration. In the case of patients receiving controlled ventilation or intermittent mandatory ventilation, inspired gas temperature, peak airway pressure, mode of ventilation, and endotracheal tube cuff pressures and volumes are noted. When indicated, expired carbon dioxide is measured.

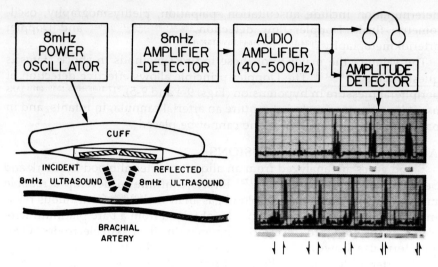

Figure 9-4.   Block diagram of the Doppler shift instrument. The relatively small motion of an uncompressed brachial artery does not generate an audible signal, but if a sphygmomanometer cuff is wrapped around the arm and inflated to a level between systolic and diastolic arterial pressure, the artery will open and close at least once in every cardiac cycle. Both movements generate distinctive Doppler shift signals with frequencies proportional to the velocity of the arterial wall. Ordinarily the artery opens much more abruptly than it closes, and this opening is indicated by a short, relatively high frequency (200–500 Hz) signal; closure is indicated by a longer, much lower frequency (30–100 Hz) signal. The Doppler shift signals can be heard through headphones.

Several important distinctions should be made between Korotkoff sounds and Doppler shift signals in indirect blood pressure measurement. First, vibratory motion in the audible range is required to produce Korotkoff sounds; however, any movement will generate a Doppler shift signal, which continues as long as the reflecting surface moves. Second, Korotkoff sounds are generated in a resonant biologic system, and their nature depends on the properties of this system (principally the functional vascular anatomy of the arm); Doppler shift signals depend in part on biologic properties but also can be altered by changing the operating frequency of the system. Third, audible Korotkoff sounds are generated only during the abrupt opening of the artery and cannot be heard during its closure; distinctive Doppler shift signals can be detected during both of these events.

The technique used to estimate arterial pressure is similar to the conventional Korotkoff technique; the cuff is inflated well above systolic arterial pressure and gradually deflated at a rate of about 1–2 mm Hg per second (0.13–0.26 kPa/s). As long as cuff pressure is above systolic, the artery remains closed and no Doppler shift signal can be detected. The first motion of the arterial wall occurs as cuff pressure falls just below systolic arterial pressure (*upper record*), and the cuff pressure at this point is recorded. Opening and closing signals cannot be differentiated at first, but as cuff pressure continues to fall, a separation between them becomes obvious (*lower record*); the closing signal appears as a broad, diffuse deflection (*downward-directed arrow*) just preceding the large, sharply defined opening signal (*upward-directed arrow*). As cuff pressure approaches diastolic levels, the closing signal falls later and later in the cycle, until it finally merges with the opening signal of a

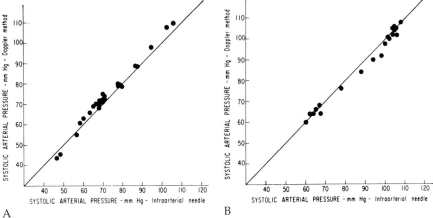

Figure 9-5. Correlation of systolic arterial pressure measurements determined with a Doppler ultrasonic flowmeter and intraarterial needle in (A) five patients in clinical shock and (B) in subjects in whom systemic pressure was lowered with amyl nitrate inhalation, Valsalva maneuver, and partial occlusion of the brachial artery. Doppler measurements have a close correlation with intraarterial measurements in hypotensive states. (From T. M. Kazamias, M. P. Gander, D. L. Franklin, and J. Ross, *J. Appl. Physiol.*[1006])

Oxygen in the gaseous phase is measurable by paramagnetic analysis, polarographic technique, a galvanic cell, a membrane electrode, and mass spectrometry.[1805,2084] We regularly use the paramagnetic and polarographic methods. The paramagnetic property of oxygen causes it to displace a glass dumbbell in a magnetic field; this results in a deflection of a light source read on a scale (Fig. 9-6).[147] Polarographic analysis relies on the same principle as the Clark electrode (Fig. 9-7).[437] Temperature stabilization of the membrane improves accuracy. The mass spectrograph is now highly

←——————————————————————————————

subsequent cardiac cycle; cuff pressure at this point is also recorded. Cuff pressure at the first signal equals systolic, and at the first merged signal equals diastolic, blood pressure. Additional opening and closing signals appear when cuff pressure is close to that associated with the dicrotic notch and wave but can be distinguished from the initial opening and final closure of the artery.

When heard through headphones the opening signal possesses a sharp, tapping quality easily distinguished from the longer drumroll character of the closing signal. This distinction suggests that three criteria may be used to identify the point at which cuff pressure equals diastolic pressure; first, the merger of opening and closing signals as outlined above; second, the disappearance of the rumbling second signal entirely; and third, a change in the character of the opening signal from a short tap to a softer, fainter signal somewhat comparable to Korotkoff sound muffling. In practice, different observers seem to use different combinations of these three auditory cues to determine diastolic pressure by the Doppler shift method. (From H. F. Stegall, M. B. Kardon, and W. T. Kemmerer, *J. Appl. Physiol.*[1841])

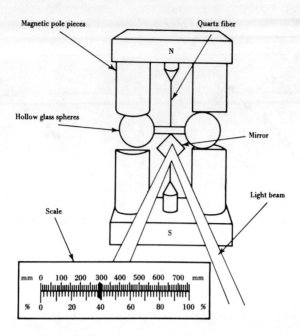

Figure 9-6. The paramagnetic oxygen (O_2) analyzer consists of a glass dumbbell containing a diamagnetic gas such as nitrogen, suspended by a quartz thread between the poles of a permanent magnet. O_2, being paramagnetic, will displace the dumbbell from the strong portion of the magnetic field. A beam of light reflected from a mirror affixed to the dumbbell onto a scale indicates the degree of rotation and thus the concentration of O_2 present in the mixture surrounding the dumbbell. (From J. W. Bellville. In J. W. Bellville and C. S. Weaver (Eds.), *Techniques in Clinical Physiology: A Survey of Measurements in Anesthesiology.*[147] Copyright © 1969 by J. Weldon Bellville and Charles S. Weaver.)

reliable (Fig. 9-8).[1401] Ionized oxygen is deflected from ions of different molecular mass by a magnetic field. Its concentration is proportional to the potential generated by the deflected ions. The unheated fuel cell consumes oxygen from its environment; the molecular oxygen reacts with the zirconium oxide cell to produce an electric current. Accuracy is reported to be ± 2 percent.

Carbon dioxide in the gas phase may be measured by infrared irradiation, thermal conductivity techniques, the Severinghaus electrode, or mass spectrometry. Different gases produce different absorption spectra with infrared irradiation, and this phenomenon forms the basis of measurement of gas concentration. By using appropriate filters, a relatively specific analysis can be performed; however, the equipment is cumbersome. The thermal conductivity of a gas mixture changes as its constituents change. This method is unreliable for carbon dioxide analysis when gases of similar thermal conductivity are present—for example, nitrous oxide.

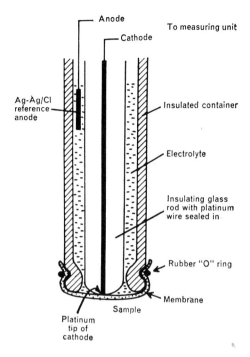

Anode

To measuring unit

Cathode

Ag-Ag/Cl reference anode

Insulated container

Electrolyte

Insulating glass rod with platinum wire sealed in

Rubber "O" ring

Membrane

Sample

Platinum tip of cathode

Figure 9-7. Diagram of Clark oxygen electrode used for the analysis of oxygen tension. When oxygen molecules diffuse to the platinum tip of the cathode, which is polarized with a negative voltage, they are very rapidly broken down. This breakdown results in a change of ionic current that is proportional to the area of platinum, the diffusion characteristics of the electrolyte, and the number of oxygen molecules surrounding the electrode. (From A. Crampton Smith and C. E. W. Hahn, *Br. J. Anaesth.*[437])

Patients are monitored for ventilator disconnection by a device that measures airway pressure or flow. Although pressure-sensitive devices continuously monitor the integrity of the ventilator-to-patient connection, they malfunction. The devices are pressure sensitive and can be deceived if the orifice of the ventilator tubing falls against the bedding. Apnea monitors usually rely on electric potential produced by muscle activity, on change in thoracic impedance, or on changes in airway pressure. Statistics about the number of patients who become disconnected from the machine while undergoing controlled ventilation are scarce. One study reported accidental disconnections in 2 of 54 patients in one year.[1934] Monitors based on expiratory flow without an on-off switch are an improvement.

VENOUS CATHETERIZATION

Right heart catheterization, first performed in 1929 and developed in the 1940's, is widely used in the monitoring of acutely ill patients.[431,657] Central venous pressure is useful as a guide to fluid therapy.[786,1180] There are,

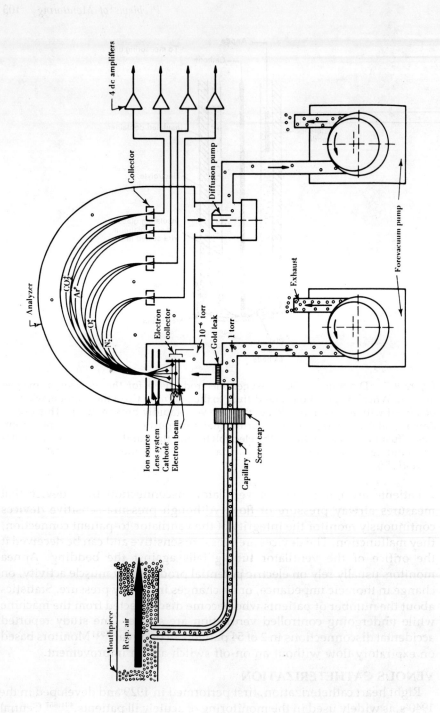

Figure 9-8. A magnetic, respiratory-gas mass spectrometer. Mass spectrometry is a technique for converting molecules into ions, which are then separated according to their mass-charge ratios. The record of the mass distribution and relative abundance of the ionic products is the mass spectrum. The ion source ionizes the molecules of the sample gas by electron bombardment. While both positive and negative ions are formed, the positive ions are more numerous. They are drawn into the accelerating system by the repulsion of a positively charged repeller plate and the attraction of the negatively charged first accelerating slit. The positive ions are then deflected in this type of mass spectrometer by application of a magnetic field. The degree of deflection depends upon the masses of the particles. The mass spectrum so produced is magnetically scanned by varying the acceleration voltage in a precise way. This causes the mass-separated ion beams to impinge upon the collector electrodes in sequential order of their mass. The mass spectrometer shown is equipped with four collector detectors arranged to be impinged upon by the ions from carbon dioxide (CO_2^+), argon (Ar^+), oxygen (O_2^+), and nitrogen (N_2^+). (From K. Muysers, U. Smidt, and G. Worth, *Bull. Physiopathol. Respir.* (Nancy).[110])

however, several problems associated with the use of this method. Successful placement of the catheter tip in the right atrium or superior vena cava is not always achieved. In 25–41 percent of attempts without x-ray monitoring the catheter tip ends up outside the thorax after insertion into the antecubital fossa.[1010,2039] Neither fluctuation of pressure with respiration nor free fluid flow is a reliable indicator of placement in the central vein. When the antecubital fossa is used, insertion through the basilic vein results in placement in the right atrium or vena cava in 65 percent of attempts, whereas insertion through the cephalic vein results in correct placement in only 46 percent of attempts. This is due either to the acute angle of entry of the cephalic vein into the axillary vein or to an inability to pass valves (Fig. 9-9).[436,975,2039] Attempts to pass a catheter for central venous pressure monitoring are more successful if the subclavian or internal jugular vein is used for insertion. However, even the subclavian route allows only 85 percent of catheters to pass into the superior vena cava or right atrium.[1423]

Since the position of the catheter tip cannot be judged by the length of catheter inserted, various means have been devised to localize the tip. These include x-ray assistance, observation of a diphasic P wave on intracardiac electrocardiograms, and insertion with the J-wire technique.[190,939]

The zero reference point for central venous pressure monitoring is the anterior or midaxillary line in the fourth intercostal space, or 3–4 cm below the sternal angle. The pressure inside the central veins is transmitted to the saline contents of the catheter and recorded either by water manometer or

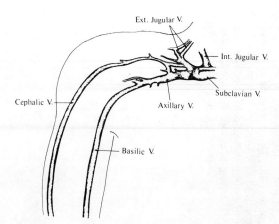

Figure 9-9. The anatomy of the venous system of the right arm and shoulder. Insertion of central venous catheters via the cephalic or external jugular veins is frequently difficult, since both veins have an acute angle of entry into the central system. (From D. R. Webre and J. F. Arens, *Anesthesiology.*[2039])

by pressure transducer.[344] The pressure transducer gives a more accurate reading.[346,347] The accuracy of the final reading will vary with the length of the catheter used and its diameter. The diameter may be significantly reduced if clots form inside the catheter. The dynamics of the catheter itself and the presence of air bubbles alter response.[610]

Complications of the subclavian route of insertion include arterial puncture, pneumothorax (in 1 percent of cases), hemothorax (1 percent), hematoma, and phlebitis.[436,682,954,1180,1423,1705,1806,2082] Complications of the external jugular approach include unsuccessful venipuncture (22 percent) and hematoma.[1180] The internal jugular approach results in arterial puncture in up to 4 percent of cases, pneumothorax (0.4 percent), hematoma (20 percent), and missed venipuncture (1–5 percent).[436,469,592,960,1264,1380,1860,1986,2143] Arteriovenous fistula,[954] air embolism,[648,960] osteomyelitis,[1135] cardiac perforation,[960,1090,1239,1666] thoracic duct injury,[1023] and brachial plexus injury[1806,2082] also have been reported as a result of attempts at central venous cannulation. The endotracheal tube cuff may be punctured.[189] Catheter breakage may require snaring the catheter under fluoroscopy or open surgical removal.[530,1108,1180,1252,1815,2020]

Substitutes for central venous pressure measurement have been proposed. Right internal and external jugular pressures are reported to have a good correlation with the central venous pressure, unless the chest is opened. Venous valves interfere with this correlation. An additional drawback to the use of the external jugular vein is the occasional necessity to rotate the head to obtain the measurement. This rotation distorts the readings.[235,436,917,1860]

SWAN-GANZ CATHETERIZATION

The central venous pressure is not always a reliable guide to circulatory hemodynamics as a whole.[236,1741,2082] In acutely ill patients the left ventricle often responds differently from the right ventricle (Fig. 9-10).[142,346,347,348,383,654,655,656,834] This is true during rapid change in blood volume, myocardial depression or stimulation, and administration of vasoactive agents.

To further evaluate cardiovascular status in such patients, a Swan-Ganz catheter is inserted through an antecubital basilic vein or through the internal jugular vein. It is guided into position by observation of a pressure tracing (Fig. 9-11). It may then be used for pulmonary capillary wedge pressure measurement, pulmonary artery pressure measurement, cardiac output determination, drawing of mixed venous blood, and angiography.[656] With fluid infusion, Starling curves of both right and left ventricles can be plotted. Complications of the catheter include atrial or ventricular arrhythmias during insertion in 1.5–11 percent of cases,[3,654,695,1885,2001] failure to achieve wedge position in up to 25 percent of cases,[1885] thromboemboli, and pulmonary infarction. Massive hemorrhage,[730,1470] perforation of the pulmonary artery,[341,1144] especially with elevated pressures, hemoptysis,[1099]

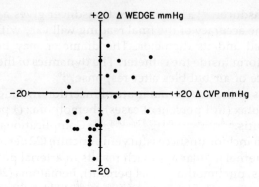

Figure 9-10. Correlation between central venous pressure (CVP) and pulmonary capillary wedge pressure (WEDGE) in 25 patients with myocardial infarction. In three patients the central venous pressure did not change despite changes in the wedge pressure. Directionally opposite changes occurred in four patients. Similar disparities occur in many critically ill patients without myocardial infarction. (From J. S. Forrester, G. Diamond, T. J. McHugh, and H. J. C. Swan.[655] Reprinted by permission from the *New England Journal of Medicine* 285:190–193, 1971.)

intracardiac knotting,[1169] balloon rupture,[1885] and endocardial thrombi[759] are less common complications.

The pulmonary artery diastolic pressure obtained from the Swan-Ganz catheter is sometimes not a reliable guide to left ventricular end-diastolic pressure (Fig. 9-12).[834,1101,1578] This is true especially when pulmonary vascular resistance is high, as with advanced emphysema, or changing rapidly, as during the onset of hypoxemia. When pulmonary vascular resistance is high, pulmonary artery diastolic pressure is a poor indicator of pulmonary

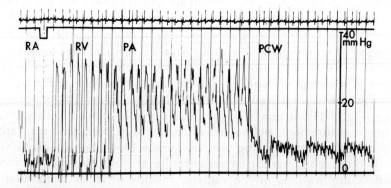

Figure 9-11. Tracing of pressures obtained during the passage of a Swan-Ganz catheter into the right atrium (RA), the right ventricle (RV), the pulmonary artery (PA), and finally into the pulmonary capillary wedge position (PCW). (From H. J. C. Swan, W. Ganz, J. Forrester, H. Marcus, G. Diamond, and D. Chonette.[1885] Reprinted by permission from the *New England Journal of Medicine* 283:447–451, 1970.)

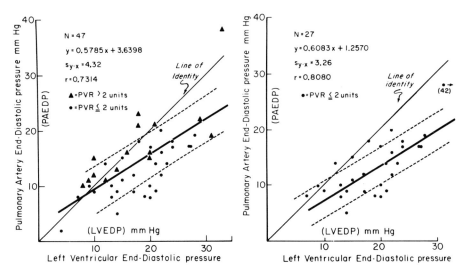

Figure 9-12. Correlation between pulmonary artery end-diastolic pressure (PAEDP) and left ventricular end-diastolic pressure (LVEDP) with changes in pulmonary vascular resistance (PVR) in 74 patients after acute myocardial infarction. The correlation is least when PVR is high (>2 units) (*left panel*). *Dashed lines* = SEM. (From S. H. Rahimtoola, H. S. Loeb, A. Ehsani, M. Z. Sinno, R. Chuquimia, R. Lal, K. M. Rosen, and R. M. Gunnar, *Circulation*.[1578] By permission of The American Heart Association, Inc.)

capillary wedge pressure.[631] During tachycardia this is also true. By contrast the pulmonary capillary wedge pressure is usually a highly reliable indicator of mean left atrial pressure, at least up to 26 mm Hg (3.5 kPa); thereafter the wedge pressure may underestimate left atrial pressure by a maximum of 3 mm Hg (0.4 kPa) (Fig. 9-13).[1101,2015] In persons with normal cardiac function the mean left atrial pressure and mean pulmonary capillary wedge pressures are closely related to the left ventricular filling pressure. In the presence of a capillary leak of the lung the pulmonary capillary wedge pressure may underestimate the left ventricular end-diastolic pressure. With endotoxin infusion there is good correlation until the wedge pressure is above 5 mm Hg (0.7 kPa). Above this level the pulmonary capillary wedge pressure underestimates left ventricular end-diastolic pressure by 3–6 mm Hg (0.4–0.8 kPa). Whether this discrepancy is due to myocardial decompensation with a left atrial boost effect or to the loss of transmission of pressure through the damaged pulmonary capillaries is not clear.[949]

The magnitude of the discrepancy between pulmonary capillary wedge pressure and left ventricular end-diastolic pressure is increased fivefold in the damaged heart. In patients with myocardial infarction the mean left atrial pressure and therefore the pulmonary capillary wedge pressure is not equal to the left ventricular end-diastolic pressure. This is due to the booster

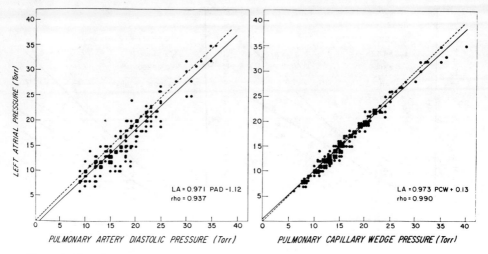

Figure 9-13. Correlation between pulmonary capillary wedge pressure (PCW) and pulmonary artery diastolic pressure (PAD) with left atrial pressure (LA). PCW is more closely correlated to LA pressure than PAD. *Dashed line* is line of identity; *solid line* is calculated regression line. (From D. G. Lappas, W. A. Lell, J. C. Gabel, J. M. Civetta, and E. Lowenstein, *Anesthesiology.*[1101])

effect of left atrial contraction, which increases the left ventricular end-diastolic pressure without increasing the mean left atrial pressure. Left atrial pressure and therefore pulmonary capillary wedge pressure just prior to atrial contraction do accurately reflect left ventricular pressure. After atrial contraction, however, the mean wedge pressure underestimates the left ventricular end-diastolic pressure (Fig. 9-14).[449,1578,2015]

The pulmonary capillary wedge pressure also underestimates the left atrial pressure after application of positive end-expiratory pressure to the airway of 10 cm H_2O (1.0 kPa) or greater (Fig. 9-15). This discrepancy can be accounted for by consideration of the rise in pleural pressure with positive end-expiratory pressure.[1192,1574]

Left atrial pressure also may be obtained by transseptal catheter perforation or by placement of a left atrial catheter during open-heart surgery. Complications include embolism and arrhythmias.[507]

TEMPERATURE

Temperature is best monitored intermittently with rectal probes using a thermistor.[527,1079,1405] Tympanic probes are difficult to manage in the awake patient and may cause membrane perforation, although their results show a good correlation with body core temperature.[160,2012,2038] Liquid crystal thermometers are useful but are still in the testing phase.[1421]

CHEST X-RAY

Chest x-ray films are taken upon a patient's entry into the intensive care unit to analyze cardiac and pulmonary status and to check the position of

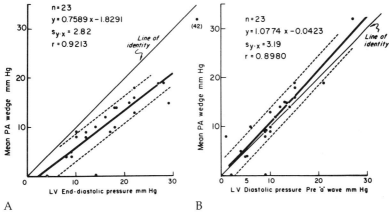

Figure 9-14. Correlation between mean pulmonary artery (PA) wedge pressure and left ventricular (LV) end-diastolic pressure and LV diastolic pressure prior to the a wave of atrial contraction. The LV diastolic pressure prior to the a wave is almost identical to the wedge pressure. (From S. H. Rahimtoola, H. S. Loeb, A. Ehsani, M. Z. Sinno, R. Chuquimia, R. Lal, K. M. Rosen, and R. M. Gunnar, *Circulation.*[1578] By permission of The American Heart Association, Inc.)

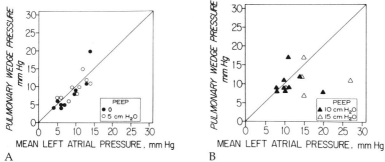

Figure 9-15. Relationship between pulmonary wedge pressure and mean left atrial pressure with (A) up to 5 cm H_2O (0.05 kPa) positive end-expiratory pressure (PEEP) and (B) 10–15 cm H_2O (0.10–0.15 kPa) PEEP.

Up to 5 cm H_2O (0.05 kPa) PEEP does not alter the close relationship between pulmonary artery wedge pressure and mean left atrial pressure (N = 18, r = 0.83, $P <$ 0.01). However, 10–15 cm H_2O (0.10–0.15 kPa) PEEP causes the pulmonary wedge pressure to deviate significantly from the line of identity in some patients (N = 14, r = 0.11, not significant). The diagonal line is the line of identity. (Reprinted from J. Lozman, S. R. Powers, Jr., T. Older, R. E. Dutton, R. J. Roy, M. English, D. Marco, and C. Eckert, *Arch. Surg.*[1192] Copyright, 1974, American Medical Association.)

the endotracheal, nasogastric, and chest tubes and the location of the central venous or Swan-Ganz catheter. Thereafter a chest x-ray examination is ordered when indicated by a change in the patient's status.

URINE OUTPUT

Urine production is measured usually on an hourly basis. The sample is analyzed as indicated for sodium, potassium, creatinine, osmolality, and routine urinalysis. Daily total intake and output is analyzed against weight gain or loss (see Chapter 6).

ELECTROCARDIOGRAM

An alarm based on rate of appearance of the R wave is used for monitoring of the electrocardiogram. Continuous computer monitoring of the electrocardiogram is rapidly being developed, however, and is more accurate in detecting arrhythmias.[1221,1652] Pacing may be indicated for patients especially prone to arrhythmias that decrease the heart rate. Electrocardiographic monitoring is continued with battery-operated units during transit to or from the intensive care unit.

ELECTROENCEPHALOGRAM

The electroencephalogram of the critically ill patient must be interpreted with caution. A single-tracing test may reflect a multitude of factors. The electroencephalogram is used to evaluate and follow cerebral status after a major insult such as prolonged hypotension or cardiac arrest, or when brain death is suspected. The determination of death in the Beth Israel Hospital in Boston is presently based on the 1968 report of the Beecher Harvard Medical School Ad Hoc Committee to Examine the Definition of Brain Death.[140] Criteria include unresponsiveness to stimulation with spinal reflexes usually absent, no movement or breathing when off the ventilator for at least three minutes, absent brainstem reflexes, isoelectric electroencephalogram at a gain of 2.5 μv per millimeter during a 30-minute recording, absence of hypothermia or central nervous system depressants, and repeat of all the above after 24 hours.[820] The declaration of death is made in consultation with a neurologist and the primary physician. The electroencephalogram is an adjunct which aids the physician in the detection of cortical dysfunction or cortical death.

CARDIAC OUTPUT

In the critically ill patient measurement of the cardiac output provides valuable information.

FICK METHOD

The direct oxygen Fick method of measurement of cardiac output relies on measurement of the uptake of oxygen by the blood flowing through the lungs.[786,1013] Under steady state conditions the mixed venous oxygen content times the flow rate is the amount of oxygen entering the lungs; the arterial oxygen content times the flow rate is the amount of oxygen leaving the lungs.[785] Oxygen uptake is measured at the mouth. The Fick equation results:

$$\dot{Q} = \frac{\dot{V}O_2}{Ca_{O_2} - C\bar{v}_{O_2}}$$

where $\dot{Q}$ = cardiac output
$\dot{V}O_2$ = oxygen consumption
Ca_{O_2} = arterial oxygen content
$C\bar{v}_{O_2}$ = mixed venous oxygen content

This can be solved so that cardiac output in liters equals oxygen consumption in milliliters per minute divided by ten times the arterial–mixed venous oxygen content difference measured in milliliters of oxygen per 100 ml of blood.

Oxygen consumption is calculated from the inspired and expired minute volumes and the fractional concentrations of oxygen in the inspired and mixed expired gas. Since these volumes and fractions are difficult to measure with the patient on a ventilator, we often substitute the carbon dioxide production for the oxygen consumption and assume a respiratory quotient of 1. Mixed venous blood for the purpose of calculating the Fick equation is obtained by a catheter from the proximal pulmonary artery. Samples from the distal pulmonary artery or right atrium are not accurate.[1882] Oxygen content is determined by the Van Slyke apparatus or other accepted techniques.

Alternatively an estimate may be made by determining the oxygen tension and saturation. In that case:

$$O_2 \text{ content} = 1.34 \times \text{saturation}$$
$$\times \text{ hemoglobin (gm/100 ml blood)}$$
$$+ O_2 \text{ solubility in blood} \times Pa_{O_2}$$

The solubility of oxygen in whole blood is 0.0223 ml dissolved O_2 per milliliter of blood at 760 mm Hg pressure at 37°C and 0.0297 at 18°C.[337,338,339]

Various modifications of the calculation of cardiac output based on the Fick principle have been reported. These include use of carbon dioxide in place of oxygen.[2129] The carbon dioxide content of mixed venous blood can be determined directly or else estimated by the carbon dioxide rebreathing technique. The methods using carbon dioxide are subject to greater error because of the relatively small venous-arterial carbon dioxide content difference.

INDICATOR DILUTION TECHNIQUES

Indicator dilution techniques are the methods that we presently use most commonly in the intensive care unit.[43,1053] Measurement of cardiac output by indicator dilution is based on the fact that after injection of a given amount of indicator the flow through the vessel is proportional to the reciprocal of the area under the curve that plots concentration against time. If one injects indicator into a stream of saline flowing through a glass tube at a given rate, then assuming that all the molecules of indicator have identical transit times, the concentration of the indicator bolus as it exits from the end of the tube is equal to the amount of indicator injected divided by the amount of fluid that passed the point of injection during the period of injection. Or put another way, the concentration of indicator bolus as it exits equals the amount of indicator injected divided by the flow rate times the period of injection. Solving the equation for flow rate, one finds that flow rate equals the amount of indicator injected divided by the concentration of indicator at the end of the tube times the period of injection. If the concentration is plotted against time, the area under the curve is equal to the denominator of the last equation. In actual practice, all particles of indicator do not move at the same rate, so that the plot of concentration versus time appears as a curve.[1584] Peripheral injection and sampling do not appreciably affect the derived flow value. Recirculation of the injectate, however, does introduce error into the calculations. This error is compensated for by the recognition that the initial downslope of the concentration-time plot (prior to recirculation) is an extrapolation of the entire indicator dilution curve without recirculation.[2033] This extrapolation is done either by manual replotting onto semilog paper, so that the downslope is a straight line, or by computer. Indicators include indocyanine green, cold saline, 5% dextrose in water, radioactive albumin, and many others.[41,424,1759] We use chiefly 5% dextrose in water or indocyanine green. Currently we employ the thermodilution technique with injection into the right atrium and sampling in the pulmonary artery by a thermistor on the Swan-Ganz catheter.[43,656] Calculations are performed by computer with digital print-out of cardiac output.[296,624,1453] This method is rapid, reliable, and can be repeated frequently.[684,2052] In critically ill patients 87 percent of the readings obtained by thermodilution are within 1.0 liter per minute per square meter of readings obtained by direct calculation using the Fick equation.[905]

PULMONARY EXTRAVASCULAR WATER MEASUREMENTS

Measurements of pulmonary extravascular water can be made by a double indicator technique using one indicator that remains intravascular and another that equilibrates with the extravascular space.[333] By calculating the mean transit times, extravascular volume is derived. Maximum accuracy is probably 70–80 percent of extravascular water under ideal conditions.[172,971,1267,1497,1585,1747] Other methods include changes in pulmonary impedance and a double gas inhalation technique.[83,720,1089,1730,1979]

PULSE CONTOUR AND OTHER METHODS

Cardiac output also may be estimated by analysis of the pulse contour.[17,983] Methods have been developed that use the change in pressure relative to time (dP/dt), mean distending pressure systolic area, and difference between systolic area and diastolic area.[174,752,1460,2030,2031,2032,2033] These methods allow beat-to-beat evaluation of cardiac output but unfortunately are unreliable when compared to indicator dilution studies and to Fick methods. Pulse contour methods lack stability and do not respond appropriately to drug infusion.[983] Correction can be made for peripheral artery tracings but is unsatisfactory.[1812] Pulse contour analysis is about as accurate as blood pressure in estimation of stroke volume.[17,983] Often systolic blood pressure has a good correlation with cardiac stroke volume, whereas diastolic blood pressure has a significantly less good correlation.[455]

Cardiac output may be determined also by indwelling electromagnetic flowmeters.[2066] Cardiac output can be measured by endotracheal phonocardiography, if there is no respiratory interference.[1871] Systolic time intervals such as the preejection period can accurately reflect the peak ascending aortic blood-flow acceleration and myocardial function.[1614,1643] An index derived from arterial diastolic pressure obtained by sphygmomanometer, from left ventricular filling pressure obtained by pulmonary artery balloon catheter, and from the preejection period determined from the phonocardiogram, carotid pulse, and electrocardiogram, provides a safe and practical means of assessing the degree of left ventricular dysfunction in patients with acute myocardial infarction.[11] Other methods of determining cardiac function include ballistocardiography, echocardiography, and cineradiography. Velocity of blood also can be determined by Doppler techniques.[149, 208,680,1023,1590,1767,1840,1853,1908,1981]

ELECTRIC HAZARD

Most monitoring systems use electricity for power. The intensive care patient is at particular risk for electric injury because of his connection to monitoring and pacemaking devices.[518,528,753,876,1146,1837] Injury by electrocution depends on the duration of exposure, voltage of the source, amount of current flowing, anatomic site of current entry and exit, type of current encountered, and current density.

Exposure to current for a period of less than 10 msec usually will not produce ventricular fibrillation. The degree of damage done by such a short stimulus is proportional to the voltage of the source. The effects of stimuli of longer than 10 msec are dependent on the quantity of current flowing into the body and on the anatomic site of entry and exit. The amount of current that flows into the body is determined by Ohm's law, which states that current equals voltage divided by resistance. Thus current flows more readily through conductors of low resistance. Skin resistance (or impedance) to current flow in the absence of a wire or catheter represents the main deterrent to flow. Skin resistance varies from 1,000 to 1,000,000 ohms, depending on its thickness and moisture content. Using Ohm's law one can calculate that currents of 110–0.1 ma can flow from a 110-volt source. When such currents are applied directly to the skin, the effects are as follows: 1.0 ma is the threshold of perception of current, 16 ma is the current above which sustained muscular contraction prevents the subject from releasing the power source, and 70–100 ma is the current associated with ventricular fibrillation. A current greater than 3 amp causes a sustained myocardial contraction during exposure, followed by resumption of sinus rhythm.[253,254,255]

The effect of current flow on the heart is dependent on the density of the current inside the heart. It is for this reason that, whereas 100 ma is required to cause ventricular fibrillation when applied peripherally, 0.02–0.1 ma (20–100 μa) is sufficient to cause fibrillation if applied directly to the heart via a wire electrode.[2018] This has significance for all intensive care patients because of the various conductors to the heart which are frequently present.[1665] Pacemaker wires, saline-filled central catheters, and serum-filled mediastinal drains represent direct conductors to the heart. A pacemaker wire has so little resistance that small currents or voltages cause fibrillation. Saline-filled catheters have a resistance of approximately 3,500,000 ohms, and therefore a source of 22 volts is required to produce a current of 10 μa.[1344] Catheters can even be used for defibrillation.[1327] Direct current is required in five times the amount of alternating current to produce equivalent damage.[1191] The source of such currents may be leakage from monitoring equipment. We take great care to prevent exposure, and periodic testing of leakage current is performed on all our electric apparatus.

COMPUTER MONITORING

Computer monitoring systems are of two main types. The first type uses on-line analysis of data; the second, off-line analysis and data retrieval. On-line display of data is accomplished by continuous monitoring of airway pressure, respiratory gas flow, oxygen, and carbon dioxide concentrations. From these data are derived respiratory rate, tidal and minute volume, oxygen uptake, lung-plus-chest compliance plus resistance, and respiratory work. A digital computer is used for analysis with television display.[1450,1459,1460,1642]

Similar methods for on-line monitoring have been developed by a number of investigators.[47,473,596,1158,1292,1749] These sophisticated systems often require highly trained personnel for equipment maintenance. A tremendous quantity of data can be generated, which may or may not be useful. The total cost compared to the benefit achieved is high.

Off-line analysis with data retrieval requires feeding into the computer each parameter as it is determined, including results determined by the nursing staff, routine laboratory results, blood gas data, and other signs and symptoms of importance. The system requires less skilled maintenance than on-line methods and can in fact be in operation 98.5 percent of the time. Such a system requires an adequate number of personnel, so that data can be entered into the computer without loss of time from routine duties (Fig. 9-16).[1443,2007]

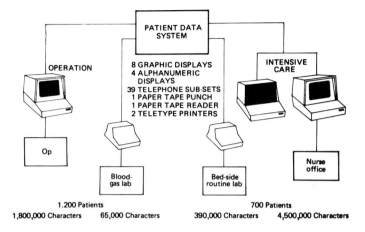

Figure 9-16. An example of a patient data retrieval system using computer technology. Other systems are capable of continuous on-line monitoring. (From O. P. Norlander, *Int. Anesthesiol. Clin.*[1443] Copyright, 1972, Little, Brown and Company, by permission.)

10

Critical Analysis of Preventive Measures

PREOPERATIVE RISK FACTORS

Prevention of respiratory complications in the postoperative patient requires recognition preoperatively of pulmonary risk factors. Acute or chronic pulmonary disease increases the respiratory complication rate three to four times.[395,1028,1472,1473,1670,1710,2063] Markedly abnormal pulmonary function increases risk by as much as twenty times.[257,395,506,1846] Cigarette smoking (10 cigarettes per day) increases risk two to seven times (Chap. 24).[395,1110,1112,1364] An age of more than 60 carries a two- to threefold increase in complications (Chap. 22).[482,543,1050,1335,1446,1919] Sepsis increases respiratory complications threefold (Chap. 5).[649,1028] Obesity (30 percent over ideal weight) doubles respiratory complications (Chap. 23).[746,1028,1112,1919] The nutritional state is also important. Men have a two to three times greater incidence of respiratory complications than women because of an increased incidence of bronchitis and smoking; if figures are adjusted for smoking, there is no difference between the complication rates.

Compensation for these risk factors may be accomplished by a program of encouraging the cessation of smoking starting at least three weeks preoperatively. A combination of stopping smoking and eliminating respiratory infection by antibiotics, as based on sputum cultures, is said to halve the number of complications.[395] Instructions in effective deep breathing and coughing are important, as is psychologic preparation for postoperative pain and the intensive care environment.[678,1616,1645,1650] Optimization of nutrition and removal of bronchial plugs and secretions by preoperative physical therapy are most valuable. Nebulized bronchodilators, we think, are of no great value.[36,329,428,429,726,1831]

INTRAOPERATIVE RISK FACTORS

An important intraoperative risk factor is the site of the surgical incision. Pulmonary complications occur most commonly after upper abdominal or thoracic surgery; thereafter the incidence of complications progressively declines through lower abdominal and extremity incisions.[19,504,580,1498] If an anesthetic lasts for longer than three hours, the risk of pulmonary complications increases, but this reflects not the effects of anesthesia but rather the nature and severity of the surgical procedure.[1413,1712] No one type of anesthesia is associated with lower postoperative respiratory complications, but the skill of the anesthesiologist is important.[207,268,1490,1597]

POSTOPERATIVE HYPOXEMIA
VENTILATION-PERFUSION RELATIONS AND SHUNTING

Arterial hypoxemia is frequently observed postoperatively without hypercapnia.[948,1212,1827] The degree of hypoxemia is dependent on the site of the procedure. The greatest impairment occurs with upper abdominal surgery, the least with peripheral surgery (Figs. 10-1, 10-2, and 10-3).[504] Hypoxemia after upper abdominal or thoracic surgery persists for five days usually and occasionally for 15 days).[1054,1212,1474,1523,2040] Clinical criteria and x-rays ideally should be analyzed together with arterial blood gases, especially in the elderly (Fig. 10-4).[282,804,2055]

Hypoxemia postoperatively is due to ventilation-perfusion abnormalities. Patients exhibit a spectrum of responses ranging from an increase in frank shunting to varying degrees of lesser ventilatory defects.[138,244,505,698] Such responses are the result of either an altered pattern of ventilation or mechanical obstruction of airways.[20,22,435,522,1120]

VENTILATION PATTERN

The effects of alteration of the pattern of ventilation by high or low tidal volumes, absence of periodic hyperinflations, and paralysis are discussed in detail in Chapter 2. In the postoperative patient the pattern of ventilation is altered by anesthetics, narcotics, and pain.[155,597,1465,1466]

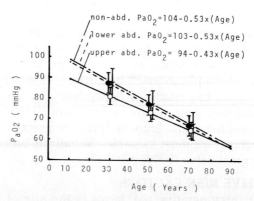

non-abd. $PaO_2 = 104 - 0.53 \times (Age)$

lower abd. $PaO_2 = 103 - 0.53 \times (Age)$

upper abd. $PaO_2 = 94 - 0.43 \times (Age)$

Figure 10-1. Arterial oxygen tension (Pa_{O_2}) with reference to site of operation in 69 patients ranging in age from 14 to 83 years. Measurements were taken while patients were breathing room air in the recovery room, as soon as they were able to respond to commands and when vital signs were stable. The oxygen tensions of the three groups (nonabdominal, upper abdominal, and lower abdominal) were not significantly different from one another at this time. (From H. Kitamura, T. Sawa, and E. Ikezono, *Anesthesiology.*[1039])

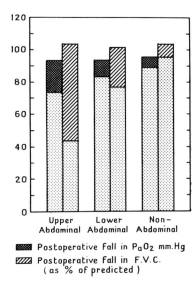

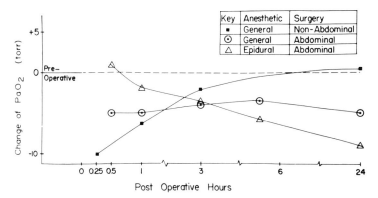

Figure 10-2. Postoperative fall in arterial oxygen tension (Pa_{O_2}) (breathing room air) and in forced vital capacity (FVC) after upper, lower, and nonabdominal surgery. The greatest reduction in both occur after upper abdominal surgery. (From M. L. Diament and K. N. V. Palmer, *Lancet*.[504])

Figure 10-3. Changes in the arterial oxygen tension (Pa_{O_2}) after general and epidural anesthesia for abdominal and nonabdominal surgery. Nonabdominal cases after general anesthesia are initially more hypoxemic but return to preoperative levels within three hours. Abdominal cases with general anesthesia continue to have lower arterial oxygen tensions than preoperatively for the first 24 hours and often for days. After epidural anesthesia the Pa_{O_2} is initially normal but within the first two hours falls to levels equal to or below the Pa_{O_2} after general anesthesia. (From B. E. Marshall and M. Q. Wyche, Jr., *Anesthesiology*.[1238])

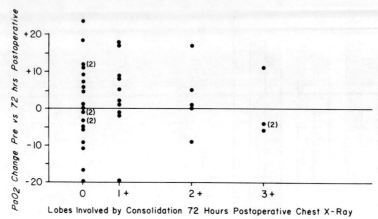

Figure 10-4.   Changes in arterial oxygen tension (Pa_{O_2}) 72 hours postoperatively with respect to the number of lobes involved by consolidation as seen on chest x-ray. As a single isolated measurement the arterial blood gas tension with the patient breathing room air may not reflect a pulmonary complication that can be detected by physical examination or by chest x-ray. (From A. E. Pflug, T. M. Murphy, S. H. Butler, and G. T. Tucker, *Anesthesiology*.[1523])

In addition obesity, pneumoperitoneum, gastric distention, pulmonary compression by retractors, effusion, or dressings, muscle spasm, straining, paralysis, or chest wall instability all cause a decrease in functional residual capacity (Figs. 10-5 and 10-6).[342,902,1118,1238,1582]

CLOSING CAPACITY

By analysis of xenon and of helium washout curves it has been shown that, at some point during exhalation to residual volume, small airways

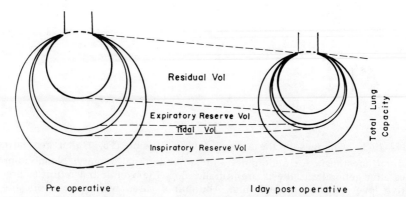

Figure 10-5.   Lung volumes on the first postoperative day. Twenty-four hours after abdominal surgery the functional residual capacity and total lung capacity are diminished due to a loss of both inspiratory and expiratory reserve volumes. The residual volume remains relatively constant. (From B. E. Marshall and M. Q. Wyche, Jr., *Anesthesiology*.[1238])

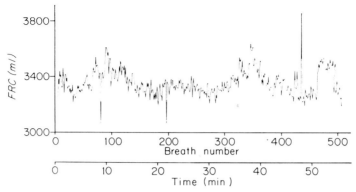

Figure 10-6. Cyclical variations in functional residual capacity (FRC) in normal man. These normal variations have to be taken into account when assessing data from patients. (From M. P. Hlastala, B. Wranne, and C. J. Lenfant, *J. Appl. Physiol.*[902])

narrow or close.[1311] Intraoperative or postoperative reduction of the functional residual capacity may shift the closure of significant numbers of airways from a point in the expiratory reserve volume to a point during the tidal volume. The functional residual capacity minus the closing capacity has a good correlation with the alveolar-arterial oxygen tension difference (Fig. 10-7).[1039] Airway closure is increased with age, smoking, and obesity. If the closing capacity is great enough to allow uninterrupted airway closure, the gas distal to the obstruction may be absorbed, creating atelectasis. Since closing capacity increases as age increases, the contribution of ventilation-

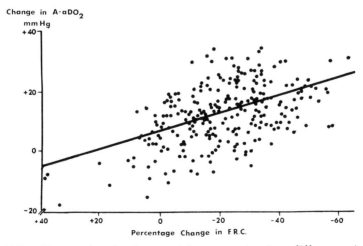

Figure 10-7. Change in alveolar-arterial oxygen tension difference ($A-aD_{O_2}$) breathing room air with reference to percentage change in functional residual capacity (FRC) after upper abdominal surgery. (From J. I. Alexander, A. A. Spence, R. K. Parikh, and B. Stuart, *Br. J. Anaesth.*[22])

perfusion abnormalities to the postoperative alveolar-arterial oxygen tension gradient on room air increases with age (Figs. 10-8 and 10-9).

PAIN

Pain promotes poor inspiratory efforts, failure to cough, and therefore respiratory complications.[580] The morphine requirement of the postoperative patient can be reduced 50 percent by instruction of the patient and by rapport with physicians, therapists, and especially nurses.[577,578]

NEUROTICISM SCORE

The personality of the patient is critical in determining the effect of the surgical incision on his perception of pain. Persons with a low "neuroticism score" are likely to have less pain, greater postoperative vital capacity, and fewer postoperative complications (Fig. 10-10).[471,1480] The neuroticism score measures emotional stability and proneness to anxiety by means of a questionnaire. Older patients are likely to have higher neuroticism scores but are more likely to respond to placebos.

NARCOTICS

Narcotics, if administered in excess of an individual patient's needs, can increase respiratory complications by a factor of 2. Narcotics also alter the respiratory pattern of breathing, such that normal sighs are infrequent or omitted.[579,630] In one study of the postoperative patient, however, patients given morphine 10 mg intramuscularly only as needed with an average dose of 50 mg over two days did not show reduced pulmonary complications as compared to patients given 10 mg morphine intramuscularly every four hours with an average total dose of 110 mg over two days.[395] Minute volume

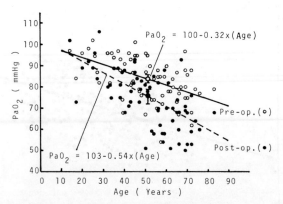

Figure 10-8. Changes in the arterial oxygen tension (Pa_{O_2}) breathing room air preoperatively and postoperatively with increasing age. A significantly greater reduction in Pa_{O_2} occurs postoperatively in older patients ($P < 0.01$). As age increases, the contribution of ventilation-perfusion abnormalities progressively increases. (From H. Kitamura, T. Sawa, and E. Ikezono, *Anesthesiology*.[1039])

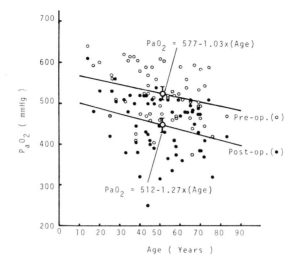

Figure 10-9. Changes in the arterial oxygen tension (Pa_{O_2}) breathing 100% oxygen preoperatively and postoperatively with increasing age. The effect of surgery is to displace the relationship without changing the slope. (From H. Kitamura, T. Sawa, and E. Ikezono, *Anesthesiology*.[1039])

and respiratory rate are decreased or unchanged by these doses of narcotics.[579,1396,1828] Narcotics in the intensive care unit are in general best given intravenously.

PERIDURAL BLOCKADE

Peridural blockade also is effective in reducing postoperative pain. Continuous peridural analgesia is said by some to allow a shorter hospital stay and earlier ambulation than when narcotics are used for postoperative pain relief.[243,1523,1785,1839] In a study in which peridural block-

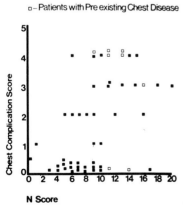

Figure 10-10. Chest complications increase postoperatively with an increasing neuroticism score (*N Score*). The severity of chest complications on a scale of 1 to 5 shows a positive correlation with the patients who have a high neuroticism score, i.e., who are more neurotic. (From D. G. Dalrymple, G. D. Parbrook, and D. F. Steel, *Br. J. Anaesth.*[471])

ade was compared to a cumulative dose of morphine 44 mg intramuscularly given over the first two days, continuous peridural analgesia provided an arterial oxygen tension 13 mm Hg (1.7 kPa) higher on room air and less alteration of pulmonary ventilation-perfusion abnormalities; but other investigators have not found these higher arterial oxygen tensions.[914,1396,1523,1828] Peridural analgesia improves vital capacity by approximately 30 percent, depending on the location of the incision, but this increase is not significantly different from that caused by morphine analgesia.[1523,1828] In another study the incidence of postoperative complications was no different in 20 patients given morphine and 20 patients given peridural analgesia. Because of problems of infection and dosage regulation and because of the equivocal results cited above we generally do not use postoperative peridural analgesia.

NITROUS OXIDE–OXYGEN

The administration of a mixture of 50% nitrous oxide and 50% oxygen intermittently significantly improves the functional residual capacity postoperatively despite an absence of change in the vital capacity. This may be due to stimulatory effects or to removal of gas from the abdomen.[21] Nitrous oxide cannot be used for prolonged periods, because leukopenia develops.

ABDOMINAL DISTENTION

Abdominal distention also causes respiratory embarrassment. Upon closure of a laparotomy, as much as 3 liters of air remain inside the abdominal cavity.[171] Meteorism is encountered occasionally in the ventilated patient. Pneumoperitoneum may occur with high airway pressures without surgical intervention usually, but not always, when there is a pneumothorax.[24,415] Abdominal distention is often overlooked and underrated. When it occurs, it should be treated as a major respiratory risk factor and corrected according to its etiology.

MANAGEMENT OF SECRETIONS

Abdominal surgery reduces the ability to cough to an average of 60 percent of preoperative values.[580] Secretions thus tend to accumulate. Suctioning must be used with caution. After 15 seconds of endotracheal suctioning, arterial oxygen may be reduced from 107 mm Hg to as little as 50 mm Hg (from 13.9 to 6.5 kPa);[219] this hypoxemia is caused by aspiration of intrapulmonary air with pulmonary collapse. Cardiac arrest due to hypoxemia occurs commonly with prolonged suctioning. Therefore suctioning is limited to 15 seconds, preferably preceded by preoxygenation. Electrocardiographic monitoring is essential. After suctioning, several large breaths are given with 100% oxygen.[1115,1963] Great care is taken to suction with aseptic technique, lest nosocomial infection occur.[1389] Selective bronchial suctioning is accomplished by contralateral turning of the head and by angled catheters.[788]

Endotracheal intubation bypasses the nose, placing the burden of warming and humidification of inspired gas onto the tracheal and bronchial epithelium.[277,508,1619,1932,1953] Dry gases slow ciliary clearance rates; in addition, secretions may build up within the tube and cause obstruction. Therefore patients with endotracheal tubes receive heated, humidified gases. Temperature at the airway is monitored with an inline thermometer and maintained as near as possible to 37°C. The dangers of nosocomial infection by humidifiers are discussed in Chapter 4. We do not often use ultrasonic nebulizers. The aerosols produce increased airway resistance due to increased bronchial tone (Fig. 10-11).[323,1215,2016,2018] Other harmful effects include water intoxication, since an ultrasonic nebulizer can produce 200 percent saturation.[4,835,1334,1801] In certain patients, in whom secretions need to be loosened and coughing stimulated, ultrasonic nebulization is used intermittently. There is some evidence that pulmonary mucus transport is increased by this method.[1486]

Patients who are dehydrated up to 0.6 kg maintain a stable vital capacity but exhibit a 7.3 percent fall in the forced expiratory volume at one second (Fig. 10-12).[82,613,750] Fiberoptic bronchoscopy can be beneficial in selected patients for diagnosis and removal of secretions.[446,2022] It must be used cautiously to minimize hypercapnia and arrhythmias. Fiberoptic bronchoscopy for two minutes produces little change in arterial blood gases or

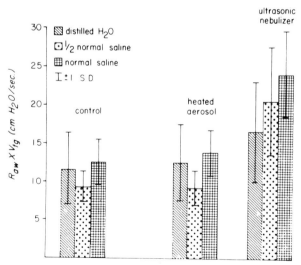

Figure 10-11. The effect of a heated aerosol and ultrasonic nebulization of distilled water, one-half normal saline, and normal saline on airway resistance (Raw) times thoracic gas volume (VTG) in normal subjects (*control*) and in patients with chronic bronchitis or asthma. Airway resistance is significantly increased by the use of the ultrasonic nebulizer. (From F. W. Cheney, Jr. and J. Butler, *Anesthesiology.*[323])

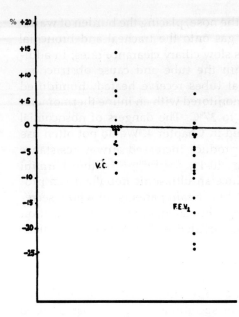

Figure 10-12. The effect of dehydration, with body weight reduced by 0.6 kg, on vital capacity (VC) and forced expiratory volume in one second (FEV$_1$). The mean FEV$_1$ is reduced by 7.3 percent; in some subjects there is a greater than 20 percent reduction. Vital capacity is not changed. The ordinate gives percent change from predehydration values. (From M. Govindaraj, *Am. Rev. Respir. Dis.*[750])

cardiac function. After ten minutes with intermittent suctioning the mean arterial oxygen tension when the patient is breathing oxygen is 58 percent of prebronchoscopy levels and tidal volume only 42 percent. Both carbon dioxide tensions and cardiac output increase by about 50 percent. If a standard fiberoptic bronchoscope is inserted through a tracheal tube of less than 8 mm internal diameter, a positive end-expiratory pressure and hypoventilation ensue.[1167] Therefore in ill patients undergoing fiberoptic bronchoscopy continuous electrocardiographic monitoring is necessary.[992]

All critically ill patients should be turned hourly from side to side to prevent pooling of secretions. Turning minimizes local pulmonary congestion by allowing redistribution of pulmonary blood flow and ventilation. In the paralyzed and mechanically ventilated patient the diaphragm moves least where the intraabdominal pressure against it is greatest. Turning allows redistribution of such pressure and therefore better ventilation of all areas.[669]

In patients who produce large quantities of sputum, the use of postural drainage, percussion, and vibration techniques along with deep breathing and appropriate antibiotics successfully reduce postoperative pulmonary complications fivefold.[5,1122,1475,1845,1919] For young patients who have no pulmonary disorders and who do not smoke, the benefits of chest physical therapy as a prophylactic measure are not as clear-cut and may be negligible.[1110,1122,1454,1523] We use physical therapy in addition to other preventive measures for all patients who have copious sputum production or infected sputum and for all patients with pulmonary disease both preoperatively and postoperatively. We use it also for all patients over 50 scheduled for abdominal surgery. Chest physical therapy is not a totally benign procedure. In adults without large amounts of sputum blood gases are not altered, but cardiac output is changed ± 50 percent (Fig. 10-13).[915,1122,1442,1523,1622]

Coughing, breath holding, and blowing into bottles or balloons are effective only insofar as the volume of inspiration is increased. The expiratory phase actually can be detrimental to the lungs, since pleural pressure may exceed airway pressure, resulting in airway or alveolar collapse.[105] Coughing is the best of this group of maneuvers and is usually associated with a deep inspiratory effort. Reports differ on the efficiency of percutaneous tracheal catheterization, but cardiac arrhythmias and bleeding into the neck and trachea are a problem.

Deep inspiration may be performed with an incentive spirometer. This procedure has reduced respiratory complications from 30 to 10 percent after laparotomy.[104,105,2024,2088] In another study respiratory complications after adrenalectomy fell from 40 to 20 percent.[1980]

OTHER PREVENTIVE MEASURES

INTERMITTENT POSITIVE PRESSURE BREATHING (IPPB)

The use of intermittent positive pressure breathing by mask or mouthpiece is not effective in preventing or improving postoperative pulmonary status as judged by clinical or radiologic criteria. Careful studies verify this fact.[113,126,256,429,658,1323,1439,1440,1697,2135]

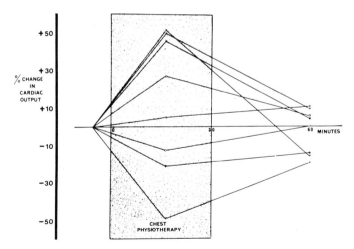

Figure 10-13. Cardiac output and physiotherapy. Cardiac output may increase or decrease by up to 50 percent. In most patients cardiac output returns to normal after 60 minutes. (From A. K. Laws and R. W. McIntyre, *Can. Anaesth. Soc. J.*[1122])

Respiratory complication rates are not reduced by its use preoperatively[429] or postoperatively[113] for nebulization of normal saline. Bronchodilators may have a beneficial effect, but we do not think they do. Intermittent positive pressure breathing by a ventilator is no more effective in delivering bronchodilators than are hand-held nebulizers.[329,726,727,1831]

PROPHYLACTIC VENTILATION

In several types of patients, the risk of postoperative respiratory failure is so great and the patients' work of breathing so large that, although an isolated postoperative examination might favor weaning, respiratory failure would ensue within hours if weaning were attempted. Such patients, as well as those who develop cardiorespiratory complications intraoperatively, are ventilated prophylactically in an effort to prevent further deterioration.[475,1517,1518,1541,1545,1565,2085] After open-heart or major vascular surgery we routinely ventilate. Patients who have been in prolonged shock also need ventilation. In addition patients who undergo upper abdominal or thoracic procedures and who are also septic, obese, hypothermic, cachectic, or have multiple trauma are ventilated prophylactically.

DOXAPRAM

Doxapram in continuous infusion has been advocated to obviate the need for controlled ventilation. We feel, however, that artificial stimulation of respiration in acute respiratory failure can be criticized on two counts. First, when the lungs are clear but the central respiratory drive is depressed, failure to intubate may result in aspiration in the comatose patient. Second, when the lungs are not clear and respiratory failure is associated with increased work of breathing and decreased compliance, stimulating already exhausted respiratory muscles only intensifies their exhaustion. Doxapram decreases cerebral blood flow and may be hazardous in patients with cerebrovascular disease.[1310,1367,2049]

PULMONARY LAVAGE

Pulmonary lavage is occasionally useful in status asthmaticus and sometimes in cystic fibrosis and alveolar proteinosis. Endobronchial tubes must be correctly placed and serial blood gases measured.[563,1649]

PREVENTION OF THROMBOSIS AND EMBOLI

Lower limb venous thrombosis and pulmonary emboli are found in 30–50 percent of necropsies.[683,706,1279,1361] Clinical signs frequently fail to provide a warning of thrombosis or embolization.[805,984,1093,1155,1950] After major surgical procedures approximately 30 percent of patients have deep vein thrombosis as noted by ^{131}I-labeled fibrinogen scanning or venography.[683,1093,1419] A variety of methods are used to reduce these complications[128,199,304,1325,1369] and include muscle stimulation, passive leg exercises, and intermittent calf compression.[251,889,1683] None, however, is as useful as administration of low-dose heparin. Many methods of giving low-dose heparin have been used.[350,683,987,1419,1426,1743,1857] We administer heparin to most major surgical candidates (excluding those awaiting open-heart surgery) two hours prior to the procedure. We give 5,000 units subcutaneously and postoperatively every 12 hours.[241] This results in a reduction of calf thromboses to 5 percent of patients from the 30 percent incidence among untreated patients. Preliminary studies indicate that the incidence of pulmonary embolism is also reduced.[986,1149,1419]

Heparin acts to alter the configuration of antithrombin, which in turn inhibits thrombin, preventing clot formation (Fig. 10-14).[1658] With low-dose heparin therapy clotting parameters are only slightly elevated and serious hemorrhage is hardly ever encountered. If pulmonary embolism does occur despite prophylaxis, full heparinization via continuous intravenous infusion is indicated.[1368,1694] We do not anticoagulate patients fully for at least a month after intracranial surgery.

Anticoagulation therapy increased survival from 42 to 92 percent in 516 patients in whom the diagnosis of pulmonary embolism was based on at least two out of the following criteria: clear symptoms and signs compatible with pulmonary embolism; abnormal lung scan; and abnormal arteriographic findings.[1540] Urokinase produces a decrease in pulmonary artery pressure and total pulmonary resistance with angiographic improvement of the pulmonary embolism, but evidence regarding improved prognosis is inconclusive.[509] Extracorporeal bypass and pulmonary thromboembolectomy in one series increased survival in massive pulmonary embolism from 61 to 71 percent,[1950] but we regard pulmonary thromboembolectomy as

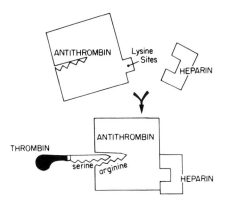

Figure 10-14. The mechanism of action of heparin is due to its ability to cause a conformational change in antithrombin; antithrombin in turn inhibits thrombin by binding with it at a serine-arginine site. Heparin causes similar inhibitions of other factors. (From R. D. Rosenberg.[1658] Reprinted by permission from the *New England Journal of Medicine* 292:146–151, 1975.)

obsolete. Long-term survival after angiographically proved pulmonary embolism depends on the cardiac status before embolism: out of 60 consecutive patients who survived an episode of acute pulmonary embolism, 36 of 42 patients without left ventricular failure, as opposed to 3 of 16 patients with failure before embolism, were alive one to seven years later.[1479]

TRANSPORTATION FROM OTHER HOSPITALS

Transportation of patients from other hospitals ideally should be accomplished without loss of physician management. Upon agreeing to accept a patient into our intensive care unit from a referring hospital, we send an ambulance which we know to be properly equipped. We also send an intensive care unit respiratory therapist, house officer, and nurse to manage the patient in transit. This system works well; with the exception of one patient who became decerebrate, we have not seen any catastrophes. A major problem after transportation is keeping the referring hospital informed of the progress of the patient.

11

Weaning from Ventilatory Support

Weaning from controlled ventilation can be a difficult task associated with numerous changes in the patient. This is especially true of patients who have been on prolonged controlled ventilation and of patients with severe underlying chronic lung disease. Weaning is generally simple when there is no underlying pulmonary disease, as in many poisoned patients. In any case of respiratory failure one must carefully consider the proper timing and method of weaning.

In this chapter the physiologic alterations that occur during weaning will be discussed. Our criteria for and methods of weaning also will be presented. Occasionally there is a patient who repeatedly fails to be weaned from controlled ventilation. The reasons for this as well as the methods of dealing with this occurrence will be evaluated.

PHYSIOLOGIC CHANGES

During the first twenty-four hours after a patient has been changed from controlled to spontaneous ventilation, several important physiologic changes occur. In patients who are successfully weaned from controlled ventilation the vital capacity increases from a mean of 10.7 ml per kilogram at the start of weaning to a mean of 16.3 ml per kilogram after 24 hours ($P <$ 0.001). Tidal volume during spontaneous breathing increases from a mean value of 4.7 ml per kilogram at the start of weaning to 5.8 ml per kilogram after 24 hours ($P < 0.001$). The maximum inspiratory force also increases significantly from -23 cm H_2O (-2.3 kPa) to -29 cm H_2O (-2.9 kPa) after 24 hours ($P < 0.001$). Changes in functional residual capacity and static compliance before and after weaning are not significantly different. Deadspace-to-tidal-volume ratio changes are also insignificant.[166,250]

CARBON DIOXIDE TENSION

Carbon dioxide tension increases in nearly all patients during weaning from controlled ventilation (Fig. 11-1). A mean increase of 8 mm Hg (1.1 kPa) is common.[166] This increase is not sustained. If the carbon dioxide tension is studied during weaning in the same patients for 10 minutes, one hour, and 24 hours, significant increases are seen in the carbon dioxide tension after the 10-minute and one-hour periods. After 24 hours the increase in carbon dioxide tension is insignificant.[250]

133

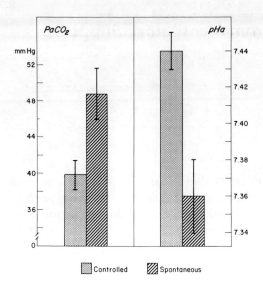

Figure 11-1. Effect of weaning from controlled ventilation on arterial carbon dioxide tension (Pa_{CO_2}) and arterial pH (pHa). Twenty-five patients in acute respiratory failure who were weaned successfully from controlled ventilation were studied, and all were found to undergo a significant increase in Pa_{CO_2} ($P < 0.003$) and a significant fall in pHa ($P < 0.001$) during the first 30 minutes of weaning. These changes returned to normal within 24 hours of the start of weaning.

RIGHT-TO-LEFT SHUNT

The majority of patients being weaned from controlled ventilation undergo a notable increase in right-to-left shunt, as indicated by an increase in the alveolar-arterial oxygen tension gradient. Even patients who are weaned successfully generally have a significant mean increase ($P < 0.05$). The increase in gradient ranges between 55 and 102 mm Hg (7.3–13.6 kPa) in different groups of patients breathing 100% oxygen. In patients who fail to be weaned successfully the mean increase in this gradient is 286 mm Hg (38.1 kPa) ($P < 0.025$). This increase occurs rapidly, usually within the first 20 minutes.[1794] Occasionally patients show a fall in oxygen gradient during weaning, which may explain why the increase in one series did not appear to be significant.[166,250]

The reason for an increased alveolar-arterial oxygen tension gradient probably is the development of rapid alveolar collapse.[1794] In several cases of such an increase we observed no change in pulmonary capillary wedge pressure or in pulmonary artery pressure. This suggests that the increase in oxygen tension gradient is not based on sudden left ventricular failure. Chest x-ray films taken of these patients also show no significant changes. Our conclusion is that certain patients develop rapid alveolar collapse when controlled ventilation is discontinued. This leads to an increase in right-to-left shunt and thus to hypoxemia, if the patient is not breathing an adequate inspired oxygen concentration. Patients who are at risk for hypoxemia and lung collapse are those with high closing capacities as well as many of those who have received prolonged ventilatory support.

PULMONARY VASCULATURE

Changes in the pulmonary vasculature following the discontinuance of controlled ventilation are poorly documented. The pulmonary vascular resistance increases in nearly all patients during weaning. This increase is slightly higher in those patients who demonstrate a fall in cardiac output during weaning.[116]

CARDIAC OUTPUT

When a patient is converted from controlled to spontaneous ventilation, one would expect to find an increase in cardiac output as well as an increase in oxygen consumption.[116] This does not happen uniformly, however. In a group of nine patients with a variety of diagnoses those patients who were weaned successfully showed no change in the cardiac index after discontinuance of controlled ventilation. Those patients who could not be weaned showed a significant rise in cardiac index from 2.4 liters per square meter per minute to 3.6 liters per square meter per minute ($P < 0.05$). This rise occurred within the first 15–20 minutes after ventilatory support was removed.[1794] In another group of postoperative cardiac surgical patients the findings were different. Half the patients showed a small but significant increase in cardiac output (19 percent). The other half had a mean fall in cardiac output of 17 percent. In the latter group there was also a significant rise in peripheral vascular resistance and a fall in the oxygen consumption. Many of these patients showed signs of restlessness, dyspnea, and diaphoresis, necessitating return to mechanical ventilation. These studies indicate that unsuccessful weaning is sometimes caused by deterioration in cardiac output.[116,715] In summary some patients who are weaned successfully show no change in cardiac output, while others show a rise. Some patients who fail to be weaned have a rise in cardiac output, while others have a fall.

OXYGEN CONSUMPTION

Oxygen consumption generally changes significantly when patients are changed from controlled to spontaneous ventilation. Patients who have a rise in cardiac output have a rise in oxygen consumption.[179] A fall in cardiac output during weaning is associated with a fall in oxygen consumption.[116]

In patients who are weaned successfully from controlled ventilation significant changes in pulse and blood pressure are rarely seen. In patients who fail to be weaned there is a significant increase in pulse from 90 to 126 beats per minute ($P < 0.05$). Blood pressure also rises, but the increase has not been shown to be significant.[1794]

SYMPATHOADRENAL STIMULATION

In most patients during weaning there is increased sympathoadrenal stimulation, demonstrated by a rise in urinary levels of epinephrine and norepinephrine.[1794] This rise may be greater in those patients who fail to be weaned, but this has not been clearly demonstrated.[116,733] The rise in catecholamine levels during weaning may explain in part the increase in oxygen consumption seen in patients with increased cardiac output during weaning.[179] Since those patients who demonstrate a rise in cardiac output often are those who cannot be weaned from controlled ventilation, the rise in blood pressure and pulse in unweanable patients can be explained by increased catecholamine levels.[1794] Certainly anxiety plays a part in sympathetic stimulation.

CRITERIA FOR WEANING

The criteria for the discontinuance of controlled ventilation are essentially the converse of the criteria for the institution of controlled ventilation.[621] The patient should have adequate pulmonary function. The vital capacity should be at least 10 ml per kilogram, or roughly twice the normal tidal volume. This is necessary to allow the patient to take deep breaths and cough effectively. The maximum inspiratory force should be at least −20 to −30 cm H_2O (−2 to −3 kPa).[589,906,1546,1688]

Alveolar ventilation during weaning is usually slightly reduced.[250] Naturally we try to avoid severe alveolar hypoventilation and respiratory acidemia during weaning. The deadspace-to-tidal-volume ratio is an accurate predictor of ability to maintain alveolar ventilation. Weaning with a deadspace-to-tidal-volume ratio of greater than 0.6 usually is not successful,[1794] although on rare occasions it has been, usually with younger patients (Figs. 11-2 and 11-3).[1913]

The ability to maintain oxygenation during weaning is also important. An alveolar-arterial oxygen tension gradient of less than 300–350 mm Hg (40.0–46.7 kPa) must be reached before weaning from controlled ventilation is begun.[621]

Cardiovascular stability is necessary prior to weaning. Hypotension and serious arrhythmias are contraindications to weaning.[1130] Since the deadspace-to-tidal-volume ratio varies inversely with the cardiac index, weaning a patient with a low cardiac index is not likely to be successful (Fig. 11-4).[572,1883] The necessity of using vasopressor drugs to maintain the blood pressure is not necessarily a contraindication to ventilator weaning, especially following cardiovascular surgery. Each case must be considered individually in terms of the stability of the cardiovascular system.

The patient's metabolic state should also be considered. Patients with greatly increased metabolic rates may be difficult to wean. Increases in oxygen consumption and carbon dioxide production secondary to fever or

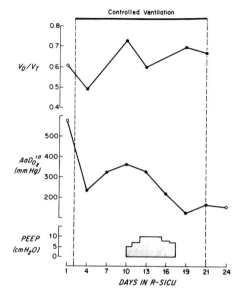

Figure 11-2. Course of a patient weaned from controlled ventilation despite high deadspace-to-tidal-volume ratios (VD/VT). A 38-year-old man was admitted to the Respiratory–Surgical Intensive Care Unit (R-SICU) with viral pneumonia. Prior to the start of controlled ventilation his alveolar-arterial oxygen tension gradient measured breathing 100% oxygen (A-aD$_{O_2}$$^{1.0}$) was 590 mm Hg (78.5 kPa) with a VD/VT of 0.6. After ten days of respiratory failure, positive end-expiratory pressure (PEEP) was necessary. During seven days of ventilation with PEEP the A-aD$_{O_2}$ began to fall, and x-rays of the chest showed improvement. The patient was totally weaned from controlled ventilation after 21 days, at which time the VD/VT was 0.67. (From D. Teres, M. F. Roizen, and L. S. Bushnell, *Anesthesiology.*[1913])

shivering prevent weaning. Whenever possible, hyperpyrexia or hypothermia is corrected prior to any attempts to discontinue mechanical ventilation.

Patients without lung disease show slight alveolar hypoventilation (Pa$_{CO_2}$ 45–50 mm Hg [6.0–6.7 kPa]) secondary to metabolic alkalemia.[1162,1746] In view of this hypercapnia every effort should be made to correct a metabolic alkalemia prior to weaning. Metabolic acidemia should also be corrected prior to discontinuance of ventilator support.

Coma has been suggested as a contraindication to weaning.[1130] This view is unfounded, except when hypercapnia would cause an undesirable increase in cerebral blood flow. Extubation, however, should be delayed until consciousness returns with the presence of an adequate gag and cough reflex.

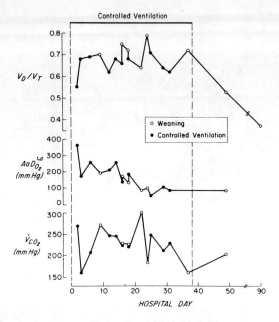

Figure 11-3.   Comparison of deadspace-to-tidal-volume ratio (Vᴅ/Vᴛ), alveolar-arterial oxygen tension difference measured breathing 100% oxygen (A-aDo$_2^{1.0}$), and carbon dioxide production ($\dot{\text{V}}$co$_2$) in a patient who was weaned from controlled ventilation despite a high Vᴅ/Vᴛ. A 32-year-old female was in acute respiratory failure due to viral pneumonia. There was no difference in $\dot{\text{V}}$co$_2$ between the weaning period and controlled ventilation. Values of Vᴅ/Vᴛ were also similar during both weaning and controlled ventilation. Note that the A-aD$_{\text{O}_2}^{1.0}$ had normalized after a month of controlled ventilation. When the patient was finally weaned completely, the Vᴅ/Vᴛ was still over 0.65. The Vᴅ/Vᴛ returned toward normal after three months. (From D. Teres, M. F. Roizen, and L. S. Bushnell, *Anesthesiology.*[1913])

METHODS OF WEANING

BRIGGS ADAPTOR OR T-PIECE

When it has been established that a patient meets the criteria for weaning, a method must be selected. Patients most commonly are weaned via a Briggs adaptor or a T-piece. Either of these allows the patient to breathe spontaneously while heated humidified oxygen is delivered via wide-bore corrugated tubing. The baseline alveolar-arterial oxygen tension gradient, arterial carbon dioxide tension, and pH are obtained while the patient is still being ventilated. Vital capacity, tidal volume, and maximum inspiratory force are also measured. If these signs confirm that the patient is ready for weaning, he is put in a sitting position and the procedures are carefully explained. Vital signs are taken and recorded, and the patient is then taken off the ventilator and connected to a Briggs adaptor. The inspired oxygen

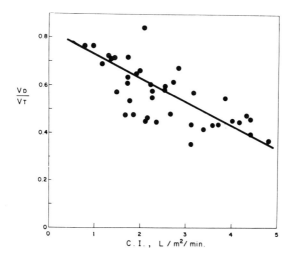

Figure 11-4. Effect of the cardiac index (CI) on the deadspace-to-tidal-volume ratio (V_D/V_T). In 14 dogs the cardiac index was obtained during infusion of trimethaphan camsylate. Simultaneous measurements demonstrated that there is an inverse relationship between V_D/V_T and CI. The lowest CI is associated with the highest V_D/V_T. All 14 dogs had measurements of V_D/V_T and CI during both controlled and spontaneous ventilation. (From K. Suwa, J. Hedley-Whyte, and H. H. Bendixen, *J. Appl. Physiol.*[1883])

concentration is set at a level slightly higher than what the patient was receiving during controlled ventilation. The use of 100% oxygen is avoided during weaning, except for the measurement of alveolar-arterial oxygen tension gradients, since it can lead to an increased intrapulmonary right-to-left shunt.[621]

Vital signs are monitored every 5 minutes until they are stable and then every 15 minutes during the weaning period. Respiratory mechanics are measured about every hour. Arterial blood gases are measured usually after 15 minutes. After that the frequency of measurement is determined by the underlying disease and the clinical appearance of the patient. Usually blood gases should be measured no less than every hour during the early stages of weaning.

If the patient develops an alveolar-arterial oxygen tension gradient of over 400 mm Hg (53.3 kPa), or if respiratory acidemia develops with a pH of less than 7.25, the patient is placed back on controlled ventilation. If the patient becomes agitated, dyspneic, cyanotic, confused, hypertensive, tachycardic, or tachypneic, a blood gas sample is drawn and the patient is placed back on controlled ventilation. These findings usually are associated with hypoxia or hypercapnia. Even if the blood gas is normal, the patient may be extremely anxious. This anxiety generally can be handled by reassurance and resumption of the weaning process.

SPONTANEOUS POSITIVE END-EXPIRATORY PRESSURE

Spontaneous positive end-expiratory pressure is beneficial for patients who have high closing capacities and patients with a history of developing rapid alveolar collapse during weaning. Patients who are weaned with 5 cm of positive end-expiratory pressure have a significantly lower mean increase in alveolar-arterial oxygen tension gradient than those who are weaned without it (Fig. 11-5).[623] In particular, patients who rapidly develop marked increases in their alveolar-arterial oxygen tension gradient during weaning without positive end-expiratory pressure are helped by institution of this method. The use of positive end-expiratory pressure during weaning also results in significant improvement in the vital capacity and inspiratory force (Figs. 11-5 and 11-6).[623]

EXTUBATION

Once the patient has been weaned for a certain period of time, consideration must be given to extubation. The exact length of time necessary depends upon the patient's underlying lung disease and the course of his

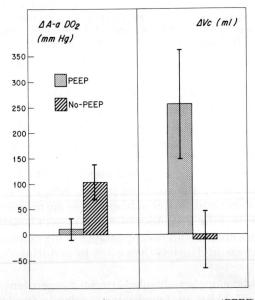

Figure 11-5. Effect of positive end-expiratory pressure (PEEP) during weaning from controlled ventilation on the alveolar-arterial oxygen tension difference measured breathing 100% oxygen (A-aD$_{O_2}$) and on the vital capacity (VC). Those patients who were weaned without PEEP (No-PEEP) (N = 13) had a significant increase in A-aD$_{O_2}$ (P < 0.01). This increase was prevented in those patients who were weaned with 5 cm H$_2$O (0.05 kPa) of PEEP (N = 12) (P < 0.03). Patients who weaned with PEEP also had a significant improvement in vital capacity during weaning (P < 0.05). (From T. W. Feeley, R. Saumarez, J. M. Klick, T. G. McNabb, and J. J. Skillman, *Lancet*.[623])

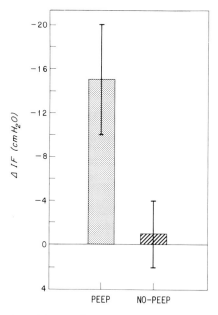

Figure 11-6. Effect of positive end-expiratory pressure (PEEP) during weaning from controlled ventilation on the maximum inspiratory force (IF). Twelve patients in acute respiratory failure were weaned with 5 cm H_2O (0.05 kPa) PEEP, while 13 patients were weaned without PEEP (No-PEEP). Those patients who were weaned with PEEP underwent a significant improvement in inspiratory force ($P < 0.01$). Patients who were weaned without PEEP did not have any improvement in inspiratory force during weaning.

weaning. The major criteria for extubation are that the patient be awake, alert, and able to cough and gag adequately. If these criteria are met, the patient's tracheal tube is removed. Oxygen is then administered by face mask at the same oxygen concentration via a heated nebulizer. The patient is closely observed for respiratory distress and laryngeal spasm.

WEANING WITH A TRACHEOSTOMY TUBE

If a tracheostomy tube is present, weaning usually proceeds with it in situ for 24 hours. If the patient's ventilatory status remains adequate after that time, and he is awake and alert with good pharyngeal reflexes, then the cuffed tracheostomy tube is replaced by a fenestrated tube. If this is tolerated, the hole of the tube at the tracheostomy site is plugged. The patient is now able to breathe through his own upper airway, talk, and cough secretions into his mouth. The fenestrated tube allows normal respiratory function while keeping the tracheostomy site open in case the patient requires the reinstitution of controlled ventilation. A tracheal button is another alternative. The fenestrated tube or the tracheal button is removed when it seems that the patient will not require further controlled ventilation. The tracheostomy site is covered with a dry sterile dressing.[621] It usually heals in one to three weeks. Occasionally a tracheostomy stoma does not close, and surgical closure is necessary.[1125]

INTERMITTENT MANDATORY VENTILATION

Intermittent mandatory ventilation has been presented as an alternative method of weaning patients from ventilatory support. This system allows the patient to breathe spontaneously in between preset ventilatory cycles. When the patient breathes, he gets his proper inspired oxygen concentration as well as adequate humidification. In order to wean a patient, the number of ventilator cycles per minute is gradually reduced, thus allowing the patient slowly to take over his own respiratory function. This system assures intermittent hyperinflation of the lungs. Positive end-expiratory pressure can be used in conjunction with it.[536,537]

Intermittent mandatory ventilation has been reported to be helpful in weaning when conventional methods have failed.[536,537] In our experience patients who are difficult to wean with conventional techniques are equally so with intermittent mandatory ventilation.[621] We often use it, however, in ventilating patients who might require sedation to bring them into phase with conventional controlled ventilation but for whom sedation is undesirable. Patients need little or no sedation when receiving intermittent mandatory ventilation, since they can safely breathe out of phase with the ventilator. Intermittent mandatory ventilation, in general, maintains patients with more satisfactory lung volumes at lower mean airway pressures.

CARDIOVASCULAR COMPLICATIONS OF WEANING

Cardiovascular collapse has been reported as a complication of weaning. It generally occurs in patients who experience a fall in cardiac output during weaning. This fall, as we have seen, is associated with a decrease in oxygen consumption and an increase in peripheral vascular resistance. The collapse seems to happen in patients who have a limited cardiac reserve and is often not associated with any changes in arterial blood gases.[116] Clinically it may be detected by evidence of peripheral vasoconstriction and, ultimately, hypotension.[715] Management consists of return to controlled ventilation and inotropic vasopressors, if necessary.

Cardiac arrhythmias can occur as complications of weaning. They are usually late complications of hypoxia and acidemia. Hypoxia usually produces tachycardia, then bradycardia, followed by conduction disturbances and idioventricular rhythm. Death occurs by ventricular standstill, but ventricular fibrillation may occur. The slowing in rate and conduction is due probably to an increase in vagal tone secondary to chemoreceptor stimulation by hypoxia. The combination of hypercapnia and hypoxia lowers the threshold for ventricular fibrillation. Hypoxia and hypercapnia can also cause pulmonary arteriolar constriction leading to pulmonary hypertension and right heart distention. This can lead to both ventricular and atrial arrhythmias. Patients being weaned from controlled ventilation should be monitored with a continuous ECG monitor. If arrhythmias develop, a blood gas sample should be drawn, the patient placed back on controlled ventilation, and specific drug treatment of the arrhythmias then begun, if still necessary.[77,1060,1503]

SPECIAL PROBLEMS

The greatest problem related to weaning patients from controlled ventilation is the patient who continually fails to be weaned successfully. The reason for repeated failure is any of three basic abnormalities: increased ventilation requirement, decreased muscle strength, and increased work of breathing. Increased ventilatory requirement is caused either by increase in deadspace-to-tidal-volume ratio or by increased carbon dioxide production.

DECREASED MUSCLE STRENGTH

Decreased muscle strength can be caused by poor nutrition during illness, neuromuscular disease, a prolonged effect of sedative and paralytic drugs, or respiratory muscle discoordination. The nutritional status of most patients can be improved. Respiratory muscle discoordination may be caused by phrenic nerve palsy, but minor degrees of discoordination may occur without phrenic nerve injury and can interfere with weaning attempts. These patients cannot coordinate chest and diaphragmatic movements. The discoordination can be detected by fluoroscopy. There is no specific treatment, and the condition disappears with time.[621,1546]

INCREASED WORK OF BREATHING

Increased work of breathing can delay weaning and is usually caused by increased airway resistance and lowered compliance. Abdominal distention also can increase the work. Upper airway obstruction from tracheal stenosis, granulation, or a small tracheal tube can increase work of breathing and delay weaning. Acute lung disease also can prolong weaning by increasing the work of breathing.[621,1543]

GRADUAL WEANING

In approaching the patient who fails to wean one must look at each individual aspect that may be contributing to his difficulty. While attempts are being made to correct those problems that are correctable, the patient is given daily trials at spontaneous ventilation. This enables him to use his respiratory muscles, even if he cannot do so for extended periods.

Whenever possible the duration of weaning is increased. When the patient tires, he is placed back on controlled ventilation. The number as well as the duration of the weaning periods is increased daily. Patients are often allowed to rest on controlled ventilation overnight. This method of weaning is tedious but is successful in most instances.[621]

INTRAAORTIC BALLOON PUMP

The intraaortic balloon pump has been effective in improving the cardiac output in certain patients with arteriosclerotic cardiovascular disease (Chap. 12). It is well recognized that the deadspace-to-tidal-volume ratio varies inversely with the cardiac index (see Figure 11-3). In patients with a low cardiac index on the basis of coronary artery disease, the deadspace-to-tidal-volume ratio may be high enough to preclude ventilator weaning. This group of patients often benefit from an intraaortic balloon pump or vasopressor agents. If an increase in cardiac index can be obtained, there is a fall in the deadspace-to-tidal-volume ratio. In cardiac surgical patients who require aortic counterpulsation, weaning from the ventilator is usually done prior to balloon weaning. This is to obtain the maximal cardiac index possible during weaning from the ventilator.[621]

II

Respiratory Consequences of Specific Surgical Problems

12

Postoperative Management of the Cardiac Patient and the Consequences of Cardiopulmonary Bypass

Specific problems related to the care of the cardiac patient in respiratory failure include inotropic and chronotropic manipulation of the cardiovascular system, management of alterations in peripheral vascular tone, and mechanical circulatory assistance. Cardiac patients are not a homogeneous group, and considerations regarding therapy differ depending upon many factors, including the type of surgery that the patient has undergone.[152]

GENERAL CONSIDERATIONS

HEMODYNAMIC DERANGEMENT

When a patient is hemodynamically compromised, optimal cardiovascular function will be achieved at a given preload, afterload, and heart rate. These can each be manipulated separately and the best combination achieved through trial and error under close monitoring. The best combination of these parameters will depend on the underlying hemodynamic derangement. Myocardial contractility can be enhanced by the avoidance of hypoxemia, hypercapnia, acidemia, hypothermia, and electrolyte imbalance and the judicious administration of beta agonists.[449,1677]

A prime consideration during hemodynamic manipulation is attention to the effect of these interventions on the balance between myocardial oxygen delivery and myocardial oxygen consumption.[1700] Myocardial oxygen delivery occurs primarily during diastole and is dependent upon the pressure difference between the aortic root and the coronary sinus. The duration of diastole is reduced during rapid heart rates. Increases in intraventricular pressure also reduce coronary blood flow, the subendocardium being at greatest risk for development of ischemic dysfunction.[228,1231] Myocardial oxygen consumption is increased by increased left ventricular work as a result of a rise in afterload or the use of most inotropic agents (Fig. 12-1).[229] The rate-pressure product, that is, the product of heart rate and systolic arterial blood pressure, is an indirect index of myocardial oxygen consumption and has good correlation with it.[1100] An increase in the rate-pressure product may cause myocardial ischemia in the presence of coronary artery disease.[2034]

In most instances after surgery on the heart we maintain controlled ventilation during the early postoperative period until satisfactory

147

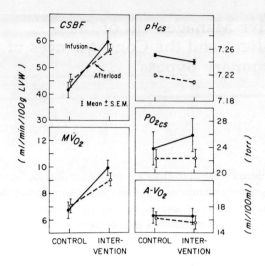

Figure 12-1.   Effect of increasing afterload or of continuous infusion of norepinephrine (3.8 μg per minute) on the coronary sinus blood flow (CSBF), myocardial
oxygen consumption (MV̇$_{O_2}$), coronary sinus pH (pHcs), coronary sinus Po$_2$
(Po$_2$cs), and arteriovenous oxygen content difference (A-V$_{O_2}$) in a dog heart-lung
preparation. Increase in afterload is achieved by increasing mean aortic pressure
from 92 to 123 mm Hg (12.2–16.4 kPa). Both CSBF and MV̇$_{O_2}$ increase significantly
with norepinephrine and with increased afterload. There are small changes in pHcs.
Data in this article suggest that there is a predictable change in coronary blood flow
with pH-induced changes in the affinity of hemoglobin for oxygen. (From H. C.
Mehmel, M. A. Duvelleroy, and M. B. Laver, *J. Appl. Physiol.*[1293])

hemodynamic stability has been achieved. The pattern of ventilation does
not differ from that used in other patients in respiratory failure. In cardiac
patients cardiac output does not invariably decrease following the application of positive end-expiratory pressure, if hypovolemia is avoided.[608,1574]
As we have mentioned elsewhere, effective circulatory volume increases
when positive end-expiratory pressure is discontinued. Circulatory failure
may ensue, if hemodynamic function is marginal.[1938]

ARRHYTHMIAS

The diagnosis and management of arrhythmias in the postoperative
cardiac surgical patient is greatly facilitated by the use of epicardial atrial
and ventricular wires, which we insert in almost every patient who has
cardiac surgery. Aggravating factors in the causation of arrhythmias include hypoxemia, acidemia, alkalemia, hypokalemia, digitalis toxicity, gastric dilatation, fever, pain, and anxiety. Premature ventricular contractions
are the most common arrhythmia, especially after aortic valve replacement
and coronary bypass surgery. Therapy consists of "overpacing," lidocaine,
or diphenylhydantoin.

If the pulse rate is less than 100 beats per minute, atrial or ventricular pacing to initiate a faster rate is a safe and effective means of suppressing ectopic ventricular activity.[141,1002] Intravenous lidocaine in doses of 50–100 mg or as a continuous infusion at 1–4 mg per minute is the next treatment of choice. In such doses intravenous lidocaine has few adverse hemodynamic effects of clinical significance in man.[1718] Diphenylhydantoin, in 100-mg increments intravenously to a total initial dose of 300–500 mg, followed by 100 mg intramuscularly or intravenously every six hours, is very effective in suppressing premature ventricular contractions due to digitalis toxicity.[862]

Supraventricular arrhythmias also occur frequently. Paroxysmal atrial tachycardia can be abolished by carotid sinus massage, pressure on the eyeball, the Valsalva maneuver, or the intravenous administration of 10 mg of edrophonium HCl. The recording of atrial activity from the atrial epicardial wire aids in diagnosis. When recording from an epicardial wire one must be careful to avoid an electric hazard that may produce ventricular fibrillation. Atrial flutter and fibrillation are treated when the ventricular response is too rapid. The ventricular rate can be reduced by digoxin,[1190] direct-current cardioversion,[2140] and propranolol.[1255] Determination of serum digoxin concentrations by radioimmunoassay helps in the control of digoxin therapy.[1813]

Sinus bradycardia and some nodal bradycardias respond to atrial pacing, atropine, or isoproterenol. Complete heart block, slow nodal rhythm, and atrioventricular dissociation are treated by ventricular or sequential atrioventricular pacing. After severe myocardial infarction coordinated atrioventricular activity results in a 24 percent increase in cardiac output over the output obtained with ventricular pacing alone (Fig. 12-2). There is an optimal P-R interval, usually around 100 msec, that provides the best augmentation of cardiac output (Fig. 12-3).[311,1863] The optimal ventricular rate and P-R interval are different in each case. Ventricular tachycardia is

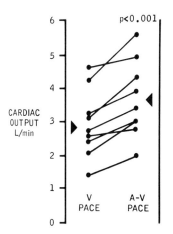

Figure 12-2. Effect of sequential atrioventricular (AV) pacing on cardiac output. Nine patients with atrioventricular block due to recent myocardial infarction had measurements of cardiac output made with ventricular (V) pacing alone and with sequential AV pacing. AV pacing resulted in a significant increase in cardiac output. *Arrows* indicate the means. (From D. A. Chamberlain, R. C. Leinbach, C. E. Vassaux, J. A. Kastor, R. W. DeSanctis, and C. A. Sanders.[311] Reprinted by permission from the *New England Journal of Medicine* 282:577–582, 1970.)

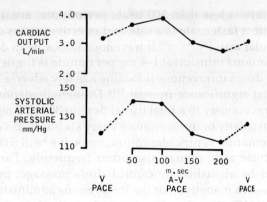

Figure 12-3.   Effect of varying atrioventricular (AV) time intervals on cardiac output and blood pressure in sequential A-V pacing of patients with recent myocardial infarction. One patient with A-V dissociation had measurements of cardiac output and systolic arterial pressure made with ventricular pacing alone and with different A-V time intervals during A-V pacing. The highest cardiac output was obtained at time intervals of 50 or 100 milliseconds. The same is true of other patients studied. (From D. A. Chamberlain, R. C. Leinbach, C. E. Vassaux, J. A. Kastor, R. W. DeSanctis, and C. A. Sanders.[311] Reprinted by permission from the *New England Journal of Medicine* 282:577–582, 1970.)

treated with intravenous lidocaine, direct-current countershock, or both.[2140]

EFFECTS OF THERAPY

DIGITALIS

We prefer to use vasopressors rather than digitalis to improve myocardial contractility in critically ill patients. Intravenous administration of a vaso-pressor can be discontinued promptly if a complication arises.[456,1814,2011] The unstable potassium balance in critically ill patients may cause therapeutic levels of digitalis to become toxic levels when hypokalemia occurs.[1190,2011] The presence of digitalis also makes accurate diagnosis of an arrhythmia difficult. Furthermore digitalis-induced arrhythmias are difficult to treat in seriously ill patients. Digitalis causes coronary vasoconstriction, an effect that appears to be neurogenically mediated through stimulation of alpha-adrenergic receptors.[685]

SHORT-ACTING DIURETICS

Furosemide and ethacrynic acid are potent short-acting diuretics used in the therapy of fluid overload and pulmonary edema and in the diagnosis of the integrity of renal function. The prompt, beneficial effect of furosemide in relieving pulmonary congestion and acute pulmonary edema frequently precedes any diuresis and is due to a decrease in the left ventricular filling pressure (Fig. 12-4).[510,1087,1104] The persistence of oliguria after adequate

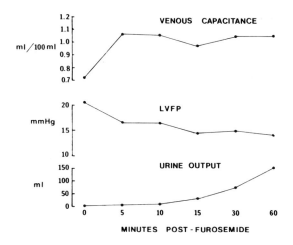

Figure 12-4. Effect of furosemide on venous capacitance, left ventricular filling pressure (LVFP), and urine output. Administration of furosemide to patients with left ventricular failure results in an increase in venous capacitance and a fall in LVFP within 5 minutes. At this time there is no significant change in urinary output. After 1 hour there is an increase in urine output which can further reduce intravascular volume. (From K. Dikshit, J. K. Vyden, J. S. Forrester, K. Chatterjee, R. Prakash, and H. J. C. Swan.[510] Reprinted by permission from the *New England Journal of Medicine* 288:1087–1090, 1973.)

volume loading, improvement of myocardial function, and trial of diuretic virtually always implies acute renal failure. The diagnostic value of urinary electrolytes and osmolarity is lost for 6–12 hours after administration of furosemide, since they interfere with sodium reabsorption and with the concentrating ability of the distal tubule. Consequently urinary sodium is high and osmolarity low after these diuretics. In acute renal failure also urinary sodium is frequently high and osmolarity low.[176,663,1026]

Nonocclusive mesenteric infarction is a serious complication of diuretic therapy.[981,1529] Furosemide has a vasodilatory effect upon the superior mesenteric artery, and thus the associated occurrence of nonocclusive mesenteric infarction is due to the secondary effects of vigorous diuresis. Digitalis decreases mesenteric blood flow. The combination of digitalis and vigorous diuresis with furosemide may worsen mesenteric insufficiency.[8]

VASOPRESSORS

Various vasopressor agents, singly or in combination, are often employed following the separation of the patient from cardiopulmonary bypass at the conclusion of surgery. The choice of agent is determined by the estimated need for beta- and/or alpha-adrenergic stimulation and by the response of the patient. Left atrial pressure monitoring is extremely useful. The benefit of improved hemodynamic function must be balanced against the cost of increased myocardial oxygen consumption. Isoproterenol and glucagon may increase myocardial injury by increasing myocardial oxygen requirements.[154,1985]

When predominantly beta-adrenergic stimulation is required, we commonly employ epinephrine. Norepinephrine and phenylephrine HCl are used when predominantly alpha-adrenergic stimulation is required. Norepinephrine increases the tone of the postcapillary sphincter more than that of the precapillary sphincter and thus promotes loss of fluid from capillary beds. Norepinephrine also causes coronary vasoconstriction and has deleterious effects on renal blood flow.[1388,1983] Isoproterenol may cause excessive tachycardia and arrhythmias and has been shown to extend infarct size after coronary occlusion; to intensify myocardial ischemia after coronary narrowing, resulting in acute cardiac failure; and to impair left ventricular function when coronary blood flow is restricted.[1232]

Dopamine

Dopamine, the third endogenous catecholamine, has hemodynamic effects not seen with the other sympathomimetic amines.[448,1177,1660] Myocardial contractility and, to a lesser extent, heart rate are increased by a direct action of dopamine on beta-adrenergic receptors. Cardiac output increases.[1203,1659,1898] Vasodilatation occurs in the renal, mesenteric, coronary, and intracerebral arterial vascular beds, probably as a result of stimulation of specific dopamine vascular receptors. The concept of specific dopamine receptors is proposed, since this vasodilatation is not antagonized by propranolol, atropine, antihistamines, or other standard antagonists but is attenuated by haloperidol and phenothiazines. Myocardial oxygen consumption does not increase unless peripheral resistance or heart rate increases. With large doses of dopamine vasoconstriction occurs in all vascular beds as a result of stimulation of alpha-adrenergic receptors. This effect is antagonized by phentolamine and phenoxybenzamine. Dopamine causes a natriuresis whether or not total renal blood flow increases.[729,1269] A redistribution of intrarenal blood flow is responsible for this, as is probably a direct action on the tubules.[811] Dopamine also may increase the efficacy of diuretics.[919] It has a lesser propensity for causing ventricular arrhythmias than has isoproterenol. At low infusion rates dopamine may cause hypotension in some patients.

Dobutamine

Dobutamine, a new synthetic cardioactive sympathomimetic amine and an analogue of dopamine, has shown encouraging results experimentally in the unanesthetized dog.[1984] In this experimental situation dobutamine augments myocardial contractility and increases cardiac output from 2.4 to 4.4 liters per minute without appreciably affecting other determinants of myocardial oxygen consumption such as heart rate or rhythm, preload or afterload. The greatest increases in flow and decreases in calculated resistance occur in the iliac and coronary beds and the least in the renal bed. Redistribution of the cardiac output tends to occur, favoring the muscular beds at the expense of the kidney and visceral beds. In patients with aortic ball-valve prostheses or coronary artery disease who are clinically stable, dobutamine increases stroke volume, cardiac output, and the maximal velocity of left ventricular shortening without significantly changing heart rate, diastolic arterial pressure, or left ventricular filling pressure. Cardiac output increases whether the resting control value is low or within the normal range.[962] The initial clinical experience of our colleague, D. J. Cullen, in three critically ill patients, however, has been disastrous (personal communication, 1975). Marked deterioration in hemodynamic function occurred with the administration of dobutamine. One patient looked as if she were having a thyroid storm.

INTRAAORTIC BALLOON COUNTERPULSATION

Indications

The intraaortic balloon pump, first introduced in 1962,[1381] is accepted as a safe and effective device for providing mechanical circulatory assistance to the failing heart.[1709] Indications for its use presently include therapy for cardiogenic shock following acute myocardial infarction. Cardiogenic shock is defined as a systolic arterial pressure of less than 80 mm Hg (10.7 kPa), cardiac index of less than 2.2 liters per minute per square meter, urine output of less than 20 ml per hour, pulmonary capillary wedge pressure of greater than 15 mm Hg (2.0 kPa), and perfusion to the brain sufficiently diminished to produce signs of mental confusion or obtundation and peripheral vasoconstriction. All possible contributory or potentiating factors, including arrhythmias, hypoxemia, hypercapnia, acidemia, and electrolyte imbalance, must be corrected before the diagnosis of cardiogenic shock is made. The mortality from cardiogenic shock when balloon counterpulsation is employed without surgery is 87 percent.

Intraaortic balloon pumping is also useful in allowing separation from cardiopulmonary bypass after open-heart surgery when left ventricular failure prevents successful weaning from extracorporeal circulation.[262,1091] Therapy for intractable ventricular arrhythmias often can be helped by intraaortic balloon pumping. Definitive therapy to abolish the arrhythmia permanently may include revascularization, infarctectomy, and aneurysmectomy. Circulatory support during coronary and left ventricular angiography and during induction of anesthesia prior to surgery for preinfarction angina or cardiogenic shock usually is best achieved with intraaortic balloon counterpulsation.[1142,1318,1895,2047] Among the surgical procedures we use to correct cardiogenic shock are aortocoronary saphenous vein bypass graft, infarctectomy, aneurysmectomy, closure of a ventricular septal defect, and mitral valve replacement following papillary muscle dysfunction or rupture.[71,468,858,1040,1393] The in-hospital mortality from true cardiogenic shock after myocardial infarction has been reduced to 53–66 percent with this approach to management.[561]

Circulatory support during emergency noncardiac surgery in patients with recent myocardial infarction or severe angina pectoris is another in- dication for intraaortic balloon counterpulsation.[376,1317] The reinfarction rate during surgery within three months of a myocardial infarct is 37–54.5 percent.[1930] The mortality rate from postoperative myocardial infarction when there is a positive preoperative history of myocardial infarction may be as high as 70 percent.[1799,1900]

Maybe reduction of infarct size following uncomplicated myocardial infarction can be achieved by intraaortic balloon counterpulsation. Some of the indications outlined above are controversial, and further clinical ex- perience is required to establish the value of the intraaortic balloon pump in various clinical situations.

Insertion and Operation

The intraaortic balloon pump can be inserted under local anesthesia via either femoral artery through an end-to-side tightly woven Teflon graft. The tip of the balloon is positioned just distal to the left subclavian artery (Fig. 12-5). The balloon has three segments and is so designed that the middle segment inflates before the other two segments. The balloon is inflated

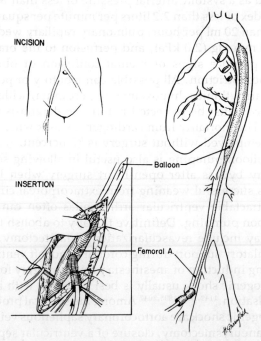

INCISION

INSERTION

Balloon

Femoral A.

Figure 12-5. Site of insertion and location of intraaortic balloon used for counter- pulsation. The intraaortic balloon is inserted through the femoral artery, utilizing a woven Teflon graft as a "side arm" of the femoral artery. The balloon lies in the descending aorta during counterpulsation. (From P. J. Ford and R. M. Wein- traub, *Intra-aortic Balloon Pumping Manual*.[653])

during diastole and deflated during systole. Helium is the gas used since its low viscosity allows it to be pumped rapidly in and out of the balloon and hence faster rates of pumping can be achieved. An isolated circuit allows the use of the same helium repetitively and reduces the hazard of embolism in case the balloon should rupture.[653] At least one such rupture has been reported.[1387]

The balloon is "driven" by the R wave of the ECG through a complex electronic console. The electrodes are positioned, and the electrocardiographic lead is chosen that provides the largest R wave. High frequency electric "noise," such as that produced by electrocautery equipment used during surgery, may interfere with the electrocardiographic signal employed to drive the balloon. The noise-signal ratio must be at least 1:2 for it to cause interference. A specially designed active notch filter eliminates some of the interference. The filter is more efficient during the "coagulation" than during the "cutting" phase of electrocautery. The console of the balloon also can be adapted to respond to the upstroke of the pulmonary or systemic arterial waveform, and the difficulties introduced by electrocautery during cycling from the electrocardiogram can be circumvented.

Therapeutic Goals

The therapeutic goals of intraaortic balloon pump counterpulsation include reduction of left ventricular work. The impedance to left ventricular outflow is reduced by deflation of the balloon shortly before the aortic valve opens. Left ventricular peak systolic pressure is lowered (Fig. 12-6). Reduction in afterload leads to a decrease of intramyocardial tension and sometimes of myocardial oxygen consumption (Figs. 12-7 and 12-8). Correct

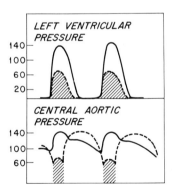

Figure 12-6. Effect of intraaortic counterpulsation on left ventricular and central aortic pressure. During counterpulsation (*dotted line*) the systolic pressure decreases in the left ventricle and aorta, while diastolic pressure increases in the aorta. *Solid line* = control values. (From C. A. Sanders, M. J. Buckley, R. C. Leinbach, E. D. Mundth, and W. G. Austen, *Circulation*.[1696] By permission of The American Heart Association, Inc.)

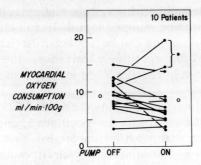

Figure 12-7.   Effect of intraaortic balloon counterpulsation on myocardial oxygen consumption in 10 patients. The majority of patients underwent no change or a fall in myocardial oxygen consumption with intraaortic counterpulsation. The two *open circles* represent the mean values. (From R. C. Leinbach, M. J. Buckley, W. G. Austen, H. E. Petschek, A. R. Kantrowitz, and C. A. Sanders, *Circulation.*[1140] By permission of The American Heart Association, Inc.)

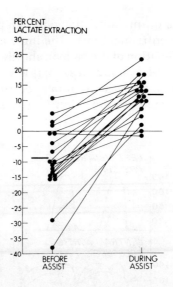

Figure 12-8.   Effect of intraaortic balloon counterpulsation on myocardial lactate extraction. Eighteen of nineteen patients in cardiogenic shock had improvement in lactate extraction with intraaortic balloon counterpulsation. The mean value increased from − 9 percent (production) before balloon assistance to +12 percent during counterpulsation. (From S. Scheidt, G. Wilner, H. Mueller, D. Summers, M. Lesch, G. Wolff, J. Krakauer, M. Rubenfire, P. Fleming, G. Noon, N. Oldham, T. Killip, and A. R. Kantrowitz.[1709] Reprinted by permission from the *New England Journal of Medicine* 288:979–984, 1973.)

timing of deflation is essential; if the balloon were inflated at any time during systole, its purpose would be defeated, and an increase in left ventricular work would occur. Systolic unloading can be enhanced by concomitant vasodilator therapy if necessary.[1696,1964]

Diastolic augmentation is another goal of intraaortic balloon pump counterpulsation. Inflation of the balloon during diastole provides the counterpulsation. Typically cardiac output increases 500–800 ml per minute with intraaortic balloon pump counterpulsation (Fig. 12-9). This increase improves tissue perfusion.[513,1824,1951] The effect on coronary flow is variable and depends on the balance between increased flow to ischemic areas, provided by increased diastolic perfusion pressure, and decreased flow to normal myocardium, in which the oxygen requirements are reduced by diminished afterload (Fig. 12-10).[951,1140,1141,1551] Intraaortic balloon counterpulsation reduces myocardial ischemic injury following acute coronary occlusion, whether counterpulsation is instituted at the time of occlusion or some hours later (Figs. 12-11 and 12-12).[1230]

Risks and Side Effects

Surprisingly intraaortic balloon counterpulsation generally has minimal risks and untoward side effects. Since it does not handle blood directly, it can be employed for prolonged periods of time. Significant depression of the platelet count can be avoided by using 10 ml low molecular weight dextran hourly. Intimal damage occurs rarely.[1211]

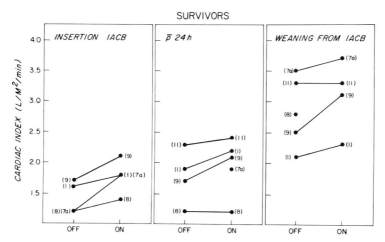

Figure 12-9. Effect of intraaortic counterpulsation balloon (IACB) on the cardiac output of five patients who survived revascularization surgery for cardiogenic shock. At the time of insertion IACB resulted in improvement of the cardiac output. Measurements were repeated 24 hours later at the time of cardiac catheterization. At the time of IACB weaning postoperatively all patients had significantly higher cardiac outputs both on and off IACB. (From M. G. Miller, R. M. Weintraub, J. Hedley-Whyte, D. S. Restall, and M. Alexander, *Lancet.*[1318])

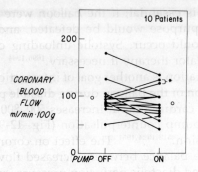

Figure 12-10. Effect of intraaortic balloon counterpulsation on coronary blood flow in ten patients with myocardial infarction. Measurements of coronary blood flow were made 14 times in ten patients on and off counterpulsation. Counterpulsation resulted in a fall or no change in coronary flow in most cases. *Open circles =* mean values. (From R. C. Leinbach, M. J. Buckley, W. G. Austen, H. E. Petschek, A. R. Kantrowitz, and C. A. Sanders, *Circulation.*[1140] By permission of The American Heart Association, Inc.)

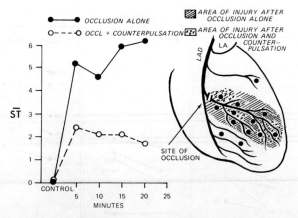

Figure 12-11. Effect of intraaortic balloon counterpulsation on the degree of myocardial ischemia. The coronary arteries of 19 dogs were occluded and the sum of S-T segment elevation ($\overline{ST}$) and myocardial injury were evaluated. The graph shows that those dogs who had coronary occlusion with aortic counterpulsation have less S-T segment elevation than dogs who had occlusion without counterpulsation. The drawing demonstrates that occlusion with counterpulsation resulted in less myocardial injury than did occlusion without counterpulsation. (From P. R. Maroko, E. F. Bernstein, P. Libby, G. A. DeLaria, J. W. Covell, J. Ross, Jr., and E. Braunwald, *Circulation.*[1230] By permission of The American Heart Association, Inc.)

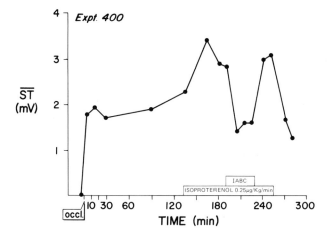

Figure 12-12.   Effect of isoproterenol and intraaortic counterpulsation on S-T segment elevation ($\overline{ST}$). A dog underwent experimental coronary occlusion. Following infusion of isoproterenol the S-T elevation increased. Counterpulsation resulted in a fall in the degree of S-T elevation, which again increased when counterpulsation was stopped. (From P. R. Maroko, E. F. Bernstein, P. Libby, G. A. DeLaria, J. W. Covell, J. Ross, Jr., and E. Braunwald, *Circulation.* [1230] By permission of The American Heart Association, Inc.)

The intraaortic balloon requires a patent aortoiliofemoral arterial tree for insertion and thus cannot be used in the presence of extensive peripheral vascular disease. A competent aortic valve is another prerequisite. The regulatory console of the balloon is complex in its circuitry and operation and requires skilled personnel to operate and service it.

Weaning

Measurements made during and without circulatory support aid in deciding whether a patient requires continued support. These include evaluation of cardiac index, mean arterial pressure, pulmonary capillary wedge pressure, and arterial oxygen tension. Weaning from the intraaortic balloon is gradual, with the number of cardiac cycles during which support is provided being reduced progressively from 1:1 to 1:8. Close monitoring with repetition of all or some of the just-mentioned measurements is essential during weaning. The balloon is removed after cardiovascular stability has been maintained for a number of hours without circulatory support.

VASODILATOR THERAPY

Satisfactory myocardial oxygenation requires that myocardial oxygen supply slightly exceed or at least equal myocardial oxygen consumption. Reduction of left ventricular work by reduction of afterload and preload through vasodilator therapy is one method of reducing myocardial oxygen consumption. Afterload represents the impedance to left ventricular outflow. Adequate aortic diastolic pressure must be maintained in order not to compromise coronary blood flow.[381] Pharmacologic means of reducing afterload include intravenous administration of sodium nitroprusside, phentolamine, and trimetaphan.

Sodium Nitroprusside

Sodium nitroprusside is a very useful agent with a specific effect on resistance vessels which results in the reduction of total peripheral resistance.[1476,1488] It has a rapid onset of action and is immediately reversible. There is no effect on other smooth or cardiac muscle systems nor on the central or autonomic nervous system. It has a high potency with a low toxic-therapeutic ratio, and no tachyphylaxis develops. In low-output states sodium nitroprusside invariably increases cardiac output (Fig. 12-13).[380,660,781] This is due to a reduction in both afterload and preload as a result of the effects of the drug on the venous and pulmonary circulation. Sodium nitroprusside also may have a direct coronary vasodilator effect.[1671] These beneficial effects on myocardial oxygen supply and demand improve left ventricular function and may abolish any signs of coronary ischemia.[382] Vasodilator therapy is also beneficial in severe mitral regurgitation.[247,319] Sodium nitroprusside has only a weak vasodilating effect on the renal vascular bed. Prolonged intravenous administration of sodium nitroprus-

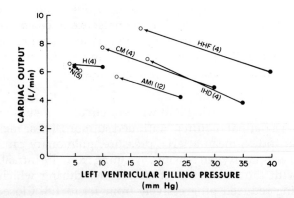

Figure 12-13.   Effect of nitroprusside in six groups of patients. N = normal individuals; H = severely hypertensive patients without heart failure; HHF = severely hypertensive patients with heart failure; CM = patients with cardiomyopathy and heart failure; IHD = patients with ischemic heart disease plus heart failure; AMI = patients with an acute myocardial infarction. The numbers of patients in each group appear in parentheses. The *asterisk* denotes normal individuals for whom the pressures given are right ventricular filling pressures. Normal individuals and patients with hypertension without heart failure show little change in left ventricular function when impedance is reduced. Those patients with heart failure all show improvement with increased cardiac output and lowering of the left ventricular filling pressure. (From J. N. Cohn, *Am. J. Med.*[380])

side is hampered by the accumulation of thiocyanate. Toxic symptoms of thiocyanate may begin to appear at plasma levels of 5–19 mg per 100 ml (0.09–0.32 mmol/l).

Phentolamine and Trimetaphan

Reduction of afterload with both phentolamine and trimetaphan has some disadvantages that have led us to favor sodium nitroprusside. Dosage control of phentolamine is more difficult. Ventricular unloading is readily demonstrable, but control of arterial blood pressure is not.[1117] Nonetheless, phentolamine has been used successfully in improving left ventricular performance.[1213,2010] A marked increase in heart rate, which would increase myocardial oxygen consumption, occurs only when phentolamine is given as a rapid bolus intravenously.[1905] Trimetaphan has undesirable ganglionic-blocking side effects and leads to tachyphylaxis.

CONSEQUENCES OF EXTRACORPOREAL CIRCULATION

Patients in respiratory failure occasionally have to be put on extracorporeal bypass as part of the treatment of cardiogenic shock refractory to conventional medical therapy. Extracorporeal bypass is also the best treatment for profound hypothermia and for heat stroke. (See Chapters 21 and 27.) Consequently we will briefly outline our present techniques.

We most frequently employ nonpulsatile roller pumps and a bubble oxygenator during cardiopulmonary bypass. A clear prime consisting of heparinized Ringer's lactate and salt-poor albumin is used in the oxygenator. Bubbles are removed from the oxygenated blood in a defoam-

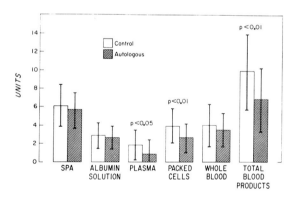

Figure 12-14. Comparison of the volume of blood products which are necessary on the day of cardiac surgery in patients who receive either fresh autologous blood or bank blood (*control*) following cardiopulmonary bypass. The use of autologous blood for transfusion following cardiac surgery results in conservation of plasma and packed red cells. The total amount of blood products used also is reduced. *SPA* = salt-poor albumin. (From P. Hallowell, J. H. L. Bland, M. J. Buckley, and E. Lowenstein, *J. Thorac. Cardiovasc. Surg.*[797])

ing chamber that contains silicone-coated, stainless steel wire mesh. Moderate hypothermia to 30–32°C and hemodilution to a hematocrit of about 20 percent are induced. Autologous blood is removed before heparinization and reinfused at the end of bypass after protamine infusion. Requirements for bank blood products are reduced by 25–50 percent without increasing overall fluid requirements (Figs. 12-14 and 12-15).[797],[1126] Flow rates are maintained at 40–60 ml per kilogram per minute at a mean arterial pressure of about 90 mm Hg (12.0 kPa). A 40 μ (40 μm) filter is used in the perfusion line.

Redistribution of organ blood flow occurs during cardiopulmonary bypass. Flow to the stomach, intestines, adrenals, and limb bones increases, while flow to the brain and kidneys decreases. Hemodilution to a hematocrit of 25 percent during normothermic bypass in monkeys maintains normal cerebral blood flow.[1673] The only consistent and significant difference between pulsatile and nonpulsatile perfusion is the difference in urinary output, although it has been suggested that pulsatile perfusion should maintain normal capillary blood flow and thus provide better cellular oxygenation and improved organ function (Figs. 12-16 and 12-17).[206],[562]

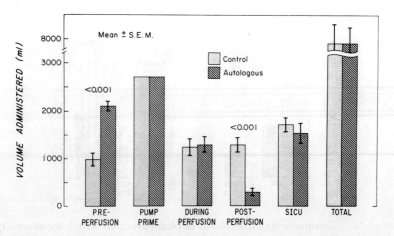

Figure 12-15.   Volume of blood components administered to patients undergoing cardiac surgery who received either autologous blood transfusions or bank blood (*control*). Those patients who received autologous transfusions required fewer blood products in the postperfusion period. *SICU* = surgical intensive care unit. (From P. Hallowell, J. H. L. Bland, M. J. Buckley, and E. Lowenstein, *J. Thorac. Cardiovasc. Surg.*[797])

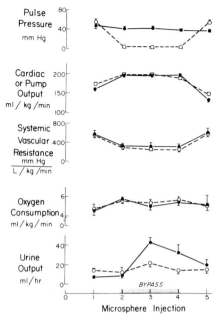

Figure 12-16. Comparison of pulsatile and nonpulsatile cardiopulmonary bypass on pulse pressure, cardiac output, systemic vascular resistance, oxygen consumption, and urinary output. To determine organ blood flow radioactive microspheres were injected into two groups of monkeys who received either pulsatile (*solid line*) or nonpulsatile (*dotted line*) cardiopulmonary bypass. The numbers on the x-axis represent: (1) before thoracotomy, (2) 5–10 minutes into bypass, (3) 60 minutes into bypass, (4) 120 minutes into bypass, (5) 60 minutes after bypass ended. Pulsatile blood flow resulted in a higher pulse pressure and higher urinary output than did nonpulsatile flow. (From J. K. Boucher, L. W. Rudy, Jr., and L. H. Edmunds, Jr., *J. Appl. Physiol.*[206])

HEMATOLOGIC COMPLICATIONS

Common causes of nonsurgical bleeding after cardiopulmonary bypass include thrombocytopenia, alteration in clotting factors, inadequate neutralization of heparin, including the heparin rebound phenomenon, and excessive protamine administration.[586,587,736,1646] Disseminated intravascular coagulation also may occur.[2097] Experimental evidence suggests that both platelet count and function are better preserved with dipyridamole, a known inhibitor of platelet function. The reduction in platelet aggregation may also reduce the sequelae of microembolization during cardiopulmonary bypass.[129,2067] Factors that increase the incidence of post-bypass bleeding include pre-bypass cyanosis, prolonged bypass time, and the use of a patch to close the ventriculotomy site. Mechanical trauma to red cells elevates serum hemoglobin and results in hemoglobinuria. Average serum hemoglobin levels after nonpulsatile and pulsatile perfusion are 40.0 mg per

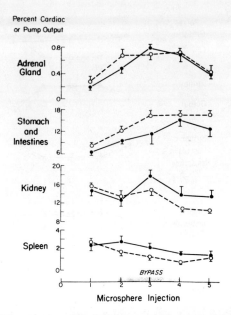

Figure 12-17.   Blood flow to selected organs during pulsatile and nonpulsatile cardiopulmonary bypass. Radioactive microspheres were injected into monkeys, who were placed on either pulsatile (*solid line*) or nonpulsatile (*dotted line*) cardiopulmonary bypass. Measurements of blood flow were made (1) before thoracotomy, (2) 5–10 minutes into bypass, (3) 60 minutes into bypass, (4) 120 minutes into bypass, and (5) 60 minutes after bypass ended. During both types of perfusion, blood flow to the intestines and adrenals increased. Patterns of blood flow were similar with each type of perfusion, except that pulsatile flow did not decrease splenic blood flow. (From J. K. Boucher, L. W. Rudy, Jr., and L. H. Edmunds, Jr., *J. Appl. Physiol.*[206])

100 ml (0.025 mmol/l) and 136.8 mg per 100 ml (0.085 mmol/l) respectively. Damage to plastic tubing in the bypass equipment and excessive suction in the coronary and left ventricular lines increase hemolysis. Potassium exchange after extracorporeal perfusion is poorly understood. Hypokalemia commonly occurs and can be avoided by frequent measurement and judicious replacement. Denaturation of plasma proteins occurs during bypass but is of minor significance. No alterations occur in the lipoprotein fraction.[963,1103]

Plasma oncotic pressure decreases from 18.0 ± 0.6 to 11.7 ± 0.5 mm Hg (2.4 ± 0.08 to 1.6 ± 0.07 kPa) during cardiopulmonary bypass with hemodilution and moderate hypothermia and returns to normal within 90 minutes after rewarming and cessation of bypass.[1247]

NEUROLOGIC COMPLICATIONS

Various types of neurologic complications of varying extent may become manifest after extracorporeal perfusion. Improved techniques of perfusion and monitoring mean that inadequate cerebral oxygenation now occurs less frequently, unless prolonged periods of aortic cross-clamping are employed. Mean arterial pressure probably should be greater than 70 mm Hg (9.3 kPa) during perfusion to avoid central nervous system dysfunction following cardiopulmonary bypass.[1858] Electroencephalographic monitoring during perfusion is of doubtful value in predicting neurologic complications.[2098]

Embolic phenomena occur as a result of platelet aggregates, air, particles of calcium, cotton fibers, or fat.[514,878] Routine use of micropore filters has reduced the incidence of cerebral nonfat emboli from 31 to 4 percent. Cerebral fat emboli are not affected by micropore filtration.[58,885]

OTHER CONSEQUENCES OF CARDIOPULMONARY BYPASS

Shivering may increase oxygen consumption nearly 500 percent (Fig. 12-18).[114,875] Circulatory failure will occur if the compromised cardiovascular system cannot compensate for this imposed stress. The danger of shivering is minimized if the muscle relaxant employed is not reversed and controlled ventilation continued into the post-bypass period.

As a result of large doses of intravenous morphine sulfate (1–3 mg/kg) given before extracorporeal bypass, marked peripheral vasodilation ensues in the early post-bypass period. Adequate fluid administration is necessary to maintain left ventricular filling pressure at a level at which the particular patient has a satisfactory cardiac output. Judicious administration of a peripheral vasoconstrictor, such as norepinephrine or phenylephrine HCl, may be needed.

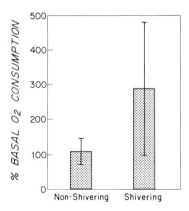

Figure 12-18. Oxygen consumption in shivering and nonshivering patients during recovery from anesthesia. Fourteen nonshivering and ten shivering patients had measurements of oxygen consumption during the immediate postoperative period. Oxygen consumption is plotted as percent of the basal value (means with range). Shivering increases oxygen consumption up to 486 percent. (Drawn from data in J. Bay, J. F. Nunn, and C. Prys-Roberts, *Br. J. Anaesth.*[114])

13

Problems of Obstetric and Gynecologic Emergencies

Deliveries and the complications of pregnancy, childbirth, and the puerperium account for over 4 million hospital admissions yearly in the United States. Dilatation and curettage and hysterectomy are the second and third most frequently performed surgical procedures in the United States (tonsillectomy is still the most common surgical procedure).[227]

Despite the numbers of obstetric and gynecologic patients admitted their morbidity and mortality are fortunately low. Maternal mortality (number of maternal deaths per 10,000 live births) varies from city to city and among socioeconomic groups. In a comparison of cities made in 1961 maternal mortality ranged from 2.6 (Chicago) to 6.2 (Philadelphia). The national maternal mortality was 2.8 deaths per 10,000 live births (as of 1967).[1096,1468]

Hemorrhage is presently the leading cause of maternal death in the United States. Toxemia is the second major cause, and sepsis is the third. The other causes of death are those related to anesthesia, cardiac disease, emboli, and several miscellaneous conditions. Nearly 80 percent of all causes of maternal death are felt to be preventable.[1097]

Since obstetric and gynecologic complications are relatively rare, physicians often are not altogether familiar with their management. In this chapter we will present the basic pathophysiology and some of our experiences with the respiratory management of major obstetric and gynecologic complications.

OBSTETRIC COMPLICATIONS

PLACENTA PREVIA

Placenta previa occurs when the placenta lies close to or over the internal cervical os. It happens in approximately 1 out of 200 deliveries. Reasons for the development of placenta previa are unclear. Since this complication occurs more frequently in multiparous women, inflammatory and atrophic changes in the decidua have been postulated as possible reasons for excessive spread of the placenta. Bleeding probably occurs as a result of the enlargement of the lower uterine segment and from dilation of the cervix.[1416]

Bleeding during the third trimester of pregnancy should be considered to be due to placenta previa until proved otherwise. The diagnosis can be made radiographically, by ultrasound, or by technetium scanning.[200] Arteriography has been used for localizing a placenta previa; however, it is probably unnecessary.[1414]

If the bleeding is excessive and pelvic examination is necessary prior to making the diagnosis radiographically, it should be done only in a delivery room with a full surgical team present and blood readily available. The following case illustrates some of the points in the perioperative management of the patient with placenta previa.

A 36-year-old gravida 4 para 3 female was admitted to the Beth Israel Hospital, Boston, at 35 weeks gestation for vaginal bleeding. She had had three cesarean sections previously because of cephalopelvic disproportion during the first delivery. At the time of admission her bleeding had stopped and she was not in labor.

The day following admission ultrasonography demonstrated an anterior placenta previa. She was scheduled for a cesarean section; however, she went into labor on that day. A cesarean section was performed under general anesthesia and a 35-week-old infant delivered without difficulty. The placenta previa was removed intact and the incision closed.

Following the procedure the patient developed profuse vaginal bleeding. The uterus remained atonic despite oxytocin, Ergotrate (ergonovine maleate), and vigorous massage. Blood pressure fell to 60 mm Hg (8.0 kPa) systolic, and blood and crystalloid fluids were infused rapidly. Because of the uncontrollable nature of the bleeding and shock the patient was anesthetized again and a hysterectomy performed. By this time the patient had received 10 units of blood and 5 liters of lactated Ringer's solution. Her blood pressure returned to 104/70 mm Hg (13.8/9.3 kPa), and she was taken to the recovery room. Shortly thereafter she again became hypotensive, and vaginal examination demonstrated a 10 × 10 cm pelvic mass thought to represent a hematoma. Platelet count at that time was 51,000 per cubic millimeter (51 10^9/l). Prothrombin time was 15.4/11.8 seconds, partial thromboplastin time was 47.7/32.1 seconds, fibrinogen level was 124 mg per 100 ml (3.6 μmol/l); and factor V was 56 percent, factor II 50 percent, factors VII and X 45 percent, and factor VIII 50 percent of normal. There were no fibrin split products. Her coagulopathy was felt to be dilutional, secondary to multiple transfusions. She had received 11 units of blood, 10 units of fresh frozen plasma, and 16 units of platelets.

She continued to bleed and was again taken to the operating room, where, under general anesthesia, bilateral internal iliac artery ligations were performed. She remained stable for two hours after the procedure but then again became hypotensive, with a blood pressure of 80 mm Hg (10.7 kPa) systolic. She continued to receive blood components. Her abdomen became distended, and by five hours after the iliac artery ligation she had received 21 units of blood. A repeat laparotomy was performed. Several liters of blood were found in the pelvis; however, no focal site of bleeding could be detected. Her pelvis was packed, and she was returned to the recovery room.

Following this procedure her bleeding apparently stopped, and she was transferred to the Respiratory–Surgical Intensive Care Unit. Six hours after the final surgical procedure she had an alveolar-arterial oxygen tension gradient of 410 mm Hg (54.5 kPa) while on controlled ventilation with an Emerson ventilator. On the first postoperative day her gradient fell to 101 mm Hg (13.4 kPa); she was weaned and had her trachea extubated. By this time her coagulation studies had returned to normal. She required no further transfusions after a total of 24 units of blood. Her abdominal packs were removed on the third postoperative day. On the twelfth postoperative day she and her baby were discharged from the hospital.

This case illustrates several important points with regard to placenta previa and obstetric hemorrhage in general. Despite the proper management of the placenta previa the patient developed massive vaginal hemorrhage secondary to uterine atony and possibly secondary to bleeding at the site of the removed placenta. The site of the implantation of the placenta has poor muscular contraction which can result in continued bleeding. When hemorrhage is severe, the only treatment is hysterectomy. By the time the hysterectomy was completed this patient had received multiple units of blood and had developed a coagulopathy secondary to massive transfusion (as described in Chapter 28). The coagulopathy led to continued pelvic bleeding. In that situation emergency ligation of the internal iliac arteries is the procedure of choice and in many patients is lifesaving.[1684] Despite this procedure this patient continued to bleed and required packing of the pelvis. Her postoperative management consisted of controlled ventilation and chest physical therapy until respiratory failure had resolved. Her acute respiratory failure may be attributed in part to the use of incompletely filtered blood (Chap. 28).

ABRUPTIO PLACENTAE

Abruptio placentae is the term for the condition which many obstetricians prefer to refer to as premature separation of the normally implanted placenta. Abruptio placentae occurs in 0.84 percent of pregnant patients in the third trimester of pregnancy. The maternal mortality is 2.8 percent with a perinatal mortality of 53 percent.[907]

The etiology of placental separation in any patient is often difficult to determine.[566] Placental separation can be produced experimentally in dogs and humans by ligation or compression of the inferior vena cava.[1298,1417] The subsequent rise in venous pressure in the uterus is thought to lead to the separation via rupture of the maternal venous sinuses. Increases in vena caval pressures commonly occur in pregnant patients, as the uterus compresses the vena cava when the patient is supine.[1811]

The fact that 42 percent of patients with premature placental separation have toxemia suggests that there may be another explanation for the pathogenesis of placental separation.[173,1737] Arterial hypertension without toxemia also is associated with a high percentage of placental separation. In this case the etiology of the separation may be related to arterial disease, since patients with toxemia demonstrate marked degenerative changes in the walls of spiral arterioles.[907]

Signs and symptoms, as well as the prognosis for the mother and child, depend upon the degree of placental separation.[1737] The most common features are vaginal bleeding, which may be massive, and absence of fetal heart tones. Abdominal symptoms are not common. Disseminated intravascular coagulation (DIC) is a frequent complication and may worsen the bleeding (Chap. 28).[109]

Treatment should be directed toward evacuation of the uterus, since this seems to control the bleeding and often reverses the DIC. Postpartum management should consist of continued evaluation for bleeding and DIC and observation of the arterial blood gases, especially when there have been multiple blood transfusions.

OTHER CAUSES OF BLEEDING

Profuse vaginal bleeding occurs occasionally from rupture of the marginal sinus of the placenta.[640] Other causes of vaginal bleeding in the third trimester are cervicitis and cervical erosions, cervical tumors, vaginal varicosities, lacerations, and foreign bodies.[1869]

Postpartum bleeding is often the result of uterine atony, which can usually be controlled with oxytocin and uterine massage. Uterine packing may be necessary occasionally. Rarely placenta accreta may be encountered. Vigorous attempts to remove the placenta manually will often result in increased hemorrhage. Hysterectomy is needed in such cases of placenta accreta.[200] Vaginal or cervical lacerations also can account for postpartum hemorrhage.

RUPTURE OF THE UTERUS

Uterine rupture is a serious complication that may be associated with massive intraperitoneal hemorrhage, especially if the placenta overlies the site of rupture. Rupture of the uterus occurs in about 1 out of 2,000 births.[776,2026] In rural countries it is more common because of a lack of medical care during labor. In Nigeria it occurs in 1 out of 112 births.[776] Respiratory failure is common after uterine rupture.

Rupture of the uterus occurs before labor in 23 percent of cases and after the onset of labor in 77 percent. The site of rupture is usually a scar from a previous cesarean section; however, an unscarred uterus can rupture.[628,1966,2026,2027,2036] Although the mechanisms of rupture of an unscarred uterus are unclear, multiparous patients and patients with histories of prolonged labor or difficult deliveries are at greater risk.[961]

The following case illustrates some of the clinical features of rupture of the uterus.

A 37-year-old gravida 5 para 4 patient had had four previous, uneventful, spontaneous, vaginal deliveries. Her antepartum course was uneventful, and she went into labor 12 days following her due date. The first stage of labor lasted six hours. Following full dilation it was noted that the baby was not descending. Shortly thereafter the blood pressure fell to 80 mm Hg (10.6 kPa) systolic, and a midforceps rotation and extraction of the baby was performed. The baby was apneic and was intubated, resuscitated, and transferred to the nursery.

The mother continued to be in shock, with profuse vaginal bleeding, and was felt to have had a uterine rupture. An emergency laparotomy was done which confirmed the diagnosis of a posterior uterine rupture. There were several liters of blood in the peritoneal cavity. A hysterectomy was performed. Immediately postoperatively coagulation studies were normal, but the patient had continued vaginal bleeding. She was returned to the operating room, where several discrete sites of bleeding in the vagina were identified and ligated. The patient received a total of 14 units of blood, 10 units of platelets, and one unit of fresh frozen plasma.

Postoperatively she was maintained on controlled ventilation for 24 hours and then weaned from ventilation and her trachea extubated. She was discharged from the hospital on the ninth postoperative day. The baby required controlled ventilation for several days but subsequently has developed normally.

COAGULATION DISORDERS

Disorders of the coagulation system frequently complicate the management of the more serious complications of pregnancy. During normal pregnancy the levels of fibrinogen and factors VII and VIII increase. Factors II, IX, and X increase less substantially.[198,467] The activity of the fibrinolytic system is decreased in pregnancy, and excessive deposition of fibrin on the placenta can be seen. These alterations make the pregnant patient vulnerable to the development of intravascular coagulation.[198]

Disseminated Intravascular Coagulation

Disseminated intravascular coagulation (DIC) occurs in conjunction with a variety of obstetric complications. Abruptio placentae is the obstetric complication that most frequently results in DIC. The damaged portion of the placenta is thought to release tissue thromboplastin, which initiates the DIC. Once the placenta is removed, the DIC usually resolves, and specific treatment is not necessary. DIC may also be seen in the infants of mothers who have abruptio placentae.[467]

Amniotic fluid embolism can initiate DIC secondary to the release of tissue thromboplastin into the circulation. Survivors of the initial embolus therefore may die of hemorrhage and respiratory failure.[467]

Toxemia is also associated with DIC. The mechanism for its occurrence in toxemia is unclear. Fetal death in utero can initiate DIC. In these patients the changes occur slowly enough for the patient to compensate, and she may not show signs of DIC until the time of delivery. The patient who has a delivery of a dead fetus should therefore be carefully monitored for the development of DIC. Pelvic sepsis can initiate DIC.[467]

Multiple blood transfusions can lead to a coagulopathy, usually on a dilutional basis. This topic is discussed fully in Chapter 28.

TOXEMIA OF PREGNANCY

Mortality

Toxemia is the second major cause of maternal death in the United States. The mortality for patients who develop acute toxemia is 4–5 percent. Cerebral hemorrhage is the most common cause of death in patients with toxemia, and cerebral edema is the second most common. Less frequently death is due to hepatic necrosis, disseminated intravascular coagulation, renal failure, airway obstruction, pulmonary edema, and drug overdosage.[871,1170]

Diagnosis

The diagnosis of toxemia of pregnancy is based upon a rise in diastolic blood pressure, hyperreflexia, edema, and albuminuria in a patient who may develop seizures or coma antepartum, intrapartum, or postpartum. The absence of retinal vascular changes and a glossy appearance of the retina aid in differentiating toxemia from hypertensive disease.[633]

Toxemia can occur in any pregnant patient but is most common in the primagravida and in the patient under 20 years of age.[633] Multiparas and patients in older age groups are the most likely to die from acute toxemia.[871]

Pathogenesis

The pathogenesis of toxemia is unknown and has been explained by numerous theories. The theory that has gained most attention centers around the uterus and placenta as excretors of a vasoactive substance. In rabbits the renin content of the placenta is three times the content of both kidneys. Evidence from nephrectomized rabbits suggests that renin is synthesized in the uteroplacental unit. Studies of toxemic patients have demonstrated increased levels of renin in the placental vein. When uterine blood flow decreases, there is a compensatory rise in systemic blood pressure. The mechanism of blood pressure control in the kidney is in some ways similar to that of the uteroplacental unit. The abnormality in toxemia may be related to an abnormality of the system that regulates uteroplacental blood flow. Defective prostaglandin production or a lack of response to prostaglandins has been postulated as the defective mechanism in the development of toxemia (Fig. 13-1).[1829]

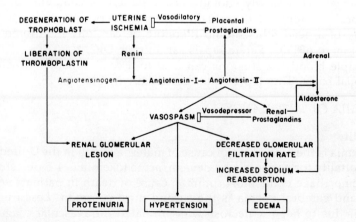

Figure 13-1. Theories as to causation of toxemia of pregnancy. (From L. Speroff, *Am. J. Cardiol.*[1829])

Management

The management of acute toxemia consists of controlling seizures and hypertension, followed by prompt delivery of the baby. Magnesium sulfate is still the drug of choice. Magnesium has a central and a peripheral effect. It acts on the neuromuscular junction by limiting the release of acetylcholine.[651,739] Magnesium sulfate also acts as a peripheral vasodilator and lowers the blood pressure. Both seizures and hypertension in toxemia can be controlled with magnesium sulfate alone. The therapeutic range is 6–8 mg per 100 ml plasma. The patellar reflex is lost at 10 mg per 100 ml plasma, and respiratory failure develops at 12–15 mg per 100 ml plasma. Despite the usually good correlation between the patellar reflex and the serum level of magnesium, complete heart block has been reported to occur with serum levels of less than 10 mg per 100 ml plasma.[739] If the diastolic blood pressure remains over 110 mm Hg (14.6 kPa) despite treatment with magnesium sulfate, antihypertensive therapy with hydralazine should be started to prevent cerebrovascular hemorrhage.[1562] Care must be taken not to lower the diastolic pressure below 90 mm Hg (12.0 kPa), otherwise a fall in uterine perfusion will occur.[1829]

When hypovolemia occurs in conjunction with acute toxemia, the use of volume expanders such as albumin is a rational form of therapy, especially when there are excessive losses of albumin in the urine.[364]

The timing of delivery in the patient with acute toxemia is controversial. Delivery of the infant is often regarded as the only definitive cure for toxemia and therefore should be achieved as soon as the blood pressure and convulsions are under control. One study suggests that delivery should be induced only in those patients who deteriorate during treatment or who fail to improve with medical management, and that the remainder of the patients should be treated with magnesium sulfate until they go into spontaneous labor. The maternal mortality in that series was 4.7 percent; however, the fetal mortality was 21.6 percent.[810]

The following case demonstrates some of the methods of respiratory management of the patient with acute toxemia.

A 25-year-old primagravida was admitted because of the spontaneous onset of labor. She was healthy except that one week prior to admission she was noted to have a blood pressure of 140/90 mm Hg (18.6/12.0 kPa). At the time of admission her blood pressure was 160/102 mm Hg (21.3/13.6 kPa) and she had 3+ peripheral reflexes and pedal edema. Because of a breech presentation she underwent a cesarean section. A healthy baby girl was delivered.

The mother awoke uneventfully from her anesthetic, but three hours after delivery she had a blood pressure of 210/130 mm Hg (28.0/17.3 kPa) with 4+ reflexes. Over the next 20 hours her eclampsia was managed with hourly doses of magnesium sulfate, which controlled her blood pressure at about 140/90–100 mm Hg (18.6/12.0–13.3 kPa). About 24 hours postpartum she became unresponsive and had a seizure. She remained comatose, probably secondary to diffuse cerebral edema. She then began to bleed massively from the nasopharynx and underwent tracheal intubation for airway protection. Her platelet count was 35,000 per cubic millimeter (35×10^9/l) with a trace of fibrin split products, probably secondary to a resolving DIC. She was allowed to breathe spontaneously via a Briggs adaptor. With 40 percent oxygen her arterial oxygen tension was 108 mm Hg (14.4 kPa), carbon dioxide tension 37 mm Hg (4.9 kPa), and pH 7.39.

Over the next 24 hours she developed diffuse edema of the head and neck and albuminuria. On the third postpartum day her alveolar-arterial oxygen tension gradient with 100% oxygen increased from 50 to 566 mm Hg (6.7–75.3 kPa), and her chest x-ray showed diffuse pulmonary edema. Controlled ventilation was begun with 10 cm H_2O (1.0 kPa) positive end-expiratory pressure, resulting in a fall in this gradient to 102 mm Hg (13.6 kPa). She was given 20, then 40, mg of furosemide with good urinary response. A Swan-Ganz catheter was inserted and showed a pulmonary artery pressure of 40/22 mm Hg (5.3/2.9 kPa) and a pulmonary capillary wedge pressure of 18 mm Hg (2.4 kPa). Her gradient rose to 350 mm Hg (46.6 kPa) despite 10 cm H_2O (1.0 kPa) positive end-expiratory pressure and continued diuresis. On the fifth postpartum day a tracheostomy was performed.

By the sixth postpartum day the patient's gradient had increased to 601 mm Hg (80.0 kPa) and she required a positive end-expiratory pressure of 15 cm H_2O (1.5 kPa). At this point she had lost 8.6 kg in weight, her peripheral edema had resolved, and her mental status had improved so that she obeyed commands. Diffuse pulmonary edema was evident radiologically. Diuresis was continued with furosemide. Daily infusions of albumin were given to maintain the intravascular volume and because the patient developed hypoalbuminemia secondary to massive losses in the urine. She remained on positive end-expiratory pressure with an increased oxygen gradient. By the eleventh postpartum day she had clearly developed bilateral pneumonia with *Pseudomonas aeruginosa,* which was treated with gentamicin. Over the next few days her peak inflation pressures on the ventilator rose to 60 cm of H_2O (6.0 kPa), at which time she developed a pneumothorax that required chest tube drainage. By the eighteenth postpartum day her pneumonia improved so that her positive end-expiratory pressure was slowly tapered down over the next four days. On the twenty-sixth postpartum day she was weaned from controlled ventilation, and her tracheostomy tube was changed to a fenestrated tube. Over the next 48 hours the fenestrated tube was plugged, then removed.

One month after admission she was discharged from the Respiratory–Surgical Intensive Care Unit. On the forty-sixth postpartum day she was discharged from the hospital, at which time her arterial blood gases on room air showed an arterial oxygen tension of 98 mm Hg (13.0 kPa), a carbon dioxide tension of 33 mm Hg (4.4 kPa), and a pHa of 7.38. Pulmonary function tests and chest x-rays following discharge were consistent with restrictive lung disease secondary to diffuse fibrosis, which gradually improved (Table 13-1).

EMBOLIC COMPLICATIONS

Amniotic Fluid Embolism

Amniotic fluid embolism is a rare but frequently fatal obstetric complication. Estimates of its incidence in all deliveries range from 1:14,000 to 1:37,000.[1760] Less than 20 reports of survivors of amniotic fluid embolism exist in the literature.[310,1722]

It usually presents as an acute onset of respiratory distress, cyanosis, shock, and coma in a patient who is having prolonged labor. If the patient survives the initial insult, seizures often develop as well as acute pulmonary

Table 13-1. Pulmonary Function Tests Following Treatment of Toxemia and Respiratory Failure

Test	July 16 (1 mo. after extubation)	Sept. 3
Vital capacity	1.8	2.1
% predicted	56	65
Expiratory reserve volume (liters)	0.940	0.746
% predicted	79	62
Residual volume (liters)	0.992	1.185
% predicted	80	96
Total lung capacity (liters)	2.809	3.285
% predicted	63	73
FEV_1 (liters)	1.699	—
% predicted	65	—
MMEFR (liters/sec)	2.9	—
Airway resistance (cm H_2O/liters/sec)	2.3	1.8
Conductance (liters/sec/cm H_2O)	0.43	0.54
Pulmonary diffusion capacity (ml/min/mm Hg)		13.7
% predicted		61

edema and disseminated intravascular coagulation. The diagnosis often can be made by aspirating blood from the right heart and centrifuging it. If amniotic fluid is present, there will be three layers instead of two.[1760] At autopsy one finds elements of amniotic fluid and meconium in the microvasculature of the lung. The elements are squamous cells, mucus, and lanugo hairs. In half the cases a tear in the myometrium is found, through which fluid may have gained access to the maternal circulation.[1216] In other cases squamous cells of amniotic fluid have been found in the placenta, suggesting the placenta as the route of transmission.[1128] Evidence suggests that amniotic fluid enters the maternal circulation only when there is an abnormality of the uterus or placenta, such as placenta accreta, ruptured uterus, placental separation, or marginal tears.[1095]

The respiratory failure is produced via occlusion of the pulmonary vasculature by substances in the amniotic fluid. Reflex vasospasm of the unaffected vessels occurs. The result is an increase in the deadspace-to-tidal-volume ratio and abnormalities of ventilation-perfusion ratios, leading to hypoxemia. The exact mechanism of the hypoxemia is not well understood, but it may result from abnormal coagulation and from venoarterial shunting through precapillary anastomoses. Shock develops because of a sudden decrease in left atrial return combined with peripheral vascular dilation.[1760] The coagulation defect is secondary to the large amount of thromboplastic material in the amniotic fluid.[2044] This initiates intravascular coagulation.[467]

Management consists of controlled ventilation via a tracheal tube and support of the blood pressure with vasopressor agents.[1760] Evidence of DIC should be sought and treatment with heparin started before signs of bleeding develop.[310]

Pulmonary Embolism

Pulmonary embolism occurs at any time during pregnancy, labor, or in the postpartum period. It is common in pregnant patients with cardiac disease. Diagnosis and management are the same as for embolism in the nonpregnant patient.[794,2087]

TRAUMA

The pregnant uterus is vulnerable to trauma, especially at term. Pelvic fracture is often of great concern to the physician caring for an injured pregnant patient. When there is no direct injury to the uterus, however, a pelvic fracture will not alter the pregnancy. About one in ten pelvic fractures will cause sufficient distortion of the pelvis to necessitate cesarean section at the time of delivery. Adequacy of ventilation must be assessed carefully in such cases.

Blunt trauma to the abdomen only rarely results in damage to the uterus and fetus. When it does, it is usually by way of uterine rupture. Penetrating injuries of the abdomen generally will involve the uterus if the patient is at term. Laparotomy, cesarean section, or hysterotomy is usually necessary.[565]

BURNS

When a pregnant patient is burned, the most frequent complication is premature onset of labor.[1715,1833] Patients who have second- or third-degree burns over 30 percent of the body will begin labor 1–7 days following the burn. Respiratory failure is common. Delivery usually can be carried out vaginally despite perineal burns. The most likely etiology of the premature labor is synthesis and release of prostaglandin E_2 from the burned skin. The fact that a burned patient is pregnant should not alter the therapy except that the physician should be aware of the probability of the onset of labor. Pulmonary problems of the burned patient are considered in Chapter 16.

PNEUMOTHORAX

Spontaneous pneumothorax is a rare complication of pregnancy and delivery. Treatment of spontaneous pneumothorax during either pregnancy or delivery should be the same as if the patient were not pregnant. The usual etiology is rupture of emphysematous blebs.[221,934]

RUPTURE OF THE DIAPHRAGM

Spontaneous rupture of the diaphragm is another rare complication of delivery. During pregnancy the diaphragm is stretched, making it vulnerable to the marked increases in intraabdominal pressure that occur during delivery. The diagnosis is sometimes difficult to make; however, one should be suspicious when a patient suddenly develops respiratory or abdominal symptoms. The diagnosis usually is confirmed by a chest x-ray film demonstrating abdominal contents in the thorax. Immediate surgical repair is necessary because of the threat of ischemia to the abdominal contents in the chest.[477]

INVERSION OF THE UTERUS

Uterine inversion is rare. Estimates suggest it occurs in 1 out of 20,000 deliveries. The diagnosis is usually obvious. There is shock with minimal hemorrhage, pain, and a mass protruding from the vagina. Inversion usually results from excessive fundal pressure, excessive cord traction, or attempts to perform a manual extraction of the placenta. Uterine inversion also can occur spontaneously. The hypotension that accompanies it is thought to be on a neurogenic basis. The blood pressure returns to normal when the uterus is replaced in the abdomen. Vasopressor support of the blood pressure may be necessary during this period.[1273]

GYNECOLOGIC COMPLICATIONS

In the nine years of existence of the Beth Israel Hospital's Respiratory–Surgical Intensive Care Unit the majority of patients admitted from the gynecology service have had acute respiratory failure because of peritonitis secondary to pelvic sepsis. Other reasons for admission following gynecologic surgery have been pulmonary edema secondary to cardiac failure, pulmonary embolism, and chronic obstructive lung disease.

PELVIC SEPSIS

Peritonitis often develops as a result of the rupture of a tuboovarian abscess. Ruptured tuboovarian abscess is a rare but major complication of pelvic inflammatory disease. Prior to 1947 the mortality for this disease was almost 100 percent; since 1947 it has fallen to 3–9 percent because of advances in management.[1309,1499] When the diagnosis of pelvic abscess is made, the patient should be operated upon as soon as any abnormalities of fluid and electrolyte balance have been corrected. Usually this can be accomplished within 24 hours.[995] This form of therapy has reduced the seriousness of peritonitis from pelvic abscess but has not eliminated the problem.

Respiratory failure occurs following hysterectomy required to manage septic abortions. In one series 40 percent of patients developed pulmonary embolism following hysterectomy and 20 percent developed pulmonary insufficiency secondary to septicemia and renal failure. All the patients in the series developed acute renal failure, which is a common complication of the respiratory management of this type of patient (Chap. 19).[107]

We have managed six patients who developed acute respiratory failure in conjunction with peritonitis secondary to pelvic abscess. There were two deaths. The following case is an example of the management of a gynecologic patient with respiratory failure caused by pelvic inflammatory disease.

A 36-year-old gravida 4 para 2 woman had a past history of pelvic inflammatory disease. One week prior to admission to the Beth Israel Hospital she noticed left lower quadrant pain. Four days prior to admission she presented at another hospital, complaining of fever and left lower quadrant pain. She underwent a laparotomy at that hospital, at which time a ruptured tuboovarian abscess was found. The abscess was treated by placing a drain in the left lower quadrant. Over the next three days the patient developed progressive tachypnea and persistent fever. She was transferred to the Beth Israel Hospital for evaluation.

At the time of admission she was in acute respiratory distress. Her blood pressure was 150/90 mm Hg (20.0/12.0 kPa), heart rate 140 beats per minute, respiratory rate 40 breaths per minute, and temperature 39°C. Her lungs had decreased breath sounds and diffuse rales. Abdominal examination revealed distention with generalized tenderness and rebound tenderness. Laboratory evaluation showed a white blood cell count of 30,000 per cubic millimeter (30 10⁹/l) with a shift to the left in the differential count. On room air her arterial oxygen tension was 52 mm Hg (6.9 kPa), carbon dioxide tension 37 mm Hg (4.9 kPa), and pHa 7.41. Chest x-ray showed bilateral pleural effusions.

The patient was transferred to the Respiratory–Surgical Intensive Care Unit, where she continued to be in respiratory distress. Breathing 100% oxygen via a face mask she had an oxygen gradient of 451 mm Hg (60.0 kPa) and a carbon dioxide tension of 48 mm Hg (6.4 kPa). Her trachea was then intubated, and she was begun on controlled ventilation via an Emerson ventilator. She was given intravenous fluids and albumin for hydration and 12 hours after admission was taken to the operating room, where a laparotomy was performed. She was found to have peritonitis with

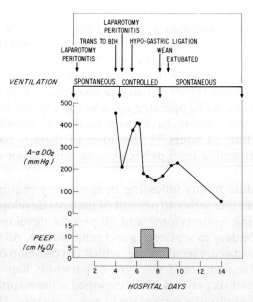

Figure 13-2. Management and course of a patient with respiratory failure caused by pelvic inflammatory disease. *BIH* = Beth Israel Hospital. A-aD$_{O_2}$ = alveolar-arterial oxygen tension gradient breathing 100% oxygen. The use of positive end-expiratory pressure (PEEP) was necessary.

over 1,500 ml of pus in her peritoneal cavity. The fluid grew *Enterococcus*. A total abdominal hysterectomy and bilateral salpingo-oophorectomy were performed. Postoperatively she developed abdominal bleeding secondary to thrombocytopenia. Disseminated intravascular coagulation could not be documented, but the bleeding did not stop with platelet transfusions. The patient therefore was brought again to the operating room, where bilateral internal iliac artery ligations were performed. There was minimal subsequent bleeding.

On the first postoperative day the oxygen gradient was 410 mm Hg (54.5 kPa) with the patient receiving 5 cm H_2O (0.5 kPa) of positive end-expiratory pressure. There was no improvement in the oxygen gradient until 13 cm H_2O (1.3 kPa) of end-expiratory pressure were applied. On the second postoperative day the patient was gradually weaned from the end-expiratory pressure without difficulty. On the third postoperative day, the patient was weaned from controlled ventilation and her trachea was extubated. Her fever gradually resolved, and she was discharged on the eighteenth postoperative day (Fig. 13-2).

Trauma and Respiratory Failure

14

High-Speed and Blunt Injuries

Accidental death is the fourth leading cause of death in the United States. It is the leading cause in persons between the ages of 1 and 35. Traffic accidents account for the majority of accidental deaths, 60,000 annually. Suicides account for 24,000 deaths annually; accidental falls, 17,000; drowning and aspiration, 9,000; fires, 7,000; and accidents with firearms, 2,500. Other miscellaneous causes of accidental deaths are carbon monoxide poisoning, 1,000; airplane accidents, 2,000; train accidents, 1,000; and explosions, 500.[1960] Accidents account for 4,224,299 potential years of life lost annually in the United States, with motor vehicle accidents accounting for one-half the total.[227] Respiratory complications are associated with over 50 percent of in-hospital deaths after trauma.[187]

THORACIC INJURIES

Of all automobile deaths, from one-quarter to one-half are associated with thoracic injury.[384,408,1513] In one study of 685 consecutive chest injuries, 73 percent of the cases were due to automobile accidents and 93 percent were blunt or nonpenetrating injuries.[51,826] Flail chest occurred in 10–20 percent, pneumothorax in 35 percent, hemothorax in 30 percent, and lung contusion in up to 30 percent. Overall mortality was 10–30 percent. Multiple system injury was common: 40 percent of the patients had other fractures, and 37 percent had neurologic injury. Abdominal injury was present in 10 percent and diaphragmatic injury in 3 percent.[51,1513]

FLAIL CHEST

Flail chest results in paradoxical movement of a section of the bony thorax with respiration. In addition there is often a contusion of the underlying lung.[459] The functional result of the trauma is an inability to inflate lung underlying the flail segment. Neither the rib cage nor the diaphragm is able to expand the underlying lung when it has such a nonrigid covering. There is a reduction of that lung's functional residual capacity, and alveolar collapse develops. The pulmonary contusion with its resulting edema further aggravates the shunting and hypoxemia.[597,674,689,1046] Initial treatment of severe flail chest consists of controlled ventilation via a tracheal tube.[73,959] Controlled ventilation by itself may be adequate to stabilize the free segment and provide oxygenation; however, if a patient remains hypoxemic despite a high concentration of inspired oxygen,[689] the application of positive end-expiratory pressure is necessary.[54,1714,2040] If a patient will require mechanical ventilation for longer than 3–6 days, a tracheostomy is performed; low-pressure cuffs are used at all times to minimize tracheal damage (see Chapter 1).[1800] The duration of mechanical ventilation is dependent on the degree of thoracic injury, the patient's pulmonary status prior to the injury, and the presence of other injuries. Often, upon improvement of the pulmonary contusion, the patient can be weaned successfully, even if a small flail segment persists. Although the death rate due to flail chest may be as high as 46 percent, the cause of death is often a concurrent brain injury or abdominal injury and not the flail chest.[51,1512,1699] A complication of controlled ventilation for flail chest injuries is the production of a hemopneumothorax when positive pressure is applied. These patients will require chest tube drainage. Bronchopleural fistulas may occur, causing substantial ventilatory problems, but do not require surgical correction unless 30 percent or more of the tidal volume escapes through the leak.

PULMONARY CONTUSION

Pulmonary contusion is one of the most common results of blunt chest trauma. It is diagnosed from the chest roentgenogram, on which it appears as an irregular opacity not following anatomic boundaries. Usually the damaged lung parenchyma corresponds to a visible area of trauma on the skin. The lesion appears within six hours of injury, and generally resolution starts within 2–3 days.[609,2068,2096] There is intraalveolar hemorrhage, atelectasis, and parenchymal edema in the lesion, causing shunting and therefore hypoxemia.[673,674,689] Mechanical ventilation usually is required for respiratory support during the first few days after the injury and has been shown to improve survival.[1654,1800]

PULMONARY LACERATION AND HEMATOMA

Pulmonary laceration and hematoma may also occur after blunt trauma. A characteristic coin-sized radiodensity appears either initially or after the local concurrent pulmonary contusion improves. Resolution of the density often is prolonged.

SIMPLE RIB FRACTURE

Simple rib fracture without a flail segment reduces ventilatory capacity because of pain. Taping of such fractures restrains not only the rib but also expansion of the underlying lung. Such fractures are usually managed with narcotics or intercostal nerve block. Rib fractures are an especially difficult problem when combined with an upper abdominal incision or when the patient has preexisting lung disease. With the institution of controlled ventilation pneumothorax frequently occurs and is dealt with by insertion of a chest tube.

AIRWAY RUPTURE

Airway rupture frequently is unsuspected. The injury usually is due to a force directed against a large segment of the thorax or more directly against the trachea. Signs and symptoms are dyspnea, pneumothorax, pneumomediastinum, subcutaneous emphysema, and inability to reexpand a collapsed lung despite chest tube suction.[274,586] In 10 percent of cases, however, no symptoms are present. Fractures of the first, second, or third rib are present in 53 percent of patients with bronchial rupture.[330] Rupture of a main-stem bronchus occurs in 80 percent of cases, and rupture of the trachea in 15 percent. While the bronchial tear is commonly horizontal and complete, the tracheal tear may be vertical and incomplete.[2096] If the diagnosis is missed, symptoms may not become apparent until bronchial stenosis occurs. In one study, one-half the cases were undiagnosed until one month after injury.[920] Confirmation of the diagnosis can be obtained by fiberoptic bronchoscopy. Although 70 percent of patients with pneumothorax will respond initially to chest tube therapy, bronchial stenosis eventually will cause pulmonary parenchymal disease distal to the site of injury unless corrective surgery is undertaken.

LARYNGEAL TRAUMA

Laryngeal trauma usually is due to a steering wheel injury or contact sports. The degree of damage depends on the extent of calcification of the thyroid cartilage. A malleable cartilage is less likely to fracture against the spine. Minor injuries should be observed closely for edema, and all patients should be examined by indirect laryngoscopy and fiberoptic bronchoscopy. Pain on swallowing and subcutaneous emphysema may be delayed symptoms. Serious injuries require prompt intervention.[463,1222]

ESOPHAGEAL RUPTURE

Esophageal rupture after blunt trauma is rare. Diagnosis can be made by fluoroscopy and dye studies, but frequently the condition is not suspected until necrosis of the esophagus has allowed massive contamination of the mediastinum.[2110] The outcome is usually fatal. A tracheoesophageal fistula after blunt trauma is quite rare.[38]

DIAPHRAGMATIC RUPTURE

Diaphragmatic rupture is also associated with major organ damage and is frequently overlooked. The majority of cases are due to automobile accidents, with the remainder due to sports and industrial causes. In 95 percent of cases the tear passes through the dome of the left hemidiaphragm; the liver seems to protect the right side.[164] In one study, of thirteen patients with diaphragmatic tears, only eight had actual herniation of abdominal contents.[2111] Frequently follow-up chest x-ray examination will reveal herniation.[37] Symptoms may be due to pulmonary compression by abdominal contents or may be entirely absent. Ninety percent of strangulated diaphragmatic hernias are traumatic in origin. Treatment consists of early repair.[886]

BLUNT CARDIAC TRAUMA

Blunt cardiac trauma can cause contusion or rupture of atrium, valves, septum, or coronary arteries.[96] An atrial rent is compatible with life, since the atria are relatively low-pressure chambers. Pericardial tamponade may occur acutely without a widened mediastinum, diminished heart sounds, or electrocardiographic voltage change. Immediate surgical intervention is needed. Mitral and tricuspid valve chordae tendineae may be ruptured, producing the murmur of insufficiency.[218,1463,2056] Coronary artery laceration is usually fatal and usually caused by penetrating injury.[1599] Cardiac contusion is seen frequently after blunt thoracic injury caused by an automobile steering wheel. It is often associated with a flail chest or fractured sternum. Electrocardiographic changes are variable and do not correspond to enzyme abnormalities. Monitoring is required until cardiac irritability subsides. Treatment is supportive, as the myocardium heals itself.[96,499] A ventricular aneurysm may occur after blunt trauma but is rare.[719]

TRAUMATIC RUPTURE OF THE THORACIC AORTA

Traumatic rupture of the thoracic aorta is the result of rapid deceleration injury. Automobile accidents account for 76 percent of these injuries, with the remaining cases the result of motorcycle collision, airplane crash, animal kicks, accidental falls, and explosion.[119,1624] Most patients with traumatic aortic rupture die prior to admission to the emergency ward.[1487] Eighty-two percent of patients die within the first hour after injury, but some may survive without surgical correction for weeks and, rarely, for years.[1624]

Diagnosis rests upon the suspicion of rupture after any high-speed injury. Hemothorax, a heart murmur, or hoarseness due to recurrent laryngeal nerve injury may be present. A widening mediastinum seen on chest x-ray examination suggests a need for immediate aortography. There must be equipment and personnel available for resuscitation. The site of aortic injury is usually at a point at which the aorta is fixed to a relatively immobile structure. The ligamentum arteriosum is the most common location, followed by the site of attachment to the heart at the pericardial reflection; these two locations account for 75 percent of the sites of ruptures. Occasionally rupture occurs at the point of aortic passage through the diaphragm. The aortic intima often is torn. Complete transection occurs in 22 percent of patients at the time of surgery. The proximal and distal ends may be as much as 7 cm apart. Surgical repair with pump bypass is undertaken at once.[120,121]

The most common postoperative complication is respiratory failure, and the next most common are mediastinal hemorrhage and vocal cord paralysis (6 percent of cases).[1624] Effects of ischemia on various organs including the esophagus and spinal cord are relatively common. Even though most patients were healthy prior to aortic injury, most have multiple system trauma and are ventilated postoperatively.[1624,1872] Massive transfusions often complicate the patient's condition.

ABDOMINAL TRAUMA

Blunt trauma to the abdomen is of concern to the intensive care physician. Limitation of ventilation by a large abdominal incision is a problem, as are the massive blood volume changes which the patient may have experienced. The development of peritonitis may pose an additional hazard.

SPLENIC RUPTURE

Splenic rupture is the most common abdominal injury.[1755] After the initial period of systemic manifestations of hemorrhage and local peritoneal irritation, splenic hemorrhage may stop temporarily, resulting in a latent period.

KIDNEY TRAUMA

The kidney is also highly susceptible to blunt trauma. In one study 80 percent of kidney injuries were due to blunt trauma, with two-thirds of these arising from automobile accidents, 23 percent from blows, and 14 percent from miscellaneous causes.[1005,2035] Unlike chest and liver trauma, trauma to the kidney may be an isolated injury. Clinical signs of flank swelling, ecchymosis, and hematuria indicate the need for an intravenous pyelogram or renal angiogram. Contusion-type injuries of the kidney account for 60 percent of all kidney injuries. They are usually managed with nonsurgical therapy. Lacerations more often require surgery.[196,1005] Postoperative complications are hemorrhage, infection, extravasation, and hydronephrosis.[1005] Ureteral blunt trauma is rare. Bladder injuries are discussed with pelvic fractures (next section), since direct blunt injury to the bladder is rare.

LIVER TRAUMA

Liver injuries account for 16 percent of the organ injuries in abdominal trauma.[1755] Blunt trauma to the liver produces an exploding type of injury with severe hemorrhage.[1209] Diagnosis may be delayed due to the presence of other major injuries. In addition to massive blood loss, biliary extravasation draws plasma into the peritoneal cavity, further decreasing blood volume. Postoperative complications include hemorrhage and infection. Mortality rates are dependent on the number and type of associated abdominal and nonabdominal injuries. If the liver is the only organ injured, the mortality is 6–30 percent.[526,1195] Blunt trauma to the biliary tree is rare and often insidious, since symptoms do not appear for days or weeks.[650]

SMALL BOWEL INJURY

Injury to the small bowel is present in 5–10 percent of patients hospitalized with blunt abdominal trauma. Steering wheel injuries are the most common cause. Injuries to the bowel occur most commonly close to the midline. The terminal ileum and the first portion of the jejunum are the most common sites of injury.[1455] Duodenal injury, although relatively rare, presents as a rupture or as an intramural hematoma.

Blunt trauma to the large bowel, mesentery, pancreas, and major vessels occurs infrequently, accounting for 3 percent or less of cases of blunt abdominal trauma.[1164]

FRACTURES

In the United States traumatic fractures and dislocations are third only to childbirth and heart disease in number of days of hospitalization per year.[227] Of primary concern to intensive care physicians are femur, rib, pelvic, and neck fractures. Pelvic fractures damage the bladder or urethra in 15 percent of cases and cause retroperitoneal hematomas.[355] Pulmonary complications result from immobilization of the patient, which makes him subject to atelectasis, pneumonia, and pulmonary embolism. To prevent these complications we roll the patient frequently from side to side on a Stryker frame. After all bleeding has stopped, usually 3–6 days after injury, we start the patient on warfarin therapy.

In all patients with multiple injuries a cervical fracture is assumed to be present until proved otherwise by cervical spine x-rays. If intubation is required, further neurologic trauma is minimized by either blind intubation or continuous cervical traction during intubation. We do not put such patients into the sniffing position. The fiberoptic laryngoscope may facilitate intubation. A traumatized patient with a full stomach, unguarded airway, and possible broken neck requires that the most experienced person immediately available perform the intubation.

Fractures of the thoracic spine may slightly modify ventilation due to loss of intercostals, but since at least 75 percent of inspiration is accounted for by the diaphragm, external intercostal loss is usually unimportant.

Cord lesions above the phrenic nerve segments (third to fifth cervical) usually are fatal if complete transection occurs. Several methods have been devised to increase ventilatory capacity in survivors; one is phrenic nerve stimulation.[721] These methods are not in routine use. Rehabilitation of such patients raises problems similar to those encountered after poliomyelitis.

FAT EMBOLISM

Fat embolism is seen most commonly after pelvic and long bone fractures but has been reported to occur without trauma.[85,261,412,534,603,1733,2050] The traumatized fatty bone marrow in the form of large droplets is forced into an open vein and trapped by the lungs.[691,1019] Adipose tissue may contribute in some cases.[670] Disseminated intravascular coagulation may be present and may also account for some of the emboli.[1029] Whether the emboli cause damage due to capillary obstruction or whether they subsequently undergo local lipolysis in the lung is not clear, although evidence favors the latter.[1504] The free fatty acids produced are toxic to the capillary endothelium, producing fluid leakage and pulmonary edema.[56] The first symptoms of fat embolism in 85 percent of cases are fever, tachycardia, dyspnea, and tachypnea. A lucid interval of up to 48 hours may occur prior to the onset of symptoms.[1733] Most patients are hypoxemic and alkalemic.[159,515,2081] Pulmonary artery pressure may not be elevated.[1483] Petechiae of the axillae, chest, flanks, conjunctivas, or soft palate occur in 87 percent of cases. Right heart strain is present in 85 percent of cases.[1496] Fat may be found in the urine and sputum.[85] The hematocrit and platelet count frequently decrease.[515]

In one-third to one-half of cases the chest roentgenogram shows numerous fluffy opacities. The disease occurs most commonly in two age groups, the young, involved in automobile trauma, and the elderly, with broken legs. Mortality is approximately 10 percent and is dependent on the duration and degree of hypoxemia and shock and the presence of multiple injuries.[52,1450,1483,1496]

The cornerstones of treatment are restoration of blood volume, oxygenation, keeping arterial oxygen tension in the 80–100 mm Hg (10.6–13.3 kPa) range, and using positive pressure ventilation with positive end-expiratory pressure as required.[52,1403,1965] The disease is self-limiting, and support over four to five days will allow recovery. Disseminated intravascular coagulation may ensue and should always be suspected (Chap. 29).

RESPIRATORY DYSFUNCTION AFTER TRAUMA

Since many trauma victims have head injuries, two other causes of acute respiratory failure are aspiration of gastric contents and massive sympathetic outflow that causes an increased cardiac afterload and failure (Table 14-1).[124,130,131,132,133,935,1109,1174,1199,1533,1940] Another consideration in the trauma patient is that pulmonary damage may be due to circulating bacteria, endotoxin, splanchnic toxins, or as-yet-undefined toxic agents (Chap. 5).[454,616,738,1450,2000] Finally, the possibility of congestive failure due to overtransfusion must be ruled out.

Whatever the etiology of the respiratory dysfunction after trauma, numerous studies have documented functional and microscopic respiratory changes even after restoration of blood volume and blood pressure. Upon rapid blood loss of 15 percent of the blood volume in healthy men, the cardiac index, left ventricular work, arterial pressure, and central venous pressure fall (Figs. 14-1 and 14-2). Minute ventilation, tidal volume, oxygen consumption, and carbon dioxide production increase (Figs. 14-3 and 14-4).[1411,1793]

During hemorrhage and prior to resuscitation the pulmonary artery pressure initially falls, then recovers slightly, and the pulmonary vascular resistance rises (Fig. 14-5).[1,384,412] Perfusion to the upper zones of the lung is markedly diminished.[1407] The physiologic deadspace increases,[665,700] and pulmonary blood volume falls.[1,700] During this hypotensive period shunting through a normal lung does not increase, whereas shunting through an

Table 14-1.   Synonyms for the Adult Respiratory Distress Syndrome

Adult hyaline membrane disease
Adult respiratory insufficiency syndrome
Bronchopulmonary dysplasia
Congestive atelectasis
Fat embolism
Hemorrhagic atelectasis
Hemorrhagic lung syndrome
Hypoxic hyperventilation
Oxygen toxicity
Postperfusion lung
Posttransfusion lung
Posttraumatic atelectasis
Posttraumatic pulmonary insufficiency
Progressive pulmonary consolidation
Progressive respiratory distress
Pulmonary edema
Pulmonary hyaline membrane disease
Pulmonary microembolism
Pump lung
Respirator lung
Shock lung
Stiff lung syndrome
Traumatic wet lung
Transplant lung
Wet lung
White lung syndrome

SOURCE: F. W. Blaisdell and R. M. Schlobohm. The respiratory distress syndrome: A review. *Surgery* 74:251–262, 1973.

atelectatic or injured lung does increase.[665,700,888,1422,2004] The water content of the lungs may increase,[144,865,924,2114] while compliance is reported to decrease or remain unchanged.[283,284,700,888,1563,1564] After resuscitation pulmonary capillary congestion may occur, with aggregates of platelets and white blood cells (Fig. 14-6);[1594,1595,2079] interstitial edema follows.[185,186,679,865,1641,1771] Shunting increases, and hypoxemia ensues.[162,888,1242] The pulmonary venular resistance may remain increased.[1398]

Pulmonary changes seen in the trauma patient in shock may also be due to pulmonary edema, caused at least in part by a reflex pulmonary venular vasoconstriction. This constriction reportedly is stimulated by perfusion of the hypothalamus with blood of low oxygen tension. The effect is blocked in a surgically reimplanted lung.[1371,1373,1374,1375,1378,1876,1878]

Treatment is similar to that detailed in Chapter 5 for pulmonary edema secondary to sepsis. We use positive pressure ventilation with optimum positive end-expiratory pressure.[54,55,1714] Diuretics are used if the cardiac output is not significantly diminished.

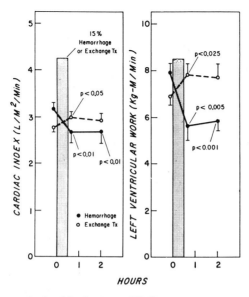

Figure 14-1. Changes in cardiac index and left ventricular work in normal, awake, young men after acute venous hemorrhage or exchange transfusion of 15 percent of blood volume over 15 minutes. Cardiac index and left ventricular work fall significantly after hemorrhage. *Closed dots* represent hemorrhage; *open dots* represent exchange transfusion. All values are mean ± SEM. (From J. J. Skillman, J. Hedley-Whyte, and J. A. Pallotta, *Ann. Surg.*[1793])

DISASTERS

Such calamities as large-scale destruction of a mass transit system, explosion and fire in a building, or a natural catastrophe will tax the ambulances and treatment facilities of many large metropolitan medical centers. Even smaller accidents can be disasters, however, if treatment facilities are limited. The simultaneous arrival of five to ten seriously traumatized patients will tax most suburban and rural hospitals. Therefore every hospital, large or small, must have a plan designed to cope with a disaster, should it occur.

DISASTER PLAN

Such a disaster plan is a detailed summary of the methods to be used to deal with a catastrophe. It designates a disaster "commander," who is responsible for coordination of the plan and who makes all final decisions including the extent of call-up of medical and paramedical personnel. Personnel must be assembled both at the site of the disaster and in the hospitals.[294] Each hospital must be prepared to convert emergency and clinic areas into receiving, triage, treatment, and morgue areas. Upon appearance at the hospital each casualty is rapidly evaluated by a triage physician as needing either immediate treatment for airway problems and

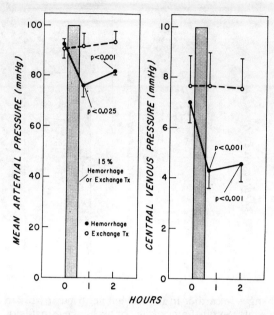

Figure 14-2. Changes in mean arterial pressure and central venous pressure in normal, awake, young men after acute venous hemorrhage or exchange transfusion of 15 percent of blood volume over 15 minutes. Hemorrhage lowers both mean arterial pressure and central venous pressure significantly. Exchange transfusion has no effect. *Closed dots* represent hemorrhage; *open dots* represent exchange transfusion. All values are mean ± SEM. (From J. J. Skillman, J. Hedley-Whyte, and J. A. Pallotta, *Ann. Surg.*[1793])

uncontrolled bleeding or delayed treatment. When facilities are in short supply, treatment may have to be directed to those patients who stand to benefit most. Similar decisions may be forced upon the physician concerning the use of blood products.

The names, addresses, and telephone numbers of physicians (by specialty), nurses, secretaries, and orderlies are held by various key members of the hospital community including the director of the intensive care unit, so that, upon the disaster commander's order, any or all of them can be mobilized. The method of contacting the acting disaster commander and his identity are posted in the emergency room at all times. The director of the intensive care unit should always know the name of the appointed disaster commander and how to contact him, as communication between the two is essential. Since the hospital switchboard may be tied up, essential personnel should communicate via the hospital's unlisted phone number.

RECORD KEEPING

A major problem is that of record keeping. Secretaries and admitting personnel are vital to the smooth flow of patients. All casualties are iden-

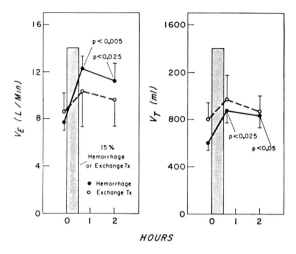

Figure 14-3. Changes in minute ventilation (VE) and tidal volume (VT) in normal, awake, young men after acute venous hemorrhage or exchange transfusion of 15 percent of blood volume over 15 minutes. Both VE and VT increase significantly after hemorrhage. The increases after exchange transfusion are insignificant. *Closed dots* represent hemorrhage; *open dots* represent exchange transfusion. All values are mean ± SEM. (From J. J. Skillman, J. Hedley-Whyte, and J. A. Pallotta, *Ann. Surg.* [1793])

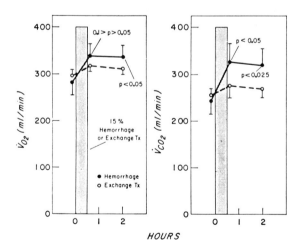

Figure 14-4. Changes in oxygen consumption ($\dot{V}O_2$) and carbon dioxide production ($\dot{V}CO_2$) in normal, awake, young men after acute venous hemorrhage or exchange transfusion of 15 percent of blood volume over 15 minutes. Both $\dot{V}O_2$ and $\dot{V}CO_2$ increase significantly after hemorrhage, whereas no significant change occurs after exchange transfusion. *Closed dots* represent hemorrhage; *open dots* represent exchange transfusion. All values are mean ± SEM. (From J. J. Skillman, J. Hedley-Whyte, and J. A. Pallotta, *Ann. Surg.* [1793])

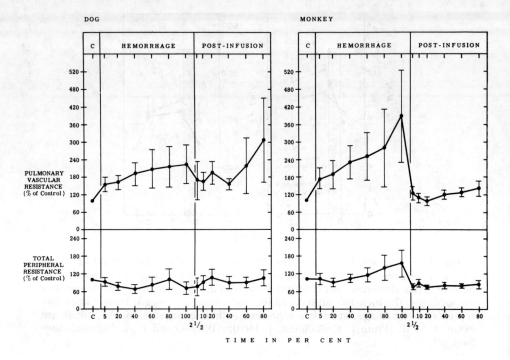

Figure 14-5. Response of pulmonary vascular resistance and total peripheral resistance in dog and monkey to hemorrhage and reinfusion. At the time of the hemorrhagic shock procedure the dogs were premedicated with morphine sulfate (3 mg/kg IM) 1 hr prior to receiving sodium pentobarbital (15 mg/kg IV). The primates received the same anesthesia except for the use of 1 mg/kg morphine and additional small doses of intramuscular methohexital sodium for transient anesthesia and handling of the animal. In all other respects the two groups of animals were similarly treated. The animals were subjected to a standardized hemorrhagic shock procedure. Following a 30-minute control period, they were given heparin (3 mg/kg) and bled from the femoral artery cannula into the bleeding bottle. The height of the bottle was adjusted as necessary to maintain the mean arterial pressure of the animal at 40 mm Hg (5.3 kPa). Bottle volumes were read at 10-minute intervals, and note made of the maximum bottle volume. When the animal had spontaneously taken back 30 percent of the maximum bleeding volume, the remaining blood was reinfused into the femoral vein and the animal was followed until death. All parameters except total blood volume were usually measured every 10 minutes in the control period, every 10 minutes after hemorrhage for 30 minutes, every 10 minutes after reinfusion for 30 minutes, and every 30 minutes throughout the remainder of the bleeding and postinfusion phases until death. Values shown are means ± SE. Time is in percent of duration of each period; C = control period. In both the dog and the monkey, PVR increases during hypotension and returns to near control levels after reinfusion. In the dog PVR later increases, whereas in the monkey it remains relatively constant. Pulmonary blood volume and pulmonary artery pressures are diminished during the hypotension. (From F. L. Abel, J. A. Waldhausen, W. J. Daly, and W. L. Pearce, *Am. J. Physiol.*[1])

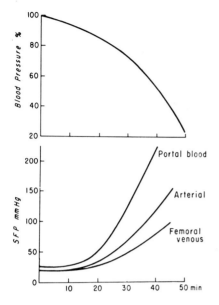

Figure 14-6. Changes in the screen filtration pressure (SFP) of blood during hemorrhagic shock. As blood pressure falls, there is a progressive rise in the screen filtration pressure, indicating formation in the blood of microaggregates composed of platelets, leukocytes, and fibrin, which are capable of releasing serotonin when lodged in the pulmonary circulation. The highest screen filtration pressures occur in the portal blood, indicating that microaggregate formation occurs to a greater degree in the splanchnic circulation. (From R. L. Swank, *J. Trauma*.[1888] Copyright, 1968, The Williams & Wilkins Co., Baltimore, with permission.)

tified by hospital number and are tagged with that number. This tag acts essentially as an attached medical record on which is also recorded all medications the patient has received, his name if known, and major problems.

In order to test the disaster plan our hospital simulates at least one unscheduled weekend disaster annually: for example, the crash of a jumbo jet in Boston.

AIRLINE CRASHES

Airline crash victims usually suffer from the consequences of fire or smoke and fume inhalation as well as from impact injury. One study of 13 crashes in which fire broke out concluded that 5 percent of the 700 passengers were killed by impact while over 40 percent were killed by fire.[575] In another crash, on take-off, fire killed all the occupants of the forward section of the cabin, and 13 of the 36 survivors were burned. In a crash in which fire did not break out and in which all passengers had seat belts on, 13 of the 16 fatally injured persons died as a result of massive brain or brainstem lesions, and the remaining 3 of ruptured great vessels. In survivors as well as nonsurvivors fractures account for 39 percent, thoracic injuries for 23 percent, spinal injuries for 18 percent, head injuries for 18 percent, and abdominal injuries for 7 percent of total injuries. Many of the fatal injuries occur not because of seat-belt failure or injury but because the entire passenger seat is ripped on impact from its attachments to the floor. The seat and the passenger in it are then propelled like a missile to the forward section of the cabin.

A triage facility should be set up at the scene by a physician, if possible. Inability of trained personnel to get to the crash site because of curious onlookers or traffic jams is often a problem, as is hampering of rescue efforts by the news media. In many crashes all the patients who arrive at hospitals alive survive.[305] Excluding crashes in which the plane disintegrates, lives may be saved by prompt, well-coordinated rescue units. Communication lines are essential, as is the presence of a traffic controller for crowd control and on-the-spot medical aid.[1349] Hypothermia may be a major problem, as in the Basle Vanguard aircrash (Chap. 27).

TRAIN WRECKS

Train wrecks also result in mass casualties and disaster situations. The London subway crash in 1975, in which a train overran a station and crashed into a dead end tunnel, produced problems not only of deceleration injuries but also of smoke inhalation and removal of victims from the wreckage. Controlled ventilation was provided at the crash scene. In all, 29 persons perished.

NUCLEAR FUEL EXPOSURE

The increasing use of nuclear fuel may present the physician with individual or mass casualties due to accidental exposure. The isotope to which the patient is exposed should be determined.[1557] Tritiated water is distributed throughout the body; its half-life is 12.3 years. Krypton 85 and xenon 133 have half-lives of 10.8 years and 5.3 days, respectively, but are relatively inert. Iodine 131, with a half-life of 8.0 days, is selectively absorbed and concentrated in the thyroid gland. Thorium products, with a half-life of 1.4 $\times$ 10^{10} years, are transferred from the lungs to the bones. Radium 226 (half-life, 1,620 years) and radium 228 (half-life, 5.7 years) are reactive with body tissues in a manner similar to that of iodine 131. The most likely modes of overexposure are breaks in technique, accidents in transportation, unknown exposure after loss or theft, and power plant mishaps.[1557] Basic therapy for topical contamination includes removal and safe disposal of exposed clothing and articles and washing of the area of exposure. Observation should be continued for bone marrow, platelet, thyroid, and skin problems and for cancer.[1740]

Plutonium accidents are still relatively rare. In 1966 in Spain the crash and burning of a United States Air Force bomber carrying nuclear devices resulted in a release of plutonium. Decontamination procedures were applied successfully, requiring removal to the United States of 604 acres of soil in 4,879 blue, metal, 55-gallon drums.[1740]

CIVIL DISTURBANCES

Violent civil disturbances produce a variety of injuries depending on the level of conflict and the weapons used. Characteristically the demonstrators are poorly equipped, using weapons such as rocks, bats, bottles, and verbal abuse, and protective devices of shields or plastic helmets. Conversely their antagonists are well equipped with tear-gas, clubs, flak jackets, and pistols or rifles. If the combating parties obtain more sophisticated weapons such as gasoline or plastic bombs, tanks, or machine guns, the conflict produces casualties more along the lines of conventional war.[422] An analysis of the 600 casualties due to civil disturbances seen at the Royal Victoria Hospital, Belfast, discloses that 70 percent of the casualties could be treated and sent home from the emergency ward.[421,1626] Of the injuries seen in the emergency room 25 percent were lacerations, 20 percent gunshot wounds, 20 percent bruises, 9 percent fractures, and 4 percent concussions. In 61 percent of these cases the cause of injury was a blow, usually to the head or neck.[1678] Peak hours of patient inflow were 11:00 P.M. to 3:00 A.M., and the maximum inflow rate was one patient every two minutes. Additional problems encountered were hospital security (identification cards were required), communication, and attacks on ambulance attendants whose uniforms resemble those of the police. (It is recommended that uniforms be changed to white coats with red crosses.[1626]) Twelve persons were admitted to the hospital because of bomb blast injuries. All had multiple abrasions and lacerations. Seven of eleven civilians injured by bomb blast lost one or more limbs. Six patients had respiratory distress, the longest period of controlled ventilation being 57 days. In-hospital mortality from bomb blasts was 33 percent and was due to aspiration, burns, shock, and renal failure. One explosion in a public house immediately killed 17 persons, with no admissions to the intensive care unit. Another explosion in a restaurant killed only 2 but hospitalized 22, with 3 admitted to the intensive care unit with multiple injuries.[609] In the same conflict, bullet wounds

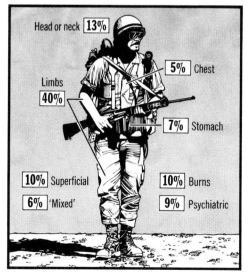

Figure 14-7. Types of wounds sustained by the Israelis in the 1973 Middle East war. There is a high incidence of extensive soft tissue injuries of the type that can later lead to respiratory failure. As in Vietnam extensive limb injuries were common and were a major cause of respiratory failure, especially after extensive blood loss. (From E. Marsden, *The Sunday Times,* London.[1235])

sustained by soldiers were primarily to the head, neck, and abdomen, since flak jackets were worn. Flak jackets can cause problems of heat stroke in climates warmer than that of Northern Ireland.

MILITARY CONFLICTS

In recent Middle East military conflicts, most casualties reported by the Israelis were due to shrapnel wounds, with wounds to the limbs in 40 percent, the head or neck in 13 percent, the abdomen in 7 percent, and the chest in 5 percent of cases. Burns accounted for 10 percent and psychiatric disorders for 9 percent of cases. There was a high percentage of injuries due to antitank missiles, with many of the armored corps sustaining eye injuries[1235] (Fig. 14-7). The Israeli authors emphasized that experienced physicians saved more lives by being in the reception areas rather than in the operating theaters or intensive care units.

15

Penetrating Injuries

The penetrating injuries that we see are most commonly the result of car accidents, stabbings, or gunshot wounds. The requirements of respiratory management encompass early recognition of life-threatening complications, maintenance of vital functions preoperatively, intraoperatively and postoperatively, and dealing with those problems arising out of massive transfusion. A careful search must be made for associated injuries. A neck fracture as a result of an assault can easily be missed. The incidence of penetrating injuries in urban areas makes triage techniques very important to the most effective use of emergency medical services.

TENSION PNEUMOTHORAX

Tension pneumothorax is an urgent, life-threatening emergency. Insertion of a chest tube, which is connected to an underwater drain, provides rapid relief. The chest tube is inserted by blunt dissection; it is not appropriate to use a trochar and cannula. If chest tube insertion cannot be performed expeditiously in a patient who is in extremis due to a tension pneumothorax, air can be "valved" out of the pleural space by intermittently applying a finger to a correctly placed plastic catheter (Fig. 15-1).[447]

Ventilation-perfusion abnormalities persist after a pneumothorax has been relieved. We rely on frequent arterial blood gas analyses to determine the need for supplemental oxygen, controlled ventilation, or both.

PENETRATING HEART WOUNDS

Cardiovascular collapse after penetrating wounds of the heart is a result of hypovolemia and interference with cardiac action, frequently due to cardiac tamponade.[1738] Injury to the coronary arterial tree and the cardiac conduction system may further complicate treatment. Initial therapy is directed toward restoration of the circulating blood volume, chest tube insertion for pneumothorax, and relief of cardiac tamponade by pericardiocentesis.[121,122,870,1258,1598]

Pericardiocentesis is best performed through the xiphisternal notch, preferably in the operating room (Fig. 15-1). Continuous electrocardiographic, intraarterial, and central venous monitoring are employed. Using the pericardial needle as chest lead the electrocardiograph provides an

199

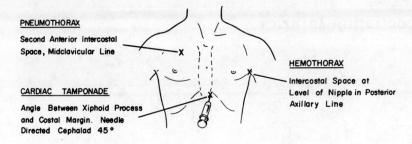

Figure 15-1. Suggested sites for needle aspiration of the pericardial and pleural spaces in the supine patient. (From O. Creech, Jr. and C. W. Pearce, *Am. J. Surg.*[447])

indication of contact with the epicardium.[178] Electrocardiographic indications of ventricular and atrial injury are illustrated in Figures 15-2 and 15-3 respectively.[743,1017]

We prepare for cardiopulmonary bypass as soon as a decision is made to perform pericardiocentesis on a patient with a penetrating wound. Early thoracotomy with cardiorrhaphy yields the best results.[123,697,1877,1916] If a coronary artery is injured, flow is reestablished by aortocoronary saphenous vein bypass graft or, occasionally, by direct surgery to the coronary artery.[1907]

AIRWAY INJURIES

Our management of airway injuries depends on the amount of bleeding into the mouth. If in our opinion the patient is likely to aspirate significant quantities of blood, we proceed to a tracheostomy after the trachea is intubated. We try to avoid intubation through an injured larynx. Tracheostomy and early reconstructive surgery provide the best results.

A massive air leak with extensive subcutaneous emphysema is an obvious indication of tracheal or bronchial rupture. In other instances, fiberoptic bronchoscopy is required to establish the diagnosis (see Chapter 14).[920] We avoid double-lumen tracheal tubes during surgery. An ordinary tracheal tube is used, which can be guided into one of the main-stem bronchi by the surgeon during thoracotomy. Immediate end-to-end anastomosis provides the best results.[1127] If the trachea is mobilized in the neck and at the pulmonary hilum, up to 5 cm of trachea can be resected.[774]

The innominate artery can be damaged following a penetrating injury to the neck.[1505] Hemostasis is achieved by external pressure exerted against the inflated cuff of a tracheal tube. We use cardiopulmonary bypass for repair.

ABDOMINAL EMERGENCIES

After abdominal injury the urgency of laparotomy is in large measure determined by the gravity of the overall clinical picture. Abdominal

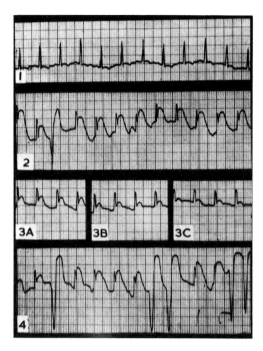

Figure 15-2. The electrocardiogram during pericardiocentesis. (*1*) Control period. In this patient the T-wave inversion is due to pericarditis. (*2*) The tip of the needle has touched the epicardium and produces a "current of injury" reflected as marked S-T segment elevation. There is one premature ventricular contraction. (*3A*) Acute "current of injury" as needle touches epicardium. (*3B* and *3C*) "Current of injury" less prominent as the needle is withdrawn from the myocardium. (*4*) Multiple premature contractions occur with a "current of injury." No attempt at aspiration should be made when there are signs of epicardial injury; the needle is slowly withdrawn into the pericardial cavity, where the aspiration is performed. (From M. S. Gotsman and V. Schrire, *Br. Heart J.*[743])

x-rays and selective angiography play a role in determining the extent of trauma when the need for surgical intervention is semiurgent.[664] Reduction in vital capacity by injury to the abdominal wall, effects of massive transfusion of blood, and right-to-left shunting seen following massive trauma often cause acute respiratory failure even preoperatively. Prophylactic short-term ventilation reduces complications after major abdominal injury.[1541]

CASE EXAMPLES

The following two case reports illustrate a number of typical problems.

Case 1. A 34-year-old female bank teller was admitted to the hospital after having been shot in the abdomen and left forearm. She arrived in very severe hemorrhagic shock and was immediately taken from the emergency ward to the operating room.

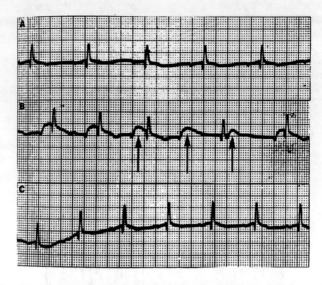

Figure 15-3.   Electrocardiogram demonstrating inadvertent atrial puncture during pericardiocentesis. *A.* Control period. There is no remarkable abnormality of the P-R segment. *B.* Immediately prior to aspiration of blood from the right atrium. There is elevation of the P-R segment (*arrows*) and intermittent atrioventricular dissociation. *C.* Following needle withdrawal the arrhythmia disappears and the P-R segment returns to normal. The S-T segment is unchanged. During pericardiocentesis the P-R segment must be observed for signs of right atrial puncture; if it occurs, the needle is withdrawn. (From R. E. Kerber, J. D. Ridges, and D. C. Harrison.[1017] Reprinted by permission from the *New England Journal of Medicine* 282:1142–1143, 1970.)

Upon arrival in the operating room she suffered respiratory arrest. She was intubated promptly with a cuffed orotracheal tube, and intermittent positive pressure ventilation was instituted. Despite rapid infusion of intravenous fluids (Ringer's lactate, 1,000 ml; Albumisol, 1,000 ml) she showed signs of virtually complete exsanguination. Laparotomy was instantly performed through a left paramedian incision extending from xiphoid to pubis and the abdominal aorta grasped below the renal arteries. Ventricular fibrillation necessitated extension of the incision through the diaphragm and pericardium to facilitate internal cardiac massage. A long intravenous catheter, which was thought to have been placed via the left subclavian vein, was found in the pleural cavity with a large amount of the transfused fluid and blood. The catheter was removed, and normal sinus rhythm was restored by further intravenous fluid replacement and administration of sodium bicarbonate and calcium chloride. Electromechanical dissociation with an electrocardiographic rate of 175 and arterial pulse rate of 70 per minute occurred during marked metabolic acidemia with a pH of 7.05. Further sodium bicarbonate administration abolished the electromechanical dissociation.

Intraabdominal injuries in the path of the single bullet included avulsion of the left common iliac artery at its origin, laceration of a branch of the superior mesenteric vein, and four perforations in the jejunum and two in the duodenum. The bullet itself had lodged in the anterior face of a lumbar vertebra, from which it was removed easily. The aortoiliac injury was repaired by oversewing both ends. Prompt refilling of the distal stump of the common iliac artery occurred upon release of the aortic clamps. The laceration in the mesenteric vein was repaired. An eight-inch segment of jejunum was resected and continuity restored by performing an end-to-end intestinal anastomosis. The perforations through the duodenum were trimmed of their ragged edges and closed with an inner layer of continuous chromic suture and an outer layer of inverting, interrupted silk sutures. The abdomen was copiously irrigated with saline and antibiotic solution. The pericardium was left open and the diaphragm closed with interrupted silk sutures. A chest tube was placed in the left pleural cavity and connected to an underwater drain. The compound, comminuted fracture of the left ulnar was immobilized in plaster. Intraoperatively the patient had received 17 units of whole blood, two units of fresh, frozen plasma, and six units of platelets.

Postoperatively, controlled ventilation was maintained in the Respiratory–Surgical Intensive Care Unit with an Emerson constant volume postoperative ventilator. Gastrointestinal function returned promptly. There was no circulatory impairment to the left lower extremity. By the eleventh postoperative day the patient was weaned from controlled ventilation and extubated. Severe laryngeal edema necessitated reintubation. Subsequent extubation in the operating room, with full preparation for immediate tracheostomy, was successful. Acute renal failure developed, and repeated hemodialyses via a Scribner shunt were required until the twenty-third postoperative day. The patient was discharged after a 41-day hospital stay.

Case 2. A 21-year-old female music student was admitted to the hospital, having been stabbed at the base of the neck on the right side with a knife after being sexually assaulted. She was awake with a blood pressure of 120/50 mm Hg (16.0/6.7 kPa), a pulse rate of 110 per minute, and cyanosis of the lips. There was a stab wound at the base of the neck on the right side, with a hematoma, and an associated hemothorax on the right. Neurologic examination was normal.

She was transferred immediately to the operating room. Arterial and venous lines were placed. Three to four minutes after induction of anesthesia and tracheal intubation there was profuse, bright red bleeding from the neck wound. The source of bleeding could not be identified through a supraclavicular incision. A lateral thoracotomy incision was performed through the right, fifth intercostal space. The chest cavity was filled with about three liters of blood. Bleeding appeared to be coming from a laceration of the innominate artery. Despite maximal attempts at fluid replacement, progressive hypotension ensued and terminated in ventricular fibrillation. The pericardium was opened and internal cardiac massage instituted. An incision was made in the right groin and partial cardiopulmonary bypass established via the femoral vessels. An attempt at electric defibrillation was unsuccessful. The heart and femoral vessels were completely empty of blood.

A median sternotomy was performed from the neck wound to the thoracotomy incision. This provided good exposure and revealed that the right subclavian artery had been severed from the innominate artery at its origin. The innominate vein was partially severed. The subclavian artery was clamped and ligated and the innominate artery and vein repaired. Partial cardiopulmonary bypass was terminated uneventfully, and two chest tubes were inserted anteriorly and posteriorly in the right pleural cavity. The patient had received 26 units of whole blood, three of these being fresh, two units of packed red cells, eight units of platelets, 6,750 ml of Albumisol, and 800 ml of Ringer's lactate.

She was transferred to the Respiratory–Surgical Intensive Care Unit. Controlled ventilation was maintained with an Emerson constant volume postoperative ventilator. The cardiovascular system was stable with the blood pressure 140/70 mm Hg (18.6/9.3 kPa). Persistent bleeding necessitated reexploration on the morning of the first postoperative day. A small bleeder was found at the angle of the thoracotomy flap and ligated. The patient was weaned from controlled ventilation and extubated the evening of the first postoperative day. A right recurrent laryngeal nerve injury was noted. A right pleural effusion developed, and needle thoracentesis on the eleventh postoperative day produced 1 liter of a bloody, sterile fluid. She was discharged on the fourteenth postoperative day.

16

Burns and Respiratory Function

The principal cause of death from burn injury has shifted from burn shock, which is now managed effectively, to respiratory failure.[6,1525,1734,1780] The mortality in patients with pulmonary complications is 80–90 percent.[1342] In the 1942 Cocoanut Grove disaster, in which 481 persons died, the Massachusetts General Hospital received 114 casualties in a period of two hours.[419] Many of these patients showed signs of respiratory distress on arrival, suggesting the possibility of a direct toxic effect from inhaled smoke and fumes.[63,139] The occurrence of pulmonary edema in the first 24 hours is common and is thought to be secondary to excessive administration of crystalloid solutions as well as a direct result of pulmonary injury.[420] The most consistent finding in the lungs is a diffuse membranous bronchitis. This lesion is seen frequently with the inhalation of toxic gases, notably nitrogen dioxide, phosgene, and mustard gas. Carbon monoxide asphyxia is also a frequent cause of death in patients who are dead on arrival in the emergency room.[1217]

The pulmonary complications of burns occur because of an interrelationship of many factors (Fig. 16-1).[6,2009] In any given patient it may be impossible to determine with certainty what role any factor plays in the development of complications. For the sake of clarity the pulmonary complications are arbitrarily divided into early, intermediate, and late. The early complications are seen immediately following the burn and are usually related to the inhalation of flames, steam, or toxic fumes into the tracheobronchial tree. The intermediate complications develop 24–72 hours following the burn. The late complications include pneumonia, sepsis, and pulmonary embolism.

EARLY COMPLICATIONS

PATHOPHYSIOLOGY

Immediate pulmonary complications generally are related to inhalation injuries. These include damage to both upper and lower respiratory tracts. The agent that produces the damage is usually difficult to ascertain, since most burn victims are exposed to heat, smoke, and many toxic fumes, all of which can cause respiratory tract damage. It is likely that direct injury to the tracheobronchial tree by heat alone is rare and that chemical damage occurs

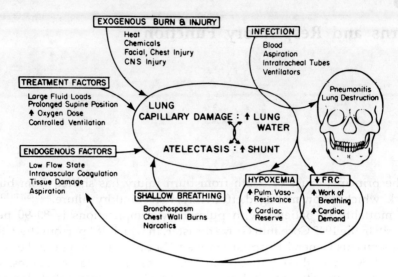

Figure 16-1. Pathogenesis of respiratory failure in burn patients. There are a multitude of interrelated factors in the production of respiratory failure after burn injury. (From B. M. Achauer, P. A. Allyn, D. W. Furnas, and R. H. Bartlett, *Ann. Surg.*[6])

much more frequently.[517] Direct damage accounts for many deaths at the scene of the fire, and few survive to receive treatment.[6]

EFFECT OF HEAT

The inhalation of flames causes massive orofacial edema, which produces airway obstruction. Inhaled heat also produces edema of the pharynx and larynx, leading to airway obstruction. Damage to the lung by inhalation of heat alone is difficult to produce experimentally. The upper respiratory tract effectively cools much of the inspired heat.[1359] There is also reflex closure of the larynx during inspiration of heat, preventing heat injury to the lung.[6] In only one patient of a series of 697 burned patients was there evidence of direct thermal injury below the larynx. In that patient there was heat necrosis extending only a few centimeters from the glottis.[1567]

EFFECT OF TOXIC PRODUCTS OF COMBUSTION

In the early postburn period pulmonary complications are caused primarily by the inhalation of toxic products of combustion. Nitrogen dioxide and carbon compounds in smoke frequently are implicated in the production of respiratory tract damage.[1862] The exact proportions of the toxic products of combustion in any given fire usually are unknown. The initial lesion most often is an acute, intense tracheobronchitis.[517,824] Later there appears edema of the tracheobronchial tree and interstitial edema. Edema is maximal 12–48 hours following the burn. After several days one sees mucosal sloughing, atelectasis, and areas of pulmonary hemorrhage. Bacterial superinfection is a late finding. Sputum frequently reveals particles of carbon.[652,1526,1861,2134]

Pulmonary function testing reveals marked abnormalities. There is a reduction in total compliance. Airway resistance is increased. As a result of these changes the work of breathing increases markedly. These changes are present for the first 10–12 days following inhalation injury and frequently return to normal a month after the injury.[690]

Blood gases reveal early arterial hypoxemia related to interstitial edema and atelectasis.[593] The combination of increased work of breathing, low total lung compliance, and high airway resistance can lead to hypercapnia and respiratory acidemia. Metabolic acidemia is frequently present and often leads to respiratory compensation and alveolar hyperventilation. The usual findings on arterial blood gases are therefore a low arterial oxygen tension, low arterial carbon dioxide tension, and near normal pH (Fig. 16-2). Oxygen consumption usually is increased.[1997]

Cardiac output is low in the early postburn period and can lead to an elevation of the deadspace-to-tidal-volume ratio. Stroke volume, left ventricular stroke work, and blood volume are usually all reduced. Peripheral vascular resistance and pulmonary vascular resistance are greatly increased (Fig. 16-3).[48] Blood pressure may be normal or low, and heart rate usually is increased (Figs. 16-4 and 16-5). These cardiovascular changes probably are related to loss of fluid at the burn site.[1763]

EFFECT OF CARBON MONOXIDE

Carbon monoxide intoxication plays a large role in the patient's clinical state in the early postburn period.[1217,2065] Carbon monoxide is a nonirritating, colorless, odorless gas that is a product of combustion of carbon compounds. Carboxyhemoglobin renders hemoglobin incapable of carrying oxygen. Since carbon monoxide has an affinity for hemoglobin several hundred times that of oxygen, carbon monoxide content increases rapidly in blood. The degree of conversion of hemoglobin to carboxyhemoglobin depends on the inspired concentration and the duration of exposure. Loss of consciousness from tissue hypoxia occurs at blood saturations of more than 30 percent carboxyhemoglobin. Death occurs frequently with blood carboxyhemoglobin saturation of greater than 50 percent.[541] During carbon monoxide poisoning with 52 percent blood saturation there is no increase in the level of alveolar ventilation in spite of elevation of the carbon dioxide tension. The level of the arterial oxygen tension is only slightly reduced at carboxyhemoglobin blood saturation of 52 percent. Carbon monoxide has little effect on the lung, and its primary toxic effect is that of producing tissue hypoxia secondary to saturation of hemoglobin with carbon monoxide.[334]

Burned patients who survive long enough to reach the hospital rarely have a carboxyhemoglobin of more than 15 percent saturation.[6] We have

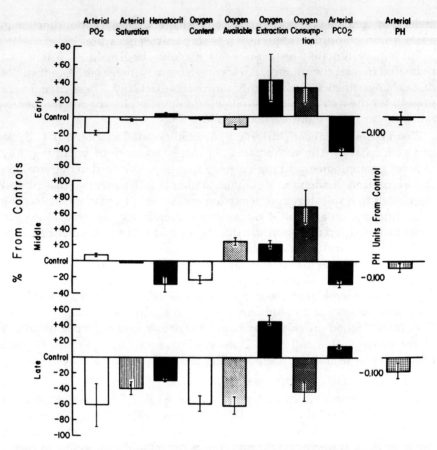

Figure 16-2.   Oxygen transport and acid-base status after severe burns. Six severely burned subjects (35–60 percent full-thickness burns) had measurements of oxygen transport and arterial blood gases in the early, middle, and late postburn periods. There were 17 healthy control subjects. The periods were divided according to the interval between the burn and recovery or death. The early period represents the first 25 percent of the interval, the late period the last 25 percent of the course, and the middle period the remaining time. In the early postburn period (*upper panel*) the oxygen availability decreased. Oxygen consumption increased. Pa_{CO_2} decreased, and pH remained normal. During the middle period (*middle panel*) blood gases normalized somewhat; pH fell slightly. Oxygen consumption increased further. In the late period (*lower panel*) arterial oxygenation and oxygen transport decreased. Pa_{CO_2} increased. The in-hospital mortality was 83 percent. Mean values are expressed as percent deviation from control. *Bars* represent ± 1 SD. (From B. C. Vladeck, R. Bassin, S. I. Kim, and W. C. Shoemaker, *J. Surg. Res.*[1997])

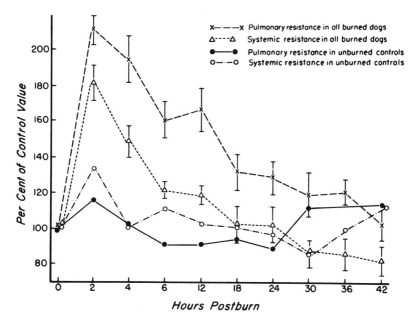

Figure 16-3. The effect of thermal injury and resuscitation on pulmonary and systemic vascular resistance. Dogs had measurements of pulmonary vascular and systemic vascular resistance done before and after severe burns were induced. Half the dogs served as unburned controls. Data were expressed as a percent of the preburn value. There was a significant difference between the increase in pulmonary vascular resistance and systemic vascular resistance. The mean pulmonary vascular resistance rose to 211 percent of preburn value 2 hours after the burn. The pulmonary vascular resistance returned to preburn levels after 42 hours. The mean systemic vascular resistance rose to 181 percent of preburn value 2 hours after the burn. (From M. J. Asch, R. J. Feldman, H. L. Walker, F. D. Foley, R. L. Popp, A. D. Mason, and B. A. Pruitt, *Ann. Surg.* [48])

seen one burned patient with more than 40 percent saturation, however. Carboxyhemoglobin saturation can be determined by analysis of muscle carbon monoxide content. Using this method it has been demonstrated that 32 percent of airline crash victims have carboxyhemoglobin saturation levels of more than 30 percent at autopsy. These findings suggest that carbon monoxide inhalation probably contributes a great deal in producing death in the early postburn period, especially when the patient is in a confined area.

DIAGNOSIS

The diagnosis of pulmonary complications in the early postburn period is made usually by careful physical examination. Evidence of upper airway obstruction secondary to massive facial edema is easily recognized. Airway obstruction secondary to pharyngeal and laryngeal edema is also obvious.

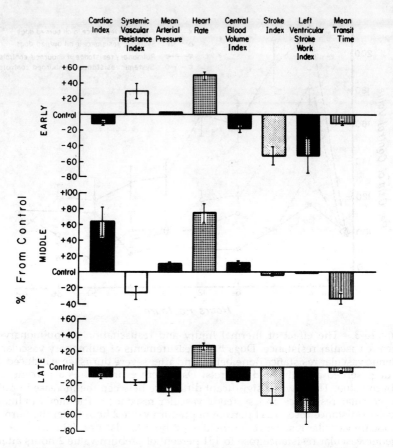

Figure 16-4. The hemodynamic pattern after severe burns. Six patients with 35–60 percent full-thickness burns had cardiovascular measurements taken in each of three periods following the injury. The periods were divided according to the interval between burn and recovery or death. The early period (*upper panel*) represents the first 25 percent of the interval, the late period (*lower panel*) the last 25 percent of the course, and the middle period (*middle panel*) the remaining time. Values are the mean ± SD expressed as percent of control values obtained from 17 healthy patients. During the early postburn period there is a fall in cardiac index, stroke index, left ventricular stroke work, and blood volume. Heart rate and systemic vascular resistance increase. Mean arterial pressure does not change. In the middle postburn period there is a marked rise in cardiac index and a fall in systemic vascular resistance. Heart rate remains increased. In the late period all values fall below normal except heart rate. The observed early fall in cardiac output probably is related to hypovolemia. The in-hospital mortality was 83 percent. (From W. C. Shoemaker, B. C. Vladeck, R. Bassin, K. Printen, R. S. Brown, J. J. Amato, J. M. Reinhard, and A. E. Kark, *J. Surg. Res.*[1763])

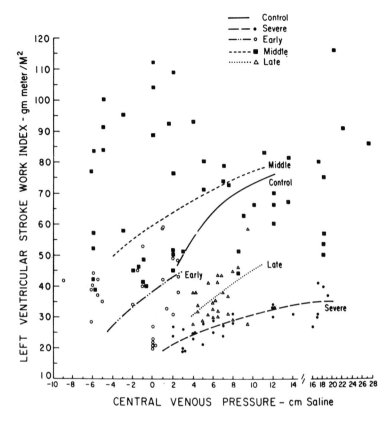

Figure 16-5. Left ventricular stroke work plotted against central venous pressure in burned patients. Six burned patients had cardiovascular studies done at three intervals following a burn injury (see definition in Figure 16-4). Two patients with severe, rapidly fatal burns also had measurements done. In the late burn period there is depression of the stroke work curve downward and to the right, which suggests decreased myocardial function. The patients with rapidly fatal burns (*Severe*) had further displacement of the curve downward and to the right, which suggests a greater reduction in myocardial performance than in the late postburn period. Five of the other six patients died within one week following the burn. (From W. C. Shoemaker, B. C. Vladeck, R. Bassin, K. Printen, R. S. Brown, J. J. Amato, J. M. Reinhard, and A. E. Kark, *J. Surg. Res.*[1763])

The presence of a severe facial burn, especially one involving the nose or mouth, should make the observer suspicious of the possibility of upper airway or pulmonary damage. Hoarseness, loss of voice, inspiratory stridor, and chest retraction also should lead one to suspect upper airway obstruction.[517]

Pulmonary damage in the early postburn period is nearly always associated with arterial hypoxemia.[593,690] This corresponds to the finding of restlessness, confusion, and panic that is common in the early postburn period. Cyanosis often is present on admission; however, its absence should not invoke a false sense of security, since high levels of carboxyhemoglobin can make the patient appear a cherry red color and mask arterial hypoxemia.[1526]

Wheezes on chest examination frequently are present when bronchospasm occurs with the pulmonary injury. Rales are an ominous sign in the early postburn period, suggesting the early development of pulmonary edema. Roentgenographic findings can be somewhat misleading, in that patients with severe pulmonary damage and hypoxemia may have a completely normal chest x-ray at the time of admission. Atelectasis or pulmonary edema may take 12–24 hours to appear on the chest x-ray. Sputum examination often reveals carbon particles in patients who have inhaled smoke. Secretions tend to increase during the 24 hours following the pulmonary injury.[29,1526]

Xenon 133 scintiphotography is a useful tool in the diagnosis of inhalation pulmonary injury. With areas of edematous tracheobronchial mucosa there is frequently gas trapping distal to the edema. These areas are detected following the intravenous injection of [133]Xe. Changes on ^{133}Xe scan can be detected before the onset of symptoms, physical findings, or even radiographic findings. The scan is easily performed, requires little patient participation, and has a low rate of false positive results. The ^{133}Xe scan may detect inhalation injury early, so that therapeutic measures may be instituted.[1384]

TREATMENT

The management of the patient who demonstrates pulmonary complications in the immediate postburn period requires attention to the upper airway. Minor degrees of airway obstruction secondary to laryngeal edema may be managed successfully with intravenous steroids while the patient is kept under observation. Although there are no controlled studies of the use of steroids in this situation, there are reports of apparent improvement in laryngeal edema following the administration of 8–10 mg of dexamethasone intravenously.

If the airway obstruction is severe, with stridor, hypoxemia, or respiratory acidemia, tracheal intubation is necessary as soon as possible. Either the oral or the nasal route is acceptable, depending upon the area of least burn involvement.[1132] If there is laryngeal as well as nasal and oral edema secondary to a severe burn, tracheal intubation may be difficult. If it is not possible to intubate the trachea either orally or nasally, then emergency access to the airway can be obtained by means of a cricothyroidotomy. A knife blade or a large-bore needle is passed through the cricothyroid membrane and the airway established. This method is easier and safer than an emergency tracheostomy.

Tracheostomy is an efficient means of relieving upper airway obstruction secondary to upper airway burn edema, but the problem of pulmonary infection that results is greatly underrated. At the Massachusetts General Hospital Shriners Burns Institute in Boston the overall rate of pulmonary sepsis in patients with thermal injuries of over 55 percent of the total body surface is 36 percent. In patients with tracheostomy the pulmonary sepsis rate is 78 percent compared with 12.5 percent for other patients.[573]

Controlled ventilation for the burn patient in respiratory failure is maintained with a volume-constant ventilator. Pressure-constant ventilators are unsuitable for use in severe pulmonary burns because of the low total lung compliance which makes the level of alveolar ventilation hard to control. Following recovery from respiratory failure the tracheostomy tube is removed as soon as possible, since the tracheal complications of tracheostomy in burn patients are greater than in any other form of acute respiratory failure.[652]

PREVENTION

The prevention of further respiratory decompensation can be achieved by proper monitoring of fluid replacement during the first 48 hours after the burn. Since burn patients require massive fluid replacement in the early postburn period, and since pulmonary edema is one of the usual accompaniments of inhalation injury, excess fluid replacement can severely impair the patient's already compromised respiratory function. In patients with an inhalation injury the central venous pressure is an unreliable indicator of left ventricular function. The Swan-Ganz pulmonary artery catheter has simplified fluid replacement. The catheter is placed, after emergency measures have been completed, in any severely burned patient with an inhalation injury. Fluids are then replaced, while the pulmonary capillary wedge pressure is kept between 10 and 20 mm Hg (1.3–2.6 kPa).[112,699]

There is no evidence that the use of steroids alters the course of the pulmonary damage, once respiratory failure has developed.[117] There is also no evidence that the prophylactic administration of systemic antibiotics lowers the incidence of acquired pneumonia. The plasma oncotic pressure should be kept as near normal as possible by use of plasma and albumin replacement.

Management of the patient with carbon monoxide asphyxia consists of controlled ventilation with maximal inspired oxygen tensions in an attempt to improve the blood oxygen content. Transfusion of packed red cells is often helpful.

INTERMEDIATE COMPLICATIONS

The second group of patients are those who are severely burned but who for the first 24–48 hours have no symptoms or signs of respiratory tract involvement. Between the first and fifth day these patients develop tachypnea, respiratory alkalemia, and, frequently, respiratory failure. The etiology of these changes probably involves many potential factors.

ATELECTASIS

Atelectasis is a common complication of burns, particularly of the chest wall.[1817] Lung volume is decreased by pain, narcotics, and immobility. Patients develop shallow respirations.[6,1764] Total lung compliance falls.[1256]

PULMONARY EDEMA

Pulmonary edema is not uncommon following a massive nonpulmonary burn. Many factors are responsible for its development. Excessive fluid administration during resuscitation can lead to pulmonary edema, especially in patients with preexisting cardiovascular or renal disease.[1567] Microembolization probably plays a large part in the development of pulmonary edema following a burn. Areas of low perfusion as well as areas of actual burn injury tend to form aggregates of platelets, thrombin, and white and red blood cells. Carbon particles may affect the development of these microaggregates.[1591] Microaggregates also may result from blood transfusion or from the disseminated intravascular coagulation seen in burn patients.[1282] Microaggregates migrate from the site of production to the pulmonary vasculature, where they are filtered from the circulation. In the lung there is a release of vasoactive kinins, which leads to pulmonary venoconstriction and bronchoconstriction. The result of this venous and bronchial constriction is pulmonary edema and further lowering of compliance. Vascular obstruction from microemboli leads to alveolar and endothelial cell damage, which produces leakage of fluid into the interstitial and intraalveolar space. The destruction is often severe enough to produce intraalveolar hemorrhage. The formation of a hyaline membrane is a late finding.[186]

INHALATION INJURY

^{133}Xe scanning has demonstrated that many patients have evidence of inhalation injury immediately but do not develop signs or symptoms for several days following a major burn.[1384]

METABOLIC ACIDEMIA

During topical therapy of the burn wound with mafenide acetate (Sulfamylon) a metabolic acidemia may develop secondary to the inhibition of carbonic anhydrase by mafenide. This acidemia is usually compensated for by a respiratory alkalemia; however, in patients with pulmonary lesions, alveolar hyperventilation may not be possible and the acidemia will have to be managed in other ways.[49,2061]

DIAGNOSIS

In the first week following a burn the patient may become dyspneic, tachypneic, restless, or agitated. Chest examination often reveals rales or signs of consolidation. Cyanosis may or may not be present. Arterial blood gases reveal hypoxemia. Respiratory alkalemia often precedes the development of respiratory acidemia. Chest x-ray reveals either the patchy infiltrates of pulmonary edema or signs of lung collapse. [133]Xe scan may be helpful in diagnosing inhalation injury that was not apparent at the time of admission.[1384] Elevation of the pulmonary capillary wedge pressure may aid in the diagnosis of increasing lung water during fluid replacement.[699] Unusual hemorrhage into the burn wound or from other sites may lead to the early diagnosis of disseminated intravascular coagulation, which usually precedes the pulmonary findings.[1282]

TREATMENT

Management of intermediate pulmonary complications involves attempts to relieve the major etiologic factors. Atelectasis is treated by vigorous chest physical therapy, coughing, deep breathing, and tracheal suction if necessary. Inspired oxygen is provided via a heated nebulizer. Pulmonary edema is managed by diuretic therapy, fluid restriction, and occasionally by digitalization of the patient.

The treatment of pneumothorax in a patient with a chest wall burn is hazardous if the thoracotomy tube has to be placed through an area of burned skin. There is a risk of empyema following this procedure. If a pneumothorax develops in a patient with a chest wall burn, and if there is no unburned skin through which to place a chest tube, then needle aspiration of the pneumothorax should be attempted. If the pneumothorax recurs, then chest tube placement is necessary in spite of the hazards.[1567]

LATE COMPLICATIONS

The two major late pulmonary complications are infection and pulmonary embolism. All burn patients are at high risk for developing pulmonary infection at any time during their hospital stay.

PNEUMONIA

Pneumonia usually does not appear until four to five days after a major burn. The control of burn sepsis with topical therapy has resulted in a lowered overall mortality rate. Rates of pulmonary infection have not changed. What has changed is the route of infection. Prior to the use of topical mafenide burned patients most often developed pneumonia via the hematogenous route (67 percent of 70 patients). Following the institution of topical therapy the airborne route has become the commonest means of transmission (65 percent of 133 patients).[1566]

The usual source of the bacteria is infection of the burn wound. The organism most commonly involved is *Pseudomonas aeruginosa*.[1909] Transmission usually occurs via the hands of personnel.

PULMONARY EMBOLISM

Pulmonary embolism is also a late complication of burns. Significant pulmonary embolism develops in 5.5 percent of burn patients and in 20.3 percent of patients with major trauma. In the majority of cases it occurs within two weeks of the burn; however, it can arise many months following injury.[1736] The cause of nearly all emboli in burn patients is deep venous thrombosis of the legs occurring secondary to prolonged bedrest and abnormal coagulation patterns.[1217]

PREVENTION

Prevention of acquired pneumonia has been discussed in Chapter 4. With regard to the burn patient, the question of the airborne route of transmission of pneumonia has become increasingly important. Since *Pseudomonas aeruginosa* is frequently a problem in burn patients, short-term topical application of polymyxin to the upper airway and trachea may be of considerable benefit in preventing acquired *Pseudomonas* pneumonia. Prophylactic administration of low doses of heparin subcutaneously reduces the incidence of pulmonary embolism and is effective in the management of the burned patient.

IV

Respiratory Management of Patients with Organ Failure

17

Respiratory Consequences of Myocardial Infarction

Acute myocardial infarction is often associated with derangements in lung function even in the absence of clinical or x-ray evidence of congestive heart failure. Arterial hypoxemia commonly occurs after myocardial infarction. Alveolar hypoventilation is uncommon; in fact arterial carbon dioxide tension is sometimes lower than normal.[1289,1471]

REGIONAL DISTRIBUTION OF PULMONARY PERFUSION

The regional distribution of pulmonary perfusion measured by the intravenous injection of 2 millicuries of ^{133}Xe in saline on the fourth day after uncomplicated myocardial infarction was shown to be abnormal.[1007] Uncomplicated myocardial infarction was defined as the absence of clinical or radiologic evidence of congestive heart failure. The average mean pulmonary artery pressure in this group was 14 mm Hg (1.9 kPa), average pulmonary capillary wedge pressure was 5 mm Hg (0.7 kPa), and cardiac output averaged 5.1 liters per minute on the fourth day after myocardial infarction. Even after uncomplicated myocardial infarction relative hypoperfusion of the lung base occurs with increased perfusion of the apex (Fig. 17-1).[12,1007] The regional distribution of ventilation as studied by inhalation of a single normal breath of oxygen containing ^{133}Xe is normal, and thus the ventilation-perfusion ratio is nearly constant from apex to base of the lungs (Fig. 17-2). The abnormal distribution of pulmonary perfusion is probably due to an increase in interstitial lung water secondary to transient left ventricular failure at the time of infarction. The perfusion abnormality returns toward normal in the third week after uncomplicated infarction.

CLOSING VOLUMES

Closing volumes, as determined by the single-breath bolus technique using 1–2 ml of the radionuclide ^{13}N, are elevated when measured 3–14 days after uncomplicated myocardial infarction (Fig. 17-3).[761,792] An increase in interstitial lung water reduces the transpulmonary pressure at the lung base, and small airway closure occurs. When the closing volume exceeds the functional residual capacity, small airway collapse occurs in the range of tidal breathing, resulting in areas of a low ventilation-perfusion ratio with hypoxemia and increased alveolar-arterial oxygen tension gradient.

219

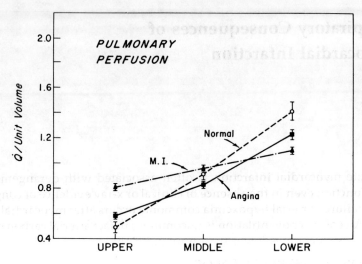

Figure 17-1. Distribution of pulmonary blood flow per unit volume of ventilated lung (Q̇/unit volume) in the upper, middle, and lower lung zones. Distribution of blood flow in normal subjects is compared to the blood flow in 15 patients following uncomplicated myocardial infarction (MI) and in 5 patients with angina pectoris. Following myocardial infarction blood flow to the lower lung regions decreases, while distribution of ventilation remains constant. The result of these changes is that, following myocardial infarction, ventilation-perfusion ratio is nearly constant from the apex to the base of the lungs. (From H. Kazemi, E. F. Parsons, L. M. Valencia, and D. J. Strieder, *Circulation.*[1007] By permission of The American Heart Association, Inc.)

Diuresis restores the high closing volumes to normal within 16 hours with an improvement in arterial oxygenation. Closing volumes return to normal 4–12 months after uncomplicated myocardial infarction. Deadspace-to-tidal-volume ratio is increased after myocardial infarction, the increase being greater when pulmonary congestion is present (Fig. 17-4).[872]

PULMONARY MECHANICS

Small, reversible abnormalities in pulmonary mechanics occur during the first three days after acute myocardial infarction. These coincide with subclinical abnormalities in pulmonary hemodynamics as reflected by a slightly increased pulmonary capillary wedge pressure (12 mm Hg ± 1.7 SE $[1.5 ± 0.2$ kPa$]$), an increased mean pulmonary artery pressure (23 mm Hg ± 3.4 SE $[3.0 ± 0.4$ kPa$]$), an increased pulmonary vascular resistance (120 dynes cm^{-5} ± 20 SE [1200 μNcm^{-5} ± 200 SE]), and a relatively normal cardiac index (3 1/min/m^2 ± 0.2 SE).The pulmonary extravascular water volume increases to 150 ± 11 SE ml per square meter from a normal of 120 ml per square meter. The radiologic criteria of the degree of pulmonary vascular congestion generally have a good correlation with pulmonary capillary wedge pressure.[1274] The vital capacity and forced expiratory volume in 1

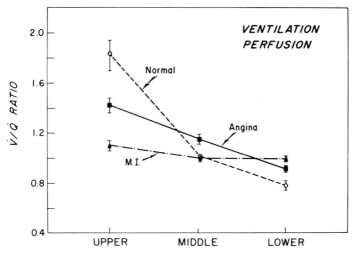

Figure 17-2. The ventilation-perfusion ratio for normal subjects, 15 patients follow-ing uncomplicated myocardial infarction, and 5 patients with angina pectoris. Following myocardial infarction the V̇/Q̇ ratio remains fairly constant from apex to base through the three lung zones shown on the abscissa. This differs markedly from the V̇/Q̇ ratio in normal subjects, which falls rapidly from apex to base. Patients with angina pectoris have a near-normal V̇/Q̇ ratio. (From H. Kazemi, E. F. Parsons, L. M. Valencia, and D. J. Strieder, *Circulation.*[1007] By permission of The American Heart Association, Inc.)

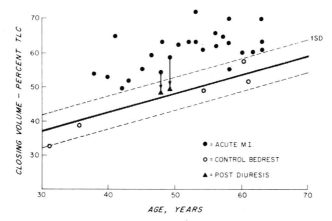

Figure 17-3. Closing volume (expressed as percent of total lung capacity [TLC]) following uncomplicated myocardial infarction. Values in 26 patients 3–14 days after myocardial infarction (*acute MI*) and in 5 patients admitted without infarction (*control bedrest*) are compared to the normal values for closing volume. The normal closing volume (*area between dashed lines* = normal ± 1 SD) increases with age. After myocardial infarction patients demonstrate an increased closing volume. In two patients (*arrows*) drug-induced diuresis had reduced the increased closing volume to normal when measured 16 hours later. (From C. A. Hales and H. Kazemi.[792] Reprinted by permission from the *New England Journal of Medicine* 290:761–765, 1974.)

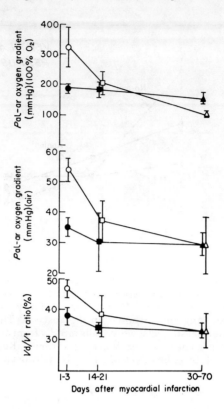

Figure 17-4. Effect of myocardial infarction on the deadspace-to-tidal volume ratio (VD/VT) and on the alveolar-arterial oxygen tension (Pal-ar) measured breathing air and breathing 100% oxygen. *Closed symbols* = patients without congestive heart failure; *open symbols* = patients with congestive heart failure following myocardial infarction. One to three days following myocardial infarction all patients demonstrate increased pulmonary venous admixture, since the alveolar-arterial oxygen tension difference measured both breathing air and breathing 100% oxygen is elevated. The deadspace-to-tidal-volume ratio is also increased. Values are highest in the patients with congestive heart failure. All values return toward normal one to two months following myocardial infarction. (From B. E. Higgs, *Clin. Sci.*[872])

second are reduced 30 percent, and the maximum midexpiratory flow rate is reduced 40 percent (Fig. 17-5).[944] Total pulmonary resistance becomes frequency dependent (Fig. 17-6). Alteration of the peripheral airways as a result of the accumulation of interstitial lung water is the most likely explanation for these changes.[908]

INDICATIONS FOR VENTILATORY AND CIRCULATORY ASSISTANCE

Oxygen administration by mask easily corrects the hypoxemia in most instances. Cautious intravenous administration of a short-acting diuretic

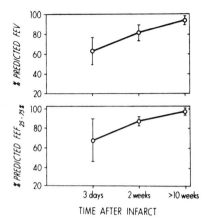

Figure 17-5. Changes in forced expiratory volume (FEV) and forced midexpiratory flow rate (FEF 25–75 percent) following uncomplicated myocardial infarction. Three days after myocardial infarction FEV and FEF 25–75 percent are both reduced. Two weeks after infarction these values begin to increase, and they are near normal ten weeks after myocardial infarction. (From B. Interiano, R. W. Hyde, M. Hodges, and P. N. Yu, *J. Clin. Invest.*[944])

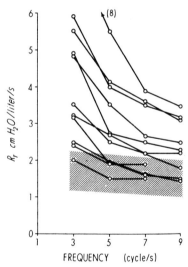

Figure 17-6. Total pulmonary resistance (R_T) measured at 3, 5, 7, and 9 cycles per second one to three days following myocardial infarction. *Shaded area* represents control subjects. Nearly all patients demonstrate increased resistance at an oscillation frequency of 3 cycles per second. This frequency-dependent rise in total pulmonary resistance is accompanied by only a small increase in total pulmonary resistance. This finding suggests that there are alterations in peripheral airways following myocardial infarction. These changes are completely reversed when measured ten weeks or more after the infarction. (From B. Interiano, R. W. Hyde, M. Hodges, and P. N. Yu, *J. Clin. Invest.*[944])

such as furosemide improves arterial oxygenation. The criteria for the diagnosis of respiratory failure are the same as for other patients. Positive end-expiratory pressure, if really needed, should be used with extreme caution.

We employ the intraaortic balloon pump when circulatory assistance is required,[1318] that is, for cardiogenic shock, intractable ventricular arrhythmias, and mechanical derangements consequent upon acute myocardial infarction.[263,1392] These mechanical derangements include papillary muscle dysfunction or rupture, ventricular septal defect, and akinesis of the left ventricle.[725,1391] Systolic unloading and diastolic augmentation also can be achieved with a combination of vasodilator therapy and external counterpulsation.[318,1488] The indications for intraaortic balloon pump counterpulsation and aggressive surgical intervention for cardiogenic shock are unclear at present.[1394] (See Chapter 12.)

18

Problems of Liver Failure and Delirium Tremens

Liver failure in patients in respiratory failure generally heralds death. Currently the mortality is greater than 95 percent. The liver has remarkable powers of regeneration, and if life can be sustained, hepatic function may be restored.[635,940] If only 10 percent of normal liver remains after major hepatic resection, it will sustain life, with full regeneration of liver mass occurring by the end of four months.[479]

HEPATIC COMA
Hepatic function is adversely affected by low perfusion pressure and a pattern of ventilation that maintains continuous positive airway pressure (Chap. 3). Hepatic coma in patients with liver disease can be precipitated by gastrointestinal bleeding, infection, sudden diuresis, and the stress of major surgery. Electrolyte imbalance and increased renal production of ammonia and amines occur as a result of a sudden diuresis.

CLINICAL CHANGES
The serum amino acid profile is altered in hepatic failure (Fig. 18-1).[639] Hyperinsulinemia due to hepatic failure results in increased uptake of branched-chain amino acids into skeletal muscle.[1397] Central nervous system uptake of amino acids is altered, and serotonin synthesis is increased, while norepinephrine synthesis is decreased.[520] Amines arising in the gut bypass the liver, where they are usually catabolized, and give rise to increased concentrations of false adrenergic neurotransmitters such as octopamine in both the brain and the urine (Figs. 18-2 and 18-3).[1339]

Some of the changes that occur during hepatic failure may be attributable to the accumulation of false neurotransmitters. Changes in the cardiovascular system include a high cardiac output, low peripheral resistance, and peripheral arteriovenous shunting (Figs. 18-4 and 18-5).[496,767,1773,1810] Accumulation of false neurotransmitters in the brain, and in the basal ganglia specifically, cause disturbances in mentation as well as asterixis due to displacement of normal neurotransmitter amines from central nervous system neurons. Some doubt, however, is cast on the false neurotransmitter theory of hepatic encephalopathy by the observation that brain octopamine levels exceeding those found in hepatic coma are present in noncomatose animals after treatment with monoamine oxidase inhibitors.[1370] Intrarenal

225

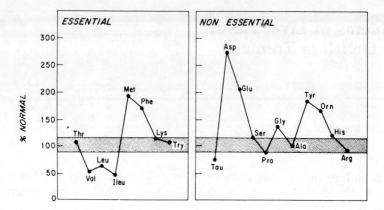

Figure 18-1. Plasma amino acid concentrations in patients with liver disease on protein-restricted diets. Excessive plasma concentrations of methionine (*Met*) and phenylalanine (*Phe*) are common in this type of patient. Aspartic acid (*Asp*), glutamic acid (*Glu*), tyrosine (*Tyr*), and ornithine (*Orn*) levels are all markedly elevated. (From J. E. Fischer, N. Yoshimura, A. Aguirre, J. H. James, M. G. Cummings, R. M. Abel, and F. Deindoerfer, *Am. J. Surg.*[639])

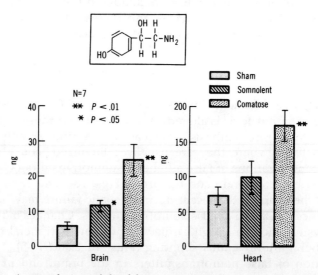

Figure 18-2. Accumulation of the false neurotransmitter octopamine in the brain and heart of animals with experimental hepatic coma. Rats had acute hepatic coma induced by gradual ligation of the blood supply to the liver over two days. The increases in brain octopamine closely parallel the state of consciousness of the animals. Values shown on the ordinate are nanograms per gram of wet tissue. (Reprinted from J. E. Fischer, *Arch. Surg.*[635] Copyright, 1974, American Medical Association.)

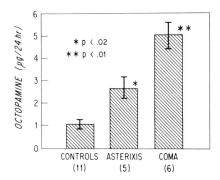

Figure 18-3. Urinary excretion of the false neurochemical transmitter octopamine is elevated in hepatic coma. Urine was collected for 24 hours and analyzed for octopamine in three groups: patients with liver disease without symptoms (*controls*), patients with "precoma" (*asterixis*), and patients in hepatic coma (*coma*). (Reprinted from J. E. Fischer, *Arch. Surg.*[635] Copyright, 1974, American Medical Association.)

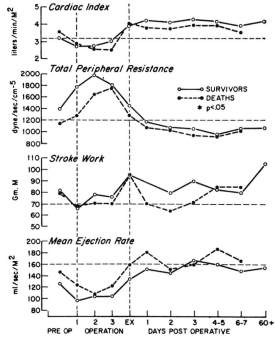

Figure 18-4. Cardiovascular changes in patients with cirrhosis undergoing elective surgery for portal decompression. Following operation the cardiac index and stroke work are elevated and the total peripheral resistance is low. These changes reflect the hyperdynamic state seen in such patients postoperatively, sometimes for as long as two years. (From M. Greenspan and L. R. M. Del Guercio, *Am. J. Surg.*[767])

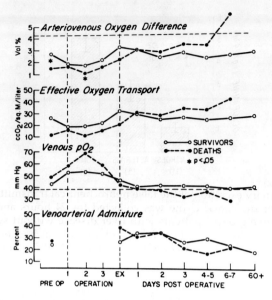

Figure 18-5. Changes in oxygenation in patients with cirrhosis undergoing elective surgery for portal decompression. The arteriovenous oxygen difference is persistently low, but venoarterial admixture is high. During surgery the nonsurvivors had increases in venous oxygen tension, suggesting that these patients have a marked degree of systemic arteriovenous shunting. (From M. Greenspan and L. R. M. Del Guercio, *Am. J. Surg.*[767])

shunting of blood away from the cortex occurs, resulting in sodium retention. Ammonia is not the sole toxin in hepatic encephalopathy; arterial ammonia levels do not have a correlation with the depth of hepatic coma. There are many possible toxic agents or deficiencies, but none successfully explain all instances of hepatic coma. Concomitant effects of liver failure include respiratory failure, hypoglycemia, hypokalemia, hypocalcemia, hypoalbuminemia, renal failure, gastrointestinal bleeding, and disseminated intravascular coagulation.[1989] Hyperventilation with respiratory alkalemia is a common early finding.

THERAPY

To preserve life long enough for hepatic regeneration to occur, supportive therapy includes correction of hypoglycemia, electrolyte imbalance, hypovolemia, and hypoalbuminemia.[478,1702,1870,1937] The need for protection of the airway and controlled ventilation is determined by the depth of coma, respiratory mechanics, and arterial blood gas measurements. The protein load is reduced by intestinal sterilization with neomycin or kanamycin, purging, and oral protein restriction. Intestinal sterilization reduces the brain content of octopamine (Fig. 18-6).

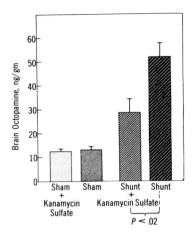

Figure 18-6. Effect of intestinal sterilization with kanamycin on brain octopamine levels in experimental animals. Either saline or kanamycin (15 mg) was given by gastric tube twice a day to rats two months after creation of a portacaval shunt. Animals that had had a sham operation were put on an identical regimen. Three days of intestinal sterilization with kanamycin results in a significant reduction in the brain concentration of the false neurotransmitter octopamine. Values shown on the ordinate are nanograms per gram of wet brain tissue. (Reprinted from J. E. Fischer, *Arch. Surg.*[635] Copyright, 1974, American Medical Association.)

PERFUSION

Perfusion techniques employed in the therapy of hepatic coma include exchange transfusion,[979,1936] plasmaphoresis,[1148] cross circulation,[982,1703,1854] and perfusion of isolated porcine, bovine, or baboon livers.[406] Dramatic awakening is produced, but survival is not affected. Asanguineous total body washout with large amounts of Ringer's lactate under hypothermic conditions is a technique requiring further evaluation.[1044] Prosthetics employing liver slices and liver cell suspensions also have been used to provide hepatic assistance.[583] Hemoperfusion through charged and uncharged resins and over albumin-conjugated agarose beads has been shown to reduce bilirubin levels in experimental animals.[94,1532, 1707,2070,2071,2072]

FALSE NEUROTRANSMITTER HYPOTHESIS

Therapy based on the false neurotransmitter hypothesis is promising. Postoperative patients in respiratory and hepatic failure respond favorably to levodopa, 250 mg orally or in daily doses of 2–25 gm by enema, or to metaraminol, 200–4,000 μg per minute intravenously (Figs. 18-7 and 18-8).[636,1485,1873] Levodopa replenishes the normal neurotransmitters, dopamine and norepinephrine. It also releases a variety of amines, which are excreted in the urine (Fig. 18-9). Hyperalimentation solutions currently in use are inadequate for patients with hepatic failure, as severe amino acid

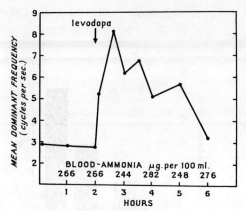

Figure 18-7. Effect of levodopa on the electroencephalogram of a patient with hepatic coma. Levodopa produced increases in the mean dominant frequency of the EEG. These changes began 5 minutes after injection and were maximal after 25 minutes. The EEG then slowly changed back to its former appearance. There were no changes in liver function tests, serum ammonia levels, or vital signs. This may reflect a defect in dopaminergic neurotransmission in patients with hepatic coma. (From J. D. Parkes, P. Sharpstone, and R. Williams, *Lancet*.[1485])

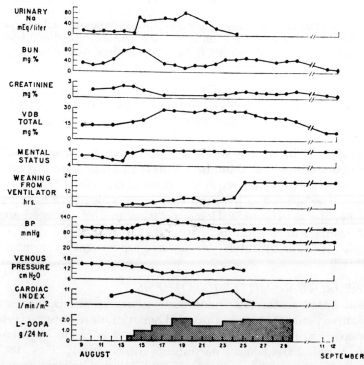

Figure 18-8. Effect of L-dopa in a patient in hepatic failure. This patient developed hemorrhagic pancreatitis and septicemia following a splenorenal shunt for portal hypertension secondary to Laennec's cirrhosis. She developed hepatic failure, coma, pulmonary edema, and respiratory failure. L-Dopa was given via a gastric

230

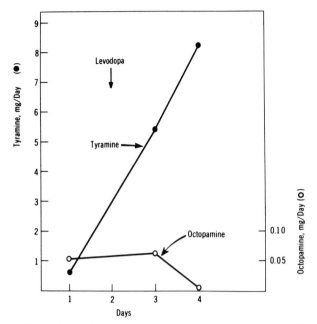

Figure 18-9. Effect of levodopa on urinary excretion of amines. A patient with hepatic coma secondary to chronic liver disease was given 500 mg of levodopa. Serial 24-hour collections of urine revealed a decrease in octopamine excretion and increased excretion of tyramine. The increased excretion of tyramine possibly resulted from displacement of amines by levodopa. (Reprinted from J. E. Fischer, *Arch. Surg.*[635] Copyright, 1974, American Medical Association.)

imbalances occur (Fig. 18-10). The intravenous administration of a special hepatic failure fluid with increased concentrations of branched-chain amino acids and very low concentrations of phenylalanine, methionine, and tryptophan normalizes plasma amino acid patterns (Fig. 18-11)[637] and probably accomplishes more efficient synthesis of normal neurotransmitters such as norepinephrine and dopamine.[639,1052] False neurotransmitters such as octopamine, present in abundance in hepatic failure, are then less likely to be taken up into the central nervous system.[638] Initial clinical trials with hepatic failure solution are producing encouraging results.

←───

tube. Within one hour she awoke and became out of phase with the ventilator. Her left ventricular failure improved, and she was gradually weaned from controlled ventilation. Weaning was complete by August 25. Her state of consciousness remained good, and L-dopa was stopped. Mental status was graded as (1) full consciousness, (2) disorientation, (3) stupor, and (4) semicoma or coma. *VDB* refers to the van den Bergh reactions for detection of bilirubin. She died of septicemia two months later. (From J. E. Fischer and R. J. Baldessarini, *Lancet.*[636])

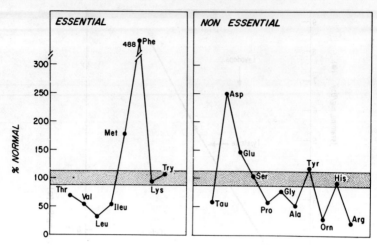

Figure 18-10. Plasma amino acids in patients who were treated with a solution of eight essential L-amino acids. The branched-chain amino acids and threonine (*Thr*) are present in persistently low concentrations. Both phenylalanine (*Phe*) and methionine (*Met*) are elevated. The majority of nonessential amino acids are present in low concentrations, which suggests that patients with liver disease are unable to convert essential to nonessential amino acids. (From J. E. Fischer, N. Yoshimura, A. Aguirre, J. H. James, M. G. Cummings, R. M. Abel, and F. Deindoerfer, *Am. J. Surg.*[639])

DELIRIUM TREMENS

Delirium tremens is characterized by profound confusion, delusions, vivid hallucinations, tremor, agitation, sleeplessness, dilated pupils, fever, tachycardia, and profuse sweating. Oxygen consumption is markedly elevated. Onset is generally three to four days after cessation of continuous drinking of alcohol. Mortalities of 15 percent are reported. Causes of death include peripheral circulatory collapse, hyperthermia, and associated injury or infection such as pneumonia, especially pneumococcal.[1991] Ethanol inhibits granulocyte adherence, one of the steps in the granulocyte response to an acute inflammatory stimulus, and may impair host defense against bacterial invasion.[1205]

An indispensable factor in the production of delirium tremens is the withdrawal of alcohol following a period of chronic intoxication. Serum hypomagnesemia and respiratory alkalemia are consistently associated with all but the mildest withdrawal symptoms (Figs. 18-12 and 18-13). No other measurements of biochemical constituents such as SGOT, SGPT, serum proteins, sodium, potassium, chloride, calcium, and glucose are consistently abnormal. The administration of intravenous magnesium sulfate raises the seizure threshold in the initial phase of withdrawal. Delirium tremens may have its onset after the serum magnesium has returned to normal, however. The occurrence of seizures and hallucinations coincides with the maximal degree of respiratory alkalemia.[2100,2101]

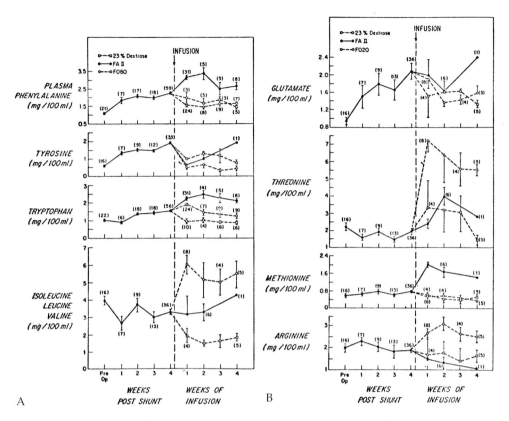

Figure 18-11. Effect of administration of amino acid solutions on the concentration of amino acids in dogs with hepatic encephalopathy. Dogs with end-to-side portacaval shunts develop a plasma amino acid pattern similar to that of a human with hepatic encephalopathy. Following creation of a portacaval shunt dogs had weekly determinations of the plasma concentrations of the amino acids shown in A and B. Numbers in parentheses are the number of measurements made. When the dogs developed encephalopathy, a central venous catheter was placed. They then received one of three fluids intravenously: an infusion of 23% dextrose and electrolytes with maintenance of serum albumin by infusion of dog plasma, an ammonia-free mixture of synthetic amino acids (Freamine II [FA II]), or an isocaloric and isonitrogenous amount of a solution F080. This latter solution has decreased concentrations of phenylalanine, tryptophan, methionine, and glycine and increased concentrations of leucine, isoleucine, and valine.

Animals that received 23% dextrose plus infusions of dog plasma developed the characteristic amino acid pattern seen in hepatic encephalopathy. Two of the five dogs in this group died. Those animals who received FA II rapidly developed hepatic encephalopathy coincident with a rise in plasma phenylalanine. Eleven of thirteen dogs in this group died. The dogs given F080 all had improvement in neurologic function within 24 hours coincident with decrease in aromatic amino acids and branched-chain amino acids. None of the eight dogs in this group died as a result of hepatic encephalopathy. (From J. E. Fischer, J. M. Funovics, A. Aguirre, J. H. James, J. M. Keane, R. I. C. Wesdorp, N. Yoshimura, and T. Westman, *Surgery.*[637])

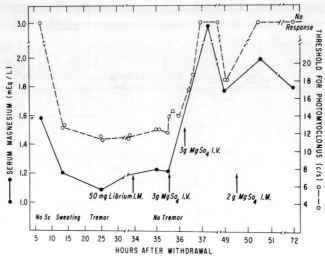

Figure 18-12. Association between serum magnesium level and photomyoclonus threshold in a patient with alcohol withdrawal. During withdrawal there is a fall in serum magnesium that closely parallels the increased response to photic stimulation. Administration of chlordiazepoxide (Librium) abolishes the tremor but has no effect on the threshold for photomyoclonus. Increasing the serum magnesium by intravenous and intramuscular injection results in a parallel increase in the threshold for photomyoclonus. The degree of hypomagnesemia in alcohol withdrawal has a correlation with the vulnerability to seizures and photomyoclonus. (From S. M. Wolfe and M. Victor, *Ann. N.Y. Acad. Sci.*[2101])

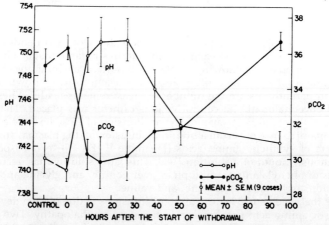

Figure 18-13. Changes in arterial pH and carbon dioxide tension in nine patients during alcohol withdrawal. Control values represent periods when the patients were not drinking, and time 0 refers to the time when patients were still intoxicated just prior to stopping drinking. Patients develop respiratory alkalemia within 8 to 10 hours after stopping heavy drinking. The severity of the blood gas changes has a correlation with the severity of the withdrawal symptoms. (From S. M. Wolfe, J. Mendelson, M. Ogata, M. Victor, W. Marshall, and N. Mello, *Trans. Assoc. Am. Physicians.*[2100])

MANAGEMENT

Management includes diagnosis and treatment of associated injuries and infections. Cardiovascular stability is maintained by adequate fluid and electrolyte replacement and judicious administration of vasopressors, if required.

Sedation is provided to reduce agitation and oxygen consumption and to facilitate nursing. Diazepam must be used with caution in patients with acute and chronic parenchymal liver disease. The half-life of diazepam is prolonged more than twofold in patients with cirrhosis as compared to age-matched controls (106 ± 15 vs 47 ± 14 hours). A decrease in the total plasma clearance of the drug is primarily responsible. The half-life of diazepam in patients with viral hepatitis is 74 ± 27 hours and in patients with chronic active hepatitis 60 ± 23 hours, as compared to a normal value in this age group of 33 ± 9 hours (Fig. 18-14).[1049]

A combination of paraldehyde and chloral hydrate appears to be superior to other forms of sedation.[204,724,1390] Hyperthermia is controlled with a cooling blanket, cool intravenous solutions, and, if necessary, muscle relaxants and controlled ventilation. Thiamine administration prevents precipitation of Wernicke's encephalopathy. Correction of respiratory alkalemia may have a salutary effect on withdrawal symptoms, but the evidence is inconclusive.[1990]

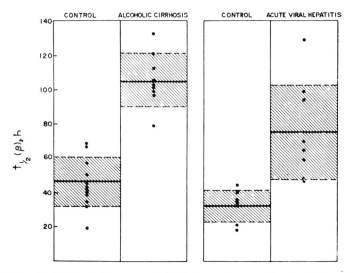

Figure 18-14. Half-life of diazepam (t ½·β) in patients with alcoholic cirrhosis or acute viral hepatitis compared to age-matched controls. *Points* represent individual patients. *Shaded area* shows the mean ± SD. Patients with alcoholic cirrhosis or acute viral hepatitis have a significantly longer half-life of diazepam than do age-matched controls ($P < 0.001$). (From U. Klotz, G. R. Avant, A. Hoyumpa, S. Schenker, and G. R. Wilkinson, *J. Clin. Invest.*[1049])

19

Problems of Renal Failure

The development of acute renal failure in a patient in respiratory failure is a serious occurrence that is still associated with a high mortality in spite of advances in methods of hemodialysis.

ETIOLOGY OF ACUTE RENAL FAILURE

Acute tubular necrosis is a syndrome of temporary loss of renal excretory function and is the most common cause of acute renal failure in patients in respiratory failure. The usual etiology of acute tubular necrosis is renal ischemia.[595] In the intensive care unit the most common reason for the development of acute tubular necrosis is a period of abnormal renal perfusion during a period of hypovolemic or septic shock. Myoglobinuria and hemoglobinuria also cause renal failure, as do toxic reactions to drugs. The mechanism of the production of acute tubular necrosis in patients exposed to nephrotoxic drugs is unclear. Renal vasoconstriction has been considered the primary mechanism, but this may not be true. Obstruction beyond the proximal tubule and leakage of filtrate probably play a greater role in producing oliguria than does vasoconstriction.[745]

RUPTURED ABDOMINAL AORTIC ANEURYSM

Renal and respiratory failure following resection of a ruptured abdominal aortic aneurysm is common. The renal failure is the result of a combination of several factors. Infrarenal cross-clamping can produce cholesterol embolization to the kidneys and turbulent flow to the kidneys. Hypotension is common in this type of patient and often occurs intraoperatively at the time of removal of the aortic cross-clamp.

GOODPASTURE'S SYNDROME

In our intensive care unit we have managed several patients with renal and respiratory failure secondary to Goodpasture's syndrome. The renal failure seen in Goodpasture's syndrome is a nephritis not unlike that seen in glomerulonephritis. Immunoglobulins have been demonstrated on the basement membranes of the glomeruli and alveoli, suggesting an immune mechanism responsible for the nephritis and the pulmonary hemorrhage.

OTHER CAUSES

The use of continuous positive pressure ventilation is associated with a redistribution of intrarenal blood flow, leading to a decreased excretion of water and sodium (see Chapter 3).[795] Acute hypoxia below an oxygen tension of 40 mm Hg (5.3 kPa) leads to a marked reduction in glomerular filtration rate, renal plasma flow, free water clearance, and sodium excretion. An oxygen tension of over 125 mm Hg (16.6 kPa) leads to significant reductions in glomerular filtration rate, renal plasma flow, free water clearance, and sodium excretion. Hypercapnia also produces similar reductions of renal function (Fig. 19-1).[1024] The use of epinephrine and norepinephrine can lead to marked reductions in renal function secondary to a worsened pattern of renal perfusion.

Obstructive uropathy is an infrequent cause of acute renal failure in patients in respiratory failure.

COURSE OF ACUTE TUBULAR NECROSIS

Oliguria occurs early in the course of acute tubular necrosis. Total anuria is uncommon. The urine is often bloody, and renal tubular cells can be seen on microscopic examination. The specific gravity of the urine is usually high. The sodium concentration of the urine is usually over 50 mEq per liter (50 mmol/l). During the first few days there is a progressive rise in blood urea nitrogen and serum creatinine. The rate of rise of blood urea nitrogen

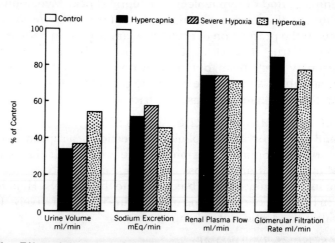

Figure 19-1.   Effect of changes in arterial oxygen tension and arterial carbon dioxide tension on renal function in patients in acute respiratory failure. Forty patients in acute respiratory failure were studied. An increase in carbon dioxide tension (hypercapnia) to a mean of 75 mm Hg (S.E. ± 1.5) (10.0 ± 0.2 kPa) resulted in marked reductions in urinary output and sodium excretion. Smaller reductions in renal plasma flow (RPF) and glomerular filtration rate (GFR) are seen. Severe hypoxia to an arterial oxygen tension of 40 mm Hg (5.3 kPa) or less resulted in significant reductions in urine volume and sodium excretion as well as lesser reductions in RPF and GFR. Hyperoxia with a Pa_{O_2} of more than 140 mm Hg (18.6 kPa) also lead to significant falls in urinary output and urinary sodium excretion. RPF and GFR were also slightly reduced. (From K. H. Kilburn and A. R. Dowell, *Arch. Intern. Med.*[1024] Copyright, 1971, American Medical Association.)

depends upon the catabolic rate of the patient. Serum potassium often increases during this time. A metabolic acidemia usually develops during the first few days of oliguria.

In the usual course of acute tubular necrosis the oliguria continues for 10–20 days. After three weeks there is rarely a return of renal function. If renal function does not return, the usual reason is that there is permanent cortical necrosis. The absence of renal function after three to four weeks does not, however, confirm the diagnosis of cortical necrosis. That diagnosis can be made only by renal biopsy. We have seen one patient who had acute tubular necrosis secondary to myoglobinuria following a crush injury and whose renal function returned to normal after five months of hemodialysis.

TREATMENT OF ACUTE TUBULAR NECROSIS

INITIAL TREATMENT

Initial treatment of acute tubular necrosis demands careful attention to fluid replacement. Since most episodes of acute tubular necrosis occur during a period of hypovolemia, the intravascular volume must be returned to normal. This must be done carefully, since excessive fluid administration will lead to pulmonary edema in a patient without renal function. For a patient in respiratory failure who develops acute tubular necrosis it is almost essential to use a Swan-Ganz catheter to monitor the intravascular volume and left ventricular function during fluid replacement.

Once the intravascular volume has been restored, the patient needs only enough fluid to replace his insensible and third space losses. The Swan-Ganz catheter is again helpful in the day-to-day fluid management of the patient in respiratory and renal failure.

Serum potassium is controlled by a potassium exchange resin (Kayexalate). To patients requiring intensive care who cannot take medication by mouth, this usually must be administered as a retention enema.

The administration of 100 gm of glucose daily prevents the breakdown of protein to a large degree. Many postoperative patients in respiratory failure and renal failure cannot be fed via the gastrointestinal tract. The intravenous use of essential L-amino acids and hypertonic glucose in patients with acute renal failure has been reported to be associated with more rapid improvement in renal function as well as with improved survival.[2,557] Silen has questioned the validity of these results.[1777] The severe complications of administration of solutions of amino acids and hypertonic glucose have been reviewed in Chapter 8. We therefore do not use this regimen routinely in the management of patients in renal and respiratory failure.

INDICATIONS FOR DIALYSIS

There are several indications for artificial dialysis in patients in acute renal failure. The major indication is the presence of uncontrollable hyperkalemia. Severe metabolic acidemia in a patient who cannot tolerate the sodium load associated with bicarbonate administration is best treated by dialysis.[595] Obtundation secondary to azotemia is another reason to begin dialysis. Pulmonary edema in renal failure is another indication. Dialysis is done as often as necessary to control the chemical abnormalities of renal failure. The patients whom we see in respiratory failure are often in a catabolic state and often require dialysis daily or every other day. Early institution of dialysis lessens mortality.

The choice of peritoneal dialysis or hemodialysis depends upon the condition of the patient. Peritoneal dialysis is often contraindicated for patients in respiratory failure postoperatively because of a recent abdominal operation or intraabdominal sepsis. In these cases, or in those in whom long-term or frequent dialysis seems likely, hemodialysis is the method of choice.

When renal function begins to return, there is usually a polyuric phase of acute tubular necrosis. During this time there must be careful replacement of urinary losses to prevent hypovolemia. During all phases of acute renal failure accurate records of daily body weights and summaries of intake and output must be kept. Care must also be taken to prevent urinary infection. This usually includes removal of the indwelling urinary catheter as soon as possible. The patient can be catheterized intermittently every 48–72 hours if necessary, as long as careful aseptic technique is used. When renal function returns, the patient usually will void spontaneously.

RESULTS OF DIALYSIS

The mortality of patients with chronic renal failure on maintenance hemodialysis is 10 percent per annum.[193,464] Acute renal failure requiring dialysis is usually associated with a higher in-hospital mortality. Postpartum acute renal failure carries a 15–20 percent mortality rate. Toxic nephropathy leading to acute renal failure has a 40 percent mortality. Renal failure developing in the postoperative period has a 47–67 percent mortality.[1036,1864]

The effect of the age of the patient on the mortality for renal failure is unclear. In our institution the mortality for patients over 60 years of age is 80 percent, but in another series of patients over the age of 70, the mortality was 57 percent.[2136]

The highest mortality for patients in acute renal failure is found in postoperative, posttraumatic, and septic patients. For patients who develop renal failure following resection of a ruptured abdominal aortic aneurysm the mortality is 94 percent.[1925] Among patients who have renal failure following major injuries there is a high incidence of respiratory failure; in this group of patients the mortality is 75 percent.

We have managed 60 patients in renal failure requiring dialysis during their stay in the Respiratory–Surgical Intensive Care Unit. Eighty-nine percent of these were postoperative or posttraumatic patients. There were three patients with Goodpasture's syndrome who were in renal and respiratory failure. All three patients underwent emergency bilateral nephrectomies. Two of the three survived. Eight patients developed renal and respiratory failure following surgery for ruptured abdominal aortic aneurysm and were treated with hemodialysis. Seven died. A ninth patient developed renal and respiratory failure following resection of a nonruptured abdominal aortic aneurysm. He also died (Fig. 19-2).

The overall mortality for patients in respiratory and renal failure is 80 percent. The most common etiology of the renal failure in this group of patients is acute tubular necrosis, which is responsible for 90 percent of the cases of renal failure. In our series the age of the patient does affect the mortality in patients with renal and respiratory failure treated with dialysis. The mortality for patients under 70 years of age is 68 percent, while the mortality for patients over 70 is 90 percent (Fig. 19-3).

TREATMENT OF THE ELDERLY

In spite of our most vigorous attempts we have made little headway in caring for elderly patients with respiratory and renal failure. The reasons for this are unclear. Elderly patients already have decreased renal function; it may be as little as 50 percent of normal function despite normal levels of

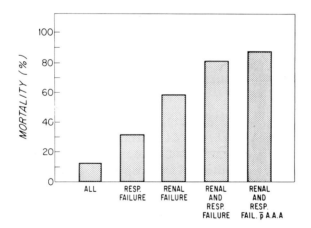

Figure 19-2. Mortality for Respiratory–Surgical Intensive Care Unit (R-SICU) patients over a period of 6½ years. *All* = mortality for all patients admitted to the unit. *Resp. Failure* = mortality for all patients treated for acute respiratory failure. *Renal Failure* = mortality for all patients in R-SICU treated with dialysis for acute renal failure. *Renal and Resp. Failure* = mortality for patients who had concurrent respiratory failure and acute renal failure requiring dialysis. *Renal and Resp. Fail. p̄ AAA* = mortality for patients with concurrent respiratory failure and acute renal failure requiring dialysis following the resection of an abdominal aortic aneurysm.

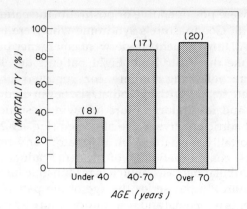

Figure 19-3. Effect of age on mortality of patients with concurrent respiratory failure and acute renal failure requiring dialysis. Of the 45 patients admitted to the R-SICU the eight patients under age 40 had the lowest mortality (36 percent). Nine out of ten patients over age 70 died. Increasing age is associated with increased mortality for patients with concurrent renal and respiratory failure. The number of patients in each group appears in parentheses.

blood urea nitrogen and serum creatinine.[1075]

Since the results of our present methods of therapy are disappointing, we should look for ways of improving the survival of these patients.[293] One answer may lie in more careful cardiovascular monitoring using the Swan-Ganz catheter, especially during hemodialysis. If the patient has an episode of hypotension during dialysis, this will contribute to further organ failure.

Since the mortality for patients in respiratory and renal failure is high, we are often faced with the question of discontinuation of hemodialysis or ventilation in this group of patients. This issue must be faced and a multitude of factors must be considered.[345,1788]

PREVENTION OF ACUTE RENAL FAILURE

The prevention of acute renal failure in the surgical patient should begin when the patient is admitted to the hospital. Correction of dehydration should start immediately. The choice of fluids is controversial. There is evidence to suggest that the use of Ringer's lactate plus red blood cells leads to less impairment of renal function than does the use of 5 percent albumin plus red blood cells in the resuscitation of hemorrhagic shock.[1770]

The patient who is not hypovolemic preoperatively should also be prehydrated to preserve renal function. Although the evidence is not clear, we feel that most patients undergoing major surgery should have several hundred milliliters of Ringer's lactate before surgery.

Careful monitoring of intravascular volume and of renal function is mandatory. The most useful guide is the hourly urine output, which should be monitored in all critically ill patients who are not anuric or oliguric.

The usual reason for a decrease in urinary output is hypovolemia. If one sees oliguria in the face of a normal or expanded intravascular volume it may be a sign of impending acute renal failure. The use of furosemide or ethacrynic acid in this situation may stimulate urinary output and possibly prevent renal failure. Incremental doses of furosemide are given up to a dose of 400 mg. If furosemide fails to produce a diuresis, it is often a sign that the patient will develop acute renal failure.[81] We have seen occasional patients in whom there is no response to 400 mg of furosemide but who have a diuresis in response to administration of ethacrynic acid.

Avoidance of potentially nephrotoxic drugs whenever possible is important in the prevention of acute renal failure. The nephrotoxic drugs most commonly used in our intensive care unit are gentamicin and kanamycin. The availability of facilities for measuring serum levels of gentamicin has decreased the incidence of gentamicin-induced acute renal failure.

Epinephrine and norepinephrine are potent renal vasoconstrictors and can lead to impairment of renal function. The frequent substitution of dopamine has decreased this problem.[728]

20

Respiratory Management of Peripheral Neurologic Disease

The respiratory management of neuromuscular disease requires considerable knowledge of neurology, although the actual respiratory management generally is relatively simple, since the lungs of the patients usually are normal. In this chapter we review those aspects of diseases of the peripheral nervous system that affect their respiratory management, and we discuss those peripheral nervous system diseases that have caused us significant respiratory problems in the last decade.

MYASTHENIA GRAVIS

Myasthenia gravis is a disease of unknown etiology, although much evidence suggests it to be an immunologic disorder involving acetylcholine receptor antibodies.[150,832] The mean age of onset is 26 years in women and 31 in men. The prognosis in general is better in women than in men. Except for congenital myasthenia, the younger the age the better the prognosis.[1511] It is essentially impossible to give an accurate prognosis, however, because we have seen old men who have required controlled ventilation for months have long-standing partial remissions later. A thymoma is present in 6 percent of cases, and then the prognosis is worsened but still not hopeless.[1511] Drug control of the disease, and thus weaning from the ventilator, generally is harder when a thymoma is present.

EMERGENCY TREATMENT

When the vital capacity of a patient with myasthenia gravis falls below 10–15 ml per kilogram of body weight or the patient is unable to generate an inspiratory force of at least −25 cm H_2O (−0.25 kPa), tracheal intubation is indicated. We feel that it is unwise to give an anticholinesterase drug such as edrophonium or neostigmine at this point, as respiratory failure may be produced, either because previous therapy with anticholinesterase drugs leads the additional drug to cause a muscarinic crisis, or because the accumulation of a serum factor renders the anticholinesterase drug ineffective.[150] Rather, the patient should have his tongue, pharynx , and larynx sprayed with a local anesthetic, and after oral or nasal intubation controlled ventilation should be started. After the patient has been moved to an area familiar with the management of respiratory failure and normal acid-base balance has been proved by blood gas measurements, then edrophonium

245

2.5 mg (per 60 kg of body weight) can be given, and vital capacity and inspiratory force serially measured.

Because of the ever-present risk of drowning from excess airway secretions due to a muscarinic crisis we feel that patients with borderline respiratory function ideally should not be given anticholinesterase drugs in doctors' offices, outpatient departments, or even emergency rooms.

MANAGEMENT OF MUSCARINIC CRISIS

Prevention

A myasthenic patient who develops an infection or who undergoes surgery frequently becomes extremely sensitive to anticholinesterase drugs. Thus it is important not to increase dosage at these times but rather to reduce it.[152] As noted above, when the respiratory status of the patient is in jeopardy, it is better to control ventilation rather than immediately give drugs. Of help in preventing muscarinic crises is the avoidance of the use of atropine in conjunction with anticholinesterase drugs.

Diagnosis

Patients with either muscarinic or myasthenic crisis have a weakness that causes pooling of secretions in the upper airway. The signs that one would expect of a muscarinic crisis from a knowledge of elementary pharmacology—namely, bradycardia, increased intestinal motility, and miosis—are almost invariably overridden by the sympathetic nervous system's response to fear and a frequently associated hypoxia.

Since administration of anticholinesterases is contraindicated in the presence of pooling of upper airway secretion, it is difficult to make a differential diagnosis between myasthenic and muscarinic crisis in patients who previously have had anticholinesterase therapy.

Differential Diagnosis

Apart from the difficulty of differentiating myasthenic from muscarinic crisis, myasthenia gravis poses other diagnostic problems. Myasthenia gravis is sometimes difficult to distinguish from pseudomyasthenia, also known as the Eaton-Lambert syndrome.[1088] This is a rare cause of muscle weakness that is associated with tumors, most commonly of the lung and large bowel. In contradistinction to myasthenia gravis, repetitive exercising of muscles by patients with pseudomyasthenia generally makes them stronger, not weaker. A test dose of edrophonium intravenously, 2.5 mg for an adult, is said to help in the differentiation, but in our experience patients with myasthenia gravis may show no improvement or worsen, while patients with pseudomyasthenia may improve their muscle strength. However, these unexpected results are rare, and at least 80 percent of the time we expect patients with myasthenia gravis, who have had no anticholinesterase drugs for at least the previous six hours, to improve their muscle strength. In our experience the use of edrophonium to diagnose pseudomyasthenia is not useful. A placebo-type response usually gives slightly increased muscle power after the intravenous injection of the edrophonium.

LONG-TERM DRUG TREATMENT

The use of alternate-day high dose corticosteroid treatment seems to have lowered the incidence of respiratory failure due to myasthenia gravis.[2029] It is not the purpose of this monograph to assess the therapeutic modalities used in the long-term treatment of myasthenia gravis.[647] Currently we employ thymectomy for most patients who have had respiratory failure or seem likely to develop it, provided they are under 60 years of age.[377] For those over 60 years of age thymectomy is of essentially no benefit except for thymoma removal, because thymic tissue is generally absent.[1510]

RESPIRATORY MANAGEMENT OF SURGERY IN
PATIENTS WITH MYASTHENIA GRAVIS

The respiratory management of a myasthenic patient undergoing thymectomy is essentially the same as for a myasthenic patient having any other type of surgery. Patients should be brought to elective surgery after the withholding of all anticholinesterase medication for at least 12 hours. The reason for this is that the tissue damage of surgery causes an unpredictable increase in sensitivity to anticholinesterase drugs.[152] Prior to the early 1960's it was fairly common to see a patient die postoperatively of a muscarinic crisis, on occasion one caused by anticholinesterase drugs given as part of the patient's premedication. Our practice is to admit patients to the Respiratory–Surgical Intensive Care Unit the night before surgery and to monitor their vital capacity. If it falls below 15 ml per kilogram of body weight, they are intubated with a tracheal tube after careful spraying of the larynx and pharynx with a local anesthetic without epinephrine. They are then ventilated with a tidal volume of 10 ml per kilogram of body weight at a frequency adjusted to maintain normocapnia until the time of surgery. Naturally the possible need for intubation and ventilation is explained to the patient beforehand.

ANESTHETIC MANAGEMENT

An intravenous thiobarbiturate provides a suitable induction. Succinylcholine is avoided, unless a life-threatening emergency occurs to block the upper airway. The reason for avoidance of succinylcholine is that its metabolites may have a curare-like action and can cause prolonged muscular paralysis. Prolonged paralysis occurs less than 10 percent of the time when succinylcholine is used on myasthenic patients.

Curare

To all intents and purposes curare should be avoided for myasthenic patients. However, good results have been claimed, with subsequent remission of myasthenic crisis, from the use of approximately a fiftieth of normal doses.[343] In our hands these results are indistinguishable from the same pattern of normal controlled ventilation without any drugs at all.

Use of Curare When the Patient Is Not Known to Be Myasthenic

Results of the use of curare-like drugs in patients who are in remission are unpredictable. In such patients we have seen 9 mg intravenous *d*-tubocurarine cause respiratory failure lasting over a week. We have also seen a normal nonmyasthenic response to 30 mg of intravenous curare. On one occasion, after a normal nonmyasthenic response to curare, a patient developed the signs and symptoms of fulminant myasthenia gravis six weeks later. In summary, we now advise our anesthetic colleagues to try to avoid the use of muscle relaxants altogether in patients with a history of myasthenia. An inhalational agent like halothane, in combination with the relaxing effect of the myasthenia, provides quite sufficient relaxation for all types of surgery.

POSTOPERATIVE MANAGEMENT

We withhold all anticholinesterase drugs until the fourth or fifth post-operative day, then if necessary restart them with extreme caution.[377] Surprisingly, when drugs are withheld, surgery of any type often seems to make the myasthenia better temporarily. If alternate-day steroid therapy is to be restarted in the immediate postoperative period, it is extremely helpful to have a sequential plot of the blood corticosteroid levels that provided optimal control of the myasthenia preoperatively. Surgery affects endogenous corticosteroid function, and the increased levels of corticosteroids followed by the postoperative decline may be the reason for the frequency of postsurgical remissions of myasthenia gravis.[1977]

In the postoperative period it is also important to avoid or at least minimize the use of antibiotics with a neuromuscular blocking action. We have seen a myasthenic crisis remit when neomycin was discontinued.

Apart from problems with anticholinesterase drugs, antibiotics, and the regulation of corticosteroid dosage, myasthenic patients after elective surgery present only the fairly simple problems of management of decreased muscle power and its effect on ventilation. Criteria for weaning are exactly the same as for other patients (Chap. 11).

EMERGENCY SURGERY

When surgery cannot be postponed for six hours from the time of the last dose of anticholinesterase drug, then one may find oneself treating a muscarinic crisis. The same principles apply as in the emergency room. Control ventilation with a tracheal tube, suction the patient, do not give atropine, and titrate levels of oxygen and ventilation by monitoring of blood gases. In the last decade we have not encountered a myasthenic patient with a need for such urgent surgery.

OBSTETRICS AND MYASTHENIA GRAVIS

Pregnancy can improve myasthenia gravis. Indeed, transfusions of pregnant women's blood once were used to treat myasthenic crises. None of the drugs used to treat myasthenia gravis is contraindicated on the grounds of teratogenicity, although germine diacetate does not appear to have been given to pregnant women, and should not be.[647]

Uterine contraction is not affected by myasthenia gravis, and labor will progress normally. Low outlet forceps are useful, however. Approximately 12 percent of myasthenic mothers give birth to a baby that is myasthenic (Fig. 20-1). Consequently facilities for intubation and ventilation of the newborn baby must be available before delivery of all myasthenic mothers.

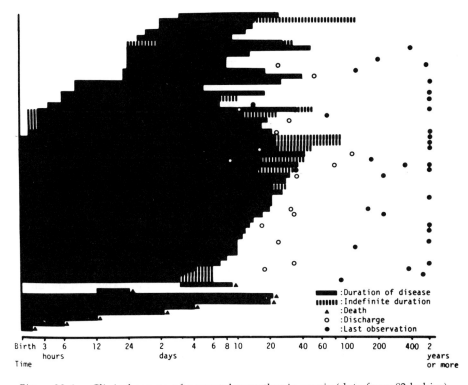

Figure 20-1. Clinical course of neonatal myasthenia gravis (data from 82 babies). Onset is often at birth. Onset on the third day after birth is uncommon, and onset never occurs after the fourth day. Length of the disease is shown by the *shaded area.* Indefinite duration means that definite information was not available as to when the baby recovered, but the *hatch marks* represent a best estimate. *Open circles* show day of discharge from hospital. Every patient who did not die recovered. Only one relapsed. The courses of those who died (*solid triangles*) are shown at the bottom of the figure. (From T. Namba, S. B. Brown, and D. Grob, *Pediatrics.*[1409])

At present we have no way of knowing which babies will be affected with myasthenia. There are two types: neonatal and, more rarely, congenital myasthenia.

NEONATAL MYASTHENIA

As we have mentioned, neonatal myasthenia is found in 12 percent of babies born to myasthenic mothers. In contrast to the situation with adult myasthenia, baby boys are as likely to get the disease as girls.[1409] In two-thirds of affected babies onset of the disease is either at birth or within a few hours of birth. The latest reported onset is 3 days of age.[1409] If the baby is kept alive, recovery from neonatal myasthenia is almost always complete within a month. The mean duration of the disease is 18 days, with a range from 5 to 47 days (Fig. 20-1). Respiratory difficulty occurs in 65 percent of babies with neonatal myasthenia.[1409] Other symptoms are similar to adult myasthenia, but ptosis occurs only in 15 percent of babies. Eighty percent of babies receive either neostigmine or pyridostigmine. These drugs are best given 15 minutes prior to feeding in a usual dose of either 0.1 mg neostigmine methylsulfate or 0.15 mg pyridostigmine bromide intramuscularly. The dose should be reduced and the interval lengthened as the baby recovers. Medication should be sufficient only to assure adequate respiration and swallowing. It is far better to resort to controlled ventilation than to overdose the baby. The mean period of need for anticholinesterase drugs is 28 ± 11 days (95 percent confidence limits).[1409]

Weakness of the baby due to anticholinesterase medication of the mother has been described.[182] According to Blackhall and her colleagues, if the baby is given edrophonium, neostigmine, or pyridostigmine under these circumstances, its weakness will increase and it will develop signs of a muscarinic (cholinergic) crisis.[182,1631] Treatment is then similar to that we have described for adult patients with muscarinic crisis. Ventilation should be controlled and secretions suctioned with careful cardiovascular monitoring. Recovery occurs within a week, and the baby will develop normally.

If doubt exists about the effect of cholinergic drugs, electromyographic tracings should document the baby's response. According to Blackhall the timing of onset of weakness is due to several mechanisms. Weakness comes on when the baby's anticholinesterase drug levels fall and the baby's cholinesterase activities have risen from low levels at birth to high levels. The neuromuscular blocking action of an anticholinesterase drug is distinct from its enzyme inhibitory action. At low drug concentrations the blocking action is overcome by the increase in neuromuscular transmission produced by the cholinesterase inhibition. At high drug levels there comes a limit to the facilitation of neuromuscular transmission but not to the neuromuscular blocking action of the anticholinesterase drugs. Recovery from the blocking action takes place much more slowly than recovery from cholinesterase inhibition. At birth, according to Blackhall and her colleagues, maternal anticholinesterase drugs have two opposing actions on the baby. They impair neuromuscular transmission but counterbalance this by inhibition of cholinesterase. Neuromuscular weakness comes on later, as the inhibition of cholinesterase wanes and the anticholinesterase-induced block persists.[182]

These theories of Blackhall's group may be valid, but none has yet shown that anticholinesterase drugs used in the treatment of myasthenia gravis cross the placenta. These drugs are quaternary ammonium compounds. Blackhall and her colleagues base their theories on indirect evidence of transfer of pyridostigmine to only one baby.[182,1631] Moreover, neonatal myasthenia is known to occur even when the mother does not receive any anticholinesterase medication during pregnancy. Babies delivered of myasthenic mothers on anticholinesterase drugs who develop respiratory failure immediately after birth should have controlled ventilation for several hours. Then the electromyographic response to 0.1 mg of intravenous edrophonium should be tested. If it is equivocal or shows a worsening of neuromuscular transmission, pyridostigmine or neostigmine is not given but controlled ventilation continued until the baby recovers. If definite improvement in strength occurs after edrophonium, then neostigmine or edrophonium can be given in the manner we have outlined. For testing it is best to transfer these babies to centers where personnel are thoroughly familiar with both neonatal controlled ventilation and electromyography. Ideally the baby should be picked up by members of the team that are to continue therapy. As we have indicated, after the initial crucial weeks the baby will have a normal life expectancy and essentially no increased risk of again getting weakness from myasthenia.[1409]

CONGENITAL MYASTHENIA GRAVIS

Congenital myasthenia gravis, by contrast with the neonatal form, occurs only in the newborn of nonmyasthenic mothers. It is a persistent disease which is probably due to a rare recessive genetic defect.[1409] The incidence of congenital myasthenia gravis is much lower than the incidence of neonatal myasthenia gravis. In one survey of over 600 myasthenic patients only 1 had congenital myasthenia.[1409] Of course this 0.2 percent incidence may have been due to lack of diagnosis and early death. The treatment of congenital myasthenia follows the principles we have outlined for other forms of myasthenia gravis.

IDIOPATHIC POLYNEURITIS

Idiopathic polyneuritis is also known as postinfectious polyneuritis, Guillain-Barré disease, and Landry's ascending paralysis. Idiopathic polyneuritis is a disease of unknown etiology.[838] It is not a common disease, the largest reported series of cases with respiratory failure being around a hundred. We have had experience in the last twenty years with controlled ventilation in 70 patients. Provided the patient is kept alive, neurologic recovery is always complete in our experience, although cases of relapse have been described. The main cause of permanent sequelae is joint contractures.

NATURAL HISTORY OF THE DISEASE

All ages and both sexes are equally susceptible to the disease. There is a suggestion that idiopathic polyneuritis is more likely to occur after viral infections such as influenza, and we have observed slightly more than the expected number of cases during influenza outbreaks. Although the paralysis is likely to be ascending and symmetric, this pattern is by no means invariable. Patients who develop the disease get an increasing paralysis for weeks, days, or even months. They then either clearly stabilize and, if kept alive, get better, or they go through an imperceptible period of stabilization and recovery follows. In our experience the time course of the worsening of the paralysis is unpredictable. For instance, we have seen a woman who had onset of paralysis in the ankles and then paralysis of the knees over a month later but who was in respiratory failure within 24 hours of her knees becoming paralyzed! Consequently we advise the hospitalization of all patients with idiopathic polyneuritis. Early in their course we tell them about techniques of artificial ventilation and that approximately half our patients with their disease go on to respiratory failure. If we think it likely that they are going into respiratory failure, then we introduce the patient to a former patient now recovered who was ventilated when he had the disease. We and our former patient stress that essentially everyone with the disease gets better, but that the disease may last many months. Once the disease starts getting better, relapses almost never occur.

INDICATIONS FOR ARTIFICIAL VENTILATION

The indications for artificial ventilation are exactly the same as in patients with other diseases; that is, vital capacity of less than 15 ml per kilogram of body weight or inspiratory force numerically less than -25 cm H_2O (-0.25 kPa). The day after tracheal intubation we perform a tracheostomy. Since the median time of ventilation in our series is a month, it is unwise to risk traumatizing the larynx by leaving in a tracheal tube.

DIAGNOSIS

The natural history of the disease is generally characteristic. In addition, in over 80 percent of our cases the cerebrospinal fluid has had elevated levels of proteins without an abnormal number of cells. If this is not found on initial lumbar puncture, it usually is true on subsequent lumbar puncture. Lack of this finding, however, does not mean that the patient does not have idiopathic polyneuritis.

MANAGEMENT OF PATIENT WITH HIGH PARALYSIS

Circulatory Problems

Hypertension is not uncommon, but in our experience blood pressure usually returns to normal as the disease progresses, and ganglionic blockers are not necessary. What is even more common and far more dangerous is the sudden hypotension caused by overenthusiastic turning of the patient. Patients with idiopathic polyneuritis have an interruption of the autonomic reflex arcs controlling the circulation.[1825,2037] The lesion is generally on the efferent side. The way we minimize these hypotensive episodes is twofold. We place a central venous pressure line and give albumin or other colloid to maintain a central venous pressure of approximately 5 cm H_2O (0.05 kPa). Nurses should be carefully instructed in the problems of circulatory homeostasis in idiopathic polyneuritis.[2037]

Sweating

Patients with this disease are usually unable to sweat except over very small portions of their bodies. They become poikilothermic because of their inability to sweat and their loss of muscle mass, which makes them susceptible to cold. Temperature should be monitored frequently or continuously and the environmental temperature changed as necessary. Loss of sweating is due to lesions either in the brainstem or in the efferent nervous pathways.[1825]

Gastrointestinal Tract

Normally patients with idiopathic polyneuritis can be fed orally either with a soft diet or by tube feedings. But as the disease progresses and muscle wasting becomes more profound, we have seen the development (in three patients) of obstruction of the third part of the duodenum by the superior mesenteric artery. The reflux can be cured by a gastrojejunostomy. Nursing the patient on one or other side continuously does not cure this.

Other problems with the gastrointestinal tract are increased gastric acidity, which is treated with antacid infusion, and fecal impaction. On occasion we have found severe circulatory disturbances during fecal disimpaction, and we have had to revert to spinal anesthesia to prevent these responses.

Sensory and Sympathetic Nervous System Lesions

Generally the sensory loss is less widespread than the motor loss, and in some patients we have seen no sensory loss whatsoever except for joint proprioception. Sympathetic nervous system lesions are most common in the sympathetic fibers that run in the involved peripheral nerves.

Joints

A relative or other interested person, such as a medical student, should be instructed by a physical therapist to take every paralyzed joint through its full range of movements as often as possible each day. Moreover each joint should be checked by a physician at least twice a week. Early in our series we forgot to passively exercise the jaw of one patient, and fusion of the temporomandibular joint was a serious sequel that required operative correction.

Idiopathic Polyneuritis Affecting the Cranial Nerves

When disease reaches this level, as it has done in 5 percent of our patients, we have found that tarsorrhaphy is the only satisfactory way to protect the eyés. We have tried cortical-evoked responses by computer scanning of electroencephalograms to provide a system of communication with the totally paralyzed patient. Results have been equivocal, but the patient seemed reassured by the monitoring of his brain waves.

Recovery Phase

Remyelination occurs from the central nervous system outward, so that the longest peripheral nerves are the last to recover. Consequently intercostal function always returns before phrenic nerve function. Patients who do not have severe preexisting lung disease generally can be weaned before phrenic function has returned, if, as is most likely, intercostal function has returned. Ankle function is generally very late in returning, and physiotherapy supervision must be excellent after discharge from respiratory care.

Drugs in Idiopathic Polyneuritis

Once respiratory failure has supervened, we find steroids have no beneficial effect on the course of the disease. The mean time of controlled ventilation is four weeks for our patients on steroids and the same for those not receiving them.[152] Since stress ulceration is more common in patients receiving steroids, the steroids should be stopped, at least by the time the patient goes into respiratory failure.

We do not routinely employ antibiotics. Chest infections should not be a problem if respiratory care is adequate, and urinary tract infections can be prevented by intermittent catheterization with small catheters. In summary the only drugs we commonly employ in the treatment of idiopathic polyneuritis are gastric antacids, if indicated. With this regimen all patients should recover, unless preexisting disease causes fatal complications (Fig. 20-2).[845]

BOTULISM

Approximately 30 patients a year in the United States develop paralytic botulism.[1494] Botulinal toxins interfere with the release of acetylcholine at the neuromuscular junction, probably by binding acetylcholine at or near the site of its release. Overall mortality in this century has been 55 percent. Recently with improved respiratory care mortality has fallen.[1957] With correct and prompt diagnosis botulism should no longer be a fatal disease.

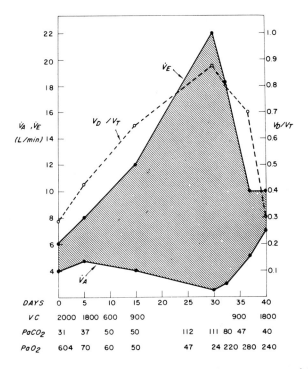

Figure 20-2. Increase in ventilation requirements in respiratory failure due to pneumonia in a 44-year-old man with idiopathic polyneuritis. On admission to hospital his vital capacity (VC) had been reduced to 2 liters by motor paralysis. Gram-negative pneumonia resistant to antibiotics supervened. On the thirtieth hospital day, despite minute ventilation ($\dot{V}E$) of more than 20 liters per minute provided by a constant-volume ventilator, alveolar ventilation ($\dot{V}A$) was only 2.5 liters per minute, and deadspace-to-tidal-volume ratio (VD/VT) rose almost to 0.9. *Shaded area* = deadspace ventilation.

For two weeks this man was ventilated with 100% oxygen and heavily sedated to decrease oxygen consumption. Even so the arterial oxygen tension (Pa_{O_2}) was consistently under 50 mm Hg (6.7 kPa). This 60 percent intrapulmonary right-to-left shunt diminished in the second month of his hospital stay, as he recovered from both pneumonia and idiopathic polyneuritis. VC (in ml) could not be measured when the patient was unconscious between the twentieth and thirtieth hospital day, but VC and polyneuritis were improving before the pneumonia worsened. (From J. Hedley-Whyte.[845] Reprinted by permission from the *New England Journal of Medicine* 279:1152–1158, 1968.)

The neurotoxins of *Clostridium botulinum* are proteins of six types, A to F. Human botulism occurs with each of the types but is commonest with A, B, and E. Antitoxin to one type is in general ineffective in neutralizing the others, but there is some cross-neutralization of types C, D, and E and of the A and B subtypes of C. The serum of patients with the disease can be injected into mice to confirm the diagnosis, the mice dying within 24 hours.

CLINICAL COURSE

After contaminated food is eaten the usual incubation period is 18–36 hours. Botulism due to wound infections and even from inhalation of the toxin has been described. Involvement of the cranial nerves often starts early in the disease. Ptosis, diplopia, and ophthalmoplegia are common. Dysphagia, dysarthria, and inability to protect the upper airway follow. Paralysis usually descends. The CSF is normal and mentation clear if normal arterial blood gases are maintained. Sensory perception is unimpaired; deep tendon reflexes become depressed but remain equal. Usually the pulse rate is normal. Nausea, vomiting, and diarrhea are quite common. Prolonged ileus is an invariable complication of severe cases. Provided adequate ventilatory support is provided and the circulation carefully monitored, recovery of spontaneous ventilation should be complete within two weeks to three months. Easy fatigability for several months is common after respiratory failure caused by botulism.[325] If joint contractures are prevented, permanent sequelae do not occur.

TREATMENT

Adequate controlled ventilation, gastric antacid therapy, blood volume replacement, and supportive management of adynamic ileus are the most important aspects of treatment. Guanidine has been used in the treatment of botulism, but in our opinion its doubtful efficacy and serious side effects do not make it a worthwhile drug (Fig. 20-3).[326,605] Guanidine must be administered orally via a nasogastric tube, as it is too irritating for parenteral use. Guanidine damages the gastrointestinal mucosa. Diarrhea and bleeding are common with its use. Hyperirritability, twitching, tremors, and even convulsions have been reported.[1494] Neurophysiologic studies of muscle response to stimuli show that respiratory muscles respond less to guanidine than do other muscles.[327]

Penicillin should be given in moderate doses to eliminate any clostridia. All antitoxins to the various types of *Clostridium botulinum* are made in horses. Thus whenever they are used in patients, there is the possibility of anaphylactic reactions. The antitoxin administered initially is usually trivalent (types A, B, and E). It is used until the specific type of *Clostridium botulinum* causing the disease is known. The antitoxins are available from the National Center for Disease Control, Atlanta, where emergency phones are manned day and night (present telephones: 404-633-3311 by day and 633-2176 by night). We recommend that antitoxins be given intravenous-

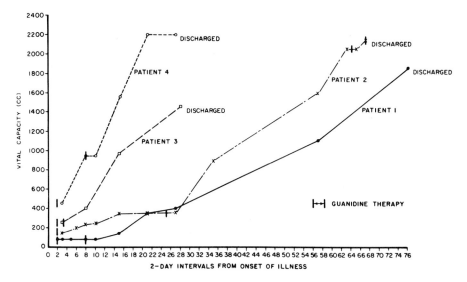

Figure 20-3. Vital capacity measurements in four family members with Type A botulism who were treated with guanidine. There is no alteration in the slope of the vital capacity curves when guanidine therapy is begun. Discontinuation of guanidine therapy did not result in a fall in vital capacity in any patient. (From G. A. Faich, R. W. Graebner, and S. Sato.[605] Reprinted by permission from the *New England Journal of Medicine* 285:773–776, 1971.)

ly and intramuscularly, 1 vial (8 ml) each, and repeated in 2–4 hours if symptoms persist. Twenty-four hours later sera should be retested for circulating toxin. If it is found at this time, the specific antitoxin should be given. With the measures that we have outlined and prompt diagnosis the mortality of botulism should, as we have mentioned, be low.

POLIOMYELITIS

Over the past few years very few cases of poliomyelitis have been reported in the developed world. There are approximately ten cases a year of paralytic poliomyelitis in Great Britain and a similar number in the United States. To maintain this satisfactory state of affairs high immunization rates should be achieved. At present they are not. In a recent survey, while 52 percent of children had received poliomyelitis vaccine, only 40 percent had antibody to all three types of poliovirus; 54 percent of children surveyed who had been immunized lacked triple immunity.[1610]

CLINICAL SIGNS

The clinical picture of acute anterior poliomyelitis is variable. Onset is more common in the summer. Initial symptoms are headache; pain in muscles, especially those of the head, neck, and back; vomiting; and fever (the minor illness). Paralyses may follow in a matter of hours to two to three days (the major illness). The paralyses develop rapidly and most commonly affect the limb muscles but of course may paralyze respiration and swallowing. The paralysis is typically flaccid of the lower motor neuron type. The full extent of the paralysis is rapidly realized, usually within 24 hours after the onset of paralysis, but in very severe cases the paralysis may continue to increase for several days.[70]

NEUROPATHOLOGIC PICTURE

Poliomyelitis affects the whole of the central nervous system, but the worst damage is concentrated in the motor cells of the anterior horn. Poliomyelitis also causes an inflammatory reaction of medullary tissue. In the acute stage of poliomyelitis the cerebrospinal fluid shows an increase in mononuclear and polymorphonuclear cells and an excess of protein. Differential blood count shows polymorphonuclear leukocytosis. After a few days inflammation of the central nervous system subsides and infected anterior horn cells show permanent damage. Paralyzed muscles begin to undergo atrophy, but neighboring muscles may be unaffected. Muscles may be partially paralyzed, some fibers being affected while others are not.

We have considered the neuropathology of poliomyelitis in some detail, because the management of the disease stems from the pathology. Another reason is that, although it is now such an uncommon disease, miniepidemics do still occur. In the last four years we have seen members of a business delegation being ventilated for acute poliomyelitis after going to Africa unimmunized. Schoolboys who had been brought up as Christian Scientists also recently required controlled ventilation for acute poliomyelitis.

TREATMENT

During the first few hours of poliomyelitis the patient may need treatment for hyperthermia and cerebral edema. The treatment of hyperthermia depends on its severity. For fever below 39°C without cerebral edema aspirin and a cooling blanket may suffice. For temperatures over 40°C, especially if cerebral edema is present, the patient should have his or her trachea intubated and should then be ventilated with a volume-constant ventilator. Steroids may have a deleterious effect on the course of acute poliomyelitis. Intravenous solutions at a temperature of 4–10°C should be started, together with a short-acting diuretic substance like mannitol. Shivering as detected by the electrocardioscope should be abolished by the use of 3–6-mg doses of *d*-tubocurarine. If controlled ventilation is started and shivering stopped, the temperature will almost certainly start to come down.

Early in the course of acute poliomyelitis clotting factors should be checked, as disseminated intravascular coagulation can be associated with medullary poliomyelitis. In addition antacid therapy should be started.

If cerebral edema and extreme hyperpyrexia are not present, the indications for tracheal intubation and controlled ventilation are the same as for any other neurologic disease. One should be prepared to intubate the trachea of a patient who, due to localized bulbar poliomyelitis, cannot swallow his saliva and upper airway secretions.[2014] Especially in children localized bulbar palsy may be difficult to spot and be manifested only by a refusal of food. The significance of the refusal may be misinterpreted.

In the majority of patients the extent of paralysis starts to diminish after the first week, as edema in the spinal cord subsides and some anterior horn cells recover function. Good function sometimes returns to patients who were hopelessly paralyzed at the height of their disease. Thus once a patient has an oral or nasotracheal tube in position, one should not rush to tracheostomy.[760] Vital capacity may recover to above 10 ml per kilogram of body weight within a few days and the patient may be able to be extubated.

If a patient is first seen unconscious due to acute poliomyelitis, it is most likely that the unconsciousness is due either to blood gas abnormalities or to cerebral edema. Appropriate treatment should be instituted at once. However, extreme medullary and other CNS invasion by poliovirus can probably on rare occasions cause unconsciousness. Such patients have marked vascular instability and require placement of intraarterial lines and Swan-Ganz catheters. Recovery of consciousness usually follows correction of blood gases, CNS edema, and circulatory instability.

CHRONIC POLIOMYELITIS

If a muscle shows signs of activity within a month of the start of the acute stage of poliomyelitis, that muscle will be useful. If no activity is apparent after three months, then that muscle will never function. Patients do not improve in muscle power in the second and subsequent years after acute poliomyelitis. These guidelines help plan therapy of the chronic respiratory cripple.

Vital Capacity Above 10 ml per Kilogram of Body Weight

If the patient has no preexisting chronic lung disease and is free of pulmonary infection the tracheostomy can be allowed to close, provided the patient's vital capacity is above 10 ml per kilogram of body weight. With this level of vital capacity alveolar hypoventilation should not be a problem. With an intact trachea the distribution of tidal volume within the lung is more favorable than through a tracheostomy. The result is that despite the increase in anatomic deadspace caused by the tracheostomy closure the level of alveolar ventilation is unchanged.[668] Thus we unequivocally suggest allowing the tracheostomy to close in patients whose total vital capacity is above 10 ml per kilogram of body weight and whose forced expiratory volume in the first second of expiration is greater than 70 percent of the total vital capacity.

Vital Capacity Below 3–4 ml per Kilogram of Body Weight

In patients whose vital capacity is below 3–4 ml per kilogram of body weight the tracheostomy should be left intact. These patients, when stable, should be given a ventilator suitable for home use. The Oxford group use a Radcliffe Respiration Pump driven by a 60 ampere-hour 12-volt storage battery that will last 24 hours.[1400,1825] Patients with vital capacities below 3–4 ml per kilogram of body weight can be cared for at home. They require a portable suction apparatus and a mobile electric battery-operated chair or bed.

Generally a few muscles below the neck can contract but not strongly enough to allow use of switches. The patient can speak, however, provided the cuff of his tracheostomy is not inflated; mouth movements and intellect generally are unimpaired. Most patients are young or middle-aged, and frequently they show incredible mental resilience in the face of their respiratory paralysis. They must be helped to earn a living if humanly possible. The first step is to teach them to use electric typewriters, computers, and touch-dial telephones by using a light hammer held in the mouth. Radio and television can also be operated in the same way but do not bolster morale as much as activities the patient does for himself.

We do not think tank respirators (iron lungs) are useful for the patient with vital capacities below 3–4 ml per kilogram of body weight, because the iron lung is terribly confining, nursing is most difficult, and mortality is higher in this group of patients than with IPPV. We have not used a tank respirator on a long-term basis in the last 15 years, but if a patient is stable in a tank we do not advocate change. Essentially all such patients whom we have seen in recent years in tank ventilators have had a vital capacity between 3 and 10 ml per kilogram of body weight.

Vital Capacity 3–10 ml per Kilogram of Body Weight

Patients with vital capacities above 3 ml per kilogram of body weight and below 10 ml are the most difficult to manage. They can be independent of a ventilator for variable periods of time but require periods of controlled or assisted ventilation. Decisions have to be made as to whether to allow the tracheostomy to close and what type of ventilator should be used. As a first step we would suggest that the tracheostomy be allowed to close in hospital and a cuirass ventilator be tried. It is generally safest to have the patient sleep in the functioning cuirass at nights. The cuirass should be set so that the patient's arterial carbon dioxide tension is maintained at between 40 and 55 mm Hg (5.3–7.3 kPa) as tested by arterial samples. If the cuirass cannot do this and arterial carbon dioxide tension rises above 55 mm Hg (7.3 kPa), then the patient has to sleep in a tank respirator and cannot be discharged from the hospital.[439] If repeated trials of a cuirass are unsuccessful, we would suggest it is better to reopen the patient's tracheostomy and give him a portable electrically driven ventilator, as described for the patient with a vital capacity below 3–4 ml per kilogram of body weight.

We do treat patients who use cuirass ventilators very successfully at home, however. Their spouses put them in the cuirass at night or when they get tired. The patient can be taught to get a pretty good estimate of a sudden rise in arterial carbon dioxide tension by evaluating changes in his own pulse, blood pressure, and subjective well-being. The patient is frequently capable of a sedentary job. Problems arise, however, when the patient gets any chest infection. The patient must then be admitted to the hospital on an urgent basis. With chest physiotherapy, postural drainage, diuretics, and antibiotics it may be possible to avoid reintubation. When lungs become stiffened by infection, cuirass ventilators are useless and dangerous, and we resort to conventional intermittent positive pressure ventilation initially by a tracheal tube. If the infection does not clear up, the tracheostomy has to be reopened.

The respiratory cripple living at home has to be taught to eat sensibly and to take antacids for heartburn;[42] otherwise gastrointestinal hemorrhage is a problem. We also teach the patient's spouse the rudiments of chest physiotherapy and respiratory care nursing.

TETANUS

Tetanus can be prevented by active immunization, but once contracted it is a difficult disease to treat adequately. More than a half century ago H. R. Dean, later Professor of Pathology at Cambridge, pointed out the overactivity of the sympathetic nervous system in tetanus.[487] His patients were mostly survivors of the battle of the Somme. Only recently have we been able adequately to treat this autonomic dysfunction.[1569] It must not be thought all patients with tetanus should be treated alike, however. The management of a severe case is very different from management of the mild form of the disease. Accordingly we will divide our discussion arbitrarily into treatment that all patients require and that is sufficient for those only mildly affected, and those regimens we recommend for mild, moderate, and severe tetanus.

SYMPTOMS AND SIGNS

Tetanus is a self-limiting disease, so if the patient can be kept alive, he or she will recover. For children and adults treated with modern methods the mortality should not exceed 20 percent. Manifestations of tetanus are probably due to overactivity of somatic motor neurons induced by the neurotoxin of *Clostridium tetani.*

GENERAL TREATMENT AND TREATMENT OF MILD CASES

In mild cases there may be only a small amount of generalized stiffness, with greater stiffness of the injured limb. Trismus may be intermittent and not severe. Opisthotonos, dysphagia, and generalized spasms are not present. In this type of case, and for all more severe attacks of tetanus, we recommend excision of the wound or puncture site. Animal experiments show that there are many times the lethal dose of toxin at the site of inoculation after the onset of symptoms.[661]

Antitetanus serum given after the onset of symptoms significantly reduces mortality, as was shown in a West African and West Indian study.[245]

In countries where many patients have received antitetanus serum, more serum may be ineffective because of antibody response to the previous inoculation.[2113] Notwithstanding this, we do suggest the use of human antitetanus serum as soon as possible in the course of the disease. Penicillin or cycline-type antibiotics should be used in large doses, as they are active against *Clostridium tetani*. All patients who develop tetanus should be anticoagulated, as otherwise the incidence of death from pulmonary embolism is 5 percent. The above measures, debridement, antitetanus serum, anticoagulation, and antibiotics should be used to treat all cases of tetanus. In addition mild cases should be admitted to the hospital, and, if needed, barbiturate sedation should be employed. Gastric antacids should be given. Patients should not be nursed in a dark room; rather, they should be where facilities for tracheal intubation are instantly available.

TREATMENT OF MODERATE CASES

Moderate tetanus is manifested by dysphagia and generalized stiffness, with moderately severe trismus and with head retraction. In treating such a case we used to employ intragastric mephenesin, but we found its use associated with gastrointestinal upsets and development of a metabolic acidemia.[33] Consequently we now sedate the patient with barbiturates, monitor arterial pressure and blood gases and, if we are at all worried about the upper airway, proceed to tracheostomy after orotracheal intubation. If at any time the patient develops hypertension or arrhythmias or acidemia, then full therapy as for a severe case of tetanus is started.

TREATMENT OF SEVERE CASES

Severe tetanus will frequently show opisthotonos and generalized spasms with cyanosis, but these severe manifestations of tetanus generally follow the development of arrhythmias and hypertension (Fig. 20-4). Ideally a patient with tetanus should not be allowed to get generalized spasms or opisthotonos. Controlled ventilation via a tracheostomy is necessary, and at least initially the increased metabolic rate requires that increased tidal ventilation be employed.[425]

The patient requires muscular paralysis. Average doses that we have used for 70-kg men are *d*-tubocurarine, 750 mg daily, or succinylcholine, 12 gm daily. The succinylcholine can be given in a dose of 500 mg intramuscularly every hour. Intravenous morphine 1 mg per kilogram of body weight over 30 minutes will generally lower blood pressure in tetanus.[1621] Presumably morphine decreases the increased peripheral vascular resistance caused by the increased catecholamine release of severe tetanus. Morphine therapy should be continued during the period of sympathetic overactivity at a dose of 1–2 mg per kilogram per 12-hour period.

In our experience morphine withdrawal symptoms are very uncommon after this treatment regimen, occurring in approximately 1 percent of patients so treated. The symptoms of morphine withdrawal, twitching, and

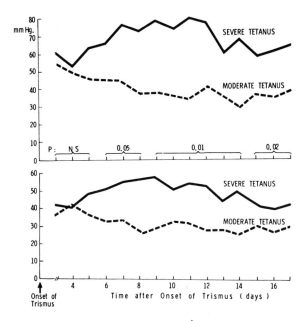

Figure 20-4.   Variability of the blood pressure in tetanus. Average variations in blood pressure are shown for 24-hour periods in patients with either severe or moderate tetanus not given beta-blockade. Systolic readings appear in upper graph and diastolic readings in lower graph. *Severe Tetanus* = patients with muscle spasms that interfere with ventilation and swallowing (15 patients). *Moderate Tetanus* = patients with less marked muscle spasms causing dysphagia (12 patients). Daily variation is calculated in each patient by taking the difference between the highest and lowest blood pressure recorded in a 24-hour period. Average variation is calculated as the mean of the values obtained on corresponding days after the onset of trismus. *P* values comparing the severe and moderate groups appear on the center line. There is a greater variability of blood pressure in patients with severe tetanus than in patients with moderate tetanus. (From J. H. Kerr, J. L. Corbett, C. Prys-Roberts, A. Crampton Smith, and J. M. K. Spalding, *Lancet.*[1018])

an increased metabolic rate are easily treated with small doses of methadone, from which, in our experience, the patient can easily be weaned over two to three days. In such cases we do not tell the patient that we made a temporary morphine addict of him. We have seen no long-term complications from this practice.

If the use of large doses of morphine does not block the sympathetic nervous system overactivity of tetanus, then beta blockers, and possibly alpha blockers, should be used also (Fig. 20-5).[423,1018]

Blockade of Adrenergic Effector Mechanisms

Propranolol should be administered intravenously in increments of 0.2 mg per 70 kg of body weight. Continuous monitoring of the electrocardiogram, arterial pressure, and central venous pressure is most important for

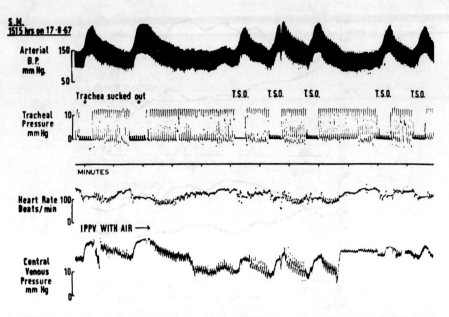

Figure 20-5. Effect of aspiration of tracheal secretions in a patient with severe tetanus who had not been given beta-blocking drugs. Tracheal suctioning during physiotherapy led to an increase in the systolic blood pressure of as much as 150 mm Hg (20.0 kPa) and in the diastolic blood pressure of as much as 60 mm Hg (8.0 kPa). Ventilating the patient with 100% oxygen did not prevent these changes. The change in heart rate was not constant. (From J. L. Corbett, J. H. Kerr, C. Prys-Roberts, A. Crampton Smith, and J. M. K. Spalding, *Anaesthesia*.[423])

titration of the propranolol. After the first 0.2-mg dose further increments should be given until normal sinus rhythm at a heart rate of about 100 beats a minute is established. The rate of administration should not exceed 1 mg per minute. The total initial intravenous dose needed probably will be around 1 mg and should not exceed 3 mg for a 70-kg patient (Fig. 20-6). Thereafter additional drugs should be given approximately every four hours. Beta-adrenergic blockade can be maintained with intragastric propranolol (10 mg every 6–8 hours) in order to maintain heart rate at 90–100 beats per minute and normal sinus rhythm. After the period of sympathetic overactivity, probably of several weeks, the propranolol should be slowly tapered.

Blockade of Postganglionic Adrenergic Activity

Blockade of postganglionic adrenergic activity is less easily achieved. After a patient with tetanus has been established on propranolol, there may, over several days, be a gradual increase in the level and variability of the blood pressure. If labile sudden hypertension appears despite the use of morphine and beta blockers, then alpha-receptor blockade with phen-

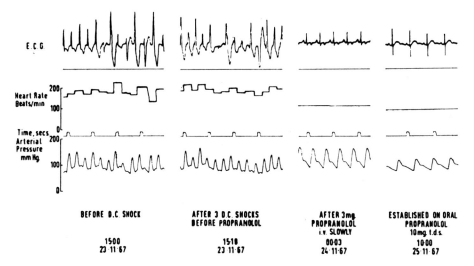

Figure 20-6. Effect of propranolol on the tachycardia and arrhythmias of a patient with severe tetanus. Signs of sympathetic overactivity in this patient were multifocal ventricular and supraventricular ectopic beats interspersed with a supraventricular tachycardia at a rate of 175 per minute. Treatment with carotid sinus massage and direct-current countershock were unsuccessful. Beta-blockade with propranolol resulted in conversion to a normal sinus rhythm at a rate of 100 per minute. This control was maintained with intragastric propranolol. (From C. Prys-Roberts, J. L. Corbett, J. H. Kerr, A. Crampton Smith, and J. M. K. Spalding, *Lancet.*[1569])

tolamine (0.5–2.0 mg intravenously) should be tried. The combination of beta and alpha blockade is undesirable, since the patient is refractory to stimulation by pressor amines. Alpha blockade should be used only for life-threatening hypertension refractory to beta blockers and morphine.

Use of Other Drugs

General anesthetics have been used in the treatment of the sympathetic overactivity of tetanus.[438] They are less effective and have even more dangerous side effects than morphine in patients with tetanus.

After large doses of chlorpromazine severe circulatory instability persists.[1012] Indeed the Oxford group could find no effect of chlorpromazine given in doses of 50 mg intragastrically. Even 1.2 gm given over 48 hours failed to control hypertension.[438] We feel chlorpromazine has no place in the treatment of tetanus.

The mortality due to tetanus has fallen in recent years.[425] It will be interesting to see if a more general use of sympathetic blocking agents can further reduce the mortality of severe tetanus (Table 20-1).[1818] It is tragic that not everyone is actively immunized against this disease, which is often so difficult and expensive to treat.[957,1975]

Table 20-1. Diagnosis and Results of the Intensive Care Unit of the Lagos University Teaching Hospital

Entity	No. Cases	No. Deaths	% Mortality
Severe tetanus	285	115	40.3
Postoperative state	138	30	21.7
Medical conditions	46	12	26.0
Cardiac arrest	35	25	71.0
Trauma and head injury	35	10	40.0
Miscellaneous	33	12	36.3
Laryngotracheobronchitis	31	10	32.2
Intoxication	13	3	23.0
Bulbar poliomyelitis	10	7	70.0
Congenital papilloma of larynx	7	3	42.8
Obstetrics	7	3	42.8
Rabies	5	5	100.0
Total	645	235	37.0

SOURCE: Modified from J. O. Sodipo, *Crit. Care Med.*[1818]

PORPHYRIA AND RESPIRATORY FAILURE

COURSE OF ACUTE INTERMITTENT PORPHYRIA

Acute intermittent porphyria is an inborn error of metabolism characterized by hepatic overproduction of delta-aminolevulinic acid and porphobilinogen.[1943] An attack of acute porphyria can be truly terrifying. Almost complete paralysis comes on rapidly, and the patient may be unable to breathe, swallow, or talk. Experiencing pain, yet mentally lucid, the patient with this form of the disease presents a considerable problem.[2008]

The respiratory failure of acute intermittent porphyria is caused by a peripheral neuropathy which is almost always preceded by abdominal pain. This pain is the initial symptom in over 85 percent of attacks. The interval from pain to paralysis is usually a matter of days or weeks, with a median time of two and one-half weeks. Motor involvement is highly variable both in degree and in rapidity of onset.[1620] Complete flaccid paralysis can develop in 72 hours. Central nervous system manifestations of the disease include bulbar paralysis, hypothalamic dysfunction, cerebellar and basal ganglion lesions, seizures, hallucinations, and coma.[1843] Hyponatremia occurs in over 90 percent of patients with severe acute intermittent porphyria due to inappropriate secretion of antidiuretic hormone.[1428] Improvement in both the hyponatremia and the renal loss of sodium usually follows fluid restriction. Vomiting may exacerbate the hyponatremia. Strict measurement of urine and gastrointestinal ion losses is important, as the fluid and electrolyte imbalances of acute intermittent porphyria are complex, variegate, and profound.[863] The glucose tolerance test is diabetic in type, and growth hormone response is often abnormal.

TREATMENT

At present there is no treatment that is always successful in ending attacks, thus the prevention of acute attacks is of the utmost importance. Barbiturates, sulfonamides, griseofulvin, meprobamate, isopropylmeprobamate, diphenylhydantoin, glutethemide, methyprylon, imipramine, and probably chlordiazepoxide are among the drugs that precipitate attacks.[163,1943] Ergot compounds also induce attacks. Chloramphenicol can induce porphyria under certain circumstances. Infections also precipitate attacks.[163,433,1943]

The abdominal pain often can be brought under control by the use of chlorpromazine.[1340] One should start with a low dose and then increase the dose as necessary. Occasionally 400 mg a day is required intramuscularly. Meperidine and propoxyphene also are useful in controlling pain. Beta-adrenergic blockade with propranolol is useful in the control of sinus tachycardia.[61] Propranolol must be used particularly cautiously on account

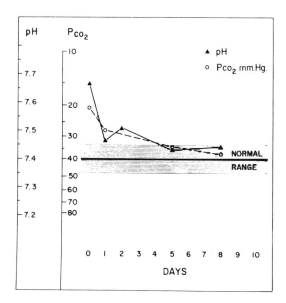

Figure 20-7. Attack of acute intermittent porphyria in a 30-year-old man. Initially there were intermittent episodes of hypoventilation, during which the patient was ventilated. Over the next few days the character of the respirations changed. As he became drowsy, episodes of hyperventilation developed, and the carbon dioxide pressure fell (see day 0). With the application of noxious stimuli he could be roused from coma, and respirations slowed and decreased in depth. All attempts at adding deadspace or impeding hyperventilation by chest strapping failed to decrease alveolar hyperventilation. Over a seven-day period this abnormality of respiration gradually and spontaneously returned to normal and remained so, even during sleep. (From N. H. Baker and B. Messert, *Neurology.*[84] Copyright, 1967, The New York Times Media Company, Inc., with permission.)

of the protean abnormalities of porphyria. In the presence of both hypovolemia and hyponatremia hypertonic saline should be given. While either propranolol or hypertonic saline is being given, pulmonary wedge pressures should be monitored in addition to right-sided filling pressures. Hypomagnesemia also may need treatment.[1428,1943] A high carbohydrate intake may be very beneficial in some patients.

Respiratory paralysis should be treated by controlled ventilation via a tracheostomy. Recovery from a severe paralytic attack requiring controlled ventilation generally starts within two weeks to two months (Fig. 20-7).[84] Recovery may be virtually complete in six weeks to over a year.[1943] Prevention of joint contractures and deformities should follow the procedures we use in treating idiopathic polyneuritis.

Published figures for death during an attack of acute intermittent porphyria that requires controlled ventilation give a rate of around 50 percent, but the prognosis for a given patient is most unpredictable.[1943]

VARIEGATE PORPHYRIA

Motor paralysis requiring controlled ventilation also can occur in variegate porphyria.[567] This disease has an incidence in South Africa of 3 per 1,000 whites. Cutaneous manifestations of photosensitivity also may be present. Increased skin fragility is of far greater importance than acute photosensitivity. Patients with variegate porphyria do not need to be nursed in the dark. Treatment is identical to that for acute intermittent porphyria; however, the mortality of an acute attack requiring controlled ventilation is only half that of respiratory failure due to acute intermittent porphyria, 25 percent versus 50 percent.

21

Applied Respiratory Physiology and Management of Cerebral Edema, Infection, and Hemorrhage

Cooperation between neurosurgeons, neurologists, and workers in respiratory intensive care units should be extremely close, because their mutual problems are complex. Cerebral trauma and stroke patients represent 10 percent of the patient days in the Respiratory–Surgical Intensive Care Unit.

BRAIN INJURY

Two-thirds of the 50,000–60,000 yearly auto accident deaths in the United States are associated with head injury. Blunt trauma to the skull causes concussion, contusion, and laceration of cerebral tissue at the site of the blow. Frequently a contrecoup injury also results. Edema of the injured tissue causes loss of autoregulation of the blood flow to the area.[1241] Vasodilatation persists at the area of injury.[1315] This vasodilatation is unresponsive to changes in arterial carbon dioxide tension.[1108,1109] Intracranial pressure increases as the brain swells within the rigid cranium, reducing cerebral blood flow and perfusion pressure to normal brain (Fig. 21-1).[763,1020,1021] Sudden rise in intracranial pressure can result in transtentorial herniation of the temporal lobe. Ipsilateral pupillary dilatation, contralateral decerebrate rigidity, and coma are the clinical signs of such herniation. We have found that, as a preliminary to rapid surgical intervention, hyperventilation in conjunction with mannitol and steroids results in clinical improvement.[1804,2130] Reduction of the arterial carbon dioxide tension results in lowering of the intracerebral pressure by reducing intracranial blood volume and cerebral blood flow (Fig. 21-2).[25,1524,2106] Because carbon dioxide production increased, however, ventilation of approximately 12 liters per minute failed to produce alkalemia in 80 percent of our patients with transtentorial herniation.[2130] Notwithstanding this, survivors resulted who were subsequently able to lead useful lives.

CEREBRAL BLOOD FLOW

Cerebral blood flow is dependent at least in part upon brain pH, which is reflected by cerebrospinal fluid pH. Any sudden change of arterial carbon dioxide tension because of hypercapnia or hypocapnia is reflected immediately in the cerebrospinal fluid by a fall or rise in pH. Since bicarbonate cannot move freely across the blood-brain barrier, the brain has additional

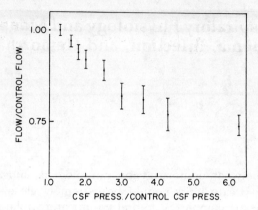

Figure 21-1. The effect on the carotid artery blood flow of acutely increasing cerebrospinal fluid (CSF) pressure in 13 patients. Carotid artery blood flow, measured by an indwelling flow probe, was significantly reduced from the control level when the ratio of cerebrospinal fluid pressure to control pressure was 1.8 or greater. The *vertical bars* represent the standard error. (From J. C. Greenfield, Jr. and G. T. Tindall, *J. Clin. Invest.* [763])

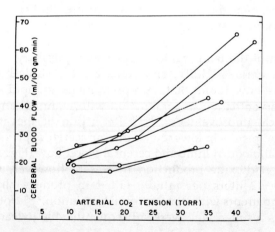

Figure 21-2. Cerebral blood flow as a function of arterial CO_2 tension (individual values in six healthy subjects). The three values obtained in each subject are connected by straight lines. The 12 cerebral blood flow values during hypocarbia were measured using [85]Kr, and the 6 values in the normocarbic range were calculated from arteriovenous oxygen content differences. (From H. Wollman, T. C. Smith, G. W. Stephen, E. T. Colton, III, H. E. Gleaton, and S. C. Alexander, *J. Appl. Physiol.* [2106])

local buffer systems that use ammonia. In the absence of injury buffer systems return the pH to normal levels in an exponential fashion over a 24- to 48-hour period. The effect of hyperventilation on the cerebrospinal fluid pH and therefore on the cerebral blood flow is limited to this 24- to 48-hour period.[1315] Thereafter, if hyperventilation is abruptly discontinued, an increase may occur in cerebral blood flow; therefore patients should be returned to normocapnia in stages over several hours.

Hypoxemia like hypercapnia increases cerebral blood flow in responsive vessels (Fig. 21-3).[1055] In one study 48 percent of patients with head trauma upon admission had arterial oxygen tensions of less than 80 mm Hg (10.6 kPa).[1787] Treatment of head trauma should start with safeguarding of the airway and prevention of hypoxemia. Respiratory management of intracranial catastrophes frequently requires an aggressive approach starting in the emergency room. Often a fast decision has to be made as to whether to treat the patient conservatively, to send him for angiographic examination or computer-assisted axial tomographic studies, or to take him directly to the operating room. In general only a patient who shows acute transtentorial herniation or has exhibited the signs and symptoms of cerebellar hemorrhage should be rushed to the operating room. On the way, as we have described, the patient is paralyzed with succinylcholine, intubated, hyperventilated, and given steroids and mannitol (Table 21-1).[926,2130]

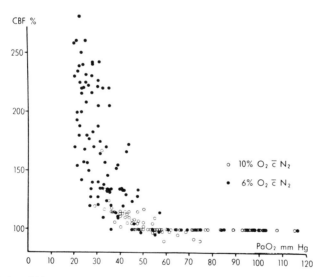

Figure 21-3. Effect of hypoxemia on cerebral blood flow. The cerebral blood flow does not increase until the arterial oxygen tension is lowered to 50 mm Hg (6.7 kPa). This increase in cerebral blood flow due to hypoxemia increases intracranial pressure. (From K. Kogure, P. Scheinberg, O. M. Reinmuth, M. Fujishima, and R. Busto, *J. Appl. Physiol.*[1055])

Table 21-1. Intervals after Onset of Intracranial Hemorrhage

Case No.	Decerebration (hr)	Medical Decompression (hr)	Surgical Decompression (hr)	Response to Verbal Command (hr)	Hospital Discharge (days)
1	0.75	1.0*	8.5	11	55
2	34.0	34.08	34.5	64.5	30
3	2.0	2.08	2.5	50.5	30
4	1.25	1.42	1.5	16.5	28
5	63.0	63.25*	63.75	67.75	69

*Pupillary dilatation & decerebrate rigidity subsided before operation.
SOURCE: N. T. Zervas and J. Hedley-Whyte.[2130] Reprinted by permission from the *New England Journal of Medicine* 286:1075–1077, 1972.

LOCALIZATION OF THE LESION

If a patient is stable or improving after an intracranial catastrophe, localization of the lesion should be attempted. Although clinical signs are often unreliable in localizing the extent of damage to the central nervous system, certain abnormal patterns of ventilation are useful in aiding diagnosis. The complete neurologic workup of a patient in coma after a cerebrovascular accident is outside the scope of this book, and the reader is referred to the most useful descriptions of Fisher,[645] and Plum and Posner.[1535]

ABNORMAL PATTERNS OF VENTILATION AFTER A CEREBROVASCULAR ACCIDENT

CHEYNE-STOKES RESPIRATION

Cheyne-Stokes respiration is most often caused by bilateral lesions deep in the cerebral hemispheres and basal ganglia. These lesions damage the internal capsules. It can also result from metabolic abnormalities that cause dysfunction of these same brain regions. Cheyne-Stokes respiration is common in patients with bilateral cerebral infarction, uremia, or hypertensive encephalopathy.[249,328]

APNEUSTIC BREATHING

Apneustic breathing suggests pontine infarction due to basilar artery occlusion, but we have seen it accompany hypoglycemic coma or profound anoxia when arterial oxygen tensions are 20–35 mm Hg (2.7–4.7 kPa). The brainstem lesions are usually extensive at autopsy, with nearly complete transection of the rostral pons and especially its dorsolateral tegmental area.[1534] If the lesion extends to the dorsolateral pontine nuclei, apneusis is more prolonged.[1535]

ATAXIC BREATHING

Ataxic breathing has a completely irregular pattern. It is caused by lesions in the dorsomedial part of the medulla.[1538] During ataxic breathing the respiratory center is hyposensitive to carbon dioxide and other regulatory ions and exquisitely sensitive to respiratory depressant drugs such as morphine or diazepam.

CENTRAL NEUROGENIC HYPERVENTILATION

The diagnosis of central neurogenic hyperventilation can be made with certainty only after it is known that the arterial oxygen tension has been above 70–80 mm Hg (9.3–10.6 kPa) for 24 hours. Central neurogenic hyperventilation can lead to arterial carbon dioxide tensions well below 30 mm Hg (4.0 kPa).[1539] We have never seen a patient survive after the arterial carbon dioxide tension has been below 25 mm Hg (3.3 kPa) due to central neurogenic hyperventilation without arterial hypoxemia.

INCREASED INTRACRANIAL PRESSURE

Increased intracranial pressure affects pulmonary function in three main ways: production of pulmonary edema;[124,465,466,1783] alteration of the pattern of spontaneous ventilation as we have described; and loss of protective airway reflexes, possibly allowing aspiration. Increasing intracranial pressure also is associated with an increase in blood pressure due to an increase in peripheral vascular resistance (Fig. 21-4).[553,1949] In some patients this causes an increase in pulmonary arterial and venous blood pressures and subsequently pulmonary edema without a significant change in pulmonary vascular resistance (Fig. 21-4).[131,551,552,553,554,1174,1415,1949]

Monitoring of intracerebral intraventricular pressure is a most useful technique for guiding therapy and suggesting prognosis.[297,977,1941,1982]

VENTRICULAR PRESSURE MONITORING

The clinical signs that normally indicate rising intracranial pressure often are unreliable or even misleading, especially after severe head injury. Monitoring of intracerebral perfusion pressure is extremely valuable under these circumstances. Johnston, Johnston, and Jennett have classified intracranial pressure into three groups: relatively normal pressures of less than 20 mm Hg (2.7 kPa), moderate elevations of pressure, and severe elevations of pressure of over 40 mm Hg (5.3 kPa).[977]

After surgical evacuation of intracranial hemorrhage, if patients, especially young patients, with low or normal intracranial pressures die or remain in coma, it is usually due to primary brainstem injury (Fig. 21-5).[297] By contrast, if a patient has a severe elevation of intracranial pressure to above 40 mm Hg (5.3 kPa), then despite prompt treatment the chances of useful recovery are less than 20 percent. Only children seem able to survive an intraventricular cerebral pressure greater than 60 mm Hg (8.0 kPa) and then only if they are treated with corticosteroids, alveolar hyperventilation to obtain an arterial carbon dioxide tension of 25–30 mm Hg (3.3–4.0 kPa), dehydrating agents, and ventricular drainage (Fig. 21-6).[977,1941] Similar measures applied to adults with ventricular pressures of over 60 mm Hg (8.0

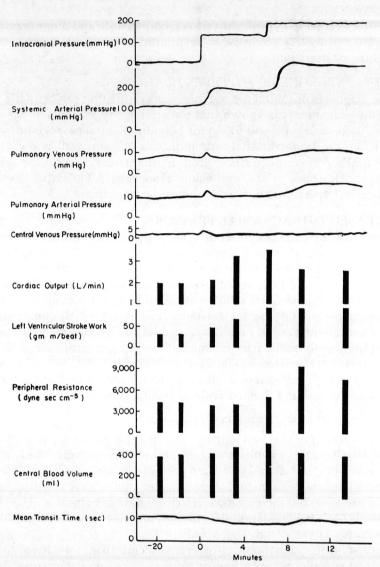

Figure 21-4. Hemodynamic response to graded increases in intracranial pressure. Seven monkeys had increased intracranial pressure induced by means of inflation of an epidural balloon. The hemodynamic pattern depicted here occurred in five of the seven animals and was not associated with pulmonary edema. When the intracranial pressure is increased to 100 mm Hg (13.3 kPa), the cardiac output and systemic arterial blood pressure increase. When the intracranial pressure is increased further to over 125 mm Hg (16.6 kPa) the cardiac output and systemic arterial pressure remain elevated, and there is also an increase in peripheral vascular resistance. The pulmonary artery pressure is moderately elevated, but pulmonary edema does not occur. (From T. B. Ducker, R. L. Simmons, and R. W. Anderson, *J. Neurosurg.*[553])

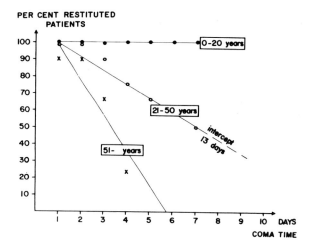

Figure 21-5. Percentage of restitution, plotted against duration of coma, of 263 initially comatose patients who survived 24 hours after head trauma and who regained full consciousness. Forty-six percent of 171 primary deaths occurred within 48 hours. Most patients who are less than 20 years old and survive the initial 48 hours after head injury recover mentally and become neurologically intact regardless of the severity and duration of coma. (From C.-A. Carlsson, C. von Essen, and J. Löfgren, *J. Neurosurg.*[297])

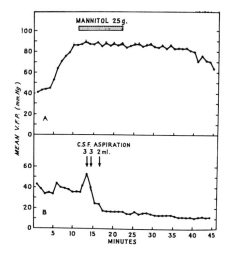

Figure 21-6. Comparison of the effects of (*A*) mannitol and (*B*) ventricular cerebrospinal fluid aspiration on ventricular fluid pressure (VFP) in a 15-year-old patient five days after head injury. (From I. H. Johnston, J. A. Johnston, and B. Jennett, *Lancet.*[977])

kPa) always fail to lead to useful survival. Though intraventricular pressure recording can predict whether survival is likely, it cannot predict the quality of survival.[1982]

Vapalahti and Troup have reported on 250 patients monitored with intraventricular pressure.[1982] They monitored other variables as well, as do we.[927] Physiologic deadspace-to-tidal-volume ratio, the alveolar-arterial oxygen tension gradient, and respiratory frequency are of little prognostic use, but there are significant differences of prognostic value in arterial blood gases of patients breathing spontaneously. The mean arterial pH and arterial carbon dioxide tension in the first 96 hours after injury of those patients who make a useful recovery is 7.41 and 36 mm Hg (4.8 kPa) respectively, while patients who go on to a vegetative existence have in these 96 postinjury hours a mean pH of 7.47 with a mean arterial carbon dioxide tension of 31 mm Hg (4.1 kPa). These differences are highly significant ($P < 0.001$). During the corresponding 96 hours the mean arterial pH and carbon dioxide tension of those patients who go on to die is 7.41 and 35 mm Hg (4.7 kPa) respectively. Mean arterial carbon dioxide tension values after brain injury are shown in Figure 21-7.[1982]

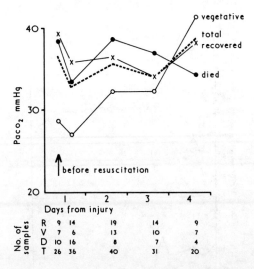

Figure 21-7. Correlation between arterial carbon dioxide tension (Pa_{CO_2}) during spontaneous ventilation and final outcome in patients with severe head trauma. R = Recovered. V = Vegetative survival. D = Dead. T = Total series. Measurements obtained before resuscitation ($P < 0.05$) and on the first day following injury ($P < 0.01$) show that there is a significantly lower arterial carbon dioxide tension in those patients with a vegetative survival when compared to patients who recover. (From M. Vapalahti and H. Troupp, *Br. Med. J.*[1982])

MEASUREMENTS OF CSF ACID-BASE BALANCE
AND BRAIN TEMPERATURE

Measurements of CSF acid-base balance usually do not help with prognosis or management, but exceptionally important results are sometimes seen.

Hyperthermia to a temperature of above 39°C occurs far more often among patients who do not recover ($P < 0.01$). Approximately 10 percent of patients with a temperature of above 39°C recover satisfactorily after being deeply unconscious from severe brain injury. Over 60 percent of those who survive in a vegetative state had a maximum temperature within two days of injury of over 39°C.[1982] Over half these vegetative patients had Cheyne-Stokes breathing within the first two days after injury. By contrast only 15 percent of patients who recover useful function have Cheyne-Stokes respiration. Over 80 percent of adult vegetative patients have extension rigidity within two days of severe brain injury, whereas less than one-fifth of useful survivors do (Fig. 21-8).[297] These survivors have almost always required muscular paralysis to allow controlled hyperventilation, diuretics, corticosteroids, and immediate successful evacuation of blood and clot, together with control of brain temperature and pressure and prevention of arterial spasm.[2131,2132] As we have mentioned, these are the important factors in treatment of brain trauma and subarachnoid hemorrhage.

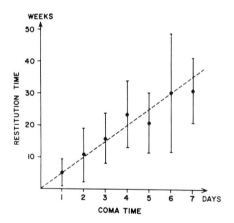

Figure 21-8. The clinical course of patients with severe head injuries. Only 5 of 320 initially comatose patients who survived severe head injury for 24 hours remained permanently unresponsive. Coma tended to be less long-lasting and restitution quicker in patients under 20 years of age. But effective restitution even followed coma of several months' duration. In patients over 20 years of age, both increasing age and a longer duration of coma worsen the outlook for normal neurologic and mental function; 57 patients had persistent dementia. Mean values ± SE are shown for 320 patients of all ages. (From C.-A. Carlsson, C. von Essen, and J. Löfgren, *J. Neurosurg.*[297])

RESPIRATORY MANAGEMENT AND PROGNOSIS OF COMA AFTER CARDIAC ARREST OR A HYPOXIC EPISODE

Consciousness is lost within six seconds after the human cerebral circulation stops or no longer supplies oxygen to the brain. Light-headedness and blindness sometimes occur within these six seconds.[1667] Generalized convulsions, pupillary dilatation, and bilateral Babinski responses ensue almost immediately. If complete oxygen deprivation lasts longer than 60–120 seconds, or if this anoxia is superimposed on preexisting cerebral disease, then confusion, motor dysfunction, stupor, or coma may last for several hours or even permanently. Total ischemic anoxia lasting longer than four minutes kills cortical neurons.[2042,2043] The hippocampus and Purkinje's cells of the cerebellum are very susceptible to anoxia. After total ischemia the astroglia swell, particularly around capillaries, and with restoration of adequate cardiac output cerebral perfusion is not restored—the no-reflow phenomenon.[30,634]

Between 5 and 45 percent of patients who are resuscitated after cardiac arrest are discharged from hospital neurologically intact. In every hospital short-term survivors outnumber those who leave the hospital alive.[1851] The electroencephalogram is of use in deciding prognosis. If there is diffuse theta and delta slow wave activity and no alpha rhythm, or if the electroencephalogram is flat and the patient has not had depressant drugs, then the prognosis after an anoxic episode is very poor.[16,771]

In dogs with total circulatory arrest for 12 minutes and consequent anoxic cerebral damage the following treatment improves neurologic outcome: heparin 150 units per kilogram of body weight intravenously, brain flushing with intraarterial injection to the brain arteries of low molecular weight dextran to a hematocrit of 25 percent, and increased cerebral perfusion pressure for six hours (mean systemic arterial pressure, 160 mm Hg [19.8 kPa]). All dogs not treated with this regimen remained comatose and spastic until death. All dogs given this regimen recovered consciousness within 24 hours, could stand, walk, and feed themselves within 48 hours, and appeared normal at one week after insult, except for very slight ataxia in 60 percent of dogs.[1687] At present we do not use anticoagulation and hemodilution after a hypoxic episode. We await with interest further studies on this treatment.

The prognosis for useful recovery cannot be accurately assessed immediately following a hypoxic or hypotensive episode. Even though they fail to awaken fully for days after the catastrophe, some patients recover completely. Others awake promptly, only to relapse and die several weeks later. Generally patients who demonstrate intact brainstem function after the hypoxic episode have a reasonable outlook for recovery of consciousness and even for total recovery. Tests that we use to assess function are pupillary and ciliospinal responses, intact doll's-eye movements, and oculovestibular caloric responses.[188] The absence of any of these responses is extremely serious.[127] Especially serious are pupils that are persistently fixed despite light stimulation. Except when the patient has severe cataracts or is drugged, this fixation implies a hopeless outlook.

DELAYED ENCEPHALOPATHY

After recovery from cardiac arrest or other hypoxic insult delayed encephalopathy with coma sometimes occurs. Plum and Posner in their now-classic description reported on 14 patients with this syndrome.[1537] Their patients resumed full activity within four to five days after the hypoxic episode. They then appeared normal for two to twenty-one days. Then abruptly the patients became irritable and confused, and agitation and mania often supervened. The worsening of the neurologic state may progress to coma or death, or the deterioration may arrest itself earlier. We have seen patients whose lucid interval was only one to four hours but who otherwise followed exactly the syndrome described by Plum and Posner. Occasionally patients have a second recovery period that leads to satisfactory function.

Delayed posthypoxic encephalopathy occurs most frequently after carbon monoxide poisoning or after asphyxiation, but hypoglycemia and intraoperative cardiac arrest also cause the syndrome. The exact mechanisms that underlie the syndrome are unclear.[1536,1537] At autopsy there is generally diffuse demyelination of the cerebral hemispheres with sparing of the subcortical connecting fibers and of the brainstem. The basal ganglia are sometimes infarcted.[716] Treatment includes prevention of cerebral edema. A guarded prognosis must always be given after a hypoxic episode. On one occasion we told the family of a 30-year-old woman that she had recovered consciousness after a cardiac arrest and would be all right. She was for a day; then she lapsed into a prolonged coma and eventually died.

RESPIRATORY MANAGEMENT AND PROGNOSIS OF VIRAL INFECTIONS OF THE CENTRAL NERVOUS SYSTEM

VIRAL ENCEPHALITIS

Only four types of viral encephalitides commonly produce coma: herpes simplex, eastern and western equine, and St. Louis. Rabies also causes coma. Occasionally patients with these encephalitides require controlled ventilation. In the last decade all such patients in our respiratory care unit have had herpes simplex encephalitis. There are a number of distinctive features of herpes simplex encephalitis which should be known to persons working in intensive care units. Hallucinations and other psychologic disturbances are extremely common in the prodromal and recovery phases of the disease. The hallucinations are often similar to those of alcoholic psychosis, and not uncommonly the clinical picture before and after frank coma is remarkably similar to delirium tremens. Headache, drowsiness, and fever occur at some time in the course of almost all cases of herpes encephalitis, as do seizures, either focal or generalized. Focal neurologic signs are generally present and include reflex asymmetry, Babinski signs, cortical sensory loss, cogwheel rigidity, and grasp reflexes.[539] Cerebrospinal fluid pressure is elevated, and there is generally an increase in protein, up to 900 mg per 100 ml. White cells, chiefly mononuclear, are found in the cerebrospinal fluid, especially late in the disease. The electroencephalogram is abnormal but without distinctive features.

During coma due to viral encephalitis the alveolar ventilation requires careful monitoring. Normally alveolar hyperventilation is present and controlled ventilation is not required, but the upper airway must be protected either by a tracheal tube or by tracheostomy. If alveolar hypoventilation suddenly ensues, controlled ventilation must be started immediately. At this time the patient will probably already be receiving diuretics and hyperosmolar agents to reduce cerebral edema.

We have tried surgical decompression of the brain at this stage but are not convinced of its effectiveness—nor indeed of whether it is ethically wise. The problem with aggressive supportive therapy of herpes simplex encephalitis is that so many of the patients are left with memory defects. These defects, which generally prevent retention of a job, are due to a remarkable predilection by the virus for the gray matter of the medial temporal lobe as well as for other limbic structures in the insula, cingulate gyrus, and inferior frontal lobe.[539] In one case that we treated viremia caused profound peripheral vascular dilatation. Colloid infusions, vasopressors, and controlled ventilation were required for resuscitation. The patient is now able to look after her family but has continued loss of memory for recent events, but not loss of distant memory. Antiviral agents are of no proved value in treating herpes simplex encephalitis.

RABIES

Recovery from rabies is possible if intensive respiratory care is given to the patient (Fig. 21-9).[828] Approximately thirty thousand persons in the United States and over one million persons worldwide are immunized against rabies each year. Over one thousand human cases are reported to the World Health Organization each year, but the United States has less than five cases each year.[861,1672]

Transmission of the RNA virus of rabies into humans almost invariably is accomplished by the bite of a rabid animal.[1016] Virus may persist at the inoculation site for up to 96 hours, but then centripetal spread occurs along nerves. In the central nervous system the virus replicates almost exclusively in gray matter before spreading along autonomic nerves to reach other tissues such as salivary glands, adrenal medulla, heart, and kidneys. Incubation periods from a week to a year have been reported. The mean incubation time is about a month.[564]

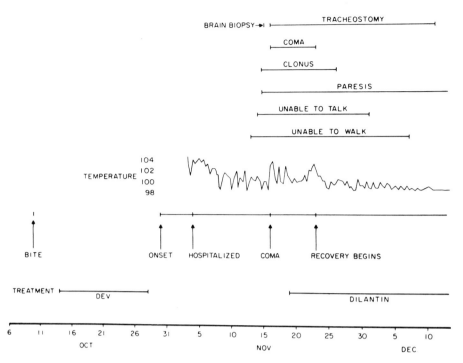

Figure 21-9. Clinical course of a 6-year-old boy who recovered from rabies. The patient was bitten by a bat that was discovered to have rabies. The boy was given a 14-day course of duck embryo rabies vaccine (*DEV*). Two days following completion of the course of vaccine treatment he developed a stiff neck, anorexia, dizziness, and vomiting. He gradually developed lethargy, which progressed to bizarre behavior and soon to coma. There were signs of increased intracranial pressure. Airway obstruction developed, requiring tracheostomy. He made a gradual improvement and was discharged three months following the bite. Four months after discharge he had no signs of neurologic or psychologic abnormality. He has continued to do well and presently is active in baseball. (From M. A. W. Hattwick, T. T. Weis, C. J. Stechschulte, G. M. Baer, and M. B. Gregg, *Ann. Intern. Med.*[828])

Stages

There are three stages to rabies: a prodromal period, a period of nonspecific encephalitis, and finally a stage of profound brainstem dysfunction. During the prodrome, malaise, anorexia, headache, fever, and vomiting are common. Hydrophobia and sensory abnormalities near the bite are absent in approximately half of all patients. Although patients with rabies may have a period of hyperactivity, paralysis occurs without this hyperactivity in 15 to 60 percent of rabid patients. Paralysis may be general, may be worse in the bitten limb, or even may ascend as with idiopathic polyneuritis. Progression to coma and respiratory arrest will then follow.

Consequently controlled ventilation via a tracheostomy is necessary at the start of paralysis. The encephalitis of rabies, besides causing coma, commonly gives rise to hemiparesis and focal seizures. Internal hydrocephalus may develop because of inflammation around the cerebral aqueduct.

Autonomic Nervous System

Abnormalities of the autonomic nervous system start relatively early in the course of rabies. Increased salivation, lacrimation, sweating, and irregular pupils are common, as are abnormalities of blood pressure. Increased alveolar-arterial oxygen tension gradients and increased pulmonary vascular markings on x-ray have been described in rabies.[828] Cardiac arrhythmias and viral myocarditis also have been reported.[1664] Rabies virus can be recovered from heart, lung, and kidney as well as from the brain. Rabies is a systemic illness.[1672]

Therapy after Exposure

Postexposure therapy aims to minimize the amount of virus at the puncture wound and then to have a high titer of neutralizing antibody present. Duck embryo–derived vaccine is given 1 ml subcutaneously daily for 14–21 days, followed by boosters 10 and 20 days after the initial series.[757,822,1508] Passive immunization with human-derived antiserum is also available. Preexposure therapy with duck embryo–derived vaccine is wise for veterinarians, Masters of Foxhounds and their hunt servants, spelunkers, and others who encounter rabid animals.

Treatment

Treatment of the established disease also consists of anticipating and trying to prevent the complications of encephalitis, myocarditis, pneumonitis, and autonomic dysfunction. Intraventricular or subdural pressure should be monitored and raised intracranial pressure treated by conventional methods and by ventricular drainage of cerebrospinal fluid if necessary (Fig. 21-6).[977] It is probably unwise to use steroids. Anticonvulsant therapy almost certainly will be needed. No specific antirabies chemotherapy is useful, although immune globulin and many other drugs have been tried. Rather, treatment depends on application of physiologic principles to keep the patient alive. Since neuropathologic changes from the virus are relatively minor and reversible, we should see an increasing number of patients survive this disease without permanent sequelae other than a tracheostomy scar.

RESPIRATORY MANAGEMENT OF BACTERIAL INFECTIONS AFFECTING THE CENTRAL NERVOUS SYSTEM

ENDOTOXEMIC COMA

Endotoxemic coma caused by bacterial infections is relatively common in most respiratory care units, but the exact mechanisms by which the bacteria cause the coma are unclear. Most commonly an elderly patient with sepsis caused by gram-negative bacillary infection of the lungs or peritoneum lapses into coma and often requires controlled ventilation. Far less commonly the major site of infection is the meninges.

The cardiorespiratory and neurologic interrelationships are complex. Let us consider an important study of these relationships. The injection into awake normal monkeys of *Escherichia coli* endotoxin led to coma, which was often reversible within 40 minutes after the end of the endotoxin infusion.[2116] Mean systolic arterial pressure fell to 94 mm Hg (12.5 kPa), significantly lower ($P < 0.05$) than in the control monkeys. The percentage of cardiac output going to heart, adrenals, and all parts of the gastrointestinal tract was significantly increased in the endotoxin-treated monkeys. However, and most importantly, the percent of cardiac output going to the brain was only 70 percent of control ($P < 0.05$) and the total flow of blood to brain was 67 percent of that in control monkeys ($P < 0.05$), although the resistance of the cerebral arteries was reduced. One day after the end of the *Escherichia coli* endotoxin infusion the resistance of the cerebral arteries was still decreased ($P < 0.05$). The monkeys seemed to feel little if any discomfort during these experiments. They lapsed into coma when blood flow to the brain fell from control values of 80 ml per 100 gm to around 60 ml per 100 gm of wet brain. They reawoke when brain blood flow returned toward control values.[2116]

The monkey's response to endotoxin is similar to what is thought to occur in patients but markedly dissimilar to nonprimate responses to endotoxemia.[1782] Consequently we feel, but without adequate proof, that a common contributing factor to coma in patients with gram-negative sepsis is a reduction in the percent of the cardiac output going to the cerebral hemispheres. Especially when an elderly patient has preexisting cerebrovascular disease, smaller reductions may produce coma.

BACTERIAL MENINGITIS

Bacterial meningitis may be difficult to detect in patients in acute respiratory failure. On at least one occasion in our hospital significant signs of unexpected bacterial meningitis have been found at autopsy in a patient who had been in coma requiring controlled ventilation.

With acute leptomeningeal infections cerebral edema is generally marked, and the swelling may become so great that the hemispheres herniate.[519] Consequently techniques for treatment of cerebral edema have great applicability to the management of meningitis.[1724] Pneumococcal and streptococcal meningitis arise secondary to infection elsewhere in the body in about 50 percent of cases of meningitis due to these organisms. Coma is common in meningitis due to these organisms and also with *Hemophilus influenzae* and meningococcal meningitis. We have had to ventilate a patient with meningitis due to *Hemophilus* but never a patient with meningococcal meningitis. Lumbar puncture must be done extremely carefully, preferably with a 25-gauge needle, in patients with meningitis who require controlled ventilation, otherwise the resultant temporal lobe or cerebellar herniation can lead to irreversible coma.[519] Patients occasionally develop the encephalopathy of meningitis before white cells appear in the cerebrospinal fluid. Bacteria can often be seen at this stage on a gram stain of the centrifuged spinal fluid. If the tap is negative and meningitis is strongly suspected, the lumbar puncture should be repeated within six hours. Bacterial meningitis may cause a severe vasculitis that produces focal or diffuse ischemia and even necrosis of underlying brain. Bacteria and their endotoxins may interfere directly with cerebral metabolism by enzymatic inhibition and substrate competition.

The interactions of bacteremia, toxemia, coma, and control of ventilation are most important in the management of infections affecting the central nervous system. At present we have little detailed knowledge of these interrelationships with which to guide our therapy. We constantly try to guard against cerebral edema, fluid overload, alveolar hypoventilation, and hypoxemia, and meanwhile we treat the sepsis vigorously. We do not even know how to prevent the changes in distribution of cardiac output produced by nonlethal endotoxemia. Here is a fruitful area for research in the next decade.

PULMONARY EDEMA DUE TO RAISED INTRACRANIAL PRESSURE

Another area of importance to management of respiratory failure is the relationship between intracranial pressure and pulmonary edema.[551,552] Pulmonary edema is most difficult to treat when caused by raised intracranial pressure.[322] Ducker reported on 11 patients with pulmonary edema associated with increased intracranial pressure in the absence of other cardiovascular or pulmonary disease. Similar cases have been noted by us and by others.[286,551,1962] Each of the patients reported by Ducker developed massive pulmonary edema while in the hospital. The patients had not received even a pint of parenteral fluid when the edema developed.[551] Characteristically the central venous pressure when measured is normal or almost normal. Cardiac arrhythmias are uncommon. The pulmonary edema does not respond to digitalis. Positive end-expiratory pressure is useful only to keep the patient alive until surgical decompression can be carried out. Even with positive end-expiratory pressure, controlled hyperventilation, treatment of cerebral edema, and almost immediate "successful" surgery, the survival rate is less than 10 percent. At autopsy the lungs are uniformly heavy with pulmonary edema foam throughout the alveoli.[551]

Pulmonary edema can be produced by inflation of a subdural balloon or by infusion of bloody saline into the cisterna magna.[552] Stimulation of hypothalamic nuclei, intracisternal injection of fibrin or endotoxin,

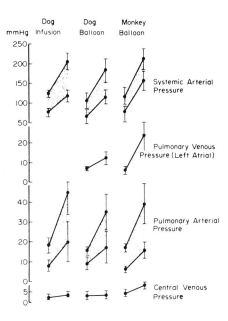

Figure 21-10. Hemodynamic response to increased intracranial pressure. Dogs and monkeys had increased intracranial pressure induced to 125–150 mm Hg (16.6–20.0 kPa) by means of infusion of blood in the subarachnoid space or inflation of a balloon in the epidural space. Results shown are the mean systolic and diastolic pressures and twice the SEM. Increased intracranial pressure results in significant increases in systemic arterial pressure, left atrial pressure, and pulmonary artery pressure. The central venous pressure is almost unaffected. (From T. B. Ducker and R. L. Simmons, *J. Neurosurg.*[552])

and destruction of the preoptic nuclei bilaterally also can cause pulmonary edema. When intracranial pressure is suddenly raised in monkeys, approximately 30 percent of the time, increases in the pulmonary arterial and left atrial pressures occur prior to and are proportionately greater than increases in the systemic pressure; 70 percent of the time they are not (Fig. 21-10). The pulse often but not invariably slows when intracranial pressure rises, and changes in pulse rate do not appear to be related to changes in pulmonary arterial and left atrial pressure. Spontaneous respiration is slowed by intracranial pressures above 100 mm Hg (13.3 kPa), and controlled ventilation becomes necessary to maintain normal levels of alveolar ventilation. Ducker, Simmons, and Anderson found that only 29 percent of chimpanzees developed pulmonary edema when their intracranial pressure was elevated above 125 mm Hg (16.6 kPa).[553] In these monkeys (Fig. 21-11) the left atrial pressure seemed to exceed the pulmonary arterial pressure for a crucial few seconds during the initial cardiovascular response to the sudden increase in intracranial pressure.[552] As the intracranial pressure was raised

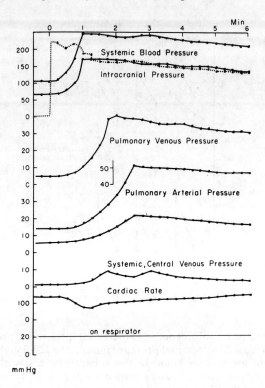

Figure 21-11.   Response of a monkey who develops pulmonary edema following induction of increased intracranial pressure (*dotted line*) by means of inflation of an epidural balloon. This response occurred in 20 percent of the monkeys and dogs studied. There is an initial systemic pressor response followed by a marked increase in the pulmonary venous pressure and distention of the left atrium. The pulmonary artery pressure rises later. This hemodynamic pattern resulted in massive pulmonary edema within 15 minutes. (From T. B. Ducker and R. L. Simmons, *J. Neurosurg.*[552])

rapidly, peripheral resistance rose and cardiac output fell, and massive pulmonary edema developed rapidly with a concomitant increase in the alveolar-arterial oxygen tension gradient (Fig. 21-12).[553] The pressure tracings made by Ducker, Simmons, and Anderson do not suggest that heart valve incompetence was responsible for the marked elevations in the left atrial pressure.[553]

In the vast majority (71 percent) of chimpanzees, however, pulmonary edema did not develop as a response to sudden rises in intracranial pressure. With intracranial pressures up to 75 mm Hg (10.0 kPa) there was no consistent significant cardiovascular change except a very slight increase in central venous pressure. At an intracerebral pressure of 100 mm Hg (13.3 kPa) cardiac output and systemic arterial pressure rise ($P < 0.01$). The total

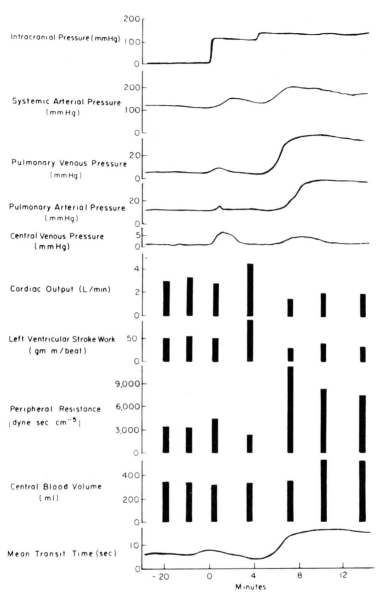

Figure 21-12. Hemodynamic response to graded increases in intracranial pressure in monkeys who develop pulmonary edema. Two of seven monkeys who had increased intracranial pressure induced by means of inflation of an epidural balloon developed massive pulmonary edema. When intracranial pressure is increased to 100 mm Hg (13.3 kPa), the cardiac output and systemic arterial pressure increase; however, no animals develop pulmonary edema at this level of intracranial pressure. Following increases in intracranial pressure to over 125 mm Hg (16.6 kPa) these animals showed a marked increase in peripheral resistance, arterial blood pressure, pulmonary arterial pressure, and pulmonary venous pressure (left atrial). As the left atrium distends, pulmonary edema develops. Cardiac output falls to 50–60 percent of normal. (From T. B. Ducker, R. L. Simmons, and R. W. Anderson, *J. Neurosurg.*[553])

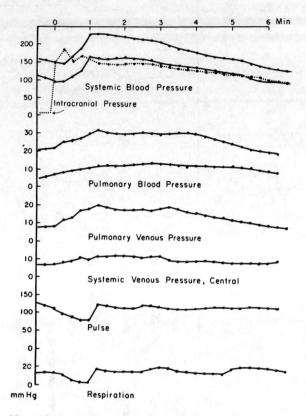

Figure 21-13. Hemodynamic response of a monkey to increased intracranial pressure. A typical response is shown of a monkey who has increased intracranial pressure induced by means of inflation of an epidural balloon. There is a rapid increase in arterial blood pressure and pulmonary artery pressure. Heart rate and respiratory rate become slower. Pulmonary edema does not appear in animals who respond in this manner. (From T. B. Ducker and R. L. Simmons, *J. Neurosurg.*[552])

peripheral resistance decreases ($P < 0.01$). After the intracranial pressure has been raised above 125 mm Hg (16.6 kPa), the mean systolic arterial pressure rises until it greatly exceeds the intracranial pressure. As this happens, peripheral resistance reaches extremely high levels and cardiac output returns to normal levels. These changes are accompanied by slight gradual increases in pulmonary arterial and left atrial (pulmonary venous) pressures but no detectable pulmonary edema (Fig. 21-13).[552,553]

RESPIRATORY MANAGEMENT OF INTRACRANIAL TUMORS

In general the principles of respiratory management of patients with cerebral tumors are the same as if the space-occupying lesion were a clot, liquid blood, or an area of cerebral edema or infarction. The degree of cerebral edema must be assessed continually. This is especially true with gliomas. The level of alveolar ventilation often needs to be increased to allow for operation or radiotherapy.

ONDINE'S CURSE

The respiratory problems of Ondine's curse are unusual. This syndrome, named by Severinghaus and Mitchell, consists of normal maintenance of alveolar ventilation when awake but alveolar hypoventilation to the point of apnea during sleep.[1732] In the last decade we have seen five cases of this syndrome, all in children and due to infiltrative disease in the floor of the fourth ventricle. One child had measles encephalitis and the other four had tumors: one medulloblastoma, one ependymoma, and two astrocytomas. Two of these patients presented after surgical exploration of the tumors. All the patients died within days or months of the onset of Ondine's curse from progression of their disease. Controlled ventilation during sleep periods is probably worthwhile if it is required to get the patient over operation or to allow radiation therapy. By day, when the child is awake, careful monitoring of consciousness and alveolar ventilation are necessary, as the carbon dioxide response curve of these patients is depressed and shifted to the right.

RESPIRATORY DYSFUNCTION AFTER CERVICAL CORDOTOMY AND ANTERIOR SPINAL SURGERY

A spectrum of respiratory and autonomic dysfunction may follow bilateral percutaneous cervical cordotomy or anterior cervical spinal surgery.[1067,1068] After the procedure the patient complains of weakness and anxiety. Sighing is common. Objective evidence of functional impairment of ventilation is not present at this time, although sometimes within the next few hours the patient may start to hypoventilate. When the patient falls asleep, apnea supervenes.[1067] If the sleep of death is not to follow, the patient must be awakened immediately. After this awakening normal breathing resumes. As hypoventilation may follow, the patient should be intubated and ventilated as soon as possible after he has been awakened.

This syndrome has been reported to last a mean of two weeks.[1067,1068] Thus tracheostomy should be performed. Approximately half of patients with this syndrome do not recover, but in the other half the sleep-induced apnea resolves.[1067,1068] All patients who have had this syndrome continue to have an exquisite sensitivity to respiratory-depressant drugs. For instance, apnea has been reported after 5 mg codeine. Response to any increase in arterial carbon dioxide tension is depressed even in the absence of any medication. Even minute quantities of narcotics and barbiturates further flatten and shift to the right the carbon dioxide response curve. Sometimes in this syndrome vital capacity is unaffected at any time; sometimes it is impaired but later recovers over a matter of months. Rarely, oxygen administration while the patient is awake may precipitate apnea.

Excessive water retention is common and probably is due to an inappropriate secretion of antidiuretic hormone. Signs of autonomic dysfunction are common. Hypotension often does not cause an appropriate increase in pulse rate. Micturition becomes difficult.

The sleep-induced apnea syndrome has many similarities to the respiratory dysfunction seen in some patients with bulbar poliomyelitis but without chest wall paralysis. These patients have major damage in the lateral reticular formation. This is the region where the spinoreticular projections of spinal afferents have been demonstrated after experimental anterolateral cordotomies.

The sleep-induced apnea syndrome after cervical cordotomy and anterior spinal surgery also has many similarities to Ondine's curse.[1732] In each syndrome conventional parameters of respiratory failure are not a reliable guide to a precarious respiratory state. Arterial blood gases and vital capacity are often deceptively normal. With each syndrome an afferent component of the central respiratory control mechanism is ablated.[1067,1068,1732]

HEAT STROKE

Extreme hyperthermia requires prompt and efficient cardiorespiratory management. Body temperatures above 42°C (about 107°F) are required to produce coma in a person with normal cerebral vasculature.[1753] Slightly lower temperatures generally cause delirium, not coma.[569] Heat stroke occurs in young people who exercise too violently in the heat and in older persons who expose themselves unduly to summer heat. Patients with heat stroke have a hot dry skin, hypertonic muscles, and usually small and reactive pupils.[1690] Tachycardia, tachypnea, and metabolic acidemia are almost invariably present.[744]

Treatment consists of copious amounts of intravenous Ringer's lactate solution cooled to about 10°C, lavage of the stomach and bladder with iced solutions, treatment of cerebral edema with corticosteroids, paralysis with pancuronium, controlled hyperventilation, and investigation of possible intravascular coagulation.[1701] Prompt cardiopulmonary bypass with a heat exchanger is also lifesaving on occasion.[1680]

Despite treatment the mortality of heat stroke is high. In one series 13 percent of patients died and another 9 percent had incapacitating neurologic sequelae.[1690] We saw a Boston marathon runner die from heat stroke several years ago. Some of these tragic deaths could be prevented if all concerned were aware of the dangers of a temperature of 42°C or over: for example, blood hypercoagulability.[79] While one organizes treatment, the patient's cerebral oxygen metabolism is decreasing and the electroencephalogram slowing.[1415] Emergency rooms and intensive care units should have Ringer's lactate solutions at 4–10°C. A large hospital should be able to place a patient on cardiopulmonary bypass within 30 minutes. Too often the initial physician does not know how to assemble the correct team.

Table 21-2. Cases of Acute Brain Swelling, 1968–1973

Etiology*	Adult	+	Pediatric	=	Total	Good Survivals	+	Deaths	+	Bad Survivals
Severe bacterial infections	14		58		72	52		18		2
Encephalitis	6		27†		33	30		2		1
Severe head injury	82		22		104	45		56		3
Convulsions and coma	2		34		36	31		5		—
Severe eclampsia	7		—		7	6		1		—
Cerebrovascular disorders	22		9		31	8		23		—
After arrest	34		20		54	29		25		—
After neurosurgery	10		3		13	8		5		—
Miscellaneous‡	27		17		44	23		20		1
Totals	204		190		394§	232		155		7

* Total of 39 individual diagnoses.
† Includes 10 who required IPPV during a 1970 epidemic.
‡ e.g., gas embolism, fat embolism, heavy metal encephalopathy, malignant hyperthermia, hepatic coma, severe gastroenteritis.
§ Represents 24% of total admissions.
SOURCE: R. V. Trubuhovich and M. Spence. First World Congress on Intensive Care.[1941] Amended as specified by authors in personal communication.

Much still needs to be learned about correct respiratory management of diseases of the central nervous system. It has been shown, however, that carefully coordinated respiratory treatment, even of decerebrating patients, can lead to most gratifying outcomes (Table 21-2).[1941] Applied respiratory physiology is especially interesting and exciting in such cases.

V

Effects of Age, Obesity, and Environment on Respiratory Function

22

Aging

An ever-increasing number of elderly patients are undergoing major surgical procedures. Since many of these patients are quite ill postoperatively, greater numbers of elderly patients requiring respiratory care are arriving in the intensive care unit. It is necessary for the physician caring for them to understand the physiologic changes that occur in the normal lung with increasing age.

This chapter will discuss the magnitude of these changes, the reasons for them, and their significance in relation to the elderly patient in respiratory failure.

PULMONARY FUNCTION

LUNG VOLUME

Vital capacity declines with advancing age.[211,989] Mean vital capacity in subjects over 50 years of age without known cardiopulmonary disease varies from 3.5 to 4 liters in males and is about 2.3 liters in females.[769] In people 60–90 years of age the mean vital capacity is 2.4 liters.[1635]

Both functional residual capacity and residual volume are increased in old lungs. The functional residual capacity in young normal subjects is 2.9 liters. In normal subjects over 50 years of age it is significantly increased to between 3.5 and 3.9 liters.[110,769] Residual volume also is increased to a mean of 2.4 liters.[769]

There is a reduction in maximum breathing capacity. Mean maximum breathing capacity for men over 50 is 44.1 liters per minute per square meter and for women is 41.2 liters per minute per square meter.[769] In spite of these changes in the subdivisions of pulmonary function there is no change in the total lung capacity in normal elderly subjects.[662] The reasons for changes in the ratio of residual volume to total lung capacity and of functional residual capacity to total lung capacity have been the subject of considerable controversy.[1640]

For the most part lung volumes are determined by the interaction of the recoil properties of the lung and the recoil properties of the chest wall.[1291] It is now well established that lung compliance increases with advancing age.[379,1640,1948] Static pressure-volume curves of lungs of elderly subjects are shifted to the left. While there is a progressive increase in static lung compliance, it appears that there is a fall in chest wall compliance.[1328,1948] In examining data related to chest wall compliance the motion of the diaphragm must be considered, since this can alter the measurements.[1326]

LUNG ELASTICITY

The elastic recoil of the lung continually declines with advancing age.[1531,1948] These decreases in lung elasticity result in the increase in static lung compliance. The increased expansibility of elderly lungs is counteracted by the decrease in chest wall compliance. The end result is that the total respiratory compliance frequently is unchanged by aging and that therefore there is little change in the total lung capacity.[1948] The alteration in the pressure-volume characteristics of the lung itself explains the increase in functional residual capacity and residual volume. As a result of this the vital capacity decreases.[1531]

The reasons for this decline in lung elasticity, which accounts for the volume changes, are not well established. The major determinant in the elasticity of the normal lung is related to the elastin in the lung.[1948] Several reports indicate that the elastin content of the lungs of elderly patients is increased.[1530,1948] The elastin content of the visceral pleura increases with age, while the ratio of collagen to elastin declines (Figs. 22-1 and 22-2). While these changes occur in the pleura, there is no change in the elastin content of the pulmonary parenchyma, although there may be a redistribution of the elastin fibers in the lung parenchyma with age.[967]

AIRWAY RESISTANCE

The changes that occur in airway resistance in aging are less well documented than the lung volume changes.[404] The resistance of peripheral airways is significantly greater in the elderly without lung disease than in young subjects. In a person without lung disease pulmonary resistance is determined largely by the mean diameter of the bronchioles rather than by changes in the larger airways.[1430]

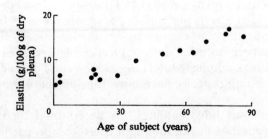

Figure 22-1. Elastin contents of the visceral pleura isolated from patients of different ages. Tissue extraction was done with 0.1M NaCl, organic solvents, and 0.1M NaOH. There is a significant increase in the elastin content of pleura with increasing age. (From R. John and J. Thomas, *Biochem. J.*[967])

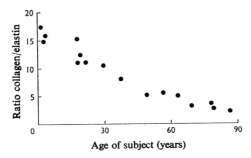

Figure 22-2. The ratio of collagen to elastin in the visceral pleurae of subjects of varying ages. The ratio falls progressively with increasing age. It is found that, since elastin content rises with age (see Figure 22-1), the collagen content remains unchanged by increasing age. (From R. John and J. Thomas, *Biochem. J.*[967])

GAS EXCHANGE

It has been suggested that normal arterial oxygen tension is 95–100 mm Hg (12.7–13.3 kPa). This is not true in the elderly. The arterial oxygen tension declines progressively with increasing age (Figs. 22-3 and 22-4).[492,1418,1823,1915] This decrease is constant and has been represented by various equations. The most reliable equation for the prediction of the arterial oxygen tension is

$$Pa_{O_2} = 109 \text{ mm Hg} - 0.43 \text{ (age in years)}$$

or,

$$Pa_{O_2} = 14.5 \text{ kPa} - 0.05733 \text{ (age in years)}$$

When this equation is used, the standard deviation is ± 4.10 mm Hg.

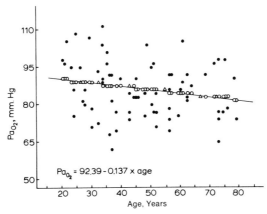

Figure 22-3. The relationship between age and arterial oxygen tension (Pa_{O_2}) in female subjects. Pa_{O_2} was measured in 84 female subjects breathing room air. *Black dots* represent each determination of Pa_{O_2}. *Circles* represent the predicted values, and *triangles* represent those patients in whom determined and predicted values coincide. There is a fall in Pa_{O_2} with increasing age; however, the range of values is wide. (From O. Neufeld, J. R. Smith, and S. L. Goldman, *J. Am. Geriatr. Soc.*[1418])

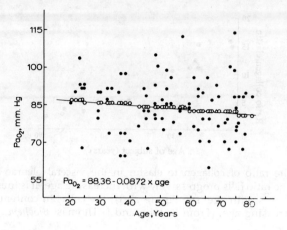

Figure 22-4. The relationship between age and arterial oxygen tension (Pa_{O_2}) in male subjects. Ninety-three male subjects had measurements of Pa_{O_2}. *Black dots* represent the individual determinations. *Circles* represent the predicted values, and *triangles* represent the points where the determined and predicted values coincide. In males the Pa_{O_2} falls with age; however, there is a wide range of values. (From O. Neufeld, J. R. Smith, and S. L. Goldman, *J. Am. Geriatr. Soc.* [1418])

The major reason for the finding of reduced arterial oxygen tension in the elderly probably is alteration in ventilation-perfusion relations.[911,1823] The alveolar-arterial oxygen tension gradient in elderly subjects is slightly greater than in young subjects, no matter what inspired oxygen concentration is used.[177] In elderly subjects the distribution of ventilation is frequently similar to that seen in young subjects. Blood flow is increased in the upper lung zones but remains predominantly in the lower zones. In many elderly patients it has been observed that there is an abnormal pattern of distribution of ventilation to the lower lung zones. This is thought to be attributable to airway closure, which would help account for the elevation in alveolar-arterial oxygen tension gradient.[911]

There is evidence of unequal distribution of gases during the quiet breathing of aged subjects.[512] During deep breathing this unequal ventilation is eliminated.[574] When the elderly subject breathes at low tidal volumes, gas is trapped in the lower lung zones because of airway closure. The volume at which this occurs, or *closing volume*, increases in a linear fashion with age.[38,1129,1544] This increase in closing volume is thought to be a consequence of the reduction in the elastic recoil of the lung. Closing volume affects oxygenation by altering the ratio of ventilation to perfusion. It has been demonstrated that higher closing volumes are associated with an increased alveolar-arterial oxygen tension gradient.[1544]

Other factors must be considered also in the etiology of the fall in arterial oxygen tension difference with age.[737] In some aged patients with elevation of the alveolar-arterial oxygen tension gradient, no elevation of the alveolar-arterial nitrogen tension gradient can be found. This suggests that other causes for elevation of the alveolar-arterial oxygen tension gradient are present besides shunting of blood and alteration in ventilation-perfusion relations. Alterations in diffusion to perfusion ratios and diffusing capacity for oxygen may be responsible for these findings.[80,378,512]

There is no evidence to suggest that there are any alterations in the carbon dioxide elimination of normal elderly lungs. The carbon dioxide tensions of the fit elderly are normal.[1635]

PULMONARY VASCULATURE

The pulmonary circulation in the aged differs from that of the young. Under conditions of rest there is no difference between pulmonary vascular pressures and resistances in the young and in the old. During exercise there is an increase in pulmonary blood flow and pulmonary artery pressure in both old and young subjects. The difference is that the pulmonary vascular resistance falls in young exercising subjects. In the elderly the change in pulmonary vascular resistance is unpredictable.[591]

VENTILATORY RESPONSE

The response of normal elderly patients to hypoxemia and hypercapnia is dramatically reduced. In patients 64–73 years old the ventilatory response to hypoxemia is decreased by 51 ± 6 percent as compared to that of patients 22–30 years old. The ventilatory response to hypercapnia is reduced by 41 ± 7 percent. The heart rate response to both hypoxemia and hypercapnia also is significantly reduced with advancing age.[511,1069]

CLINICAL IMPLICATIONS

Elderly patients are at increased risk for development of acute respiratory failure, especially in the postoperative period.[852] The lowered vital capacity is further reduced by abdominal or thoracic surgery. The development of acute lung disease can further increase the risk of respiratory failure.

In elderly patients with respiratory failure lung volumes are significantly higher than in young patients with respiratory failure (Fig. 22-5).[847] The functional residual capacity in elderly patients is increased to a greater degree than it is in young patients with acute respiratory failure.

The increase in closing volume in elderly patients can increase the difficulty of weaning old patients from controlled ventilation. During weaning there is a tendency to ventilate at low tidal volumes. With increased closing volumes this pattern of ventilation can lead to airway collapse, elevation of the alveolar-arterial oxygen tension gradient, and subsequent hypoxemia during weaning. This can be minimized by the use of positive end-expiratory pressure during weaning, as is discussed in Chapter 11.

To summarize, the physiologic changes that occur in the aged lung are a decreased vital capacity, increased functional residual capacity, and in-

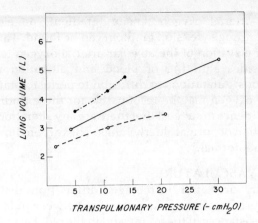

Figure 22-5.   Effect of age on relationship between lung volume and transpulmonary pressure. Changes in lung volume with changes in transpulmonary pressure were studied in ten patients in respiratory failure and in healthy patients. *Solid line = fit adults; broken top line* = patients over 54 years of age with bronchopneumonia; *broken bottom line* = patients under 42 years of age with bronchopneumonia. Mean values are shown. Young patients can survive a large amount of pneumonic consolidation. By contrast, in older patients respiratory failure due to bronchopneumonia is often associated with relatively normal lung volumes. (From J. Hedley-Whyte, P. Berry, L. S. Bushnell, H. K. Darrah, and M. J. Morris. In T. B. Boulton et al. (Eds.), *Progress in Anaesthesiology.*[847])

creased residual volume. Chest wall compliance decreases, and static lung compliance increases. Arterial oxygen tension declines linearly and closing volume increases linearly with age.

23

Obesity

One out of every five American males above 20 years of age is at least 10 percent overweight. One out of every twenty is 20 percent overweight. Obesity is more common in American women, with one out of four 10 percent overweight and one out of every nine over 20 percent overweight.[23] For overweight individuals mortality ranges from 131 to 180 percent of the predicted rate.[1229]

In this chapter we discuss the effect of obesity on various aspects of pulmonary function. In order to describe the result of obesity on pulmonary function, we arbitrarily divide the effect produced on the so-called complete Pickwickian patient from the effect on the non-Pickwickian patient.

PICKWICKIAN SYNDROME

The complete Pickwickian syndrome consists of massive obesity, somnolence, alveolar hypoventilation, periodic respiration, hypoxemia, secondary polycythemia, and right heart failure.[1755] In the management of obese patients the complete Pickwickian syndrome is most unusual; however, one or more of the above signs may be found in any obese patient.

The syndrome was named by Burwell in 1956. He felt that the first adequate description of this type of patient had been made in 1837 by Charles Dickens in *The Posthumous Papers of the Pickwick Club*, in which he described an obese, somnolent boy named Joe.[278]

The most common abnormality of blood gas exchange in Pickwickian patients is elevation of the arterial carbon dioxide tension secondary to alveolar hypoventilation. This is accompanied by hypoxemia, which eventually leads to a secondary polycythemia.[278,789,1004,1755] The abnormalities can be corrected in these patients simply by weight reduction (Fig. 23-1). This implies that there is no preexisting lung disease and that the Pickwickian syndrome is related to obesity alone.[278,599,1755]

Since the complete syndrome occurs in an extremely small percentage of obese patients, its pathogenesis is still somewhat unclear. Abnormalities in pulmonary function in the Pickwickian patient include a decrease in total lung volume and a decrease in expiratory reserve volume, which produce a small functional residual capacity. Vital capacity and maximum breathing capacity also are reduced. This is attributed to an increase in intraabdom-

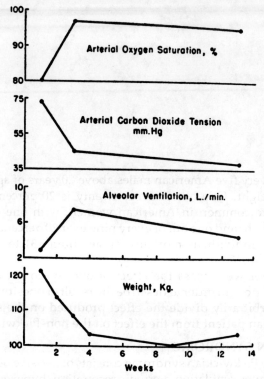

Figure 23-1. Changes in arterial blood gases and alveolar ventilation with loss of weight in a patient with the Pickwickian syndrome. Following weight reduction the arterial oxygen saturation rose and the carbon dioxide tension fell to normal. Alveolar ventilation of 2.7 liters per minute before weight reduction was barely compatible with survival. Following weight reduction alveolar ventilation rose to 4.4 liters per minute. (From C. S. Burwell, E. D. Robin, R. D. Whaley, and A. G. Bickelmann, *Am. J. Med.*[278])

inal pressure.[278,458,599] The deadspace-to-tidal-volume ratio is normal (Fig. 23-2). The timed vital capacity and the maximum midexpiratory flow rates usually are normal.[1004] These changes in pulmonary function are reversible in the Pickwickian patient (Fig. 23-3), again suggesting that such patients have no underlying lung disease.[278,599] A decrease in total compliance produces an increase in the work of breathing and eventually leads to alveolar hypoventilation.[789,1004] In obese patients without underlying lung disease the compliance of the lung itself is completely normal. The decrease in total compliance is related to decreased compliance of the chest wall.[1406]

It has been theorized that respiratory center disease is the basis of hypoventilation in obese subjects. Pickwickian patients, while overweight, have a decreased response to breathing carbon dioxide; however, no good evidence exists to suggest a central cause for this syndrome.[789]

The pulmonary vascular changes in the Pickwickian syndrome are

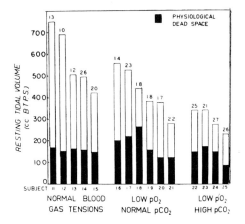

Figure 23-2. Tidal volume and physiologic deadspace in 15 obese patients (mean weight, 113 kg) grouped according to their blood gases. Patients with low arterial oxygen tensions (Pa$_{O_2}$) and a high arterial carbon dioxide tension (Pa$_{CO_2}$) had the lowest tidal volume. In all patients the physiologic deadspace was normal. (From B. J. Kaufman, M. H. Ferguson, and R. M. Cherniack, *J. Clin. Invest.*[1004])

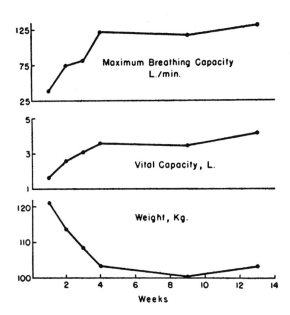

Figure 23-3. Improvements in vital capacity and maximum breathing capacity with weight loss in a Pickwickian patient. (From C. S. Burwell, E. D. Robin, R. D. Whaley, and A. G. Bickelmann, *Am. J. Med.*[278])

marked pulmonary hypertension, right axis deviation on the electrocardiogram, and evidence of right ventricular hypertrophy.[789,1163,1755] The reasons for these changes are thought to be chronic hypoxemia and polycythemia, which have led to right heart failure.[64,1163] Left heart failure can complicate the clinical course, but the usual finding is a normal pulmonary capillary pressure.[1755]

OBESE NON-PICKWICKIAN PATIENTS

Following Burwell's initial description of the Pickwickian syndrome there appeared numerous reports of obese patients with hypoxemia and polycythemia. Most of these patients, however, were not true Pickwickian examples but obese patients with underlying chronic lung disease. As more obese patients were studied, it became clear that obese patients with alveolar hypoventilation usually had intrinsic lung disease.[134]

There is evidence that obese non-Pickwickian patients, without intrinsic lung disease, do have abnormalities of pulmonary function. As with Pickwickian patients these abnormalities include a reduction in functional residual capacity without any change in residual volume, producing a fall in the expiratory reserve volume.[325,1945] Many patients also demonstrate a low maximum breathing capacity.[458]

ABDOMEN AND CHEST WALL

The abdomen and chest wall play a major part in altering the pulmonary function of obese patients. Because of an increased resistance to expansion of the thorax the compliance of the total respiratory system of obese patients is significantly lower than the compliance of normal subjects. This effect of subcutaneous fat is accentuated by recumbency in overweight patients. The decrease in compliance has a correlation with the decrease in lung volumes seen in obese patients.[1406] This correlation is supported by the fact that mass loading of the chest wall of normal individuals produces total respiratory pressure-volume curves similar to those produced by obese individuals (Fig. 23-4).[1744,2017] At any lung volume the compliance of the obese or the mass-loaded individual is roughly half the normal compliance (Fig. 23-5).[2017]

During exercise ventilation and oxygen consumption increase twice as much in obese patients as in normal individuals,[497] owing to high respiratory rates and low tidal volumes.[1947] This increase is consistent with the increased weight, suggesting that there is no inefficiency of oxygen utilization.[809] Obese patients with normal alveolar ventilation often demonstrate mild carbon dioxide retention during the first two minutes of exercise, but usually there is a return to normal after these two initial minutes of exercise.[66]

HYPOXEMIA

The most common abnormal blood gas finding in the obese patient is hypoxemia. Although hypoxemia can occur as a result of hypercapnia, most

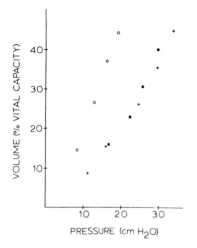

Figure 23-4. Pressure-volume curves of individuals of normal weight (*open circles*), obese individuals (*crosses*), and mass-loaded individuals of normal weight (*black circles*). The abscissa gives the airway pressure. Total respiratory compliance is decreased in obesity. Mass loading by placing 23-kg sand bags on the thorax and abdomen of normal individuals results in a fall in compliance similar to that seen in obesity. The decreased compliance in obesity is related chiefly to the weight of fat on the chest and abdomen. (From C. L. Waltemath and N. A. Bergman, *Anesthesiology.*[2017])

often it is a result of abnormal relationships between ventilation and perfusion.[1689] Arterial oxygen tensions in obese patients breathing air frequently are in the range of 60–80 mm Hg (8.0–10.6 kPa).[498,1689] Elevations in alveolar-arterial oxygen tension gradients have been demonstrated in many obese patients, reflecting an increase in venous admixture. In most instances this is due to low ventilation-perfusion ratios. In obese subjects perfusion to dependent areas is often great but is accompanied by little or no ventilation in those areas.[100,913] This decrease in ventilation to dependent areas of lung is probably secondary to closure of small airways,[432] which is a tendency most often found in obese patients with low expiratory reserve volume. It is this dependent airway closure combined with the normal gravitational increase in blood flow to dependent areas that causes marked abnormalities in ventilation-perfusion ratios and therefore hypoxemia in the obese patient.[99,532]

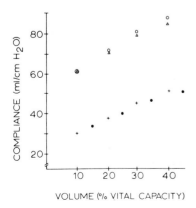

Figure 23-5. Comparison of respiratory compliance and respiratory system volume. *Open circles* and *triangles* (data of Kallos, Wyche, and Garman[988]) represent individuals of normal weight. *Black circles* indicate mass-loaded individuals of normal weight, and *crosses* represent obese individuals. The compliance of obese and mass-loaded individuals is about one-half the compliance of normal individuals at any respiratory volume. (From C. L. Waltemath and N. A. Bergman, *Anesthesiology.*[2017])

CARBON DIOXIDE RETENTION

Abnormalities of carbon dioxide elimination are less frequent than abnormalities of oxygenation in the obese patient. In patients without the Pickwickian syndrome who develop carbon dioxide retention the usual mechanism is some form of superimposed chronic or acute lung disease. With the imposition of acute or chronic lung disease obese patients are more likely to develop carbon dioxide retention. There are several reasons for this. The first is that these patients often are functioning at low lung volumes, and any further reduction may lead to alveolar hypoventilation. Secondly, obese patients have markedly reduced total respiratory compliance, and any further reduction of lung compliance can increase the work of breathing to such an extent that alveolar hypoventilation develops.[710] Obese patients also show evidence of being unable to increase the activity of the diaphragm sufficiently during acute lung disease to maintain alveolar ventilation.[1184] All these factors play some contributory role in the development of respiratory failure. An obese patient faced with a relatively minor pulmonary infection can be at great risk for the development of respiratory failure. The obese patient also is at much greater risk of developing respiratory failure postoperatively.

PULMONARY VASCULATURE

There is little change from normal in the pulmonary vasculature of obese patients without lung disease. Pulmonary artery, pulmonary capillary, and pulmonary venous pressures are normal in obese patients without heart or lung disease. There is little evidence to suggest that cor pulmonale occurs in non-Pickwickian patients without lung disease. The most common cause of right heart failure in the obese patient is left heart failure. Isolated right heart failure does occur in cases of severe chronic lung disease associated with obesity.[23]

TREATMENT OF RESPIRATORY FAILURE IN THE OBESE PATIENT

The usual etiology of respiratory failure in extreme obesity is the superimposition of some form of acute lung disease, either pneumonia, congestive heart failure, or atelectasis. Since ventilatory reserve is marginal in obese patients, it takes a very small insult to produce respiratory failure. Treatment should be aimed at correcting the underlying lung disease.[134]

Once conservative treatment has failed and the diagnosis of respiratory failure is made, a tracheal tube is placed. Orotracheal intubation is preferred, with the patient breathing spontaneously, since laryngoscopy in the obese patient is often difficult. If orotracheal intubation cannot be accomplished, blind nasotracheal intubation should be performed. The use of muscle relaxants should be avoided if possible, unless it is known that intubation will be possible without undue difficulty.

Following intubation the patient is placed on controlled ventilation with a volume-constant ventilator, since obese patients have a low respiratory compliance even prior to development of respiratory failure. With the superimposition of acute lung disease there is a further fall in compliance. A chest x-ray is performed to determine the position of the tracheal tube. The tip of the tracheal tube should be at least 3–4 centimeters above the carina. This serves to prevent streaming of gases into the right main-stem bronchus.

Obese patients should be weaned from controlled ventilation as soon as possible. Weaning is best accomplished with the patient in the sitting position. When an obese patient is recumbent, he has greater abnormalities of ventilation-perfusion relations and a lower arterial oxygen tension.[1945]

The following case report illustrates many of these points.

A 69-year-old, 305-pound female, 4 feet 6 inches tall, was admitted to Beth Israel Hospital because of increasing shortness of breath. The patient had been obese for many years. Three years prior to admission she had been hospitalized because of gastrointestinal bleeding secondary to a gastric ulcer. At that time pulmonary function tests had shown evidence of chronic lung disease. At the time of her admission for shortness of breath her total vital capacity was 1,540 ml, 67 percent of predicted; timed vital capacity was 1,050 ml, 68 percent of predicted; maximum midexpiratory flow rate was 33 liters per minute, 26 percent of predicted; and maximum breathing capacity was 50 percent of predicted. Arterial carbon dioxide tension was 46 mm Hg (6.1 kPa) with a normal arterial oxygen tension and pH. Hematocrit was 28 percent secondary to gastrointestinal bleeding. She complained of many years of shortness of breath but denied somnolence.

Three weeks prior to her next admission she developed an upper respiratory tract infection consisting of sneezing, rhinorrhea, and malaise. Over the next week she developed a cough productive of yellow sputum and increased shortness of breath. One week later she came to the emergency ward, where she was found to have an acute respiratory acidemia with blood gases on room air showing arterial oxygen tension of 48 mm Hg (6.4 kPa), arterial carbon dioxide tension of 53 mm Hg (7.0 kPa), and a pHa of 7.27. The hematocrit was 67 percent and the electrocardiogram showed right axis deviation. Chest examination was normal, and no pulmonary infiltrates were seen on x-ray examination. She refused hospital admission at that time, only to return two weeks later in acute respiratory distress.

Physical examination revealed a short, massively obese female in acute respiratory distress. Blood pressure was 180/90 mm Hg (23.9/12.0 kPa), heart rate was 120 per minute, respiratory rate was 40 breaths per minute, and temperature was 37.5°C. There was cyanosis of the lips and nails. Her pharynx was markedly inflamed, and her neck veins were distended. Chest examination revealed decreased breath sounds at the left base with coarse rales in all lung fields. Heart sounds could not be heard. There was massive pitting edema of the legs extending above the knees.

Laboratory evaluation revealed a hematocrit of 63 percent; arterial blood gases on room air showed an arterial oxygen tension of 42 mm Hg (5.6 kPa), an arterial carbon dioxide tension of 74 mm Hg (9.8 kPa), and a pHa of 7.15. Chest x-ray showed no infiltrates, but there was a question of upper zone redistribution. The electrocardiogram showed right axis deviation. Sputum gram stain showed many polymorphonuclear leukocytes but few organisms. Subsequent culture revealed no growth.

Blood urea nitrogen was 50 mg per 100 ml (17.8 mmol/l) with a serum creatinine of 1.8 mg per 100 ml (159.1 μmol/l).

On the first hospital day a central venous catheter was placed and revealed a central venous pressure of 25 cm H_2O (2.5 kPa). She was phlebotomized of 800 ml of blood, and her arterial blood gases improved on room air to an arterial oxygen tension of 50 mm Hg (6.6 kPa), an arterial carbon dioxide tension of 58 mm Hg (7.7 kPa), and a pHa of 7.23. Over that night she was phlebotomized of an additional 700 ml of blood, and the arterial blood gases continued to improve.

On the second hospital day her shortness of breath worsened. Blood gases on an inspired oxygen concentration of 28% were: arterial oxygen tension, 44 mm Hg (5.8 kPa); arterial carbon dioxide tension, 73 mm Hg (9.7 kPa); and pHa, 7.09. Tidal volume was 200 ml and vital capacity 250 ml. At that time orotracheal intubation was performed, and she was placed on controlled ventilation via an Emerson ventilator. The alveolar-arterial oxygen tension difference on 100% oxygen was only 76 mm Hg (10.1 kPa). Effective compliance was reduced to 25 ml per cm H_2O. At that time there was no evidence of bacterial infection, and the reason for her acute decompensation was unclear.

A Swan-Ganz catheter was passed on the third hospital day and revealed a right ventricular pressure of 92/0 mm Hg (12.2/0 kPa), a pulmonary artery pressure of 100/38 mm Hg (13.3/5.1 kPa), and a pulmonary capillary wedge pressure of 18 mm Hg (2.4 kPa). She was thought to have left heart decompensation as well as cor pulmonale and was treated with phlebotomy of an additional 1,500 ml of blood, which brought her hematocrit down to 48 percent. She was begun on digoxin and furosemide. Her deadspace-to-tidal-volume ratio was 0.51. Carbon dioxide production was 223 ml per minute.

Over the next two days weaning from controlled ventilation was attempted but was unsuccessful due to the rapid development of respiratory acidemia on each occasion. A tracheostomy was performed after three days of orotracheal intubation.

On the sixth hospital day the patient developed hypotension to a systolic blood pressure of 50–60 mm Hg (6.7–8.0 kPa) associated with a fall in CVP to 3 cm H_2O (0.3 kPa), a rise in blood urea nitrogen to 60 mg per 100 ml (21.4 mmol/l), and the development of a hypochloremic, hypokalemic, metabolic alkalemia. During her hospital stay she had lost over 13 pounds. She was thought to be depleted of water, potassium, and chloride secondary to diuretic therapy. Her fluid deficit was replaced with 4 liters of normal saline and 50 gm of albumin with return of blood pressure to normal levels. Her renal function never improved. She developed progressive azotemia secondary to acute tubular necrosis and required daily peritoneal dialysis for the next week. The excessive phlebotomy may have contributed to her renal failure.

On the ninth hospital day the patient again became hypotensive with a fever of 39°C. No site of infection could be determined. At that time the pulmonary artery pressure was 42/18 mm Hg (5.6/2.4 kPa) with a pulmonary capillary wedge pressure of 13 mm Hg (1.7 kPa). The cardiac index was 2.4 liters per minute per square meter. Isoproterenol was begun to maintain her blood pressure.

She continued to spike fevers to 39–40°C daily; however, physical examination and blood, sputum, and cerebrospinal fluid cultures never revealed the source of the sepsis. She required isoproterenol to maintain her blood pressure. On the twelfth hospital day she developed ventricular tachycardia and then asystole. Resuscitation attempts were unsuccessful, and she was pronounced dead. A postmortem examination was not obtained.

PREVENTION OF RESPIRATORY FAILURE

The need for the prevention of obesity is obvious.[1218] It would be desirable if all obese patients who were to undergo major surgery would reduce their weight to within normal limits. In practice this is impossible, and we must concentrate on the prevention of respiratory complications in these high-risk patients.

PULMONARY FUNCTION TESTS

All obese patients should have pulmonary function tests periodically and especially prior to elective surgery. It is important to determine the extent of impairment of pulmonary function as well as to determine the presence of chronic lung disease. It is also important to follow blood gases in the obese patient, particularly prior to any surgery. Knowing the level of oxygenation and alveolar ventilation facilitates the preoperative and postoperative management of the obese patient.

CHEST PHYSICAL THERAPY

Chest physical therapy is important preoperatively for two reasons. It enables the patient and therapist to know each other and gives the therapist time to instruct the patient in methods of coughing and deep breathing. It also enables the therapist to help the patient clear his lungs of any secretions that may be present preoperatively.

WEANING

The postoperative management of the obese patient is of great significance in the prevention of respiratory failure. When the patient is fully awake and the conditions for weaning are met, the patient is placed on a Briggs adaptor, and blood gases and vital signs are followed. The patient is encouraged to ambulate as soon as possible following surgery. Prolonged recumbency is avoided because of its adverse effects on ventilation-perfusion relations.[1945]

RELIEF OF PAIN POSTOPERATIVELY

Relief of pain in the postoperative obese patient is important. The use of too small an amount of narcotics can lead to increased splinting due to pain and a fall in vital capacity. Insufficient narcotic administration also can result in the patient's being intolerant of attempts at chest physical therapy. Excessive administration of narcotics obviously can lead to respiratory depression.

In view of the difficulties of using narcotic analgesics for postoperative pain relief, we employ thoracic epidural analgesia for postoperative pain relief of obese patients. Patients receiving thoracic epidural analgesia can be mobilized much earlier than those receiving morphine.[1523] In the very obese patient thoracic epidural analgesia is an important mode of therapy.

INTESTINAL BYPASS

In the Respiratory–Intensive Care Unit at Beth Israel Hospital we have managed massively obese patients who have undergone jejunoileal bypass as treatment of morbid obesity. Intestinal bypass has been shown to be an effective method of producing weight loss in massively obese patients.[897,1495,1719,1720,1721] As well as producing weight loss the operation has improved the psychologic state of many patients.[1820] The major complications seem to be related protein malnutrition and subsequent hepatic dysfunction.[918,1383] We have managed these patients by using thoracic epidural analgesia for pain relief in the postoperative period. They were able to ambulate freely on the night of surgery.

In summary, most obese patients have some impairment in pulmonary function. The most common abnormality is arterial hypoxemia. Lung volumes are also diminished, as is total respiratory compliance. Alveolar hypoventilation is usually secondary to the imposition of some form of intrinsic lung disease. The complete Pickwickian syndrome of hypoventilation, hypoxemia, polycythemia, somnolence, and right heart failure is unusual and is a rare primary cause of respiratory failure in the obese patient. Respiratory failure in the obese patient usually results from a combination of factors: decrease in lung volume, decrease in compliance, and the effect of chronic or acute lung disease, especially in the postoperative patient.

24

Smoking, Air Pollution, and Contamination of Medical Gases

SMOKING

Smoking has been repeatedly shown to increase mortality.[34,1955,1956] One of every three deaths of middle-aged males in the United States is caused by a disease associated with smoking.[411] For the intensive care patient with a history of smoking the most serious problems are respiratory and cardiac.

The extent of respiratory dysfunction is related to the total number of cigarettes smoked and the number of years of habitual smoking.[807,1077,1955,1956] Chronic cigarette smoke inhalation is associated with obstructive pulmonary disease, progressing to emphysema.[67] The ratio of forced expired volume in one second to vital capacity is significantly reduced in smokers (Fig. 24-1).[372,1070,1515] Closing volume also increases in smokers (Figs. 24-2 and 24-3).[264,265,1261] These changes are due to increased bronchiolar sensitivity, resulting in constriction, and to loss of small airway elasticity, with collapse.[1431,1727,2144] The pathologic condition of the airway results in a worsening of ventilation-perfusion relationships of the lung and an increase in the alveolar-arterial oxygen tension gradient on room air (Fig. 24-4).[1867] The acute effects of smoking one cigarette are an increase of airway resistance of approximately 30 percent and a decrease of dynamic compliance of 20 percent.[476,1316,1404,1613]

Cigarette smoking causes ciliary paralysis acutely and loss of ciliated cells with chronic smoking.[68] This results in a reduction in the tracheobronchial mucociliary clearance rate such that after three months of smoking, clearance rates are 10 percent of presmoking values.[13,1185,1944]

Smoking increases the amount of pulmonary fibrosis and alveolar septal rupture and causes thickening of small arterial and arteriolar walls (Fig. 24-5).[69] Bronchial glands and goblet cells increase up to 15 times above their number in nonsmokers.[68] Clara cells are significantly reduced in number in heavy smokers.[571]

The alveolar macrophages of smokers develop heterogeneous, pleomorphic inclusions.[1219,1431,1556,2118] Lavage fluid from smokers' lungs yields four to five times the number of macrophages obtained from the lungs of nonsmokers. The macrophages from smokers are different in that their resting glucose utilization is four times that of nonsmoker macrophages.[823]

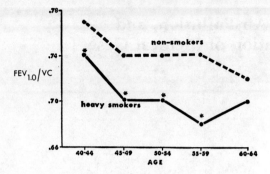

Figure 24-1. The ratio of forced expiratory volume in one second to vital capacity ($FEV_{1.0}/VC$) is significantly lower in smokers than in nonsmokers. Data were collected from 1,584 postal employees over 40 years of age who worked in the same metropolitan building. (From E. O. Coates, Jr., G. C. Bower, and N. Reinstein, *J.A.M.A.* 191:161–166, 1965.[372] Copyright, 1965, American Medical Association.)

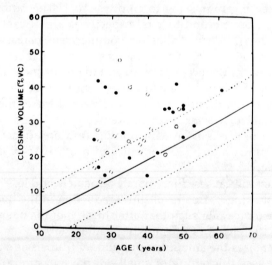

Figure 24-2. The closing volume as percent of vital capacity in 39 smokers and 66 nonsmokers while supine. *Solid line* = average relationship ± 2 SD between closing volume and age in the nonsmokers. *Open circles* = asymptomatic smokers; *closed circles* = smokers with chronic bronchitis by history. In nine asymptomatic smokers closing volume was above normal limits. (From D. S. McCarthy, R. Spencer, R. Greene, and J. Milic-Emili, *Am. J. Med.*[1261])

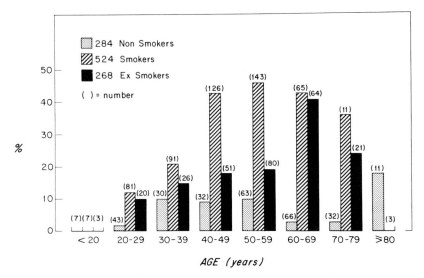

Figure 24-3. Percentage of abnormal closing volume to vital capacity ratios in smokers as compared with nonsmokers. This percentage increases with age until the 50–59-year age group. Exsmokers have fewer abnormal ratios than smokers but a greater percentage compared with persons who have never smoked. The results were obtained from 1,073 persons attending an emphysema screening center. (From A. S. Buist, D. L. Van Fleet, and B. B. Ross, *Am. Rev. Respir. Dis.*[265])

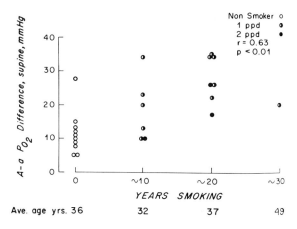

Figure 24-4. The increase in alveolar-arterial oxygen tension gradient on room air with increasing duration of smoking. All 24 volunteers had normal chest films and denied respiratory symptoms. *ppd* = pack per day. (From D. J. Strieder, R. Murphy, and H. Kazemi, *Am. Rev. Respir. Dis.*[1867])

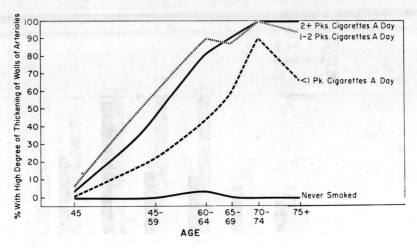

Figure 24-5.   Thickening of the walls of small arteries in cigarette smokers. Results obtained from microscopic analysis of lung tissue from approximately 1,000 persons are plotted against age and the amount of cigarette smoking. (From O. Auerbach, A. P. Stout, E. C. Hammond, and L. Garfinkel.[69] Reprinted by permission from the *New England Journal of Medicine* 269:1045–1054, 1963.)

In addition the ability of the smokers' alveolar macrophages to adhere to glass is increased by a factor of 10.[1219] Oxidative phosphorylation is depressed, as is protein synthesis.[1082,1187] The ability of macrophages to phagocytose and kill bacteria is markedly depressed in the presence of smoke (Figs. 24-6 and 24-7).[755] In the absence of smoke, however, macrophages lavaged from smokers do not differ in phagocytic ability from those of nonsmokers (Fig. 24-7). The pinocytic activity of smokers' cells is less than that of nonsmokers.[2118] The combination of increased secretions, failure to clear secretions, airway damage and irritability, and macrophage dysfunction leads to bronchospasm and even pneumonia in sick patients.

Although the surfactant system has been reported to be adversely affected by cigarette smoke,[88,197,632,703] these changes probably are due to the method of analysis.[359]

The effects of smoking are partially reversible.[405,806,1071,1519,2064] Therefore smoking should be minimized prior to a surgical procedure. The sputum is cultured, and if it proves purulent, antibiotic coverage is provided. Maintenance of adequate hydration, along with chest physiotherapy, helps to mobilize secretions. Effective coughing and breathing techniques are taught. These methods and the role of other methods are discussed in Chapter 10.

The effects of smoke inhalation are not restricted to the cigarette smoker. As is discussed in the next section, fire fighters, smog victims, and persons in the same room as cigarette smokers may all suffer ill effects.[1516,1676,2128]

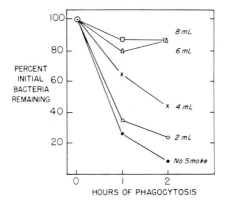

Figure 24-6. Inhibition of the bactericidal ability of alveolar macrophages by cigarette smoke. Macrophages were lavaged from normal rabbits and then exposed to a strain of *Staphylococcus albus*. The percentage of initial bacteria remaining was determined after two hours of incubation either with no smoke or in the presence of 2, 4, 6, or 8 ml of cigarette smoke in a 125-ml Erlenmeyer flask. (From G. M. Green and D. Carolin.[755] Reprinted by permission from the *New England Journal of Medicine* 276:421–427, 1967.)

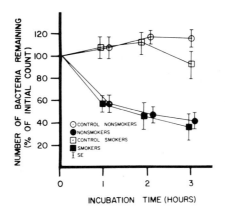

Figure 24-7. The phagocytic and bactericidal capacity of alveolar macrophages of smokers and nonsmokers. Alveolar macrophages were obtained by lavage from six cigarette smokers and from five nonsmokers. Macrophages of smokers and nonsmokers were incubated with *S. albus*. The alveolar macrophages of smokers and nonsmokers have the same phagocytic and bactericidal capacity. (From J. O. Harris, E. W. Swenson, and J. E. Johnson III, *J. Clin. Invest.*[823])

AIR POLLUTION

Atmospheric air pollution usually is composed of smoke, sulfur dioxide, hydrocarbons, carbon monoxide, nitric oxide, nitrogen dioxide, lead, and ozone.[1412] The worsening of atmospheric air pollution is known to cause increased morbidity and mortality due to aggravation of chronic lung disease.[308] Examples include the 1952, 1957, and 1962 London smog disasters. The oxidizing group of atmospheric pollutants (nitrogen dioxide, nitric oxide, or ozone) produces destruction of alveolar type I cells and stimulates proliferation of type II cells.[602,1752,2123] These effects closely resemble the effects that are produced by high partial pressures of oxygen (Chap. 31).

CARBON MONOXIDE AS A POLLUTANT

Carbon monoxide has an affinity for hemoglobin 210 times that of oxygen. Patients in the intensive care unit may manifest carboxyhemoglobinemia for a variety of reasons. Cigarette smokers inhale smoke that contains 4.2 percent carbon monoxide, resulting in the conversion of as much as 20 percent of all hemoglobin into carboxyhemoglobin.[411,1955] The average nonsmoker has less than 2 percent carboxyhemoglobin, depending on his environment. Carboxyhemoglobin saturation in smokers, therefore, ranges between 2 and 10 percent and possibly reaches as high as 20 percent. Carbon monoxide also is elevated in heavy traffic, which can raise the carboxyhemoglobin level to over 5 percent.[46,1706,2145] Even a nonsmoker in a cigarette smoke–filled conference room is noted to increase his level of carboxyhemoglobin to that of a smoker (Fig. 24-8).[1676]

The oxygen-carrying capacity of the blood is reduced by carboxyhemoglobin, and there is a left shift of the oxyhemoglobin dissociation curve (Fig. 24-9).[59,531,791,1312,1669] A value of 5 percent carboxyhemoglobin saturation is equivalent to the anoxia produced by an elevation of 8,000 feet.[1501,1956,2128] Even slight anoxia is particularly important to patients with coronary artery disease or cerebral vascular insufficiency.[331,375,734,1706] Low levels of carboxyhemoglobin do cause slight cerebral malfunction such as in visual acuity and discrimination of time intervals.[125,2145] Cerebral blood flow increases.

Care must be taken to locate the air-conditioner intake vent for the intensive care unit away from automobile exhaust fumes.

CONTAMINATION OF MEDICAL GASES

Nitrous oxide has been reported on different occasions to be contaminated by nitric oxide, nitrogen dioxide, nitrogen, or carbon monoxide. Nitric oxide (NO) is a colorless gas with an affinity for hemoglobin 10^6 times greater than that of oxygen.[1929] Nitrogen dioxide (NO$_2$) is a reddish brown gas. Both cause methemoglobinemia with cyanosis. Clinically the onset of cyanosis is followed by wheezing. Coughing and pulmonary edema should

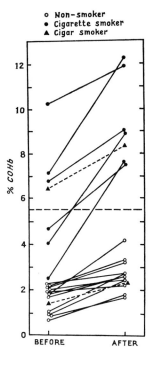

○ Non-smoker
● Cigarette smoker
▲ Cigar smoker

Figure 24-8. Venous carboxyhemoglobin (% *COHb*) in twelve nonsmokers, six cigarette smokers, and two cigar smokers before and after spending a mean of 78 minutes in a smoke-filled room with average carbon monoxide concentration of 38 parts per million. The mean carboxyhemoglobin of the nonsmokers increased to 2.6 percent, from a preexposure level of 1.6 percent, while that of the smokers increased from 5.9 percent to 9.6 percent. The mean increase of 1.0 percent in the nonsmokers was similar to the mean increase of the smokers after smoking one cigarette, 0.7 percent. Therefore, nonsmokers in a smoke-filled room increase their carboxyhemoglobin levels as much as if they had actively smoked one cigarette. The *horizontal line* shows the approximate equilibrium saturation for carbon monoxide at 38 parts per million (38 p/10^6). (From M. A. H. Russell, P. V. Cole, and E. Brown, *Lancet*.[1676])

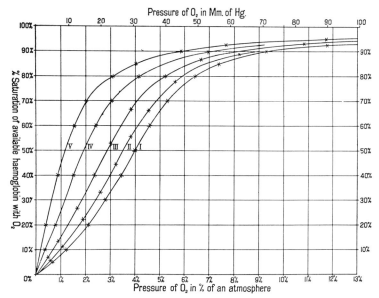

Figure 24-9. The shift in the oxyhemoglobin dissociation curve in the presence of carboxyhemoglobin (COHb). *Curve I* = 0% COHb; *Curve II* = 10% COHb; *Curve III* = 25% COHb; *Curve IV* = 50% COHb; and *Curve V* = 75% COHb. (This work was published by J. B. S. Haldane when he was 19 years old. His father J. S. Haldane was of course Professor of Physiology at Oxford. [From J. B. S. Haldane, *J. Physiol*.[791]])

317

suggest the diagnosis. Other more likely causes of cyanosis should be ruled out first, however. The arterial blood may be a deep blue or brownish color. If cyanosis is suspected, the offending tank should be kept for future analysis by a gas chromatograph–mass spectrometer linkup, preferably by an independent laboratory. If the diagnosis is confirmed by the presence of methemoglobin in the blood, treatment consists of oxygen administration. Controlled ventilation is used when indicated by arterial blood gases and pulmonary function tests.[1568] Methemoglobin is slowly reduced to hemoglobin by methemoglobin reductase. The hexose monophosphate shunt and glutathione also may play a role. Methylene blue, 2 mg per kilogram (1% solution), given intravenously as an initial dose, aids reconversion of methemoglobin to hemoglobin. Thereafter the methylene blue dose is

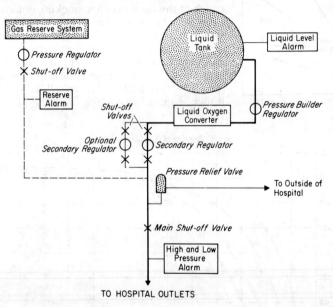

Figure 24-10.   Schematic representation of a typical bulk oxygen supply system with a reserve supply. *Dotted lines* = reserve supply system. The arrangement of the valves, regulators, and supply tanks may be varied, as long as they provide equivalent safeguards. Shut-off valves permit manual closing of either the main supply, the reserve supply, or the entire system. Additional shut-off valves are located within the hospital at the base of each rising pipeline. Location of shut-off valves and regulators should be known by hospital personnel. The pressure builder regulator controls the tank pressure. The secondary regulator maintains line pressure at 55–60 PSIG (379.2–413.7 kPa). The emergency alarm system should be activated if there is (1) low supply in either the main or reserve tanks or cylinders, (2) operation of the reserve supply, and (3) high or low pressure in the main hospital pipeline. A pressure relief valve is required to vent pressures in excess of 50 percent of normal pipeline pressures and must exhaust this gas outside the hospital. (From T. W. Feeley, K. J. McClelland, and I. V. Malhotra, *Lancet.*[622])

monitored, lest overdosage produce hemolysis and reconversion to methemoglobin.

Compressed air for use in the intensive care unit is often contaminated with oil or grease. This problem can be solved by the use of a compressor that does not allow the air to contact the lubricant. We use a clinical pump with a carbon seal.

Oxygen is rarely contaminated in the intensive care unit. Errors usually are those of faulty connection of gas lines; therefore all wall outlets must be checked prior to use in any newly installed system. Many deaths still occur each year in North America from failure to check oxygen lines. Oxygen line pressure is maintained at 55–60 pounds per square inch (379–414 kPa) in the United States (Fig. 24-10).[622]

VI

Special Problems

25

Management of Poisoning

INCIDENCE

Approximately a quarter of a million United States citizens take an overdose of hypnotic drugs each year, and approximately 24,000 succeed in committing suicide. In many large hospitals over 1 percent of admissions are due to drug overdosage.[44] Women are far more likely than men to use drugs for suicidal purposes, men preferring firearms.[2059] Hypnotic drugs are not a particularly effective way to kill oneself, since even if one goes into respiratory failure, the chances of dying should be less than 1 in 10 after arrival in the hospital. In some centers, however, one in four such patients die, so careful management does make a considerable difference to outcome.

GENERAL MANAGEMENT OF OVERDOSAGE WITH BARBITURATES AND OTHER HYPNOTICS

The management of patients poisoned with barbiturates is similar to that of poisoning with nonbarbiturate hypnotics.[1768] We will first consider general principles that we have found useful in the management of all patients poisoned with hypnotics.[1434] Later we consider special problems posed by drugs other than the barbiturates.

If the poisoned patient is unresponsive to verbal command and is comatose but will respond to painful stimuli, we intubate the trachea by using cricoid pressure and succinylcholine. Suction and mouth gags should be available, and an intravenous cannula should have been put in already and be working.[1436] When the cuffed orotracheal tube is secured and the patient oxygenated, the trachea should be aspirated. The pH of the aspirate should be determined, as pulmonary aspiration remains one of the main causes of death after suicidal overdosage. The chance that aspiration has taken place also can be assessed by chest x-ray and measurement of the alveolar-arterial oxygen tension gradient.[306]

After the patient is intubated, the stomach may be lavaged. The return from this is very unpredictable. In over 90 percent of poisonings the return as measured by gas chromatography of the aspirate is not sufficient to decrease the length of coma, but in 10 percent of lavages we found sufficient return that it was likely the length of coma was reduced by several hours.

Hypoxic episodes prior to entering the hospital are probably the most common cause of failure to resuscitate a patient after an overdose of hypnotic drugs. After intubation each patient should have a central venous pressure catheter inserted and a funduscopic and neurologic examination. If there is evidence of raised intracerebral pressure, then appropriate treatment should be started. The patient is stabilized, if necessary by colloid infusion. When the patient is on controlled ventilation in an intensive care unit, comparison of the EEG, neurologic examination, and plasma drug levels can help decide prognosis (Fig. 25-1).[790,2095] At this stage it is also wise to perform a full physical examination. Many patients attempt suicide because they are worried about their general health. We estimate that this is true of about 10 percent of our suicide patients over 50 years of age. We have found analyses of cerebrospinal fluid and stool guaiacs to be useful tests. It should also be remembered that a patient who is found on the floor has to get there; each patient should be examined for trauma. In a number of cases of poisoned patients in the last ten years we have found subdural hematomas.

The management of ventilation follows the same principles outlined in Chapter 2, except that the metabolic rate of the patients is often depressed by up to 20 percent and mechanical deadspace almost invariably has to be added to maintain normocapnia. Unless we think that the patient has aspirated, we do not give antibiotics. If a patient has aspirated, we give moderate doses of a penicillin-like drug until we know the sensitivity of the tracheal organisms.

DIALYSIS

We regard the indications for dialysis for a patient poisoned with hypnotic drugs as being exactly the same as for a nonpoisoned patient. We know of no hypnotic drug that is not best and most safely eliminated by the patient's own metabolism and urinary excretion.[790] (Lithium poisoning may prove to be an exception.) Dialysis for poisoning was in vogue in the 1960's, probably because colorimetric methods for measuring drug clearance rates were inaccurate and the amount of drug not cleared by the patient's natural kidney during dialysis was not taken into account.[849]

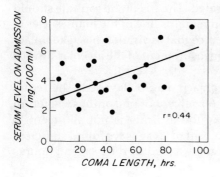

Figure 25-1. Relationship between length of coma and serum level of short-acting barbiturates. A regression analysis was done to examine the correlation between coma length and the serum level of secobarbital or pentobarbital at the time of admission. Increasing serum levels resulted in a significantly longer duration of coma. (From J. Hadden, K. Johnson, S. Smith, L. Price, and E. Giardina, *J.A.M.A.* 209:893–900, 1969.[790] Copyright, 1969, American Medical Association.)

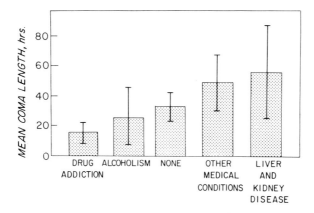

Figure 25-2. Relationship between length of coma and underlying medical condition. Five categories of preexisting medical illness were determined by examination of records of patients poisoned with short-acting barbiturates or with a mixture of secobarbital and amobarbital. After corrections for serum level have been made, it is found that the underlying illness does affect the length of coma ($P < 0.025$). Alcoholics and drug addicts have shorter comas than do normal patients. The patients with liver and kidney disease or with the other medical conditions studied have longer comas. (From J. Hadden, K. Johnson, S. Smith, L. Price, and E. Giardina, *J.A.M.A.* 209:893–900, 1969.[790] Copyright, 1969, American Medical Association.)

Although we have strong negative feelings (now shared by many centers) about peritoneal dialysis and hemodialysis, if the patient has been hypoxic or in shock then renal damage may make dialysis necessary and lifesaving (Fig. 25-2).[790] A prospective study was carried out on a rotational basis, comparing supportive care alone, forced diuresis, and dialysis in patients with barbiturate overdose.[790] According to length of coma, slope of the disappearance of serum barbiturate, and clearance data, which were used as indicators of the effectiveness of treatment, the three treatment forms did not differ. Supportive care alone was associated with less morbidity. By supportive care is meant frequent and careful attention to changes in vital signs and fluid and electrolyte balance.[790] Protection of the airway with an endotracheal tube and controlled mechanical ventilation to produce and correct alveolar ventilation are also essential. Prevention of respiratory infection with frequent turning and suctioning also must be employed. Central monitoring catheters guide electrolyte and on occasion colloid therapy. Dopamine may be necessary to maintain the systolic pressure at a level for adequate renal function. Attention to eye care, pressure sores, and sterile catheter technique is important. Analeptics should be avoided.[1768]

FORCED DIURESIS

Only two controlled clinical studies show that length of coma is decreased by forced diuresis. In both studies long-acting barbiturates had been ingested, and urine flow rates of over 500 ml per hour were produced. The forced diuresis did not lower mortality, and 1.3 percent of patients died from pulmonary edema.[1107,1403] If a long-acting barbiturate has been ingested, our practice is to allow forced alkaline diuresis if the patient appears to have a healthy heart but concurrently to monitor serial alveolar-arterial oxygen tension gradients. If they increase, we stop the fluid infusion and use short-acting diuretics.

As we have already mentioned, no controlled trial has shown that either forced diuresis or peritoneal dialysis significantly decreases the length of coma caused by ingestion of short-acting barbiturates; hemodialysis, when the patient's kidneys are working, increases morbidity and mortality. We recommend the supportive therapy that we have outlined.

GLUTETHIMIDE OVERDOSAGE

The course of patients who take an overdose of glutethimide is often complex (Fig. 25-3).[320] The coma may be long-lasting and its depth variable

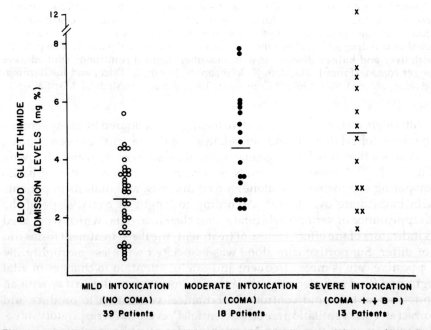

MILD INTOXICATION   MODERATE INTOXICATION   SEVERE INTOXICATION
(NO COMA)   (COMA)   (COMA + ↓ B P)
39 Patients   18 Patients   13 Patients

Figure 25-3. Relationship between blood glutethimide level and degree of intoxication at the time of admission of 70 patients. Patients without coma (mild intoxication) had a significantly lower ($P < 0.01$) mean blood level than the other two groups. There was no significant difference in blood levels between the patients with coma and hypotension (severe intoxication) and the patients with coma but without hypotension (moderate intoxication). There was considerable overlap of the blood glutethimide levels and the degree of intoxication possibly reflecting different levels of the coma-causing metabolite 4-hydroxy-2-ethyl-2-phenylglutarimide (4-HG). (From J. A. Chazan and S. Garella, *Arch. Intern. Med.*[320] Copyright, 1971, American Medical Association.)

(Fig. 25-4).[320] 4-hydroxy-2-ethyl-2-phenylglutarimide (4-HG)., a metabolite of glutethimide, accumulates in the plasma of patients who have ingested glutethimide. This metabolite, 4-HG, has been tested for pharmacologic activity and found to be twice as potent as its parent compound both in ability to kill and, in lower doses, in producing ataxia.[808] If the levels of both glutethimide and 4-HG are measured by gas chromatography and allowance made for the double potency of 4-HG, a reasonable correlation with coma level is found (Fig. 25-5).[808] Levels of 4-HG in the brain may be ten times the glutethimide level (Table 25-1).[707] Measurements should be made promptly, as levels fall if determinations are delayed by storage of the plasma sample syringe. Not only are there problems with correlating plasma levels and coma in glutethimide poisoning, but management tends to be difficult and patients are often hypotensive on admission. Apart from circulatory depression the main reasons for difficulty are viscid secretions, sudden hyperpyrexia, variable levels of coma, and convulsions on awaken-

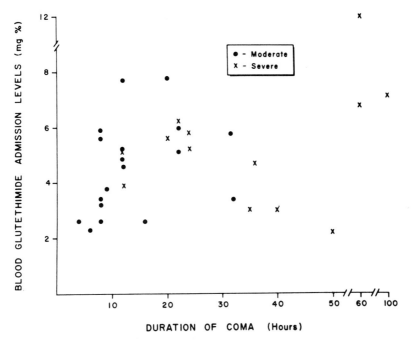

Figure 25-4. Relationship between length of coma and blood level of glutethimide. Admission blood levels of glutethimide of 18 patients with moderate intoxication (coma without hypotension) and 13 patients with severe intoxication (coma with hypotension) showed no correlation with the duration of coma, probably because of different rates of metabolism of glutethimide. The chief metabolite 4-hydroxy-2-ethyl-2-phenylglutarimide (4-HG) is more potent than glutethimide in causing coma. (From J. A. Chazan and S. Garella, *Arch. Intern. Med.*[320] Copyright, 1971, American Medical Association.)

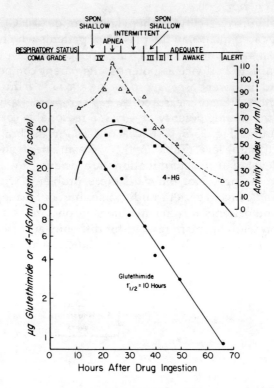

Figure 25-5. Concentration of glutethimide and its metabolite 4-hydroxy-2-ethyl-2-phenylglutarimide (4-HG) in a patient poisoned with glutethimide. A 22-year-old male was admitted in coma following ingestion of 12 gm of glutethimide. His respiratory status and coma level are shown. *I* = drowsy but responsive to verbal commands, *II* = responsive to mildly painful stimuli, *III* = minimally responsive to severely painful stimuli, *IV* = totally unresponsive. Concentrations of glutethimide and 4-HG are plotted on a semilog scale. The activity index (--Δ--) is an estimate of the total drug activity in plasma. The activity index is obtained at each sampling time by multiplying the concentration of 4-HG in plasma by its relative potency in mice (i.e., 2). This number is then added to the concentration of glutethimide at the time of the determination. The clinical course of the patient corresponds best to this activity index. There is no correlation between the patient's course and the plasma glutethimide concentration. The level of coma in patients who are poisoned with glutethimide therefore is related to the accumulation of the metabolite 4-HG in plasma. (From A. R. Hansen, K. A. Kennedy, J. J. Ambre, and L. J. Fischer.[808] Reprinted by permission from the *New England Journal of Medicine* 292:250–252, 1975.)

Table 25-1. Concentrations of Glutethimide and 4-HG in Postmortem Tissue Samples in Cases of Fatal Glutethimide Poisoning

Autopsy Case No.	Age (yr)	Sex	Tissue	Concentration (μg/gm of tissue)*	
				Glute-thimide	4-HG
1	34	F	Brain	6	44
			Kidney	10	37
2	29	F	Brain	3	33
			Liver	5	53
3	45	F	Kidney	17	41
			Blood	6	18
4	86	F	Liver	13	69
			Brain	61	†
5	19	M	Liver	514	†
			Brain	72	5
6	76	M	Liver	190	8
			Blood	27	17
			Liver	189	52

* Data shown are means of duplicate assays.
† None detectable.
SOURCE: A. R. Hansen, K. A. Kennedy, J. J. Ambre, and L. J. Fischer.[808] Reprinted by permission from the *New England Journal of Medicine* 292:250–252, 1975.

ing. Dialysis after glutethimide ingestion is valuable only in treating renal failure. We will discuss each of these problems in turn.

SECRETIONS OF THE UPPER AIRWAY

After glutethimide ingestion the secretions of the upper airway, including the salivary glands, become viscid and hard to aspirate. Segmental collapse of the lungs is more common than with other forms of drug overdosage. This collapse predisposes to gram-negative bacterial superinfection. Ileus is present at lighter levels of coma than it is after barbiturate poisoning.

SUDDEN HYPERPYREXIA

Sudden hyperpyrexia is rare after poisoning with hypnotic drugs other than glutethimide. By contrast we have found that after suicidal attempts with glutethimide approximately 25 percent of patients develop fever spikes to over 39°C. The fever will respond to infusion of 10–20°C intravenous solutions and hyperventilation with added mechanical deadspace to maintain normal arterial carbon dioxide tension. The fever may be due to segmental atelectasis, which because of the viscid secretions does not respond to chest physical therapy alone but must be managed with fiberoptic bronchoscopy as well.

GRAND MAL SEIZURES

Grand mal seizures occur in approximately 10 percent of patients awakening after suicidal ingestion of glutethimide who have previously been on regular glutethimide dosage to aid sleep. The danger of convulsions is sufficient indication to give diphenylhydantoin during awakening and for several days thereafter. If a seizure does occur, the patient should be paralyzed and anticonvulsants given immediately intravenously.

COMA

Patients with glutethimide ingestion not uncommonly awaken and then, probably due to the potency of 4-HG as a hypnotic, relapse into coma (Fig. 25-6).[320] Very occasionally this happens more than once.[489] Patients have been described who awoke 24 hours after glutethimide ingestion, went back into coma about 12 hours later, and awoke again 40 hours after ingesting the glutethimide.[489] Such cyclical coma presents a problem in

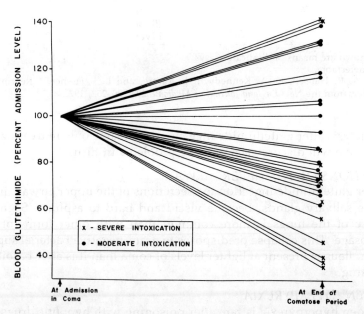

Figure 25-6. The percent change in blood glutethimide levels at admission and at the end of the period of coma in patients with moderate (coma without hypotension) and severe (coma with hypotension) intoxications. Most patients regained consciousness when the blood level of glutethimide was still over 50 percent of the admission value. Several patients awoke when the blood level was higher than it was at the time of admission. This extraordinary finding probably reflects the complex metabolism and enterohepatic recirculation of the drug. Note also that patients after awakening frequently relapse back into coma for a second and even third time. (From J. A. Chazan and S. Garella, *Arch. Intern. Med.*[320] Copyright, 1971, American Medical Association.)

management, and we do not hesitate to paralyze the patient with pancuronium during awakening from glutethimide ingestion.

One suggested reason for the cyclical level of coma after glutethimide ingestion is enterohepatic recirculation. In experimental animals 60–85 percent of ^{14}C-labeled glutethimide is excreted in bile.[1009] No such direct evidence exists in man. Possibly rising levels of the metabolite 4-HG and enterohepatic recirculation both contribute to cyclical coma. We favor the importance of 4-HG, because neither duodenal aspiration, induction of diarrhea, forced diuresis, hemodialysis, nor peritoneal dialysis reduce significantly either coma time or the cyclical nature of the coma. These complex techniques increase morbidity. Patients also may complain of hallucinations after awakening.[2139]

PHENOTHIAZINE POISONING

With the closing of many state mental hospitals and the increasing outpatient treatment of chronic schizophrenics, phenothiazine poisoning is becoming increasingly common. Phenothiazine poisoning is characterized by tachycardia, tachypnea, a fall in diastolic blood pressure, and to a lesser extent a fall in systolic blood pressure.[101] Patients frequently become hypothermic. It is extremely uncommon for patients to be put into frank acute respiratory failure by phenothiazines, although aspiration into the lungs can occur if a tracheal tube is not used.

ALPHA-ADRENERGIC BLOCKING AND ANTICHOLINERGIC EFFECTS

The phenothiazines possess marked alpha-adrenergic blocking and anticholinergic effects, which cause the hypothermia, tachycardia, and reduction in diastolic blood pressure. The hypothermia responds to conventional therapy (Chap. 27). The decreased blood pressure responds to raising the legs, volume expansion, or in very extreme cases direct-acting alpha stimulators. Vasopressors with a beta-stimulating action do not help. The Q-T interval is prolonged in approximately one-sixth of patients who have an overdosage of phenothiazines. Persistent widening and QRS changes can be reversed with diphenylhydantoin.[101] Patients who have ingested large quantities of phenothiazines have small pupils 75 percent of the time, not dilated as one might expect. Athetoid movements and ataxia after awakening are especially common with prochlorperazine, thioridazine, and trifluoperazine. The reported incidence of extrapyramidal activity ranges up to 33 percent.[101]

TRICYCLIC ANTIDEPRESSANTS

Acute poisoning by tricyclic antidepressants such as amitriptyline and imipramine is also common (Fig. 25-7).[1437] A typical neurologic pattern is seen. There is coma after large doses, although respiratory depression is uncommon.[1437] More common is restless agitation with twitching movements, hyperreflexia, extensor plantar responses, and extrapyramidal signs

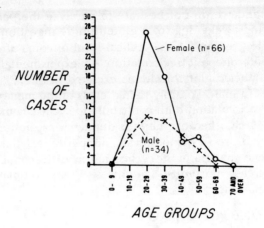

Figure 25-7. Incidence of poisoning with tricyclic antidepressants according to age and sex. In this series of 100 patients women outnumber men by nearly 2 to 1. One-third of the patients were between 21 and 30 years of age, and nine out of ten were under 50 years of age. (Reprinted from J. Noble and H. Matthew, *Clin. Toxicol.*[1437] By courtesy of Marcel Dekker, Inc.)

(Fig. 25-8).[484] The anticholinergic actions of these drugs often lead to pyrexia, urinary retention, constipation, mydriasis, and absence of bowel sounds (Fig. 25-9).[1437] Convulsions may develop, and bizarre visual hallucinations develop in about 5 percent of patients. Blisters may develop over pressure points, especially when amitriptyline has been ingested.

CARDIOVASCULAR EFFECTS

Approximately one-third of patients show a systolic hypotension below 100 mm Hg (13.3 kPa) after suicidal ingestion of antidepressants. The maximal fall in systolic pressure generally occurs in the first four hours after ingestion. Tachycardia occurs in nearly all patients, and in comatose patients the average pulse rate is approximately 120 beats per minute. This tachycardia tends to subside as the patient recovers, but a striking clinical feature of tricyclic antidepressant poisoning is the reappearance of tachycardia 24 hours after its subsidence. It is postulated that this is due to persistent vagal blockade after the myocardium has recovered from the direct toxic effects of the drug.[1437]

Probably the most dangerous complication of poisoning with tricyclic antidepressant drugs is arrhythmias. Atrial tachycardia, nodal tachycardia, atrioventricular block, ventricular tachycardia, and asystole may occur. Myocardial damage and congestive heart failure have been reported. As long as a week after ingestion of the antidepressant drugs death may occur due to sudden arrhythmias.[1437]

These arrhythmias, conduction blocks, and S-T segment and T-wave changes are not due to the atropine effect of the antidepressants. Rather, tricyclic antidepressants are bound by heart muscle. This blockade of ad-

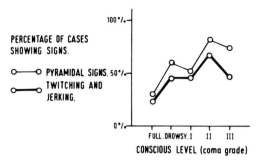

Figure 25-8. Incidence of pyramidal signs and jerking movements related to depth of coma due to tricyclic antidepressant poisoning. Coma was graded in 100 patients as follows: *Full* = fully awake and responsive, *Drowsy* = sleepy but responsive to verbal commands, *I* = responsive to mild pain only, *II* = minimally responsive to maximal pain, *III* = totally unresponsive. Jerking movements and pyramidal signs were seen most frequently in patients with grade II coma and least frequently in those patients who were fully awake. (Reprinted from J. Noble and H. Matthew, *Clin. Toxicol.*[1437] By courtesy of Marcel Dekker, Inc.)

renergic receptors in the heart prevents release of stored norepinephrine.

The tricyclic antidepressant drugs are absorbed rapidly from the gastrointestinal tract. They are bound to proteins in serum and tissues. Less than 3 percent of an ingested dose is excreted unchanged in urine. Metabolism is chiefly by the liver and glucuronides are excreted in the urine. Desmethylimipramine is a long-acting breakdown product. The activity of other metabolites is not known.[1437]

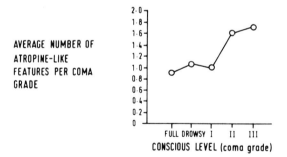

Figure 25-9. Incidence of atropine-like (anticholinergic) features related to depth of coma due to tricyclic antidepressant poisoning. Coma was graded in 100 patients as follows: *Full* = fully awake and responsive, *Drowsy* = sleepy but responsive to verbal commands, *I* = responsive to mild pain only, *II* = minimally responsive to maximal pain, *III* = totally unresponsive. Patients received one point for each of the following anticholinergic features: dry mouth, pyrexia, urinary retention, constipation, ileus, mydriasis. The peak number of anticholinergic signs is seen in the patients who are in the deepest coma. (Reprinted from J. Noble and H. Matthew, *Clin. Toxicol.*[1437] By courtesy of Marcel Dekker, Inc.)

TREATMENT

Both the central nervous system and cardiac effects of tricyclic antidepressants can be treated with physostigmine.[1803] Three milligrams intravenously is a suitable dose for a 70-kg patient. The physostigmine should be given in 1-mg increments. We now use it whenever a patient presents with the triad of agitation, peripheral signs of atropinism, and cardiac arrhythmias. Prompt response to physostigmine suggests the ingestion of tricyclic antidepressants or other drugs with anticholinergic properties.

Early administration of physostigmine awakens a comatose patient within 5–20 minutes, but the dose may need to be repeated every six hours for the first 24 hours. Electrocardiographic control should be used. If the patient is convulsing, physostigmine probably will stop the seizure, but if it does not, intravenous diazepam should be added.

The early administration of physostigmine also prevents cardiac arrhythmias.[1803] Sodium bicarbonate and potassium chloride are useful adjuvants to physostigmine in the treatment of conduction defects. Tricyclic antidepressants may impair the action of the sodium pump, and intracellular potassium is often low.

Digitalis and similar cardiac glycosides increase the tendency to heart block and should be avoided at all costs. Propranolol, however, may be most useful in preventing late deaths (up to one week after ingestion) from arrhythmias. Hospital surveillance for a week after severe tricyclic antidepressant ingestion is probably indicated.

Because of tissue binding neither forced diuresis nor dialysis is useful. Acidemia enhances the cardiotoxic effects of the tricyclic antidepressants, and alveolar ventilation should never be allowed to become depressed.

Determination of amitriptyline, nortriptyline, and their metabolites can be done by the method of Wallace and Dahl.[2013] Other tricyclic antidepressants can be detected and roughly quantitated by thin-layer chromatography. An ingested dose of over 30 mg of amitriptyline per kilogram of body weight can give rise to coma and initial blood levels of 0.5 mg per 100 ml.

MEPROBAMATE OVERDOSAGE

Meprobamate overdosage is encountered often but rarely causes significant problems in management. Coma lasting over 36 hours is unusual.[1210] Gas chromatography provides by far the best way of determining plasma meprobamate levels and levels thus obtained have a good correlation with depth of coma (Fig. 25-10).[1210] Serious intoxication is associated with plasma levels of over 10 mg per 100 ml.[137] If no complications supervene, a patient with a plasma level of 20 mg per 100 ml can be awake within 12 hours. Ileus or severe hypotension, however, slows the uptake of meprobamate from the gut and prolongs coma. Under these circumstances plasma meprobamate levels may not peak for 12 hours.

Only approximately 20 percent of plasma meprobamate is bound to

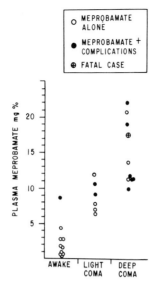

Figure 25-10. Relationship between plasma meprobamate level and degree of coma. Ten patients with meprobamate poisoning were divided into three levels of coma as follows: *Awake* = alert and oriented, *Light Coma* = unintelligently responsive to stimulation, *Deep coma* = totally unresponsive. The state of consciousness has a good correlation with the level of plasma meprobamate. Patients were usually awake at concentrations of less than 5 mg per 100 ml of plasma. Light coma occurred in patients with plasma concentrations of 6–12 mg per 100 ml. Deep coma was seen in patients having meprobamate concentrations over 10 mg per 100 ml. (From R. K. Maddock, Jr., and H. A. Bloomer, *J.A.M.A.* 201:999–1003, 1967.[1210] Copyright, 1967, American Medical Association.)

protein. Renal elimination plays a greater role in disposal of meprobamate than it does for other hypnotics or sedatives. Excretion rates vary with urine flow. As urine volume rises, tubular reabsorption of meprobamate falls and excretion increases. At urine flow rates of over 8 ml per minute, 40 percent of meprobamate filtered by glomeruli appears in the urine. In clinical practice 10–20 percent of meprobamate is excreted in the urine, hepatic metabolism presumably disposing of the majority of the rest.

Meprobamate is a neutral compound, and alteration of plasma pH does not affect its urinary clearance. Hemodialysis has been advocated for patients with levels of over 20 mg per 100 ml of plasma as measured by gas chromatography. In contradistinction to nearly all other situations of drug overdosage, hemodialysis of severe meprobamate poisoning does shorten coma time. We have never found it necessary, however, and it has not been shown to lessen either morbidity or mortality from meprobamate ingestion. The overall mortality with supportive therapy without dialysis is 0.75 percent, but deaths have been reported after ingestion of as little as 12 gm.[194] With carefully monitored forced diuresis, however, patients can survive oral ingestion of 50 gm with only supportive therapy.[1726]

POISONING WITH LIPOPHILIC NONBARBITURATE HYPNOTICS SUCH AS ETHCHLORVYNOL

A great number of lipophilic nonbarbiturate hypnotics have been marketed in the last twenty years. Treatment of patients who have ingested these drugs is harder than treatment of equipotent barbiturate ingestion.[849] Metabolism of these drugs is slow, excretion is poor, and circulatory depression is often profound (Fig. 25-11).[849] Hepatic damage probably prolongs coma caused by ethchlorvynol.[298] Dialysis should be used only if the patient is in renal failure. Our data show that in man almost all ethchlorvynol is metabolized.[849]

NARCOTICS

Patients who have taken an overdose of heroin, morphine, or methadone usually do not need admission to an intensive care unit.[2059] Intravenous naloxone and careful safeguarding of the upper airway generally provide satisfactory treatment (Fig. 25-12).[601] The total dosage requirement of intravenous naloxone for a 70-kg man comatose due to heroin overdosage can range from 0.4 to 20 mg given in 0.4-mg increments (Fig. 25-13).[601] For patients who require controlled ventilation and subsequent admission to an intensive care unit, the average dosage requirement of naloxone (for a young adult) is 5 mg (Fig. 25-14).[601] We have recently had to use 40 mg of

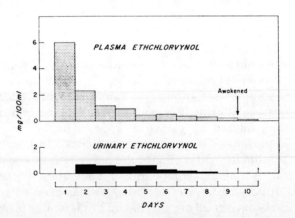

Figure 25-11. Mean plasma and urine levels of ethchlorvynol in a 36-year-old man poisoned with ethchlorvynol. The patient underwent peritoneal dialysis at an outside hospital and suffered a cardiac arrest. He was transferred to us and awoke on the ninth hospital day. He was discharged five days later. The drug was identified by using gas-liquid chromatography. Only 59 mg of ethchlorvynol was excreted in 13.5 liters of urine. (From J. Hedley-Whyte and L. H. Laasberg, *Anesthesiology.*[849])

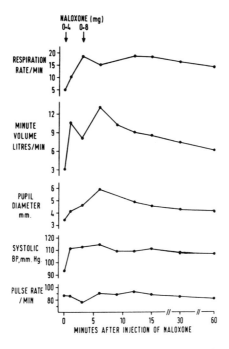

Figure 25-12. Effect of naloxone on the vital signs of four patients with overdosages of narcotics. Intravenous naloxone results in an increase in respiratory rate, minute ventilation, pupil size, and systolic blood pressure in patients with narcotic overdosages. (From L. E. J. Evans, P. Roscoe, C. P. Swainson, and L. F. Prescott, *Lancet.*[601])

naloxone to maintain blood pressure in a patient who had suffered cardiac arrest due to methadone overdosage. He made a full recovery.

We have found that the most common reasons for admission to an intensive care unit after narcotic overdosage are pulmonary edema, pulmonary aspiration of gastric contents, sepsis, and central nervous system complications.

PULMONARY EDEMA

Pulmonary edema is present in as many as 50 percent of patients who render themselves unconscious with heroin.[1848] Severe pulmonary congestion or even frank edema may develop from 2 to 18 hours after recovery from coma. Ideally all patients who have been unconscious with acute heroin overdosage, even if they have responded rapidly to naloxone, should be observed closely for 24 hours. During heroin pulmonary edema, pulmonary artery pressures and cardiac output usually are normal. Congestion of the lungs and pulmonary edema may progress over a day to lobar pneumonia or bronchopneumonia.

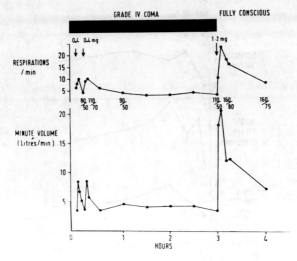

Figure 25-13. Effect of intravenous naloxone on consciousness and respirations in a male with an overdosage of dipipanone. Dipipanone is structurally and therapeutically allied to methadone.[1134] Larger doses are occasionally necessary as in this patient, who had minimal responses to two doses of 0.4 mg. When 1.2 mg was given, the patient awoke fully and his minute ventilation increased dramatically. Note that blood pressure also increased. (From L. E. J. Evans, P. Roscoe, C. P. Swainson, and L. F. Prescott, *Lancet.*[601])

The pathogenesis of the pulmonary edema in acute heroin intoxication is still unclear. Allergy or hypersensitivity, neurogenic stimuli, and hypoxia all have been suggested as the chief cause of the pulmonary edema. There are arguments for and against each suggestion.[1848] Despite our inadequate understanding of how heroin pulmonary edema is produced, there is a satisfactory treatment for it. Naloxone and controlled ventilation via a tracheal tube are given. If necessary, short-acting intravenous diuretics are also used. If leukopenia has been caused by adulterated heroin, pneumonia seems more likely to develop. Bone marrow aspirations are nondiagnostic, and the granulocytopenia nearly always disappears within 48 hours.

SEPSIS

Sepsis is a major problem after heroin overdosage and a major cause of admission to intensive care areas.[1186] The usual practice of heroin addicts, at least in Boston, is to make up their injections with any convenient liquid. Spit, tap water, and even wine are used as mixers. Skin sepsis and joint effusions are fairly common. Staphylococcal septicemia may lead to pneumonia and lung abscesses. Empyema, bronchopleural fistulas, and tension pneumothoraces may result. Often there is little abnormality in the initial chest x-ray. Blood cultures should be taken from any addicts with fever or with signs of pulmonary congestion before antibiotic treatment is

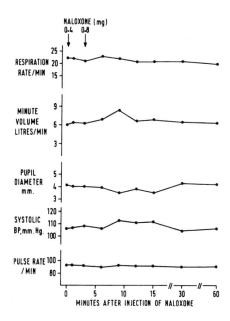

Figure 25-14. Effect of intravenous naloxone on vital signs in patients with nonnarcotic central nervous system depressant poisonings. Use of naloxone in patients comatose secondary to overdosage with hypnotics, tranquilizers, or antidepressants does not result in any change in mean levels of respiratory rate, minute ventilation, pupil size, blood pressure, or heart rate, nor is level of coma altered. (From L. E. J. Evans, P. Roscoe, C. P. Swainson, and L. F. Prescott, *Lancet.*[601])

started.[1186] Septicemia occurs with beta-hemolytic streptococci, *Hemophilus influenza,* or staphylococci. *Candida albicans* often appears in the sputum of these patients after antibiotic therapy is started. Hepatitis and tetanus are other infections related to narcotic addiction that we have seen cause respiratory failure. Over 40 percent of endocarditis in drug addicts is due to staphylococci.[1186] Both right- and left-sided endocarditis often develop. Tricuspid endocarditis is often diagnosed from the venous pressure wave and the chest x-ray. Cardiac murmurs usually are absent. In a heroin addict with severe infection it is hard to know whether to continue with narcotics. Normally we try to withdraw them, but if signs of withdrawal develop, we counteract these effects with the lowest possible dose of methadone.

DRUG DETECTION

Seven years ago, by writing to drug houses around the world, we collected pure samples of over 250 prescription drugs that cause coma in overdosage. We have since used these samples to provide standards for our gas chromatographic identification and quantification of hypnotic drugs in the plasma of unconscious patients. Approximately 85–90 percent of the time the drug or drugs can be identified with near certainty by gas chromatography alone, using a temperature-programed oven and a flame-programed ionization detector.[238]

DRUG IDENTIFICATION SYSTEM

Since we are unable to identify 10–15 percent of the drugs that cause coma by gas chromatography, we have cooperated with Professor Klaus Biemann's group of the Massachusetts Institute of Technology in establishment of a drug identification system.[900] The system consists of a mass spectrometer, which can quickly identify atoms, organic compounds, or metabolic byproducts in a sample of the patient's blood or urine; a computer with a memory of more than 8,000 mass spectrograms of organic compounds, and a gas chromatograph.[901]

To identify a drug, 20 ml of blood is drawn from the patient and heparinized with 0.2 ml of heparin (8,000 units). The blood is centrifuged at 3,000 g for 15 minutes. The plasma is separated into 2 aliquots. One aliquot is used for immediate gas chromatography, and the other is kept for possible later combined gas-chromatographic–mass-spectrometric analysis. The plasma for immediate gas chromatography is extracted with spectral grade $CHCl_3$ at pH 7.8. Normal HCl is then added to the residual plasma to pH 2.0, and further extraction is carried out with $CHCl_3$. The extracts are combined and the $CHCl_3$ evaporated. The residue is then redissolved in 50–100 μl spectral grade $CHCl_3$.[1918] A 5-μl sample is injected into a gas chromatograph fitted with dual 6-foot columns packed with 3.5% w/w OV 17 silicone rubber gum on Chromosorb AW (siliconized). A hydrogen flame ionization detector is used. The carrier gas is helium at a flow rate of 60 ml per minute. The oven is temperature programed from 80 to 290°C per minute with a hold at 290°C for 25 minutes. Quantitative analyses of all drugs that cause coma and can be vaporized below 290°C without change in their chemical structures are possible with this program.[1484] A list of coma-causing drugs that do not fill these requirements has been compiled. The residual plasma is alkalinized with 2N NaOH to pH 13.0. The plasma layer is then extracted twice with a triple volume of ether. The ether is then separated by centrifugation and evaporated to dryness. The residue is dissolved in 50 μl ether, and 5-μl samples are injected into the gas chromatograph as just described.

Further analysis of unknown drugs has employed the gas chromatograph–low resolution mass spectrometer–computer system mentioned earlier in conjunction with high and low resolution data. The computer data acquisition system searches a "library" of mass spectra of 250 drugs known to cause coma. The extraction procedure is as described above. High- and low-resolution spectra are obtained on each of the fractions by introduction into a gas chromatograph attached to a mass spectrometer. Mass spectra of the gas stream effluent from the chromatograph are scanned every 3 seconds, and a digital computer performs the following functions: (1) peak center and intensity calculations proceed, while each spectrum is scanned; (2) peak positions in time units are converted to masses using an external mass standard; and (3) the spectra are correlated with the gas chromatogram by a plot of the total mass spectrometer ionization against the spectrum index number. The relationship of the various components generally indicates a mixture of drug (or drugs) and metabolites. If necessary, an elemental composition of the ions of relevant components is obtained by high resolution mass spectrometry. High resolution measurements are obtained on a spectrometer with photoplate recording. By these techniques we have identified within a day the initial plasma levels of patients admitted to our hospital after suicidal ingestion or accidental overdosage of drugs.[900]

Since the management of overdosage with hypnotic drugs is now relatively standardized, the chief use of the gas chromatograph–mass spectrometer system has been to exclude drugs as a cause of flaccid coma. We have seen cases of acute multiple sclerosis, encephalitis, and even idiopathic polyneuritis in which the patient was found at home in coma and the exclusion of poisoning was most valuable. Accurate drug identification

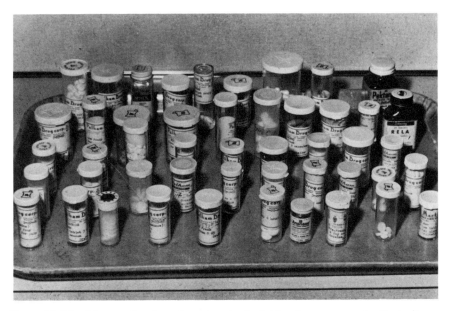

Figure 25-15. The medications found at the bedside of a woman admitted after an attempt at suicide. The wide variety of drugs found made treatment difficult. Almost every Boston teaching hospital had contributed to this patient's loot. Eleven different drugs were found in her bloodstream. (From L. S. Bushnell, *Clin. Trends Anesthesiol.*[280])

and plasma levels are valuable in deciding whether to give naloxone, as after propoxyphene or narcotic overdosage. For forensic purposes drug identification and plasma levels are also extremely valuable.[1008]

Our record number of different hypnotic drugs identified in the blood of a would-be suicide is 11. A neighbor of the woman who tried to commit suicide found that she had 48 different hypnotics beside her bed at home as a result of prescriptions issued by physicians associated with five different Boston hospitals (Fig. 25-15).[280] The wanton prescribing of hypnotics is a major disgrace of current therapeutics.

26

Pulmonary Aspiration and Near-Drowning

Aspiration of gastric contents accounts for up to 12,000 deaths per year in the United States. Of patients who aspirate, 61 percent do so in association with an operative procedure.[45] Inhalation of gastric contents occurs in 7 percent of surgical patients during anesthesia.[167,460,1976] Aspiration causes between 11 and 14 percent of anesthetic deaths.[90,576]

LARYNGEAL FUNCTION

Laryngeal ability to exclude from the lungs any vomited or regurgitated material is a major factor in aspiration. The older the patient, the less his ability to detect and respond to laryngeal irritation (Fig. 26-1).[1542] Drugs such as diazepam, atropine, ketamine, and any general anesthetic depress laryngeal function.[303] The use of a combination of fentanyl and droperidol fails to prevent aspiration, although the cough reflex persists.

Topical anesthesia to the hypopharynx and superior laryngeal nerves delays or abolishes reflex glottic closure.[349,803,892,1061] The laryngeal reflex is often depressed or lost after poisoning, central nervous system damage, or laryngeal surgery.[148] The presence of a tracheostomy favors aspiration even if the cuff is inflated. After Evans blue dye is placed onto the tongue, 67 percent of patients with inflated cuffed tracheostomy tubes show aspiration of the dye, while 73 percent with uncuffed tracheostomy tubes aspirate the dye. In these studies the cuffs were briefly deflated every two hours. Of patients with inflated cuffed orotracheal tubes, none show evidence of aspiration.[290] The prolonged presence of an orotracheal tube renders the glottis incompetent following extubation.[483]

PATHOPHYSIOLOGIC CHARACTERISTICS

Once aspiration occurs, the extent of pulmonary damage depends on the acidity of the aspirated fluid.[18,75,91,442,765] Mendelson noted the similarity of effect on lungs of acid gastric juice and of an acidic solution. He also noted the difference between the effects of acidic fluid and the effects of neutral solutions. Maximum pulmonary damage is achieved at an aspirate pH of 1.5. Above pH 2.5 the response is similar to that of distilled water.[75,1906] The effect of acidic aspirate has been compared to that of a chemical burn, since atelectasis appears within three minutes of aspiration.[802] Bronchial pH returns to normal within 30 minutes of acid aspiration (Fig. 26-2). The

343

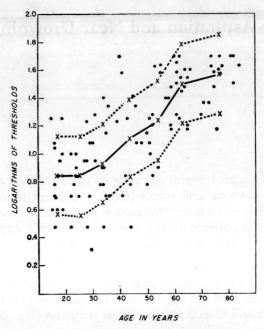

Figure 26-1. The threshold of laryngeal sensitivity to ammonia gas increases with age. Therefore there is a greater probability that aspiration will be undetected by symptoms of cough or airway irritation. *Dotted line* shows range defined by 1 SD. (From H. Pontoppidan and H. K. Beecher, *J.A.M.A.* 174:2209–2213, 1960.[1542] Copyright, 1960, American Medical Association.)

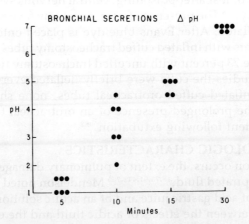

Figure 26-2. Relation between pH of bronchial secretions and acidity of aspirate. Ten minutes after aspiration of 0.1N HCl, 4 ml per kilogram, the pH of bronchial secretions no longer reflects the acidity of the aspirate. Bronchial acidity is progressively buffered, until a pH of 7.0 is reached at 30 minutes. (From W. C. Awe, W. S. Fletcher, and S. W. Jacob, *Surgery*.[75])

acidity of the stomach contents, normally pH 1.3–2.0 in fasting individuals, is increased by stress, peptic ulcer disease, cholecystitis, and alcohol ingestion.[1745]

Acid aspiration produces pathologic changes, often in the portion of the lungs most dependent at the time of aspiration. The lungs become two to three times heavier than normal, with patchy consolidation and hemorrhage. There is necrosis of the capillary endothelium as well as alveolar cells, with outpouring of fluid into the pulmonary interstitium and migration of white blood cells into alveoli.[18,287,535,765,2094]

In addition to the effect of the acid, the composition of the aspirate affects the degree of pulmonary insult. Fecal-contaminated gastric juice produces 100 percent mortality in dogs.[802] Possible explanations include mechanical obstruction of airways by proteinaceous material and effects of endotoxin.[1992] Food particles, especially vegetable fibers, cause some pulmonary reaction regardless of pH.[1906] Aspiration of blood, saliva, or alcohol does not produce a severe reaction if not accompanied by acid.[800] The aspiration of tube feeding, pH 5.5, does not produce the hypoxemia and pulmonary edema seen with acids.[75,1456]

Aspiration of large chunks of food allegedly accounted for 2,641 deaths in the United States in 1969.[1959] These unfortunate victims usually are not seen in the intensive care setting, since without appropriate treatment they usually die at the scene.[585] In fact, of patients hospitalized for aspiration, 81–92 percent aspirated liquid material rather than food.[75,576,1297]

Upon aspiration of liquid there is a brief apneic period with an immediate fall in arterial oxygen tension.[75,799,801,1159,1477] This initial episode may produce cardiac arrest due to hypoxemia. If the patient survives, apnea gives way to tachypnea. The arterial oxygen tension may be as low as 25 mm Hg (3.3 kPa) at this point. The arterial carbon dioxide tension will be the result of a balance between the degree of lung damage and the degree of tachypnea due to hypoxemia.[765] The aspirate causes constriction of bronchioles as well as mucosal edema with filling of alveoli by plasma. Compliance falls.[388,389,801] The systemic and pulmonary circulations are both immediately affected by aspiration. There is a fall in systemic blood pressure and cardiac output without compensatory tachycardia.[75,765,1477] Sometimes the initial episode is so severe as to cause immediate cardiac arrest or ventricular fibrillation. The hypotension may persist due to plasma loss into the lung.[75,288,802] The pulmonary vascular resistance is increased, with an elevated pulmonary artery pressure, if hypoxemia is present. The elevation of pulmonary artery pressure is usually abolished by the administration of 100% oxygen or mechanical ventilation.[288,1157,1477] Occasionally pulmonary hypertension can persist due to irritation of small airways and vagal stimulation of pulmonary vasculature.[388,389,801] Poor tissue perfusion may produce metabolic acidemia in addition to the respiratory alkalemia. Intrapulmonary shunt may rise to as high as 50 percent of cardiac output.[288]

PREVENTION

In 88 cases of aspiration at the Mayo Clinic, risk factors were as follows: operation, 61 percent; nasogastric tube, 42 percent; impaired consciousness, 40 percent; no operation, 39 percent; tracheostomy, 28 percent; debilitation, 25 percent; recovery from anesthesia, 14 percent; esophageal disease, 14 percent; anesthetic induction, 6 percent; seizure, 1 percent; and other, 1 percent. The mean age of patients in this study was 53 years. If patients who aspirate are analyzed by site of surgery, upper abdominal cases account for 25 percent; thoracic, 20 percent; lower abdominal, 19 percent; otolaryngeal, 10 percent; neck, 10 percent; and extremities, 10 percent. Neurosurgical patients comprise the remaining 6 percent.[45,1926]

Always position an unconscious patient on his side. Several positions have been advocated for patients at risk of aspiration including elevation of the foot of the bed, full prone position, and fully supine position.[60,1386] The best compromise is that of nursing a patient on his side with periodic turning. The patency of nasogastric tubes must be verified repeatedly.

OBSTETRIC PATIENTS

Obstetric patients have long been recognized as a high-risk group for aspiration.[273,317,445,516,793,898,1105,1297] Aspiration is responsible for 2 percent of all maternal deaths.[1301] It is the leading cause of maternal anesthetic mortality, accounting for 52 percent of such deaths.[443,444] At least 1 in every 430 mothers aspirates during general anesthesia for cesarean section.[1064,1350,1633] All obstetric patients who are to undergo cesarean section or who may receive a general anesthetic are given 30 ml of antacid orally at least 30 minutes prior to induction of anesthesia. The oral administration of 14 ml of a mixture of magnesium trisilicate, magnesium carbonate, and sodium bicarbonate (BPC) 15–45 minutes prior to the administration of a general anesthetic to emergency, unfasted obstetric patients is successful in raising the pH of gastric contents to above 2.5 in 100 percent of patients. Only 60 percent of untreated patients have a pH above 2.5. The lowest pH for the antacid group is 4.6, while the lowest pH for the untreated group is 1.2 (Fig. 26-3). The effectiveness of prophylactic antacids diminishes progressively with time.[1903] Analysis of the gastric contents of patients under general anesthesia at cesarean section show 44 percent have a pH of 2.5 or less. The preoperative administration of magnesium trisilicate reduces this incidence to 8.5 percent.[1514]

The amount of magnesium absorbed into the maternal blood during the course of prolonged labor only slightly raises the concentration of the magnesium ion in the fetal blood.[74] Studies are not available to decide whether administration of an oral antacid prior to anesthesia can contribute to an increased frequency of regurgitation or vomiting, but gastric alkalinization does increase lower esophageal sphincter tone.[873] Titration data have led to the suggestion that 14 ml magnesium trisilicate, magnesium carbonate, and sodium bicarbonate (BPC) should be given each mother every two

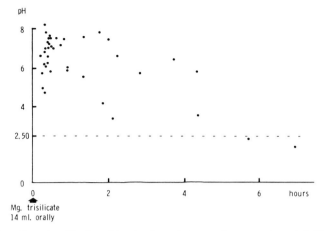

Figure 26-3. Gastric pH after 14 ml of a mixture of magnesium trisilicate, magnesium carbonate, and sodium bicarbonate (BPC). Gastric pH is increased to above 2.5 for nearly five hours. When gastric fluid of pH 2.5 or lower is aspirated, pneumonitis results. (From G. Taylor and J. Pryse-Davies, *Lancet*.[1903])

hours.[2069] Other regimens include sodium citrate or 15 ml aluminum or magnesium hydroxide every three hours and at least 30 minutes prior to induction.[1085,1632] The sodium load of multiple doses may have to be taken into account in preeclamptic patients. No investigation has yet determined whether oral antacids would be useful in other high-risk groups prior to general surgery.

TREATMENT

MANAGEMENT OF HYPOXEMIA

Hypoxemia is the most dangerous abnormality initially after aspiration and is best treated by administration of oxygen. Tracheal intubation is almost always required for prevention of further aspiration, for suctioning, and for positive pressure ventilation. The patient must be observed closely for cardiorespiratory failure for at least 12 hours following aspiration, since the pulmonary response is often progressive.[535,765] Respiratory failure may not become manifest for over five hours.[831]

MECHANICAL VENTILATION

Mechanical ventilation, if instituted within 24 hours after aspiration, improves blood gases, reduces mortality,[291] and may prevent elevation of pulmonary arterial pressure and formation of clots in the pulmonary arteries.[201] Positive end-expiratory pressure is used if hypoxemia persists despite temporary ventilation with 90–100% oxygen.[315] The initial aspirate, excluding feculent aspirate, is usually sterile and remains so for the first 24 hours.[765,802,1159,1906] Thereafter cultures demonstrate gram-positive or gram-negative superinfection or both, usually with *Escherichia, Klebsiella,*

Staphylococcus, Pseudomonas, Bacteroides, or anaerobes.[103,704,1183,1859] No prophylactic antibiotic has been shown to improve mortality or reduce secondary infection rates, but we often use a penicillin-like drug.[289,1159] Cultures are taken as soon as possible after aspiration and thereafter as clinically indicated. The antibiotic regimen is changed according to the sensitivity of the predominant organism. Broad-spectrum antibiotics are not given prophylactically, since one-third of cultured organisms are resistant to the antibiotics chosen.

SYSTEMIC STEROIDS

The value of systemic steroids after aspiration is controversial.[205] An experimental study in 1966 on mongrel dogs given dexamethasone 0.4 mg per kilogram of body weight intravenously at the time of aspiration and 8 mg intramuscularly in divided doses daily for two days supported the use of steroids in aspiration pneumonitis.[1124] Subsequent studies in New Zealand white rabbits given methylprednisolone 40 mg per kilogram of body weight intraarterially within 60 seconds of aspiration showed some microscopic improvement at 48 hours after aspiration.[555] Further studies in dogs given dexamethasone 0.4 to 0.8 mg per kilogram intravenously 15 minutes before aspiration and 0.2 to 0.4 mg per kilogram intravenously two hours after aspiration or methylprednisolone 30 mg per kilogram or 0.3 mg per kilogram as a single dose or 30 mg per kilogram every eight hours, have shown that steroids have no effect on the course of experimental aspiration pneumonitis as judged by radiologic examination, arterial oxygen tensions, and lung weights.[75,315,535,2077]

BRONCHOSCOPY

Bronchoscopy in general is not indicated; however, if a major bronchus is obstructed, bronchoscopy should be carried out with a fiberoptic bronchoscope. Large volumes of lavage fluid are not used. Volumes of less than 10 ml of lavage fluid are acceptable. Lavage with fluid containing steroids is not indicated.[75,555,1156,1904] Methods of decreasing lung water by diuretics should be used cautiously to avoid hypovolemia and hypoperfusion.[1742] Complications of aspiration in all types of patients include pneumonia in 46 percent, myocardial infarction in 10 percent, gastrointestinal hemorrhage in 10 percent, and pulmonary abscess in 3 percent, as well as septicemia and empyema.[45,92,842,1802]

NEAR-DROWNING

Drowning is responsible for over 6,000 deaths a year in the United States.[1959] It ranks as the second leading cause of death of children ages 5 to 14.[1618] While technically it is a form of aspiration, its pathophysiologic features are somewhat different from aspiration of gastric contents and deserve separate consideration. Upon sudden immersion in water the initial response is voluntary apnea followed by intermittent uncontrollable swallowing.[1330] Ninety percent of deaths are due to aspiration of water. The remaining 10 percent are due to asphyxia without fluid aspiration.[1358] Over 70 percent of drowning victims aspirate mud, vomitus, or algae in addition to water.[672] Upon the aspiration of sea water the lungs increase to three times their normal weight, whereas no increase is detectable after fresh water aspiration.[798] After aspiration of sea water more fluid is obtained by gravity drainage of the lungs than was aspirated, whereas after fresh water aspiration no significant amount of fluid can be obtained.[672,1338,1601,1602] These results indicate that hypertonic sea water (sodium, 509 mEq per liter [509 mmol/l]; potassium, 11.3 mEq per liter [11.3 mmol/l]; chloride, 56 mEq per liter [56 mmol/l]) draws even more fluid into the lungs, whereas hypotonic fresh water is absorbed into the circulation.[798] Hypoxemia in fresh water aspiration persists because some fluid persists in the alveoli and because heart failure ensues with circulatory overload, but hypoxemia is more prolonged after sea water aspiration.[702,1338]

HYPOXEMIA

In both sea and fresh water near-drowning, hypoxemia is the primary and most important abnormality. Changes in blood gases and acid-base balance account for the deaths of 85 percent of drowning victims.[1332,1338] With filling of alveoli with water, hypoxemia immediately ensues, with a large alveolar-arterial oxygen tension gradient. Pulmonary compliance falls significantly after aspiration of 1 ml per kilogram of body weight of water. Arterial carbon dioxide tension increases initially but then falls gradually, depending on the amount of fluid aspirated regardless of the type of water aspirated. A metabolic acidemia is found in 78 percent of near-drowning cases. It persists when severe hypoxemia remains uncorrected (Fig. 26-4).
[671,1333,1892]

INCREASED BLOOD VOLUME

The absorption of fluid in fresh water near-drowning can increase the blood volume by 60 percent within three minutes (Fig. 26-5).[1329] Blood volume may return to normal within one hour.[1336] The blood volume generally decreases when sea water is aspirated (Fig. 26-6).[1337,1338,1893]

SERUM ELECTROLYTES

Electrolytes also exhibit changes within three minutes after aspiration, returning to normal spontaneously within two hours.[1336] Changes depend on the amount and type of fluid aspirated (Fig. 26-7). Serum sodium, chloride, and calcium increase after sea water near-drowning and decrease after fresh water near-drowning. Potassium increases in both types of near-drowning. With fresh water drowning the increase is due to hemolysis by the fresh water. In salt water the increase is due to absorption of sea water. Although electrolytes may change significantly, such changes are not the cause of death.[1330,1331]

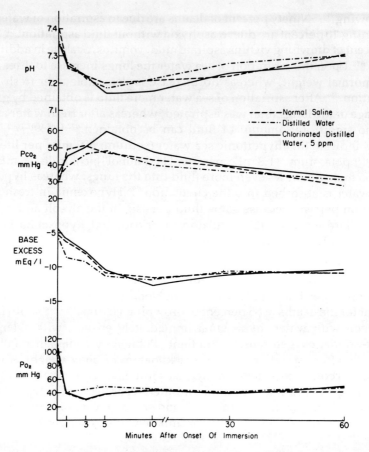

Figure 26-4. A comparison of arterial blood gas and acid-base values at various intervals after aspiration of 22 ml per kilogram of normal saline, distilled water, or chlorinated distilled water, 5 ppm. The primary problem after near-drowning is that of hypoxemia. (From J. H. Modell, M. Gaub, F. Moya, B. Vestal, and H. Swarz, *Anesthesiology*.[1333])

CARDIOVASCULAR AND CEREBRAL EFFECTS

The most common response of the cardiovascular system to hypoxemia is hypotension and bradycardia with progression to ventricular fibrillation. Alternatively hypertension and tachycardia may result. The response is related to the amount of fluid aspirated.[1333,1336]

Cerebral edema secondary to the hypoxemia of near-drowning is sometimes a major problem. Disseminated intravascular coagulation may be present. Platelets have been shown to aggregate in the lungs of drowning victims.

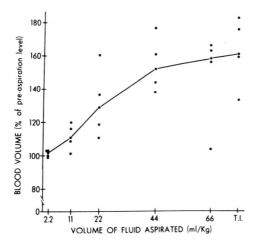

Figure 26-5. Increase in the blood volume three minutes after aspiration of different volumes of fresh water. Continuous total immersion (*T.I.*) was carried out until the onset of ventricular fibrillation. (From J. H. Modell and F. Moya, *Anesthesiology*.[1336])

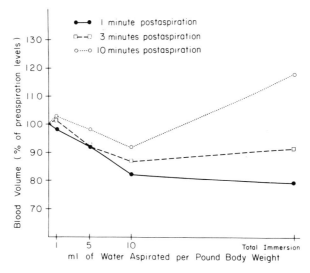

Figure 26-6. The effect of aspiration of sea water on blood volume. Blood volume initially decreases, unlike the initial increase in blood volume after fresh water aspiration. (From J. H. Modell, F. Moya, E. J. Newby, B. C. Ruiz, and A. V. Showers, *Ann. Intern. Med.*[1337])

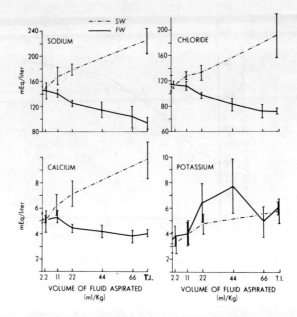

Figure 26-7. Electrolyte changes three minutes after aspiration of various quantities of fresh water (*FW*) and sea water (*SW*). Although the changes shown are significant, they are of relatively short duration. Continuous total immersion (*T.I.*) was carried out until the onset of ventricular fibrillation. (From J. H. Modell, *Pathophysiology and Treatment of Drowning and Near Drowning*.[1330] Courtesy of Charles C Thomas, Publisher, Springfield, Illinois.)

TREATMENT

Since apnea and hypoxemia are the primary abnormalities, ventilation is initiated as soon as possible. Mouth-to-mouth ventilation is indicated in the absence of equipment. Ventilation can be initiated in the water, if both rescuer and victim are kept afloat by an object.[1601] One hundred percent oxygen should be given as soon as possible. Closed chest cardiac massage is employed when indicated.[890] Metabolic acidemia is corrected with bicarbonate. Electrolyte abnormalities seldom require therapy.[1331] Diuretics may be effective in fresh water aspiration. In sea water aspiration, however, the decreased blood volume must be restored if likelihood of survival is to be increased.[1602] As much as 25 percent of blood volume is lost into the lung. Hemolysis, although present, is rarely significant enough to require specific therapy. Since, as noted previously, over 70 percent of victims aspirate material other than water, such as algae or vomitus, the mouth and tracheal fluid are examined and appropriate treatment instituted.[672] Isoproterenol is used to relieve bronchospasm, if present, although its effectiveness is only temporary.[387] Vigorous chest physical therapy is instituted and arterial blood gases noted for at least 48 hours, since sudden death has been reported up to 48 hours after aspiration, even after return of consciousness.[1332] These deaths may be due to unrecognized respiratory failure with hypoxemia. Survival may occur even after total submersion under cold fresh water for up to 40 minutes, if patients are young and are treated correctly.[1080,1625]

27

Accidental Hypothermia

Mortality for patients whose body temperatures have accidentally fallen below 35°C varies but averages 50 percent.[560,1558] The prognosis is worst for those patients whose temperatures fall below 32°C, especially when they are elderly. Diseases in which accidental hypothermia commonly occurs include myxedema, pituitary insufficiency, Addison's disease, hypoglycemia, cerebrovascular disease, myocardial infarction, near-drowning, cirrhosis, and pancreatitis.[604] Elderly, bedridden patients in cold rooms and babies, whether under the influence of alcohol or drugs or not, when exposed to extremely cold temperatures, also cool easily. Experimental evidence suggests that intoxicated animals fibrillate at lower temperatures but we have no clinical evidence to suggest a favorable effect of alcohol on patients suffering from accidental hypothermia.[1204,2060]

DIAGNOSIS

Those who work in emergency wards and intensive care units must have a high index of suspicion and use low-reading thermometers. A coarse background tremor, bradycardia or slow atrial fibrillation, and a characteristic J wave (which occurs at the junction of the QRS complex and S-T segment) on the electrocardiogram are very helpful clues (Fig. 27-1).[1457,1928]

PHYSIOLOGIC EFFECTS

CIRCULATION

The physiologic effects of moderate hypothermia are illustrated in Figure 27-2.[1884] A linear relationship exists between cardiac output and oxygen consumption during cooling (Fig. 27-3).[183] If active external warming is instituted, oxygen consumption increases more rapidly than cardiac output, and circulatory failure may occur (Fig. 27-4).[1072] If this circulatory stress is imposed in the presence of coronary artery disease, fatal ventricular fibrillation may result.[1933] Successful electric defibrillation is extremely difficult below 28°C.[1942]

RESPIRATION

Arterial oxygen tensions may be lowered in hypothermia by dependent atelectasis. The oxyhemoglobin dissociation curve is moved to the left by

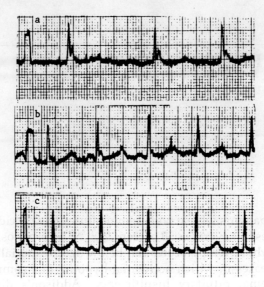

Figure 27-1. Effect of hypothermia on the electrocardiogram. A man was found unconscious lying under a bridge and was immediately brought to the hospital. At the time of admission his temperature was 20.5°C. Lead 2 of his electrocardiogram is shown in *a* and demonstrates a background somatic tremor, slow atrial fibrillation, and J waves. Four hours following admission his temperature was 27°C and his electrocardiogram (*b*) demonstrated a background tremor, normal sinus rhythm, and J waves. By 16 hours following admission his temperature was 35.5°C and his electrocardiogram (*c*) was normal. (From K. G. Tolman and A. Cohen, *Can. Med. Assoc. J.*[1928])

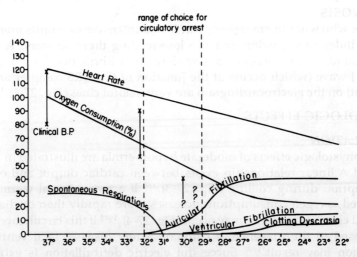

Figure 27-2. Physiologic effects of moderate hypothermia in man. Early experience with hypothermia for open-heart surgery led to this representation of the effects of hypothermia. Both heart rate and oxygen consumption fall linearly with the rectal temperature in °C until about 26°C, where the oxygen consumption plateaus. Ventricular fibrillation and coagulopathy do not become important until the temperature is below 27°C. (From H. Swan, *Surgery.*[1884])

356

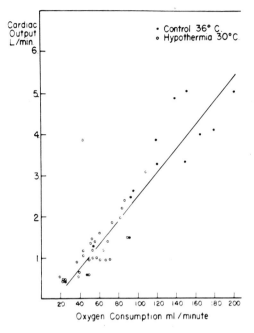

Figure 27-3. Relationship between oxygen consumption and cardiac output during hypothermia. There is a linear correlation between normal and hypothermic animals. Since both variables decrease simultaneously, it appears that the cardiac output is adequate for the oxygen needs of the tissues. There is a wider scatter in the normothermic state than in the hypothermic state. (From E. Blair, A. V. Montgomery, and H. Swan, *Circulation.* [183] By permission of The American Heart Association, Inc.)

hypothermia (Fig. 27-5).[1461] Oxygen delivery to tissues is further compromised by lowered cardiac output and increased blood viscosity.

Respiratory stimulation occurs at the onset of hypothermia but is soon followed by respiratory depression. Arterial pH and carbon dioxide tensions reflect these changes. Respirations generally cease at a rectal temperature of 24°C. During rewarming, increased carbon dioxide production and a high deadspace-to-tidal-volume ratio make ventilatory requirements unpredictable.[1729] Unexpectedly high minute ventilation thus may be needed. A metabolic acidemia develops due to mobilization of lactic acid from the periphery, and the impairment of hepatic function attendant upon hypothermia impairs lactate catabolism. It is essential to use temperature correction factors when making blood gas measurements in hypothermic patients, unless the blood gas electrodes are kept at the patient's temperature.[337,338,339,850,856] Cold injury to the lung does not occur; hypothermia per se has been shown to have no effect on alveolar-arterial oxygen tension gradients.[853]

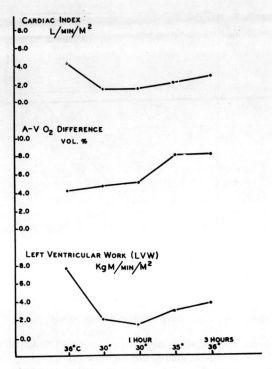

Figure 27-4. Effect of hypothermia and rewarming on the cardiac index, arteriovenous oxygen difference, and left ventricular work. During rewarming the cardiac index remains low, while the arteriovenous oxygen difference increases. The left ventricular work increases slightly but remains below normal. (From E. Blair, A. V. Montgomery, and H. Swan, *Circulation*.[183] By permission of The American Heart Association, Inc.)

BLOOD

Blood viscosity varies inversely with temperature, a 2 percent increase occurring for every 1°C decrease in temperature (Fig. 27-6).[1300,1588,1668,1713] Blood flow in small vessels is markedly reduced, and there is a greater likelihood of thrombosis.[1201,1587] The effect of pH changes on viscosity are negligible.[1586] We recommend that as soon as possible the hematocrit of the patient be adjusted to the same numerical value as the core body temperature in degrees Celsius. This can generally be done within 30 minutes to an hour by exchange transfusion of Ringer's lactate solution against blood.

A bleeding tendency becomes manifest at body temperatures below 28°C, an acute reversible thrombocytopenia being a frequent finding (Figs. 27-2 and 27-7).[2002] Other coagulation factors are probably also adversely affected.

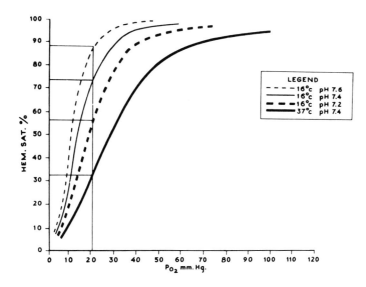

Figure 27-5. Variation of the oxyhemoglobin dissociation curve with temperature and pH. Hypothermia lowers the P_{50} of hemoglobin, as indicated by a shift in the oxyhemoglobin dissociation curve to the left. Alkalemia shifts the curve further to the left. (From J. J. Osborn, F. Gerbode, J. B. Johnston, J. K. Ross, T. Ogata, and W. J. Kerth, *J. Thorac. Cardiovasc. Surg.*[1461])

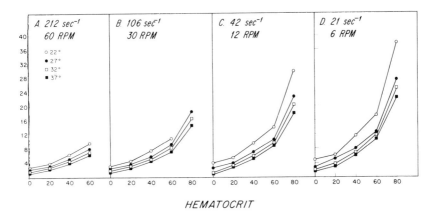

HEMATOCRIT

Figure 27-6. Relationship between viscosity and hematocrit of blood at different temperatures and shear rates. At high shear rates, above 32°C, there is a linear rise in viscosity with increasing hematocrit between 0 and 40 percent. At lower temperatures there is a linear segment between hematocrits of 20 and 60 percent, which is more marked at the low shear rates. In all curves there is a rapid rise in the viscosity when the hematocrit is above 50 percent. (From P. W. Rand, E. Lacombe, H. E. Hunt, and W. H. Austin, *J. Appl. Physiol.*[1588])

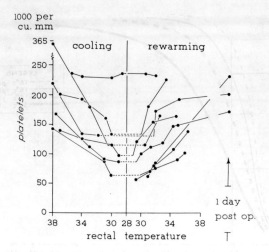

Figure 27-7. Platelet counts in hypothermia. Eight of nine patients developed significant thrombocytopenia during surface hypothermia. The largest depression occurs at the lowest temperature. During rewarming the platelet count returns to near normal. (From W. G. Waddell, H. B. Fairley, and W. G. Bigelow, *Ann. Surg.*[2002])

CEREBRAL EFFECTS

A progressive deterioration occurs in the state of consciousness with a fall in body temperature, most patients being unconscious below 26°C. Muscle rigidity is profound below 32°C.[1290]

The cerebral effects of rewarming after prolonged hypothermia are unexpected. Relapse into coma or confusion can occur with rewarming, but improvement occurs if the temperature is allowed to fall again. These changes appear to be the result of an increase in cerebrospinal fluid pressure. Patients who become increasingly drowsy during rewarming promptly become more alert when cerebrospinal fluid pressure is reduced by lumbar puncture with removal of cerebrospinal fluid.[191] Some patients who develop acute pulmonary edema during rewarming experience dramatic relief within a few minutes of reduction of cerebrospinal fluid pressure. The cerebral effects of rewarming play a role in any neurologic deterioration that may occur during rewarming.[191]

HYPOVOLEMIA

Hypovolemia is associated with accidental hypothermia. A diuresis caused by cold inhibition of tubular reabsorption occurs. We have seen 7 liters of urine produced during this phase. During rewarming an increase in plasma volume takes place due to transfer of fluid into the intravascular space. Renal function remains abnormal for some time after normothermia has been restored. Fluid therapy must reflect these changes in renal and cardiovascular function.[999]

PANCREATITIS AND OTHER DISEASES

Pancreatitis is a known accompaniment of hypothermia, but diagnosis is difficult.[1600,1704] There is often a vague tenderness in the epigastrium and a raised serum amylase. Although hypothermia may occur in conjunction with myxedema and pituitary insufficiency as described earlier, thyroid function is relatively unaffected by hypothermia per se. There is gastrointestinal bleeding in patients with severe hypothermia.[416] Gangrene of the limbs may occur as a result of frostbite, intense peripheral vasoconstriction, increased blood viscosity, and hypovolemia.

MANAGEMENT

We employ external passive rewarming in the majority of patients with temperatures over 30°C. These patients need to be insulated from further heat loss in a comfortably warm room and covered with a light blanket. Rapid external rewarming by the application of surface heat, although it has been used with success, is dangerous; it must be avoided especially in the elderly patient who may have coronary artery disease.[35,486,629] External rewarming releases peripheral vasoconstriction and increases peripheral metabolic demand. The hypothermic heart is unable to increase its output, and circulatory failure ensues. For this reason shivering, which may cause a 200–500 percent increase in oxygen consumption, must be prevented, if necessary, with the use of muscle relaxant drugs.[114]

When a patient's temperature is under 30°C, or if the circulation becomes ineffective, as happens when ventricular fibrillation complicates profound hypothermia, "core" rewarming must be employed while the circulation is supported. Core rewarming is achieved by cardiopulmonary bypass, taking blood from the inferior vena cava via the femoral vein and returning it to the aorta via the femoral artery.[480,626] Heparinization is essential. A Ringer's lactate–albumin pump prime is the most appropriate in view of the increased blood viscosity. A heat exchanger in the extracorporeal circuit is used to raise the temperature. Electric defibrillation is performed once the temperature is greater than 34°C. Peritoneal dialysis[1106] and open thoracotomy with bathing of the heart with warm saline[1168] also have been used with success to provide "core" rewarming. Peritoneal dialysis remains relatively effective in the clearance of urea and potassium during hypothermia.[1492] We prefer a heart-lung machine, since it provides the control of the circulation essential for patients whose temperatures are below 30°C.[1131,1491]

If cerebral edema occurs during rewarming, intracranial pressure may be reduced by aspiration of CSF, production of hypocapnia, administration of an osmotic diuretic, and administration of corticosteroids.[2130]

We employ antibiotics only when a specific indication exists. There is no evidence to support the prophylactic use of antibiotics in accidental hypothermia.

CONTROLLED VENTILATION

Protection of the upper airway is very important in hypothermic coma, as the patients are likely to aspirate. Controlled ventilation is necessary when hypoxemia or hypercapnia supervenes or when muscle relaxant drugs are used to abolish shivering. Since the increase in deadspace-to-tidal-volume ratio due to hypothermia cannot be predicted, frequent blood gas measurements must be made to ensure that the correct minute ventilation is being employed.[1545] If cerebral edema supervenes during rewarming, hypocapnia will reduce cerebral blood flow. When arterial carbon dioxide tension is reduced from 39 to 19 mm Hg (5.2 to 2.5 kPa), cerebral blood flow is reduced by 43 percent.[2106] A dangerous reduction in cardiac output as a result of raised airway pressure must be avoided.[855] The inspired oxygen concentration is regulated to provide adequate oxygenation.

POTASSIUM REPLACEMENT

Potassium loss during the diuresis associated with hypothermia may total over 37 gm (500 mEq [500 mmol]). Intravenous potassium therapy is almost always needed in the treatment of accidental hypothermia. We try not to exceed a replacement rate of 20 mEq (20 mmol) potassium an hour given "piggyback" to crystalloid infusion through a central venous line. Judicious bicarbonate administration is sometimes needed to correct metabolic acidemia partially. To prevent a metabolic alkalemia after the patient has been rewarmed, we never correct more than half the base deficit.

FROSTBITE THERAPY

Once the core temperature has been corrected, a frostbitten limb can be warmed in water, starting at a temperature of 10–15°C and increasing by 5°C every 5 minutes to a maximum of 40°C. Elevation of the injured part is also important. Reduction of blood viscosity is helpful. Low molecular weight dextran is recommended by some authors, but we do not employ it, as the evidence for its use is inconclusive. Regional sympathectomy performed 24–48 hours after thawing may reduce the extent of the cold injury. Amputation is required for gangrene.[731,1506]

PREVENTION

Elderly survivors of accidental hypothermia have an impaired temperature regulation mechanism and are at high risk.[1208] In our experience social agencies do not remember this. Prevention of accidental hypothermia is much cheaper than its acute treatment.

28

Massive Transfusion

MICROAGGREGATE FORMATION
AND RESPIRATORY FAILURE

Microaggregates of leukocytes, platelets, and fibrin accumulate in stored blood. If allowed to remain in transfused blood these aggregates are filtered by the lung and cause pulmonary dysfunction.[156,410,899,1285,1575] Microaggregate formation in stored blood can be detected and evaluated by measurement of the screen filtration pressure of blood. Measurements of blood viscosity are not capable of easily detecting changes due to microaggregate formation. Screen filtration pressure is a sensitive indicator of the presence of substances that may occlude the microvasculature. The device used measures the resistance to flow as blood is passed through a screen with 20-μm square multiple openings.[1891]

During the storage of blood in acid citrate dextrose (ACD) solution the screen filtration pressure is low for the first five days. After five days the mean screen filtration pressure increases markedly (Fig. 28-1), and it continues to increase gradually from that point on.[821,1284] The reason for this sudden increase in microaggregate formation is unknown; it is possible, however, that it is due to fibrin formation.[821] After one week of ACD storage there are over 140,000 microaggregates per milliliter of stored blood, ranging in size from 10 to 164 μm.[410]

Experimentally, infusion of stored blood with high screen filtration pressures results in increases in pulmonary vascular resistance, end-inspiratory bronchial pressure, and lung water.[156,1285] There is also a rise in pulmonary artery pressure and evidence of pulmonary edema both grossly and microscopically.[156,899] A rise in deadspace-to-tidal-volume ratio also follows massive transfusion and suggests an increase in alveolar deadspace consistent with pulmonary microvascular occlusion. During shock these areas of occlusion may be enlarged by fibrin formation secondary to the release of serotonin.[1889,1890]

Significant pulmonary venoconstriction occurs following induction of platelet aggregation in dogs, suggesting that this aspect may be of greater importance than the actual mechanical obstruction from microaggregates. Serotonin may be an important mediator in this response.[1575] After infusion of stored blood in the dog, microemboli in the lung are seen with electron

363

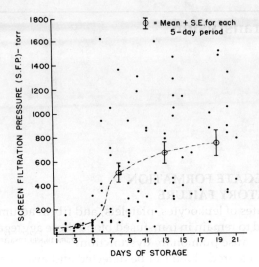

Figure 28-1. Screen filtration pressures (SFP) during 21 days of storage of whole blood. Measurement of the screen filtration pressure gives an accurate estimate of the amount of microaggregate formation in stored blood. During the first five days of storage of blood there is little change in SFP. After five days there is a sudden rise in SFP, which continues during the entire storage period. The sudden rise seen around the sixth day may represent fibrin formation. (From J. R. Harp, M. Q. Wyche, B. E. Marshall, and H. A. Wurzel, *Anesthesiology.*[821])

microscopy. These emboli are associated with marked changes. Cellular swelling, vacuolation, and lysis of capillary endothelial, type I, and type II alveolar epithelial cells are found.[410]

Infusion of blood with high screen filtration pressure also causes peripheral vascular occlusion during extracorporeal circulation. In cats whose heads are perfused with blood having high screen filtration pressures, the electroencephalogram soon decreases in activity and then becomes flat, suggesting occlusion of brain capillaries by microaggregates.[896] In humans who have undergone cardiopulmonary bypass, emboli can be found in many systemic arterioles and capillaries at autopsy.[956]

There is a definite correlation between the amount of stored blood infused and the degree of postoperative hypoxemia in combat casualties, irrespective of the degree of shock or trauma.[1287] In combat casualties requiring massive transfusion respiratory failure has been noted in the absence of any known pulmonary injury. At autopsy many microemboli have been identified in the pulmonary arterioles and capillaries. Their diameter ranges from 10 to 100 μm. Although there are several possible explanations for these emboli, it is likely that emboli from stored blood is a major factor in the development of posttraumatic respiratory failure.[1283,1366]

DIAGNOSIS

The effect of microaggregate embolization to the lung may be difficult to distinguish from other etiologic factors in the patient who requires massive blood replacement. The first signs usually appear within three days following blood replacement.[1319]

Pulmonary artery pressure usually rises. In the patient breathing spontaneously there may be an increase in minute ventilation to compensate for the increase in deadspace. Patients receiving mechanical ventilation generally will need an increase in their minute ventilation because of increased deadspace-to-tidal-volume ratios. As interstitial edema and intraalveolar fluid accumulate, the alveolar-arterial oxygen tension gradient rises. Chest x-ray reveals diffuse increase in lung markings, often without appreciable increase in heart size. The radiographic findings occur relatively late and often lag 6–12 hours behind deterioration in arterial blood gases. Sputum may reveal evidence of alveolar hemorrhage.

TREATMENT

There is no really satisfactory treatment, once microembolization has occurred. Mechanical ventilation is instituted if respiratory failure develops. Diuretics are necessary if lung water is increased. There is no evidence to suggest that steroids prevent or alter the embolic complications of massive blood replacement.

PREVENTION

Microaggregates must be filtered prior to infusion. Conventional blood filters are designed to filter out particles larger than 170 μm in diameter. If two conventional filters are used in succession, the second filter removes 8.6 gm of particulate matter for every 10 units of average age bank blood infused.[1365] Conventional filters are therefore not adequate for filtration of blood during massive blood replacement.

Dacron wool filters (Swank filters) effectively remove microaggregates during infusion of stored blood (Fig. 28-2).[410,1286,1616,1819,1866] Filtration of blood with high screen filtration pressures through Dacron wool filters returns the screen filtration pressure to normal.[410] Dacron wool filters are designed to take advantage of the adhesiveness of aging platelets and leukocytes. Dacron fibers of 10–12 μm form pores in the range of 20–30 μm. Microaggregates are filtered by becoming stuck to the Dacron wool fibers. Once aggregates surround a fiber, they are difficult to dislodge.[1886]

Filtration depends upon the adhesiveness of the filtered substance rather than the pore size. During experimental exsanguination platelets develop increased adhesiveness. If blood is then filtered through a Dacron wool filter, these adhesive platelets are removed.[1887] This situation is quite different from the removal of old aggregates from stored blood. Normally functioning platelets can be removed by Dacron wool filtration, which accounts

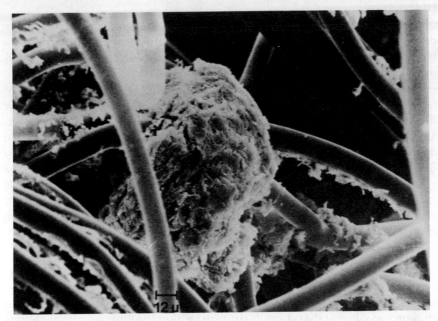

Figure 28-2. Effective filtration of blood with Dacron wool. Scanning electron micrographs of a Dacron wool filter after filtration of 5-day-old canine ACD-stored blood. There are large amounts of adhesive debris caught on the fibers. This debris includes platelets and leukocytes. (From R. S. Connell and R. L. Swank, *Ann. Surg.*[410])

partially for the thrombocytopenia seen following massive transfusion when Dacron wool filters are used.

Mesh filters (Pall filters) have also been developed which have uniform pore sizes of 40 μm. As compared to the Dacron filter (Swank filter) the mesh filter is much less effective. During filtration the Pall filter removes 45–78 percent of debris, while the Swank filter removes 96–100 percent of debris.[1286] The efficiency of the Pall filter increases as consecutive units of blood are infused. With the Swank filter, screen filtration pressures may increase to 1,320 mm Hg (171.3 kPa) after the second unit. Up to 7 units of blood can be infused through a Pall filter, whereas the Swank filter always obstructs flow by the fourth unit.

Clinically, micropore filtration of blood decreases the incidence of respiratory failure following massive blood replacement. In a prospective evaluation of the 40-μm filter, 13 patients received massive blood transfusion (10–63 units per patient) through the filter. The control group of 16 patients received 10–40 units of blood per patient through the standard 170-μm filter. Fifty percent of the control group developed respiratory failure, in contrast to only 15 percent of the group who received micropore-filtered blood.[1616] Similar results are found when Dacron wool filters are used during procedures involving cardiopulmonary bypass.[26,58,409,877,1462]

Micropore filtration of blood should be employed whenever 3 or more units of stored blood are to be administered over 24 hours. Because of micropore filters' high affinity for platelets these filters should not be used when platelet concentrates or fresh whole blood are administered.

DEPLETION OF 2,3-DPG AND THE OXY-HEMOGLOBIN DISSOCIATION CURVE

Red blood cell hemoglobin stored in ACD or citrate phosphate-dextrose (CPD) solutions for one week has a markedly increased affinity for oxygen.[1739,1973,1974] This increased oxygen affinity is related to depletion of red cell 2,3-DPG, which occurs with storage.[314,1593,1874] Although this depletion has been well documented in both in vitro and in vivo studies, the clinical significance remains controversial.

2,3-diphosphoglycerate (2,3-DPG) and adenosine triphosphate (ATP) cause increased dissociation of oxyhemoglobin.[1969] During storage of blood in ACD solution at 4°C there is a rapid depletion of 2,3-DPG during the first seven days. Levels of 2,3-DPG fall from 0.88–1.0 mol per mol of hemoglobin at the time of collection to 0.22–0.44 mol per mol of hemoglobin at seven days. After that point there is a slower but continual depletion of 2,3-DPG, so that by 21 days the levels are less than 0.11 mol per mol of hemoglobin (Fig. 28-3).[269] Decreases in ATP concentrations also appear to be significant.[102] The shift of the oxyhemoglobin dissociation curve to the left closely parallels the fall in 2,3-DPG.[314,1874,1967]

CLINICAL IMPLICATIONS

Patients requiring massive blood replacement of 2,3-DPG–depleted blood will undergo a fall in P_{50} from the normal of 27 mm Hg (3.6 kPa) to as low as 15 mm Hg (2.0 kPa). In theory oxygen unloading at the tissue level, which occurs on the steep portion of the curve, should be impaired in patients with a left shift of the curve. Whether patients suffer any harm from this effect is not clearly established.[314]

The military forces have wide experience with transfusion of massive amounts of whole stored blood. In these young healthy males no evidence of alteration in mortality could be found with the type of blood used.[314] In a more recent evaluation of surgical patients at the Massachusetts General Hospital no correlation could be found between total number of units infused, 2,3-DPG levels, P_{50} of hemoglobin, and ultimate survival.[1119]

Following transfusion of 3–5 units of 2,3-DPG–depleted blood to anemic patients there is no immediate change in oxygen consumption. An initial fall in arterial pH occurs, as well as a fall in the arterial–mixed venous oxygen content difference. At this time circulating levels of red cell 2,3-DPG are low. After four hours the arterial pH and arteriovenous difference return to normal. After 24 hours the 2,3-DPG levels and P_{50} of hemoglobin fre-

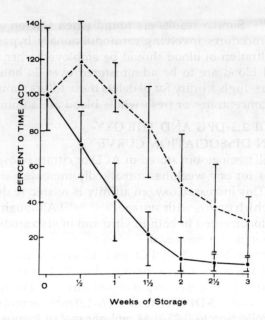

Figure 28-3. Depletion of 2,3-DPG during storage of blood in acid citrate dextrose (ACD) or citrate-phosphate-dextrose (CPD) solutions. Blood was obtained from six normal donors and stored in either ACD or CPD solutions. (--------) = blood stored in CPD; (———) = blood stored in ACD. The concentration of 2,3-DPG in the ACD blood at time 0 is taken as 100%. The means and ranges are shown. During all phases of storage the blood stored in CPD has higher concentrations of 2,3-DPG; however significant depletion of 2,3-DPG does occur regardless of the type of storage solution. The range shown for time zero represents the range for CPD blood. (From A. W. Shafer, L. L. Tague, M. H. Welch, and C. A. Guenter, *J. Lab. Clin. Med.*[1739])

quently become normal, but complete restoration of levels of 2,3-DPG may take up to 11 days (Fig. 28-4).[170,1967,1968,1969] After red cell levels of 2,3-DPG reach normal, they often continue to rise, possibly reflecting a compensatory mechanism for delivery of more oxygen to the tissues.[242,1062]

Another clinical point should be remembered. In patients who are undergoing massive blood replacement there may be a marked metabolic acidemia. If the oxyhemoglobin dissociation curve is determined in vitro at a pH of 7.40, the dissociation curve will be shifted to the left. If it is replotted at the patient's pH—say, 7.11—it will be shifted to the right. One should be careful, therefore, to evaluate the P_{50} of hemoglobin in an in vivo situation (Fig. 28-5).[1119]

PREVENTION

As we have mentioned, there is at present no definite clinical evidence of any adverse effects of massive transfusion of 2,3-DPG–depleted blood, but we think that ideally attempts should be made to prevent depletion of

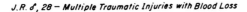

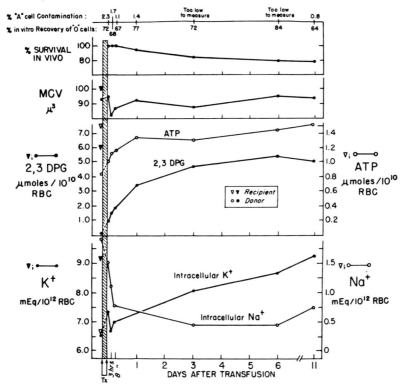

Figure 28-4. In vivo restoration of red cell 2,3-DPG. Following transfusion of four units of O-positive red cells in a 2¾-hour period to a patient with multiple trauma the restoration of 2,3-DPG and ATP was observed in the patient's red cells. These red cells had been stored as whole blood for 16 days. Concentrations of ATP and 2,3-DPG were restored rapidly in the first 24 hours following transfusion. Levels continued to rise for 11 days. Intracellular sodium fell rapidly. Intracellular potassium increased slowly for 11 days. MCV = mean corpuscular volume. (From C. R. Valeri and N. M. Hirsch, *J. Lab. Clin. Med.*[1969])

2,3-DPG during red cell storage. Since levels of 2,3-DPG usually are well maintained for the first 4–5 days of storage, ideally we would like to transfuse only blood that is less than 5 days old. This is impossible, so one must use methods of storage that protect 2,3-DPG.

The addition of sodium chloride to red blood cells to a concentration of 0.45% can increase the P_{50} of ACD-stored blood.[1973] Since the rate of 2,3-DPG depletion is higher at low pH, a higher pH is desirable. Storage of blood in CPD results in a higher pH and therefore slower depletion of 2,3-DPG.[169,314] Normal levels of 2,3-DPG cannot, however, be maintained by storage in CPD.

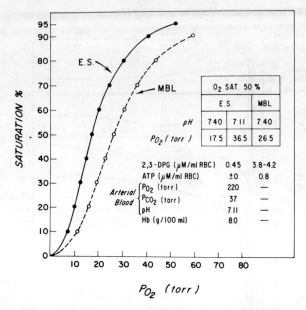

Figure 28-5. Oxyhemoglobin dissociation curve following massive transfusion. The dissociation curve of a patient who received 52 units of ACD-stored blood (E.S.) is plotted beside the curve of MBL. At a pH of 7.40 the patient's P_{50} was 17.5 torr (2.3 kPa), however, at the patient's actual arterial pH of 7.11 the P_{50} is 36.5 torr (4.8 kPa). Red cell 2,3-DPG concentration was 10 percent of normal. (From M. B. Laver, M. Broennle, B. Trichet, C. Tung, and E. Jackson. In H. Chaplin, Jr., et al. (Eds.), *Preservation of Red Blood Cells.*[1119])

Additives

Additives to the storage solution have been proposed to limit the depletion of 2,3-DPG. Addition of inosine to 21- to 28-day-old ACD-stored blood to a final concentration of 10 mmol/l raises the 2,3-DPG concentration from an average of 176 nmol per milliliter of red blood cells to 1,395 nmol per milliliter. Addition of a combination of inosine, pyruvate, and phosphate to a final concentration of 10 mmol/l of each substance increases 2,3-DPG levels to 6,637 nmol per milliliter of red blood cells.[1464] The addition of dihydroxyacetone and ascorbic acid is also effective in reducing the depletion of 2,3-DPG.[314] All these additives are still in the experimental stage.

Freezing

Freezing is an excellent method of storage of red blood cells.[1946] The levels of 2,3-DPG and the characteristics of the oxyhemoglobin dissociation curve do not seem to change, once the red cells are frozen.[1449] Red cell 2,3-DPG depends upon the length of time the cells were stored in ACD or CPD prior to freezing (Figs. 28-6 and 28-7).[242,1119] There is also evidence that 2,3-DPG–depleted red cells, when treated with pyruvate, inosine, glucose,

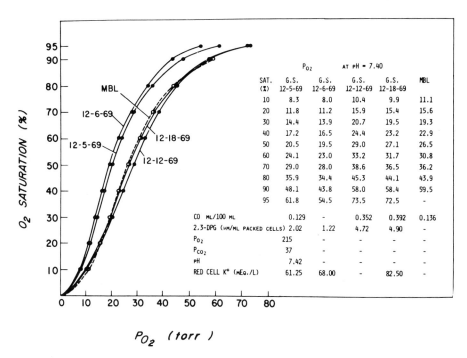

SAT. (%)	G.S. 12-5-69	G.S. 12-6-69	G.S. 12-12-69	G.S. 12-18-69	MBL
10	8.3	8.0	10.4	9.9	11.1
20	11.8	11.2	15.9	15.4	15.6
30	14.4	13.9	20.7	19.5	19.3
40	17.2	16.5	24.4	23.2	22.9
50	20.5	19.5	29.0	27.1	26.5
60	24.1	23.0	33.2	31.7	30.8
70	29.0	28.0	38.6	36.5	36.2
80	35.9	34.4	45.3	44.1	43.9
90	48.1	43.8	58.0	58.4	59.5
95	61.8	54.5	73.5	72.5	-
CO ML/100 ML	0.129	-	0.352	0.392	0.136
2,3-DPG (μM/ML PACKED CELLS)	2.02	1.22	4.72	4.90	-
P_{O_2}	215	-	-	-	-
P_{CO_2}	37	-	-	-	-
pH	7.42	-	-	-	-
RED CELL K+ (mEq./L)	61.25	68.00	-	82.50	-

(P_{O_2} AT pH = 7.40)

Figure 28-6. Response of red cell 2,3-DPG content and oxyhemoglobin dissociation curve after massive transfusion. A patient (G.S.) required 35 units of frozen packed red cells for hemipelvectomy and insertion of a prosthesis. The oxyhemoglobin dissociation curve shifted to the left one and two days postoperatively. At one week the curve returned and exceeded the normal P_{50}. After two weeks the P_{50} returned to the level of the control. All changes were related to changes in red cell 2,3-DPG. The patient recovered uneventfully. (From M. B. Laver, M. Broennle, B. Trichet, C. Tung, and E. Jackson. In H. Chaplin, Jr., et al. (Eds.), *Preservation of Red Blood Cells*.[1119])

phosphate, and adenine and then frozen and stored for a prolonged period, will have near-normal oxyhemoglobin dissociation curves when thawed for use. This process provides a means of rejuvenating outdated red cells and storing them for prolonged periods of time.[1970]

COAGULATION DISORDERS

Coagulopathy is a frequent complication of massive blood replacement. Thrombocytopenia, loss of factors V and VIII, hypocalcemia, fibrinolysis, and disseminated intravascular coagulation all lead to its development.[1509,1751]

Thrombocytopenia

Thrombocytopenia is probably the most frequent posttransfusion coagulation disorder.[1319,1320] The actual number of platelets declines gradually

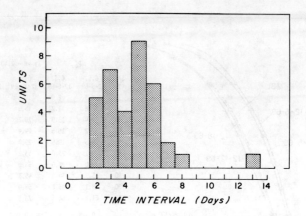

Figure 28-7. Duration of storage of blood in ACD solution prior to freezing at −80°C for units given to patient illustrated in previous figure. Freezing of blood results in a 2,3-DPG concentration at time of thawing equal to the 2,3-DPG concentration at time of freezing. This explains why the frozen blood transfused into the patient in Figure 28-6 resulted in a shift of the oxyhemoglobin dissociation curve. (From M. B. Laver, M. Broennle, B. Trichet, C. Tung, and E. Jackson. In H. Chaplin, Jr., et al. (Eds.), *Preservation of Red Blood Cells.*[1119])

over the course of storage in ACD solution, and there is a rapid reduction in the in vivo viability of the platelets that remain. After storage at 4°C platelets are damaged sufficiently so that after transfusion they are rapidly removed from the circulation by the reticuloendothelial system. After three hours of storage only 60 percent of platelets are viable, after 24 hours only 12 percent are viable, and after 48 hours only 2 percent are viable.[1319] Following the infusion of more than 10 units of ACD-stored blood there is nearly always a significant reduction in the number and function of circulating platelets, so that abnormal bleeding results.[1509] When the platelet count is below 65,000 per cubic millimeter (65 10⁹/l), abnormal bleeding frequently occurs in surgical patients.

Factors V and VIII

Both factor V (proaccelerin) and factor VIII (antihemophilic factor) are depleted slowly during the storage of blood (Fig. 28-8). The normal circulating concentrations of these two factors are considerably greater than what is needed for hemostasis: only 5 to 20 percent of the normal concentration of factor V is necessary, and 30 percent of the normal concentration of factor VIII. These factors are decreased usually to 20–50 percent of the initial value by the end of 21 days of storage.[1319] Loss of these factors hardly ever significantly contributes to posttransfusion coagulopathy, except in patients with a preexisting coagulation disorder. Patients with a posttransfusion bleeding diathesis often do not respond dramatically to the administration of fresh frozen plasma containing all the coagulation factors except platelets.[1319,1509] Fibrinogen as well as the remaining coagulation factors is quite stable during storage (Fig. 28-8).

Disseminated Intravascular Coagulation

Disseminated intravascular coagulation, and far less commonly primary fibrinolysis, do occur during massive transfusion of blood.[1319,1509,1751] We consider them in Chapter 29.

Ionized Calcium

Ionized calcium is necessary for the adequate coagulation of blood. Transfusion of citrated blood lowers the serum ionized calcium, but hypocalcemia is of little or no significance in terms of hemostasis, because very low calcium levels stop the heart before impairing hemostasis.[1509] The role of ionized calcium will be discussed further under Metabolic Effects.

DIAGNOSIS AND MANAGEMENT

If a patient develops excessive bleeding during or following a massive blood transfusion, several evaluative steps are necessary. Blood should be sent for a platelet count and estimate of prothrombin time, and partial thromboplastin time. Blood should also be collected to determine the degree of clot formation and the stability of the clot. Patients who are having a dilutional thrombocytopenia will demonstrate a low platelet count, usually below 65,000 per cubic millimeter (65 10⁹/l). Prothrombin and partial thromboplastin times usually will be normal.[1320]

Treatment of thrombocytopenia is best accomplished by the administration of fresh whole blood without the use of a micropore filter.[1320] Very often fresh whole blood is not available for use in the treatment of throm-

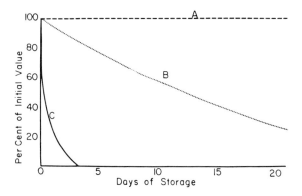

Figure 28-8. Changes in hemostatic factors during storage of blood in ACD solution. *A* = levels of fibrinogen, factor IX (Christmas factor), factor X (Stuart factor), factor VII (proconvertin), and prothrombin expressed as percent of initial value at time of collection of blood. *B* = factor VIII (antihemophilic factor) and factor V (proaccelerin). *C* = platelet viability after transfusion. (From H. A. Perkins, *Anesthesiology.*[1509])

bocytopenia. In such cases platelet concentrates have to be used. For the bleeding thrombocytopenic patient the platelets from 8–10 units of blood should be administered.[1319] An average unit of whole blood contains 1×10^{11} platelets. In a patient with a body surface area of one square meter, this single unit should increase the platelet count 12,500 per cubic millimeter $(12.5 \ 10^9/l)$. The incidence of survival of platelets immediately after transfusion is only 25 percent, and few of these platelets survive more than one to two days.[2142] Platelet counts should therefore be monitored for several days after transfusion to ensure that adequate marrow production is taking place.

In patients who have become depleted of factors V and VIII there will be an increase in the prothrombin ($> 2 \times$ control) and partial thromboplastin times ($> 2 \times$ control), often associated with a dilutional thrombocytopenia. These patients require platelet transfusion as well as the administration of fresh frozen plasma. Fresh frozen plasma is given until the prothrombin and partial thromboplastin times return to the normal range.

Patients who demonstrate thrombocytopenia and prolonged prothrombin and partial thromboplastin times may have disseminated intravascular coagulation. The character of the clot can be used to exclude fibrinolysis. Patients with disseminated intravascular coagulation will have fibrin split products present.[1319] Further evaluation and treatment is discussed in Chapter 29.

PREVENTION

Coagulation disorders can be prevented by careful attention to the blood products used. Fresh blood or platelet concentrates should be administered for every 5 –10 units of stored blood transfused. Pletelet count and evaluation of the clot for lysis should be done after every five units of blood. Prothrombin and partial thromboplastin times should be measured after transfusion of every ten units of stored blood.[1319]

HYPOTHERMIA

Blood is normally stored at 4°C. If several units of cold blood are infused slowly, there is little effect. If massive blood replacement is required, there will be a fall in body temperature which is directly proportional to the number of units of blood transfused (Fig. 28-9). The transfusion of 25–30 units of stored blood at 4°C results in reduction of core body temperature to 26–29°C; ventricular arrhythmias and cardiac arrest follow. The incidence of cardiac arrest in patients receiving over 3,000 ml of blood at 4°C at a rate of greater than 50 ml per minute is 58 percent. When blood is warmed to body temperature prior to transfusion and administered at the volumes and rates described above, the incidence of cardiac arrest is significantly reduced to 6.8 percent ($P < 0.01$).[212]

Blood that is to be transfused should be warmed whenever more than four units are to be given over several hours.[1319] Various methods of warm-

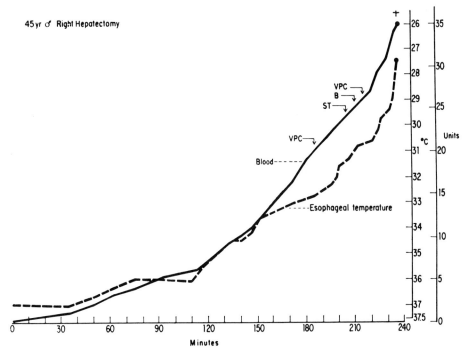

Figure 28-9. Effect of massive transfusion of cold blood. A patient received 35 units of cold (4°C) whole blood during the course of a right hepatectomy. The esophageal temperature is plotted with the number of transfusions given over a four-hour period. Ventricular premature contractions (*VPC*) appeared after 20 units when the temperature of the patient was 31°C. Prolongation of the S-T segment (*ST*) developed after 25 units, when the body temperature was slightly over 29°C. Bradycardia (*B*) then followed. Cardiac arrest (†) occurred at an esophageal temperature of 26°C after 35 units of blood. (From C. P. Boyan, *Ann. Surg.*[212])

ing have been described. The early devices for warming blood merely consisted of water baths, into which a 24-foot coil of plastic tubing was placed. Blood was transfused from the storage bottle, through the bath, and into the patient. The water bath was maintained at 37°C by continual addition of warm water.[212] This system works well but requires the continual addition of warm water. Other warming devices we use have electric coils surrounding the warming bath, which keep the water at a constant temperature.

Microwave blood warmers can warm an entire unit of blood prior to transfusion. A single microwave warmer can be used by multiple operating rooms. With this type of warmer there is a definite danger of overheating of blood and subsequent hemolysis.[1836] If this type of warmer is used, the unit must be equipped with a means of determining the actual temperature of the warmed blood.

Other devices have been developed which pass blood through a plastic packet enclosed in a dry warming device. This system has a high temperature alarm to prevent overheating.

METABOLIC EFFECTS

ACID-BASE BALANCE

The pH of blood collected in ACD solution is 6.9–7.0 immediately after collection.[266] The pH of blood collected in CPD is 7.2.[707] The pH falls over three weeks of storage to 6.4–6.5 for ACD-stored blood, due to production of lactic and pyruvic acid by red cell metabolism.[1319]

A 500-ml unit of whole blood contains the equivalent of 14 mmol of hydrogen ion. Unbuffered, this acid load results in a fall in pH when infused. In actuality most of this acid load is buffered by bicarbonate and hemoglobin. On infusion there is a reduction in the circulating bicarbonate and an initial fall in pH. This fall is usually transient, due to renal production of more bicarbonate as well as metabolism of citrate to bicarbonate.[266,1172]

The usual clinical picture following massive blood replacement is an initial transient metabolic acidemia. The degree of the acidemia does not have a correlation with the number of units transfused but depends upon the presence or absence of shock.[1321] The acidemia often disappears after several hours, and a metabolic alkalemia develops for the reasons mentioned above. The alkalemia is usually most marked by the third posttransfusion day.[1172]

The acid-base management of the patient who receives multiple transfusions should consist of careful monitoring of the acid-base status. If a severe metabolic acidemia develops, it should be corrected. Bicarbonate should not be given routinely for every 4 or 5 units transfused. This practice causes the supervening metabolic alkalemia to be even more severe. Alkalemia in a patient who has had multiple transfusions is important in terms of the oxyhemoglobin dissociation curve. As described previously, depletion of 2,3-DPG leads to a left shift of the dissociation curve. Metabolic alkalemia tends to increase this left shift. One should therefore attempt to limit the degree of metabolic alkalemia as much as possible.[1321]

IONIZED CALCIUM AND SODIUM CITRATE

The rapid infusion of sodium citrate in man results in circulatory depression manifested by hypotension, decreased pulse pressure, fall in cardiac output, decreased left ventricular work, and a prolonged Q-T interval on the electrocardiogram.[267] These are findings similar to those seen in marked hypocalcemia and are probably secondary to the binding of ionized calcium by citrate.[1319] When ACD-stored blood is infused in man, the level of serum ionized calcium falls approximately 0.6 mg per 100 ml (0.15 mmol/l) after 1,000 ml of blood. This level returns to normal after 10 minutes.[891] In order to produce significant circulatory depression from citrate-induced hypocalcemia, one would need to infuse blood at a rate of 500 ml every 3 to 4 minutes into a 70-kg man or 360 ml into a 50-kg woman.[267] Tolerance to the effects of sodium citrate is caused by its rapid metabolism to bicarbonate in the Krebs cycle.[1319]

Calcium is rapidly mobilized from bone when ionized calcium falls. During rapid blood replacement one should measure the level of ionized calcium and manage the patient accordingly.[266] Routine administration of calcium during blood replacement is unnecessary, since clinical manifestations of citrate intoxication rarely occur.[1319] During periods of rapid blood replacement, however, one should watch for signs of hypocalcemia, notably prolongation of the Q-T interval. If signs of hypocalcemia result, calcium chloride (100 mg every three minutes) should be given intravenously until the ECG changes return to normal. The cardiovascular depression is usually responsive to this measure.[267,1319]

Storage of blood in CPD solution makes calcium chloride even less necessary. Storage in CPD solution results in 20 percent lower citrate levels than storage in ACD solution. Use of CPD-stored blood therefore results in less depression of serum calcium than does an equivalent transfusion of ACD blood.[267,707]

POTASSIUM

During storage red blood cells lose potassium into the plasma. After seven days of storage in ACD solution the serum potassium is 12 mEq per liter (12 mmol/l). After three weeks of storage it can be as high as 32 mEq per liter (32 mmol/l). Occasional cases of hyperkalemia have been reported following massive transfusions, but infusion rates must be over 120 ml per minute to cause persistent hyperkalemia.[1319] Following massive blood transfusion there is usually little change in the patient's serum potassium. This stability is possibly related to the fact that once red cells are rewarmed, they are again able to maintain their normal gradient of potassium across their cell walls.[266] Red cells after transfusion take four days to regain their intracellular potassium concentration completely.[414]

In managing patients undergoing rapid transfusion the electrocardiogram is helpful in detecting hyperkalemia. Early signs of hyperkalemia include peaking of the T wave and prolongation of the QRS complex. Hyperkalemia can be managed acutely by the intravenous administration of insulin and glucose.

OTHER COMPLICATIONS

POSTTRANSFUSION HEPATITIS

Nearly 30,000 patients get posttransfusion hepatitis every year. Fifteen cases are reported for every 1,000 patients who have at least one blood transfusion.[1319] Patients receiving multiple transfusions are at greater risk for developing hepatitis.

The correlation of positive hepatitis-associated antigen with posttransfusion hepatitis has accounted for a marked reduction in the incidence of posttransfusion hepatitis.[997] If blood that is positive for hepatitis-associated antigen is not transfused, 25–37 percent of posttransfusion hepatitis can be prevented. Further reduction in the incidence of posttransfusion hepatitis can be accomplished by the elimination of paid donors of blood and by accepting only volunteer donations.[723,1319]

HEMOLYSIS DURING INFUSION

Hemolysis following massive blood replacement is related to many different factors, such as a mismatched transfusion or overheating during warming of blood. Both the pressure at which blood is infused and the size of the cannula through which it is infused influence the degree of hemolysis.

Although it is often claimed that blood tends to hemolyze more when it flows through a narrower needle, this is untrue.[1372] Needles with smaller internal diameters cause less hemolysis than do needles with larger internal diameters.[600]

Blood administered rapidly is usually pumped in via a pneumatic device. The higher the pressure applied to the blood, the greater the degree of hemolysis. In an evaluation of the effect of both needle size and infusion pressure, administration of blood through an 18-gauge needle under 300 mm Hg (40.0 kPa) infusion pressure resulted in the greatest degree of hemolysis (44.5 mg hemoglobin per 100 ml plasma [27.6 μmol/l]). Hemolysis in the infused blood of less than 75 mg per 100 ml (46.5 μmol/l) is not considered to increase morbidity or mortality.[600]

AUTOTRANSFUSION OF BLOOD

Before present-day blood banking techniques were available, autotransfusion of blood was occasionally a lifesaving procedure. Autotransfusion has been successfully applied to obstetric hemorrhage, vascular trauma, vascular reconstructive surgery, plastic surgery, neurosurgery, thoracic and cardiovascular surgery, and transurethral prostatectomy. In view of the large number of complications that occur due to transfusion of bank blood, there has been a recent resurgence of interest in the use of autotransfusion.[453,1098,1441,1834,2076]

In most methods of autotransfusion the patient is fully anticoagulated with heparin.[1581] Blood is suctioned from the patient by use of a roller pump suction apparatus,[1043] filtered through some form of reservoir filter, and reinfused into the patient.

Experimentally autotransfusion produces changes in the circulating blood components. Platelets decrease in number, and free plasma hemoglobin rises. Other clotting factors are unchanged. Screen filtration pressures are high but can be reduced by using a micropore filter.[157] Dacron wool is effective in removing microaggregates from autotransfused blood.[2112]

Perfusion with autotransfused or fresh whole blood causes no change in pulmonary vascular resistance and endobronchial pressure. Perfusion with autotransfused or fresh whole blood minimizes intraalveolar edema.[158] One criticism of autotransfusion is that it cannot be used when there is bacterial wound contamination.

There have been reports of over 1,000 cases of successful use of autotransfusion.[1045] Disposable units are now available for autotransfusion and have been employed in combat situations with excellent results.[1043] Complications reported in man include coagulation disorders. Thrombocytopenia and hypofibrinogenemia as well as the presence of fibrin split products have been seen following autotransfusion, suggesting an ongoing defibrination process. However, it is unclear what role autotransfusion plays in this process.[1580,1581] Microemboli from platelet aggregates can be a complication, and therefore micropore filtration should be used. We find autotransfusion of definite but very limited value.

29

Disseminated Intravascular Coagulation

Disseminated intravascular coagulation is a disease process in which thrombin or thrombin-like substances induce fibrin deposition in the vascular tree. Paradoxically systemic coagulation is inhibited by circulating degradation products of fibrin and fibrinogen and by the consumption of circulating clotting factors. The clinical result is intravascular thrombosis with concurrent systemic bleeding.

MECHANISM

This pathologic coagulation is a complication of the cellular injury sustained in many diseases (Table 29-1).[1047,1849,2058] Although diverse in nature, these diseases have in common the ability to expose plasma to a substance that initiates reactions culminating in the conversion of fibrinogen to fibrin and subsequent fibrinolysis.[402,1303] This substance may be tissue thromboplastin, which initiates the clotting cascade via the extrinsic system; exposed collagen, which initiates clotting via Hageman factor XII and the intrinsic system; or phospholipids from red blood cells and platelets, which will catalyze clotting via both systems (Fig. 29-1).[399] The final event of all stimuli is the production of thrombin.

Thrombin formed by these stimuli converts fibrinogen to fibrin monomer by cleaving from it peptides A and B, and it also activates factor XIII, which forms stable fibrin polymers. Thrombin also causes release of platelet factor 3, phospholipid necessary for prothrombin activation, and platelet factor 4, which can neutralize heparin. Thrombin activates factors V, VIII, and plasminogen and causes irreversible platelet aggregation.

Sepsis may cause capillary endothelial damage with exposure of collagen to plasma. This exposure activates factor XII, the intrinsic cascade, and the kallikrein systems of fibrinolysis (Fig. 29-1).[427,1559,2121] Endotoxin also activates factor XII.[146,1248,1278] Trauma and shock with massive transfusion can cause disseminated intravascular coagulation due to endothelial damage or tissue thromboplastin release.[62,812,813,1276,1644,1868] Transfusion reactions cause hemolysis with release of phospholipids and thromboplastins and platelet aggregation.[1066,1181,1182] Extracorporeal circulation with exposure of plasma to foreign surfaces and hemolysis activates factor XII and ruptures platelets.[213,1776] Disseminated intravascular coagulation also oc-

Table 29-1.   Diseases Associated with Disseminated Intravascular Coagulation

Infections
   Gram-negative septicemia
   Gram-positive septicemia
   Viremia
   Aspergillus septicemia
   Rocky Mountain spotted fever
   Acute histoplasmosis
   Cytomegalic disease
   Malaria
   Tuberculosis
   Hepatitis, acute fulminant
Vascular (endothelial) damage
   Heat stroke
   Transplant rejection
   Thrombotic thrombocytopenic purpura
   Glomerulonephritis
   Hyaline membrane disease
   Malignant hypertension
Surgical conditions
   Extensive surgical trauma
   Extracorporeal circulation
Miscellaneous
   Giant hemangioma (Kasabach-Merritt syndrome)
   Prolonged hypotension
   Dog bite
   Pulmonary embolism
   Pancreatitis
   Snake bite
   Burns
   Fat embolism
   Brain destruction
Malignancies
   Prostatic, stomach, colonic, bronchogenic
   Acute promyelocytic leukemia
   Acute myelogenous leukemia
   Acute lymphatic leukemia
   Rhabdomyosarcoma
   Breast, pancreatic, gallbladder, ovarian
Obstetric conditions
   Abruptio placentae
   Amniotic fluid embolism
   Hydatidiform mole
   Retained dead fetus
   Eclampsia
   Septic abortion
Hemolysis
   Transfusion reaction
   Glucose 6-phosphate dehydrogenase deficiency

Table 29-1 (continued)

Paroxysmal nocturnal hemoglobinuria
March hemoglobinuria
Sickle cell crisis
Malaria
Hemolytic uremic syndrome

SOURCE: Reproduced and modified from D. Steinberg. In E. A. Stiene (Ed.), *Hematology Laboratory Medicine.*[1849]

curs in fat embolism, due to fat activation of factor XII.[79,1507] Head injury with brain destruction also leads to disseminated intravascular coagulation.[740]

CLINICAL PICTURE

Fibrin thrombi can be found in 90 percent of diagnosed cases, most often in the kidney, lungs, skin, and testes.[1628,1629] Red blood cells damaged by passage through partially thrombosed capillaries are indicative. Helmet

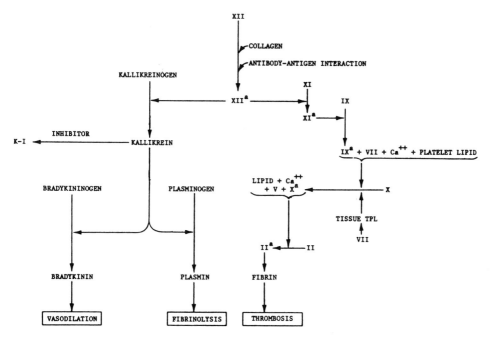

Figure 29-1. Thrombosis, fibrinolysis, and vasodilation are triggered by a variety of pathways utilizing the activation of factor XII (Hageman factor) or tissue thromboplastin (TPL). *K-I* denotes the kallikrein inhibitor complex. Roman numerals refer to factor numbers. [a] = activated. (From R. W. Colman. In W. S. Beck (Ed.), *Hematology.*[399] Copyright, 1973, M. I. T. Press, by permission.)

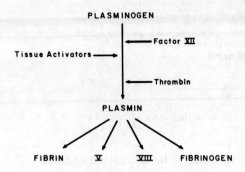

Figure 29-2. The fibrinolytic system can be activated by tissue activators, thrombin, or activated factor XII to produce plasmin. Plasmin acts on fibrin, factor V, factor VIII, and fibrinogen. (From R. W. Colman. In W. S. Beck (Ed.), *Hematology*.[399] Copyright, 1973, M. I. T. Press, by permission.)

cells or schistocytes are supportive of a diagnosis of disseminated intravascular coagulation.[216,398,1662] A microangiopathic hemolytic anemia may result.[1662]

Bleeding is seen in 88 percent of cases, usually at multiple sites.[402] The lung is a site of hemorrhage in 18 percent of cases.[1628,1629] The same processes that stimulate thrombosis also initiate fibrinolysis. Tissue substances, thrombin-activated factor XII via kallikrein, and urokinase stimulate the conversion of plasminogen to plasmin (Fig. 29-2). Plasmin is responsible for fibrinolysis but in addition inhibits coagulation directly by destroying factors V and VIII and prothrombin and by releasing fibrin split products. Fibrinogen, molecular weight 320,000, and fibrin, when exposed to plasmin, are broken down progressively into several smaller fragments (Table 29-2).[1063,1225,1226] In addition to the direct effects of fibrin split products on the coagulation cascade, there is formation of faulty fibrin gels by the reactions of fibrin monomer with the fibrin split products (Fig. 29-3).[502] The thrombosis occurring in the body consumes circulating coagulation factors,

Table 29-2. Properties of Fibrinogen and Its Digestion Products

Component	Mol. Wt.	Clotted by Thrombin	Effect on Hemostasis
Fibrinogen	330,000	Yes	Is essential component
Fragment X	270,000	Slowly	Slows clotting
Fragment Y	155,000	No	Is antithrombic
Fragment D	90,000	No	Delays polymerization of fibrin
Fragment E	50,000	No	Is weakly antithrombic
Small fragments	<10,000	No	Inhibits platelet aggregation

SOURCE: R. W. Colman. In W. S. Beck (Ed.), *Hematology*.[399] Copyright M.I.T. Press, 1973, by permission.

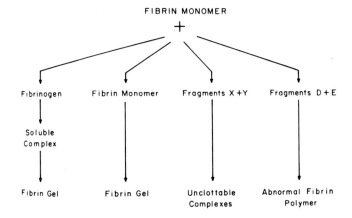

FIBRIN MONOMER

Fibrinogen Fibrin Monomer Fragments X +Y Fragments D + E

Soluble
Complex

Fibrin Gel Fibrin Gel Unclottable Abnormal Fibrin
Complexes Polymer

Figure 29-3. The formation of fibrin monomer complexes inhibits the production of a stable clot. (From D. Deykin.[502] Reprinted by permission from the *New England Journal of Medicine* 283:636–644, 1970.)

reducing their plasma concentration.[1644] Activated factor V and probably factor VIII break down rapidly in the presence of thrombin, as happens in disseminated intravascular coagulation (Fig. 29-4).[397] Platelet and fibrinogen destruction and turnover occur concurrently (Fig. 29-5).[818] The platelet and fibrinogen turnovers do not show a correlation with decreased circulating concentrations, however, because there is a compensatory increase in their production (Fig. 29-6).

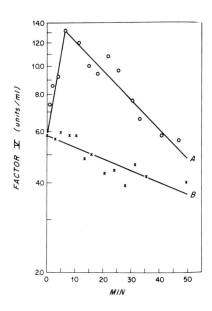

Figure 29-4. Loss of factor V activity following thrombin activation (*A*) and in the absence of thrombin (*B*). Thrombin probably catalyzes the formation of an altered form of factor V with higher activity but a decreased inherent stability compared with native factor V. In disseminated intravascular coagulation thrombin may be responsible for depletion of factor V by formation of an unstable form. (From R. W. Colman, *Biochemistry.*[397] Reprinted with permission. Copyright, 1969, by the American Chemical Society.)

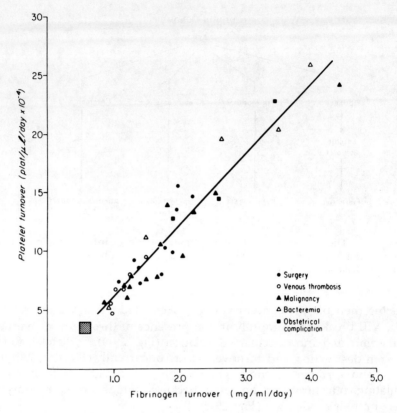

Figure 29-5. Correlation between the rates of platelet turnover and fibrinogen turnover in patients with disseminated intravascular coagulation due to bacteremia, trauma, thrombosis, and obstetric complications. The correlation coefficient is 0.942 ($P < 0.001$). Normal values ± 1 SD are shown in *shaded block.* (From L. A. Harker and S. J. Slichter.[818] Reprinted by permission from the *New England Journal of Medicine* 287:999–1005, 1972.)

Bleeding therefore is the result of many factors, including decreased circulating coagulation factors, increased fibrinolysis, the presence of coagulation inhibitors such as fibrin split products, and the formation of faulty fibrin gels.

DIAGNOSIS

The diagnosis of disseminated intravascular coagulation rests on the presence of bleeding or thrombosis with laboratory confirmation. Three screening tests that we use are platelet count, prothrombin time, and fibrinogen level.[402] If the platelet count is less than 60,000 per cubic millimeter (60 10⁹/l), the prothrombin time greater than 18 seconds (if control time is 12 ± 1 sec), and the quantity of fibrinogen less than 160 mg per 100 ml (4.7 μmol/l), then we feel that the diagnosis of disseminated intravascular

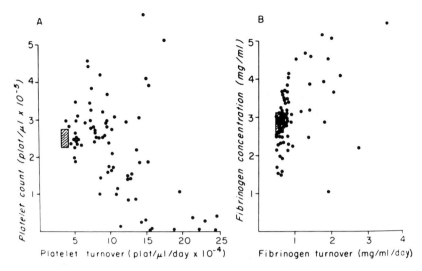

Figure 29-6. Platelet count vs. platelet turnover (A) and fibrinogen concentration vs. fibrinogen turnover (B) during intravascular coagulation. Platelet count and fibrinogen concentration may not reflect the increased turnover rate. Normal values ± 1 SD are in *shaded areas*. (From L. A. Harker and S. J. Slichter.[818] Reprinted by permission from the *New England Journal of Medicine* 287:999–1005, 1972.)

coagulation is confirmed. If, however, only two of the three screening tests are abnormal, then the diagnosis must be substantiated by abnormal results from at least one confirmatory test. A thrombin time of more than 25 seconds (if control time is 15 ± 1.6 sec), a euglobulin lysis time of less than 120 minutes (normal time is greater than 120 minutes), and a fibrin degradation products assay of greater than 80 μg per milliliter by the staphylococcal clumping test, are positive confirmatory tests.[833] These tests measure the consumption of coagulation factors. As noted previously the platelet count may be normal, even though platelets are rapidly being removed from the circulation as evidenced by increased platelet turnover time; the same applies to fibrinogen (Fig. 29-6). Fibrinogen levels are usually increased postoperatively, in pregnancy, and with fever.[474,1855] Fibrin degradation products tests (Table 29-3) are based on the fact that in disseminated intravascular coagulation serum from clotted blood contains fibrin split products or fibrin-related antigen. These substances retain the antigenic properties of fibrinogen and will react with specific antifibrinogen serum. The fibrin split products or fibrin-related antigen products will cause clumping of staphylococci. When exposed to cold, protamine, or ethanol, the split products polymerize.[502,588,1038,1224,1304]

TREATMENT

As disseminated intravascular coagulation is triggered by a specific disease, therapy is first directed to that disease process.[890] Correction of low flow states, hypoxemia, and acidemia is of foremost importance.

Table 29-3. Soluble Complexes Detected by Various Laboratory Tests

Laboratory Test	Complexes Detected
Immunologic	
"Fi test"	Fibrin monomer + X, Y, D, E
Immunodiffusion ± electrophoresis	
Precipitin test	
Tanned red cell agglutination	
Staphylococcal clumping	Fibrin monomer + X, Y, D, E
Paracoagulation	Fibrin monomer + Fragment X
Protamine sulfate precipitation	+Fibrinogen
Ethanol gelation	
Cryoprecipitation	

SOURCE: D. Deykin.[502] Reprinted by permission from the *New England Journal of Medicine* 283:636–644, 1970.

There are different degrees of intensity of disseminated intravascular coagulation.[502] Mild forms or compensated forms, in which there is neither bleeding nor thrombosis but laboratory evidence of intravascular coagulation, usually are best managed indirectly by treatment of the underlying disease only.[1220,1223,1294]

HEPARIN

In acute disseminated intravascular coagulation improvement of the triggering disease may not be possible without concurrent therapy of the coagulation process.[426] In such severe cases, once the diagnosis is made, we give heparin by continuous intravenous infusion.[754,1302] Heparin binds to antithrombin, causing a change in its conformation that renders the antithrombin's reactive site more accessible to the active site of thrombin. This conformational change accelerates the interaction and therefore the inhibition of coagulation (Fig. 10-14).[1657,1658] In a similar fashion heparin inhibits factors X and XI and probably other factors as well.[2120] Heparin therapy is monitored by partial thromboplastin, clotting, or accelerated clotting times. Although the partial thromboplastin time is sensitive to heparin, it also responds to fibrin degradation products and of course to coagulation factors.[108,407,882,884,930,937,1445,1694]

Heparin therapy in sufficient dosage stops intravascular coagulation and allows plasma factor concentrations to recover. Usually the prothrombin time responds within one day and falls by at least five seconds.[402,839] The fibrin split products assay takes several days to return to normal. Fibrinogen rises in one to three days, and the euglobin lysis time is normalized within 72 hours. Platelet counts are not indicative of successful heparin therapy, since they may remain low, requiring platelet concentrates.

FACTOR REPLACEMENT

Once heparin therapy has been started, factor replacement may be initiated, although usually deficits are corrected by the body within three days. Administration of fibrinogen concentrates is not necessary and is hazardous due to the risk of transmitting hepatitis. Serum fibrinogen increases 25 mg per 100 ml (0.7 μmol/l) for each unit of fresh frozen plasma given.[402] Heparin therapy is continued until clotting parameters return to normal and until the disease process is partially under control. If the intravascular coagulation is severe, attempts to replace coagulation factors prior to heparinization may exacerbate the problem.

SPECIAL PROBLEMS

HEPARIN RESISTANCE

Antithrombin is deficient in 0.05 percent of the population.[1658] The presence of platelet factor 4 neutralizes heparin. These two abnormalities cause resistance to heparin therapy. The dose of heparin must be increased when either of these abnormalities is present.

LIVER DISEASE

In the presence of liver disease the normal mechanism of removal of fibrin, endotoxin, procoagulants, and activated clotting factors is malfunctioning. The diagnosis of disseminated intravascular coagulation then requires a platelet count of less than 50,000 per cubic millimeter (50 10⁹/l), a prothrombin time of more than 25 seconds, a fibrinogen level of 125 mg per 100 ml (3.7 μmol/l) or less, and a fibrin split products titer of 1:64 or greater.[1220]

FIBRINOLYSIS

Fibrinolysis in disseminated intravascular coagulation is secondary to intravascular clotting.[1627] Systemic primary fibrinolysis, if it occurs at all, is very rare. Selective fibrinogen destruction has been shown, however, in urokinase infusion[818] and may also occur with certain snake venom extracts. Local primary fibrinolysis caused by urokinase may occur after prostatic surgery.[666] Only in this unique circumstance do we infuse epsilon-aminocaproic acid into the bladder via irrigation or intravenously, since it is excreted through the kidney.[1750] Otherwise there is no indication for this drug in disseminated intravascular coagulation;[502,1596] its administration may precipitate massive thrombosis or arteritis.[316,1822]

PULMONARY HEMORRHAGE

The clinical presentation of pulmonary hemorrhage in disseminated intravascular coagulation is that of sudden dyspnea, wheezes, rales, hemoptysis, and tachypnea, with diffuse infiltrates appearing on chest x-ray films.[1572,1628,1629] If the underlying triggering disease is not apparent after the initial evaluation, heparin therapy cannot be delayed. Patients with disseminated intravascular coagulation have abnormal lung scans.[175] Platelet thrombi due to disseminated intravascular coagulation frequently contribute to or cause the adult respiratory distress syndrome and respiratory failure.[195,533,814,815,1452,1575,1692,2078]

In summary, heparin therapy usually will remedy the intravascular coagulation, but often the patient will not survive his underlying disease state.[427,1868] Mortality is not improved if the primary disease state is not treated or is irreversible upon initiation of heparin therapy.

30

Miscellaneous Special Problems

INTRACARDIAC SHUNTING

Intracardiac right-to-left shunting occurs in about 1–2 percent of patients in acute respiratory failure. An increase in pressure on the right side of the heart is caused by a worsening of pulmonary disease or the application of positive end-expiratory pressure. A persistent foramen ovale may then be reopened.[845] Analysis of dye curves for cardiac output measurements will provide the diagnosis. If dye is injected into the superior vena cava, detection may be difficult, as most of the blood shunted through the foramen ovale comes from the inferior vena cava. Treatment consists of lowering right heart pressure, if it is possible to do so safely.

100% OXYGEN AND THE ALVEOLAR-ARTERIAL OXYGEN TENSION GRADIENT

A significant increase in right-to-left shunting occurs after breathing pure oxygen.[386,1546,1881] Absorption atelectasis and pulmonary flow redistribution resulting from the vasodilating effect of an increase in oxygen tension in hypoxemic lung segments are possible mechanisms for this increase (Figs. 30-1 and 30-2).[612,2003,2055] Having critically ill patients breathe pure oxygen to measure the alveolar-arterial oxygen tension difference thus can be misleading and possibly detrimental. We estimate the required inspired oxygen concentration from the alveolar-arterial oxygen tension difference measured on 100% oxygen, because the hazard of breathing pure oxygen for short periods of time is unproved and the cost for using special oxygen-nitrogen mixtures would be huge. When the estimated required inspired oxygen concentration is being administered, we determine the adequacy of oxygen dosage by another set of arterial blood gas measurements.

CONTROL OF METABOLIC RATE

Oxygen consumption increases up to 500 percent during shivering (Fig. 12-18)[114] or hyperthermia. The cardiac output in patients in respiratory failure almost invariably cannot increase sufficiently to compensate for this increased demand, and the mixed venous oxygen content falls. The increased cardiac output may also cause less favorable distribution of pulmonary blood flow.[947,1545] Respiratory efforts against the ventilator due to

391

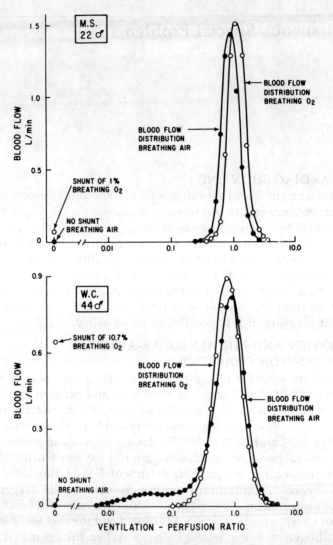

Figure 30-1. In a 22-year-old normal man (M.S.) breathing air the distributions of both ventilation and blood flow with respect to ventilation-perfusion ratio were approximately symmetric on a log scale and were very narrow. Ninety-five percent of the ventilation and blood flow falls in a ventilation-perfusion ratio of 0.3–2.1. Notice particularly that this man has no blood flow to unventilated areas (shunt), a typical finding in this age group. Pure oxygen breathing caused a small shift to the right of the main body of the distribution of blood flow. This was caused by the increased ventilation that usually occurs when normal subjects are given oxygen to breathe at rest. Since there was no significant change in cardiac output in this 22-year-old man, there was an increase in the overall ventilation-perfusion ratio. A small shunt of 1 percent developed.

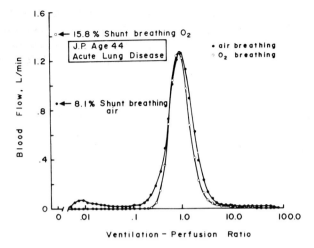

Figure 30-2. The use of 100% oxygen can result in an increase in the intrapulmonary right-to-left shunt in patients receiving intermittent positive pressure ventilation. The blood flow distributions of a 44-year-old man (*J.P.*) in acute respiratory failure following an automobile accident are shown. During controlled ventilation with air there is a considerable amount of blood flow to lung units with ventilation-perfusion ratios between 0.01 and 0.1 with a shunt of 8.1 percent. When the same patient is ventilated with 100% oxygen for 30 minutes, blood flow to lung units with low ventilation-perfusion ratios disappears, and the shunt increases to 15.8 percent. (From J. B. West, *Crit. Care Med.*[2055])

uncontrolled bodily activity cause a Valsalva effect with decreased venous return. All these factors cause oxygen delivery to the tissues to become inadequate.

Reduction of oxygen consumption must then be brought about immediately by reassurance, sedation, and, if necessary, paralysis to stop shivering. We reduce oxygen consumption and bodily activity with intravenous morphine, curare, or pancuronium; controlled ventilation; and normothermia; or, on extremely rare occasions, moderate hypothermia to 30°C.

ACUTE PANCREATITIS

Over half of all patients with acute pancreatitis develop some degree of pulmonary insufficiency during the course of their illness. The commonest

←───────────────────────────────

This small change can be contrasted with the dramatic alteration in the blood flow distribution shown in the 44-year-old man (*W.C.*). After 45 minutes of pure oxygen breathing the lefthand shoulder of the distribution to units of ventilation-perfusion ratios between 0.01 and 0.1 was abolished, and in its place a shunt of 10.7 percent of cardiac output appeared. (From P. D. Wagner, R. B. Laravuso, R. R. Uhl, and J. B. West, *J. Clin. Invest.*[2003])

finding is arterial hypoxemia and respiratory alkalemia, usually occurring in the first 48 hours of the attack of pancreatitis.[1589] Acute respiratory failure occurs in approximately 5 percent of all patients with acute pancreatitis.[1425] Respiratory failure contributes to or is the major cause of death in 60 percent of deaths related to acute pancreatitis.

ETIOLOGY

The etiology of respiratory failure in acute pancreatitis probably depends on the interaction of several factors. Patients with pancreatitis have abdominal pain and distention, which result in a reduction in vital capacity. Pleural effusions, which often are present, can also decrease vital capacity. There is an increase in the metabolic rate in patients with pancreatitis, which necessitates an increase in alveolar ventilation.[1011]

Patients who have acute pancreatitis have increased activity of serum phospholipase A. This lecithinase splits a fatty acid off the lecithin molecule.[696,2133] When phospholipase A extracted from cobra venom is infused into dogs, there is a rapid development of acute respiratory failure. Lungs of dogs infused with phospholiphase A for more than 10 hours have elevations of surface tension, suggesting that the phospholipase A causes damage to the surfactant system. A similar process may occur in the human with pancreatitis.[1352]

Compromised cardiac performance secondary to pancreatitis also may result in pulmonary insufficiency. During experimental pancreatitis a myocardial depressant factor is released into the circulation by the pancreas. This myocardial depressant factor is a peptide with a molecular weight of 800–1,000.[1137] In patients with pancreatitis compromised myocardial function can result in pulmonary edema.[945] Patients who develop respiratory failure with pancreatitis usually demonstrate an increase in pulmonary capillary wedge pressure, suggesting decreased myocardial performance even without preexisting cardiovascular disease.[837]

Direct pulmonary damage from other circulating enzymes released by the pancreas also has been postulated as the cause of respiratory failure but has not been adequately proved. The administration of excessive volumes of intravenous fluid to patients with acute pancreatitis may also further compromise pulmonary function.[1589]

MANAGEMENT

Optimal management of the patient with pancreatitis and respiratory failure requires an understanding of the factor or factors contributing to the pulmonary insufficiency in that particular patient. Most patients have a low serum albumin level and require large amounts of albumin replacement to maintain the intravascular volume. Since these patients also have markedly increased lung water, the combination of albumin and a diuretic is effective in lowering the intrapulmonary right-to-left shunt.[837,1011] Steroids do not improve the degree of intrapulmonary shunt. Positive end-expiratory pressure is needed frequently.

Thermodilution Swan-Ganz catheters have greatly improved the management of this type of patient. Myocardial performance can be judged accurately by analysis of the cardiac output and the pulmonary capillary wedge pressure and so can the use of colloid, diuretics, and vasopressor agents. When acute respiratory failure and pancreatitis are managed with the early institution of controlled ventilation, PEEP, albumin, diuretics, and careful monitoring of the cardiac output and pulmonary artery pressure, over two-thirds of patients survive.[837]

31

Pulmonary Oxygen Toxicity in
Respiratory Management

Oxygen can produce toxicity when given in a large dosage for prolonged periods of time.[675,941] Pulmonary symptoms in normal man are progressive. Substernal pain and an occasional cough progress to a burning pain on inspiration, an uncontrollable cough, and dyspnea.[111] Unfortunately these symptoms cannot be described by a sedated, acutely ill patient on controlled ventilation. The degree of toxicity is related to the tension but not to the percentage of oxygen inspired, as shown by toleration of 100% oxygen for two to four weeks at a tension of 250 mm Hg (33.3 kPa) during U.S. space flights.[403,521,547,864] The onset of symptoms is related to the duration of breathing oxygen at a given tension.[351,352,2048,2051]

PULMONARY CHANGES

Microscopic pulmonary changes of fibrin membranes, alveolar and septal thickening due to edema, cellular proliferation, and collagen deposition occur with prolonged controlled ventilation with increased oxygen but not with controlled ventilation with air.[1410]

The effect of 100% oxygen at 1 atmosphere on alveolar type II cells is one of an initial slight depletion of numbers during the first two days of exposure, followed by a marked, progressive (up to nine times) proliferation. Eventually, with continuous oxygen breathing, the type II cells line the alveoli (Fig. 31-1).[7,210,370,747,993,994,996,1638,1639] Their subcellular structure also changes. In rats, after 48 hours of 100% oxygen at 1 atmosphere, the number of lamellar bodies per cell is unchanged, but their size is smaller. After 96 hours of exposure the lamellar bodies are larger than in controls.[1250,1251] Mitochondria also are unchanged in size after 48 hours but enlarge after 96 hours. Mitochondrial cristae lose their perpendicular arrangement, and there is a loss of mitochondrial granules.[1249] This proliferation of type II cells is a nonspecific response to pulmonary injury, since it is seen also after oleic acid, nitrogen dioxide, and ozone injury.[209,451,602,1752,2123] It may represent a mechanism of pulmonary protection against oxidants. Treatment with an immunosuppressant, which blocks type II cell proliferation, also blocks the induction of oxygen tolerance.[1478]

The type I alveolar cell, the membranous pneumocyte, is more sensitive to destruction by oxygen than the type II cell; after four days of oxygen, more of the type I cells have become swollen.[747,993,1469] They later fragment.

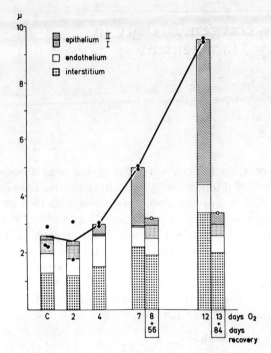

Figure 31-1.   Changes in alveolar type I and type II cells and interstitium with increasing duration of exposure to pure oxygen. Pure oxygen destroys alveolar type I cells and stimulates type II cell growth, as shown by changes in the air-blood tissue barrier thickness. *Closed circles* = monkeys sacrificed immediately after exposure; *open circles* = monkeys allowed to recover. C = control monkeys. (From Y. Kapanci, E. R. Weibel, H. P. Kaplan, and F. R. Robinson, *Lab. Invest.*[994] Copyright, 1969, U.S.-Canadian Division of the International Academy of Pathology through The Williams & Wilkins Company, by permission.)

After seven days the number of type I cells in lung is markedly depressed (Fig. 31-1).

The effect of oxygen on the pulmonary capillary endothelium is one of destruction with an increase in capillary permeability (Fig. 31-2).[748,993,994,1735,1971,2102] Capillary blood flow to the lung is maintained despite widespread endothelial destruction, leukocyte infiltration, and fibrin thrombi.[747,1728] Continued flow is promoted by capillary proliferation, repair, and vasodilation.[1554,1555,1573]

The alveolar septum thickens (Fig. 31-3), initially because of fluid transudation from damaged capillaries, then later because of type II cellular proliferation (Fig. 31-1). Septal cells also proliferate, and collagen fibers appear in the interstitium. This septal edema, cellular proliferation, and collagen deposition persist if oxygen is administered for several weeks.[1521,1821]

The alveolar macrophage is the principal cell responsible for destruction

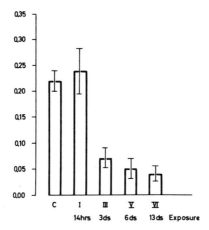

Figure 31-2.   Reduction in the total volume of endothelial cells per cubic centimeter of alveolar tissue (on the ordinate) with increasing duration of exposure to pure oxygen. C = control; *ds* = days. (From Y. Kapanci, R. Tosco, J. Eggermann, and V. E. Gould, *Chest*.[993])

of bacteria in alveoli.[735,756] One hundred percent oxygen depresses the ability of alveolar macrophages to kill phagocytosed *Klebsiella pneumoniae, Proteus mirabilis,* and *Staphylococcus aureus*.[936,1084] The degree of inhibition is to 60 percent of control values after 48 hours of oxygen and to 40 percent of control activity after 72 hours oxygen (Fig. 31-4).[641,642,846] The alveolar lining fluid is essential to the killing of bacteria, and its character is altered by oxygen.[1084] In alveolar macrophages oxygen is said to block pyruvate decarboxylation and the subsequent metabolism of pyruvate by the tricarboxylic acid cycle. An increase in the activity of the pentose pathway occurs. Glucose consumption rises.[641,1769,1784]

Pure oxygen probably causes marked depression of ciliary activity. Mucus flow is impaired.[1113,1166,1196,1228,2103,2104] Tracheitis, as noted by bronchoscopy, is apparent after only six hours of 100% oxygen.[644,1198,1444,1571,1624,1685,1808,1972]

EFFECTS ON THE PULMONARY CIRCULATION AND PULMONARY FUNCTION TESTS

In normal man, breathing of 100% oxygen for up to 12 hours causes no change in pulmonary artery pressure, cardiac index, or pulmonary extravascular water volume.[113,1978] Only a respiratory alkalemia without an increase in respiratory rate is noted. Human diffusing capacity decreases by 19 percent after 30–74 hours of 100% oxygen breathing at 1 atmosphere.[285]

In patients with irreversible brain damage, a progressive fall in arterial oxygen tension occurs after 41 hours in patients ventilated with 100% oxygen as compared with controls ventilated with air (Fig. 31-5).[97]

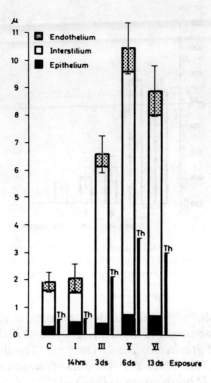

Figure 31-3. Changes in the thickness of the endothelium, interstitium, and epithelium in a patient with increasing duration of exposure to higher than 60 percent oxygen. The increase in thickness of the air-blood tissue barrier is due chiefly to interstitial edema. The harmonic mean (*Th*) is measured directly and represents the mean of different tissue thicknesses through which diffusion takes place. *C* = control case; cases *I*, *III*, *V*, and *VI* were exposed to higher than 60 percent oxygen for 14 hours, 3 days, 6 days, and 13 days respectively. (From Y. Kapanci, R. Tosco, J. Eggermann, and V. E. Gould, *Chest*.[993])

After open-heart surgery 100% oxygen by intermittent positive pressure ventilation for 15–48 hours (mean 24 hours) produces no change in physiologic shunt, deadspace, or compliance, in contrast to what happens under similar conditions in patients exposed to concentrations of oxygen limited to that required to prevent hypoxemia.[1786] Other studies also have shown a slight decrease or no change in compliance with 100% oxygen at 1 atmosphere for 48 hours.[285,773]

In normal man, breathing of oxygen for 10 hours causes a decrease in vital capacity (Fig. 31-6).[2092] Decreases in vital capacity that occur during the first seven hours of breathing 100% oxygen are said to be due to absorption atelectasis.[493,984] Such early decreases are prevented by addition of 5% nitrogen to the breathing mixture and by deep breathing.[271,272,548] Persons with low lung volumes are particularly subject to absorption atelectasis.

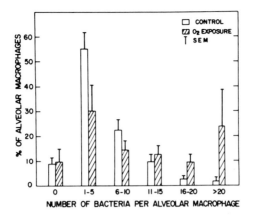

Figure 31-4. Phagocytosis of heat-killed *Staphylococcus albus* by alveolar macrophages obtained by lavage from four control and four oxygen-exposed rabbits. Phagocytosis was measured by the percentage of macrophages that contained the indicated numbers of bacteria. In the oxygen-exposed group there is an increased number of bacteria per cell, indicating an inability to digest phagocytosed bacteria. (From A. B. Fisher, S. Diamond, S. Mellen, and A. Zubrow, *Chest.*[642])

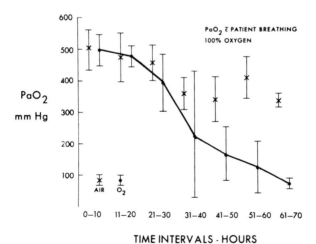

TIME INTERVALS - HOURS

Figure 31-5. Changes in arterial oxygen tension (Pa_{O_2}) during intermittent positive pressure ventilation with air or with 100% oxygen in patients with irreversible brain damage. Measurements of arterial oxygen tension were made with the patients normally ventilated with air, breathing 100% oxygen for 20 minutes. After 41 hours of continuous 100% oxygen the Pa_{O_2} is significantly decreased. No such reduction occurs in patients ventilated with air. (From R. E. Barber, J. Lee, and W. K. Hamilton.[97] Reprinted by permission from the *New England Journal of Medicine* 283:1478–1484, 1970.)

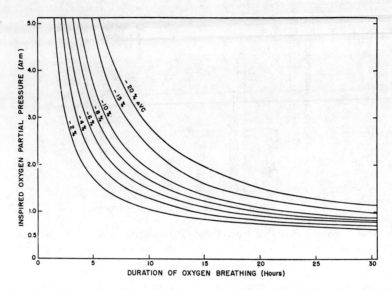

Figure 31-6. Pulmonary oxygen tolerance curves for normal men. The vital capacity of normal subjects decreases progressively in proportion to the duration of oxygen breathing and the partial pressure of inspired oxygen. (From J. M. Clark and C. J. Lambertsen, *Pharmacol. Rev.*[353] Copyright, 1971, The Williams & Wilkins Co., Baltimore, by permission.)

This absorption atelectasis is reversible and distinct from later pulmonary pathology.

EFFECTS ON OTHER SYSTEMS

Oxygen has a marked effect on the eye. Its role in retrolental fibroplasia in the premature infant is well known.[40,87] It also affects the cornea and lens in adults, causing tearing and edema.[1424,1866]

The effect of oxygen on red blood cells is one of destruction of a select population of the cells, possibly the oldest and the youngest. This destruction is associated with hydrogen peroxide accumulation in the red cell.[973,974,1102] There is a synergism between lead ingestion and susceptibility to oxygen toxicity.[980]

The effects of oxygen at 1 atmosphere on the central nervous system are limited to anorexia, nausea, and paresthesias. Such central effects are probably due to sympathetic stimulation, which is known to increase with pure oxygen breathing.[452,501,523,606,1092,1145,1809]

MECHANISMS

In oxygen toxicity enzymes containing sulfhydryl groups are inactivated by oxygen.[28,313,481,641,1299] Glutathione, when oxidized, attacks sulfhydryl groups; however, reduced glutathione may reactivate those groups. Inactivation of glyceraldehyde phosphate dehydrogenase interferes with glycolysis.[923] Mitochondrial electron transfer is impaired by decreased levels of ATP and succinic dehydrogenase activity.[313,461,1921] The integrity of lysosomes is lost as cells are disrupted, but this is probably not the primary defect caused by oxygen toxicity.[1896] Enzymes involved in the production and transport of surfactant are depressed.[713]

Exposure to toxic tensions of oxygen is found to increase the activity of several biochemical pathways. In rats exposed to 85% oxygen at 1 atmosphere, significant increases in glucose-6-phosphate dehydrogenase occur, reflecting an increase in activity of the hexosemonophosphate shunt.[79,1351,1923] Such an increase in the hexose shunt produces increased nicotinamide adenine dinucleotide phosphate, which can be used for oxidation-reduction, oxidation of glutathione, or repair of tissues.[450] Glutathione can help to protect the lung against oxidant damage, and its levels are increased after low doses of ozone for 24–48 hours.[336,943] During oxygen exposure alveolar type II cells, epithelial cells of terminal airways, and alveolar macrophages all exhibit increased pentose shunt activities.[450,1952]

The superoxide anion (O_2^-), a highly destructive oxidizing free radical, may be increased with exposure to pure oxygen.[28,202,373] Oxidation of lipids and enzymes occurs with exposure to high oxygen concentrations.[829,830,1651,2092] Superoxide dismutase (SOD), a metaloprotein, antagonizes the action of superoxide anion by catalyzing the reaction

$$O_2^- + O_2^- + 2H^+ \xrightarrow{\text{SOD}} O_2 + H_2O_2$$

SOD protects certain bacteria from the toxic effects of oxygen.[768,1266,1691] Rats made oxygen-tolerant have increased levels of SOD, and SOD levels fall as tolerance is lost (Fig. 31-7).[72,440] The role of superoxide dismutase in pulmonary oxygen toxicity in man is not yet clear.[1265]

A great number of conditions provide partial protection from oxygen toxicity. These include adrenalectomy, antioxidants,[1648] hypophysectomy, thyroidectomy, sympathectomy, anesthesia, prior injury by oleic acid,[1809,2093] previous hypoxemia,[223,225,226] and intermittent exposure to low tensions of oxygen.[93,353] None has proved useful in clinical practice, however. In some instances after lung injury the administration of 100% oxygen may actually worsen the pulmonary status; one such condition is paraquat poisoning.[72,1502] The use of intermittent positive pressure ventilation does not worsen oxygen toxicity.[232,493,2105]

Although pretreatment with hypoxic breathing mixtures for at least 120 hours does increase oxygen tolerance, systemic hypoxemia produced by right-to-left shunts, resulting in large alveolar-arterial oxygen tension differences, does not protect against pulmonary oxygen toxicity at 1 atmosphere (101 kPa).[50,1324] At hyperbaric pressures, (2.5 atmospheres [252.5 kPa] and 3.0 atmospheres [303 kPa] oxygen) systemic cyanosis does protect against pulmonary oxygen toxicity.[356,1609,1917,2090]

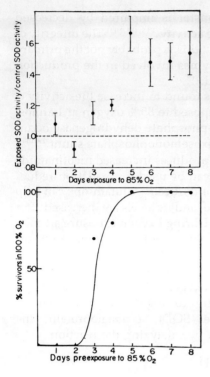

Figure 31-7. Increase in pulmonary superoxide dismutase (SOD) activity during the development of oxygen tolerance in rats. Rats were exposed to 85% oxygen and sacrificed 1–8 days later. SOD activity in the lungs is expressed as the ratio of SOD activity in exposed animals to SOD activity of control rats not exposed to oxygen. During the development of oxygen tolerance there is an increase in pulmonary SOD activity, which occurs between days 3 and 5 of oxygen exposure (*upper panel*). This increase in SOD activity correlates well with the survival of oxygen-tolerant rats placed in 100% oxygen (*lower panel*). We wonder if SOD will come to have a therapeutic use in intensive care units. (From J. D. Crapo and D. F. Tierney, *Am. J. Physiol.*[440])

SURFACTANT CHANGES

Oxygen toxicity does produce changes in the surfactant complex after endothelial capillary damage.[358,1357,1432,1433,1972] After 48 hours of oxygen there is decreased production of the proteins of the surface active complex. Synthesis of these proteins increases after 96 hours.[677] Lecithin synthesis from palmitic acid decreases. This correlates with inhibition of acylation activity; in addition oxygen inactivates N-methyltransferase which has a role in lecithin synthesis.[1356] Prior exposure to hypoxemia alters the composition of endobronchial lavage phospholipids upon oxygen exposure.[222] The importance of the surfactant-complex alteration is probably minor since the microscopic changes of pulmonary oxygen toxicity can be noted without any surfactant decrease.[1603]

TREATMENT

After pulmonary oxygen toxicity occurs, no specific therapy is yet available to counteract the effects. Steroids have no beneficial effect and may actually be harmful.[2091] Interruption of exposure to high oxygen tensions prolongs life but is not possible in an acutely ill patient. We monitor inspired oxygen concentrations at least every 6 hours and after every change in oxygen flow rate or ventilator settings. Inspired oxygen percentage is kept no higher than the level that produces an arterial oxygen tension of 70–100 mm Hg (9.3–13.3 kPa).[361,857,2109] If pulmonary disease is so severe as to require over 60% oxygen, a trial of positive end-expiratory pressure is instituted and maintained if the inspired oxygen concentration can thereby be reduced.

32

Extracorporeal Membrane Oxygenation

Certain patients in acute respiratory failure, despite maximum efforts of conventional ventilatory care, succumb due to hypoxemia and hypercapnia. Maximum conventional ventilatory care as defined here includes tracheal intubation, constant volume-controlled ventilation with 10–15 cm H_2O (1.0–1.5 kPa) positive end-expiratory pressure, diuresis, chest physical therapy, antibiotics, normothermia or mild hypothermia (32–37°C), sedation, paralysis, and increased oxygen.[1544,1615]

Despite the many hazards entailed, selected patients receiving maximum conventional care may benefit from prolonged extracorporeal oxygenation. This additional therapy provides time and better conditions for recovery of the diseased lungs.[749,883,1161]

Extracorporeal oxygenation was first proposed by Ludwig in 1865 [1197] and was made practicable by Gibbon in 1937.[705] The Mayo-Gibbon pump oxygenator as well as the rotating disc and bubble oxygenators have a limited duration of use because of blood element destruction.[1037] A device that permits prolonged extracorporeal oxygenation is the membrane oxygenator, described by Clowes [367] and developed by Bramson.[217]

SELECTION OF PATIENTS

Patients in acute respiratory failure with reversible lung disease, who are dying of hypoxemia despite maximal conventional ventilatory care, are candidates for the artificial lung. To determine whether lung disease is reversible or not may be difficult. The clinical history, x-ray appearances, and lung biopsy may be of help in making this determination. A decision to use the artificial lung is preferably made early in the course of the disease, before prolonged high inspired concentrations of oxygen and high inflation pressures have caused irreversible pulmonary damage.[880,1138]

Active bleeding is the only absolute contraindication to the use of the artificial lung. Recent surgery, trauma, or renal failure are not contraindications. The artificial lung has been used successfully under these circumstances. Patients with advanced chronic obstructive pulmonary disease, metastatic carcinoma, and major neurologic damage, including cerebral hypoxic death, must be excluded.[2126]

METHODS OF USE

The artificial lung must provide safe and efficient gaseous exchange while allowing the diseased lungs time to recover. There are a number of membrane oxygenators available.[542,2024] The Bramson membrane lung and Kolobow spiral membrane lung are most often used clinically for prolonged periods (Fig. 32-1).[1056,1058] The Landé-Edwards membrane lung has been used mostly during open-heart surgery.[1094] Large-bore cannulas are used to avoid high pressures in the oxygenator circuit.[1057]

Different routes of perfusion have been employed during extracorporeal oxygenation. The venovenous route is from the inferior vena cava via the femoral vein to the superior vena cava (Fig. 32-2). Maximum bypass flow with this route is 50 percent of the cardiac output. The route allows uniform distribution of arterial blood but requires two incisions and does not reduce pulmonary blood flow. Reduction of pulmonary flow is desirable, especially in the presence of right heart failure, to allow optimal conditions for healing of the diseased lungs. If balloon cannulas are used, and a double-lumen

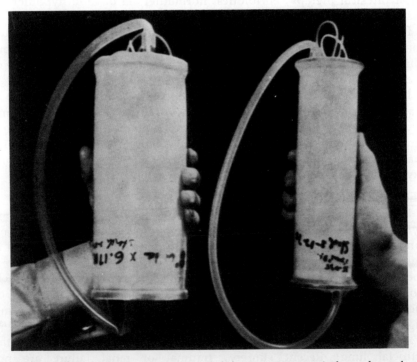

Figure 32-1. The spiral membrane lung. A 2½ square-meter spiral membrane lung is shown on the left and a 1.1 square-meter unit is on the right. The membrane envelope is wound around a spool and covered by a tight silicone rubber jacket. (From T. Kolobow and W. M. Zapol, *Adv. Cardiol.* 6:112–132, 1971.[1058] By permission.)

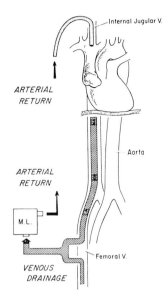

Figure 32-2. Diagram of the venovenous perfusion route for extracorporeal membrane oxygenation. Blood is removed from the femoral vein, pumped through the oxygenator, and reinfused into the internal jugular vein. M.L. = membrane lung. (From W. M. Zapol, R. Schneider, M. Snider, and M. Rie, *Int. Anesthesiol. Clin.*[2127] Copyright, 1976, Little, Brown and Company, by permission.)

cannula is placed in the superior vena cava, 80–90 percent of the cardiac output can be diverted to the oxygenator (Fig. 32-3). Extracorporeal flows of this magnitude are required if there is total pulmonary failure.[879]

The venoarterial route uses the femoral vessels only (Fig. 32-4). Maximum bypass flow can be increased to 60–70 percent of the cardiac output. Pulmonary blood flow is reduced, promoting recovery of the diseased lungs. The distribution of arterial blood is inappropriate, however, as most of it goes to the lower half of the body. The technique can be modified with return of some of the oxygenated blood via the superior vena cava to improve oxygen delivery to the head and heart (Fig. 32-5).[2127]

Venoarterial perfusion with aortic arch return allows for more appropriate distribution of oxygenated blood (Fig. 32-6). The arterial return cannula, which needs to have a very large bore, is inserted via the femoral artery into the aortic arch to the level of the left subclavian artery. Cerebral oxygenation is significantly improved.

Optimal heparinization is difficult to achieve. Heparin is used to prevent the thrombosis that inevitably occurs in the extracorporeal circuit, since no truly nonthrombogenic surface has yet been devised despite recent progress in this area.[881,1693,2124] On the other hand uncontrollable bleeding must be avoided. Maintaining the activated clotting time at 100–240 seconds provides the best results. (The activated clotting time is the time taken for 1.5 ml blood to clot in a prewarmed glass tube containing 12 mg of diatomaceous earth.[882,1961]) An average initial heparinization dose is 100 units per kilogram of body weight before cannulation and 5,000 units per liter added to the priming volume in the extracorporeal circuit. Further

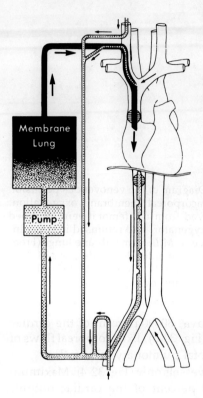

Figure 32-3. Cannulation system which is designed to bypass 80–90 percent of the cardiac output. The system employs balloon cannulas and a double-lumen tube, so that nearly all the venous return is pumped through the membrane lung. Blood flows in the direction of the arrows. (From J. D. Hill, R. Fallat, K. Cohn, R. Eberhart, L. Dontigny, M. L. Bramson, J. J. Osborn, and F. Gerbode, *Trans. Am. Soc. Artif. Intern. Organs.*[883])

heparin is administered by constant infusion to maintain the desired activated clotting time (Fig. 32-7).

During extracorporeal oxygenation ventilator settings should be changed to provide a 50% inspired oxygen concentration and peak airway pressures of 20–30 cm H₂O (2.0–3.0 kPa). Thus further pulmonary damage from oxygen toxicity and high inflation pressures is avoided. Positive end-expiratory pressure of 5 cm H₂O (0.5 kPa) should also be maintained and vigorous chest physical therapy with tracheal suctioning continued to promote healing of the damaged lung.

Pulmonary arterial pressure, pulmonary flow, and total pulmonary resistance are all significantly reduced by extracorporeal oxygenation employing the venoarterial route rather than the venovenous route (Fig. 32-8). An increase in arterial oxygen saturation occurs with both routes of perfusion (Fig. 32-9). These changes are important in providing favorable conditions for pulmonary healing.[880]

HEMATOLOGIC EFFECTS

The platelet count falls appreciably after the institution of extracorporeal oxygenation (Fig. 32-10).[192,494,1500,1544] The white cell count falls initially as well but promptly returns to normal. This phenomenon is also observed

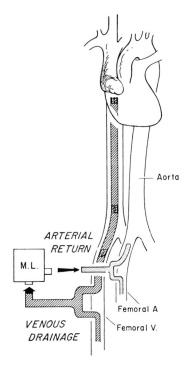

Figure 32-4. Diagram of the venoarterial perfusion route for extracorporeal membrane oxygenation. Blood is removed from the femoral vein, oxygenated, and reinfused via a cannula in the common femoral artery, which provides return to the distal aorta. *M.L.* = membrane lung. (From W. M. Zapol, R. Schneider, M. Snider, and M. Rie, *Int. Anesthesiol. Clin.*[2127] Copyright, 1976, Little, Brown and Company, by permission.)

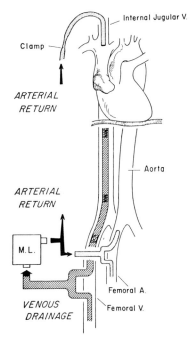

Figure 32-5. Diagrammatic representation of the venovenous arterial perfusion route for membrane oxygenation of patients in respiratory failure. Venous blood is removed from the femoral vein and passes through the membrane oxygenator. Blood is then perfused into both the internal jugular vein and the femoral artery. *M.L.* = membrane lung. (From W. M. Zapol, R. Schneider, M. Snider, and M. Rie, *Int. Anesthesiol. Clin.*[2127] Copyright, 1976, Little, Brown and Company, by permission.)

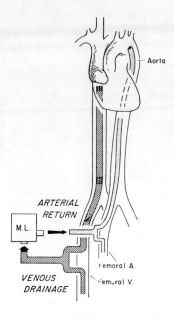

Figure 32-6. Diagram of the venoarterial arch perfusion route for extracorporeal membrane oxygenation. Blood is removed by the femoral vein cannula and reinfused via a cannula lying in the aortic arch. This cannula is inserted through the femoral artery. *M.L.* = membrane lung. (From Case records of the Massachusetts General Hospital.[307] Reprinted by permission from the *New England Journal of Medicine* 292:1174–1181, 1975.)

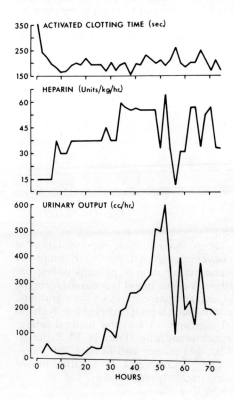

Figure 32-7. Heparin requirements during extracorporeal membrane oxygenation. This patient's requirement for heparin varied to a large degree, depending upon the urinary output. Despite these wide variations the clotting time could be maintained within the desired limits. (From J. D. Hill, L. Dontigny, M. R. deLeval, and C. H. Mielke, Jr., *Ann. Thorac. Surg.*[882] Copyright, 1974, Little, Brown and Company, by permission.)

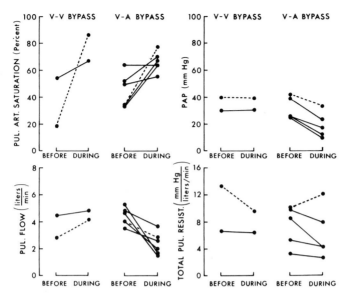

Figure 32-8. Comparison of venovenous (V-V) and venoarterial (V-A) perfusion routes on pulmonary dynamics before and during bypass. Each line represents a separate patient. Pulmonary artery saturation increased with either perfusion route. Pulmonary artery blood flow increased slightly in those patients having venovenous perfusion and decreased in those having venoarterial perfusion. Venoarterial perfusion decreased pulmonary artery pressure (PAP) but venovenous perfusion did not affect pulmonary artery pressure. Total pulmonary resistance fell in one patient during venovenous perfusion but was unchanged in another. Venoarterial perfusion resulted in a fall in pulmonary resistance in four of five patients. One patient demonstrated a rise in pulmonary resistance. This patient had severe disseminated intravascular coagulation. (From J. D. Hill, M. R. deLeval, R. J. Fallat, M. L. Bramson, R. C. Eberhart, H. D. Schulte, J. J. Osborn, R. Barber, and F. Gerbode, *J. Thorac. Cardiovasc. Surg.*[880])

during hemodialysis when margination of white cells occurs in the pulmonary circulation.[252,1931] Platelet function may also be disturbed, although this is difficult to assess (Fig. 32-11). A controversy exists regarding the fate of the platelets. A slow regeneration of platelets probably occurs, although it has been suggested that reversible sequestration of platelets in the liver may explain the rapid return of platelet count to pre-bypass levels that has been observed in splenectomized dogs.[494]

Disseminated intravascular coagulation can be another serious problem, as in all critically ill patients. Disseminated intravascular coagulation, however, is not caused by prolonged extracorporeal circulation per se.

Blood replacement to maintain a hematocrit of 30 percent and blood element replacement as indicated are both accomplished through a micropore filter, so that microaggregates found in stored blood can be removed (see Chapter 28).

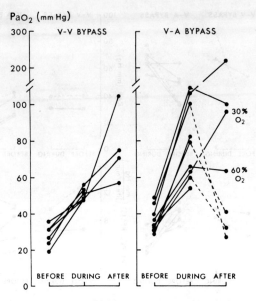

PaO$_2$ (mm Hg)

Figure 32-9.   Comparison of the effect of venoarterial (V-A) and venovenous (V-V) perfusion on arterial oxygen tension (Pa$_{O_2}$) before, during, and after extracorporeal membrane oxygenation in 51 patients. Three patients (*dotted lines*) had Pa$_{O_2}$ measured after stopping perfusion but prior to death. Those patients had shown no improvement of acute lung disease. The arterial oxygen tensions after perfusion were taken on an inspired oxygen concentration of 100% (except where indicated otherwise) to show the improvement in oxygenation after perfusion. (From J. D. Hill, M. R. deLeval, R. J. Fallat, M. L. Bramson, R. C. Eberhart, H. D. Schulte, J. J. Osborn, R. Barber, and F. Gerbode, *J. Thorac. Cardiovasc. Surg.*[880])

COMPLICATIONS

Serious hemorrhage occurs in 20 percent of patients on prolonged extracorporeal circulation. This is a result of the anticoagulation required to prevent thrombosis in the extracorporeal circuit and a reduction in platelet count with or without concomitant platelet dysfunction.[881]

Sepsis in patients undergoing prolonged extracorporeal oxygenation is a major hazard, as it is in all critically ill patients. In fact major sepsis, as in patients with extensive burns, is considered a relative contraindication to extracorporeal oxygenation. Frequent blood cultures may be required. These should be taken from the extracorporeal circuit rather than by repeated venipuncture. Specific antibiotics as determined by culture and sensitivity tests should be given in adequate dosages.[2127]

Patients with chronic obstructive pulmonary disease in acute respiratory failure are not candidates for the artificial lung. Some diseases are more destructive of lung parenchymal tissue than others. Diseases from which

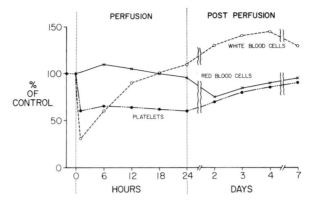

Figure 32-10. Effect of membrane oxygenation on blood cells. Initially there is a slight increase in red cells, which is probably related to release from the reticuloendothelial system. Following this rise there is a gradual fall in red cells, related to injury and hemolysis. In the postperfusion period the red cells continue to decline slightly as damaged red cells are removed from the circulation. There then follows gradual restoration of red cells. White blood cells decrease in number right after perfusion is begun. White blood cell numbers quickly return to normal, and a postperfusion leukocytosis, probably secondary to a release of immature cells, is not uncommon. Platelet counts fall immediately after perfusion is begun and remain depressed during perfusion. After perfusion the platelet count slowly returns to normal. (From E. C. Peirce II, *Mt. Sinai J. Med. N.Y.*[1500])

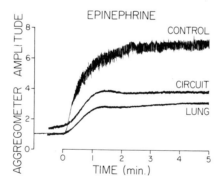

Figure 32-11. Effect of membrane oxygenation on platelet aggregation. Platelet aggregation was measured after six hours of use of an in vitro test perfusion circuit with epinephrine to induce aggregation. Nonperfused platelets (*control*) demonstrate rapid aggregation. Platelets in the circuit but not perfused through the lung (*circuit*) show less aggregation. Platelets perfused through the lung circuit (*lung*) show the least aggregation. (From E. C. Peirce II, *Mt. Sinai J. Med. N.Y.*[1500])

patients have recovered after having required extracorporeal oxygenation for survival include traumatic shock lung, fat embolization, pneumocystis carinii, Goodpasture's syndrome, influenza-A pneumonia, and gram-negative pneumonia. The high inspired concentrations of oxygen and high inflation pressures required to keep patients with extensive pulmonary disease alive are capable of themselves causing further irreversible pulmonary damage, especially if used for prolonged periods of time. Thus an early institution of extracorporeal oxygenation, to minimize lung damage before perfusion is started, has great advantages.[884]

FACILITIES REQUIRED

Patients who require extracorporeal oxygenation are critically ill and have other medical and surgical problems. Thus these patients should be cared for in specialized centers staffed by people familiar with the problems of caring for the critically ill.[1961] An example of a patient–artificial lung circuit is shown in Fig. 32-12.

Many measurements need be made to ensure optimal care. These include continuous pressure measurements in the arterial system and pulmonary artery, flows through the perfusion circuit, and repeated measurements of cardiac output. Arterial blood gas tensions must be

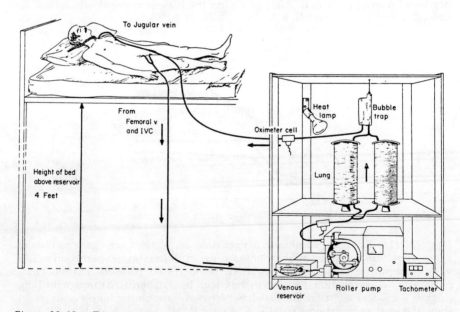

Figure 32-12. Diagrammatic representation of a patient undergoing venovenous perfusion for extracorporeal membrane oxygenation. Venous blood drains by gravity, hence the need for the 4-foot elevation of the bed. (From Case records of the Massachusetts General Hospital.[307] Reprinted by permission from the *New England Journal of Medicine* 292:1174–1181, 1975.)

measured frequently. Oxygen content measurements from the pulmonary artery, radial or temporal arteries, and across the oxygenator give an assessment of oxygen transport when correlated with cardiac output and flow measurements. The contribution of the patient's own lungs to gas exchange can then be calculated. If there is minimal transpulmonary gas exchange and the lungs are completely opacified on chest x-ray for more than 12 hours, the chances of recovery are remote.[2127]

WEANING

The timing and method of weaning from extracorporeal oxygenation present many problems. The effect on arterial oxygenation of reduction of flow rates through the oxygenator provides a means of determining whether a patient can be weaned from the oxygenator or not. Controlled ventilation, positive end-expiratory pressure, and an inspired oxygen concentration of 60% are continued. If an arterial oxygen tension of greater than 50 mm Hg (6.7 kPa) is maintained for a number of hours, perfusion probably can be stopped, provided the cardiovascular system remains stable. During weaning, flow through the extracorporeal circuit should not be stopped completely until the cannulas are removed; otherwise thrombosis may occur.[2127]

This mode of therapy, although fraught with many hazards, is indicated for patients in acute respiratory failure who are dying of hypoxemia and hypercapnia despite maximum conventional ventilatory support. Early institution of extracorporeal oxygenation, before irreversible pulmonary damage has occurred, is desirable.[2125] More than 150 patients have now undergone prolonged extracorporeal oxygenation, and there are more than 18 long-term survivors.[307]

Appendix

Normal Laboratory Values of Tests Frequently Used in Respiratory Care

Conversion of Traditional Units to SI Values for Normal Laboratory Tests

Constituent	Traditional		Multiplication Factor	SI	
	Units[a]	Range		Range	Units[a]
Arterial Blood Gases (Sea Level)					
Carbon dioxide tension, arterial blood	mm Hg	35–45	0.1333	4.7–6.0	kPa
Carbon dioxide content, serum	mEq/l	24–30	1.0	24–30	mmol/l
Oxygen tension, arterial blood					
breathing air	mm Hg	75–100	0.1333	10.0–13.3	kPa
breathing 100% oxygen	mm Hg	610–670	0.1333	81.1–89.1	kPa
Oxygen saturation, arterial blood					
breathing air	%	96–100	0.01	0.96–1.00	*
Oxygen content, arterial blood					
breathing air	—	—	—	18–21	ml/100 ml
breathing 100% oxygen	—	—	—	19.5–22.5	ml/100 ml
Alveolar-arterial oxygen tension gradient					
breathing air	mm Hg	2–30	0.1333	0.27–3.99	kPa
breathing 100% oxygen	mm Hg	10–60	0.1333	1.33–7.98	kPa
pH, arterial blood	—	7.35–7.45	1.0	7.35–7.45	*
Blood, Plasma, and Serum Tests					
Ammonia, blood	µg/100 ml	80–110	0.5872	47–65	µmol/l
Ascorbic acid, blood	mg/100 ml	0.4–1.5	56.77	23–85	µmol/l
Barbiturate, serum	mg/100 ml	0	43.06	0	µmol/l

Conversion of Traditional Units to SI Values for Normal Laboratory Tests (*Continued*)

Constituent	Traditional		Multiplication Factor	SI[a]	
	Units[a]	Range		Range	Units[a]
Bilirubin (direct), serum	mg/100 ml	≤0.4	17.10	≤7	μmol/l
Bilirubin (total), serum	mg/100 ml	≤0.7	17.10	≤12	μmol/l
Blood volume, patient	% body weight	8.5–9.0	9.4	80–85	ml/kg
Calcium, serum	mg/100 ml	8.5–10.5	0.2495	2.1–2.6	mmol/l
Carbon monoxide, blood	% saturation	0	0.01	0	*
Chloride, serum	mEq/l	100–106	1.0	100–106	mmol/l
Cholinesterase, serum	pH units	≥0.5/hour	1.0	≥0.5	arb. unit
Creatine phosphokinase, serum	mU/ml	5–35	0.01667	0.08–0.58	μmol.s^{-1}/l
Creatinine, serum	mg/100 ml	0.7–1.5	88.40	60–130	μmol/l
Cryoglobulins, serum	—	0	1.0	0	arb. unit
Diphenylhydantoin, serum	μg/ml	0	3.964	0	μmol/l
Glutethimide, serum	mg/100 ml	0	46.03	0	μmol/l
Ethanol, blood	%	0	217.1	0	mmol/l
Gastrin, serum	pg/ml	0–200	1.0	0–200	ng/l
Glucose, blood	mg/100 ml	70–100	0.05551	3.9–5.6	mmol/l
Iron, serum	μg/100 ml	50–150	0.1791	9.0–26.9	μmol/l
Lactic acid, blood	mEq/l	0.6–1.8	1.0	0.6–1.8	mmol/l
Lactic dehydrogenase, serum	mU/ml	60–120	0.01667	1.00–2.00	μmol.s^{-1}/l
Lead, blood	μg/100 ml	≤50	0.04826	≤2.4	μmol/l
Lipase, serum	units/ml	≤2	1.0	≤2	arb. unit
Cholesterol, serum	mg/100 ml	150–280	0.02586	3.9–7.2	mmol/l
Cholesterol esters, serum	% total	60–75	0.01	0.60–0.75	*
Phospholipids, serum	mg/100 ml	9–16	0.3229	2.9–5.2	mmol/l
Fatty acids, serum	mg/100 ml	190–420	0.01	1.9–4.2	g/l
Total lipids, serum	mg/100 ml	450–1,000	0.01	4.5–10.0	g/l
Triglycerides, serum	mg/100 ml	40–150	0.01	0.4–1.5	g/l
Magnesium, serum	mEq/l	1.5–2.5	0.5	0.8–1.3	mmol/l
Osmolality, serum	mOsm/kg	280–295	1.0	280–295	mmol/kg

Test	Units	Reference range	Factor	Reference range (SI)	Units (SI)
Phenylalanine, serum	mg/100 ml	0–2	60.54	0–120	μmol/l
Phosphatase (acid), serum	Sigma	0.13–0.63	278.4	36–175	nmol.s^{-1}/l
Phosphatase (alkaline), serum	Bodansky	2.0–4.5	0.08967	0.18–0.40	nmol.s^{-1}/l
Phosphorus (inorganic), serum	mg/100 ml	3.0–4.5	0.3229	1.0–1.5	mmol/l
Potassium, serum	mEq/l	3.5–5.0	1.0	3.5–5.0	mmol/l
Protein (total), serum	g/100 ml	6.0–8.0	10	60–80	g/l
Albumin, serum	g/100 ml	4.0–5.0	10	40–50	g/l
Globulin, serum	g/100 ml	2.0–3.0	10	20–30	g/l
Protein, mass fraction (paper electro-phoresis), serum Albumin	% total	50–60	0.01	0.50–0.60	*
Globulin α 1	% total	4.2–7.2	0.01	0.04–0.07	*
α 2	% total	6.8–12	0.01	0.07–0.12	*
β	% total	9.3–15	0.01	0.09–0.15	*
γ	% total	13–23	0.01	0.13–0.23	*
Pyruvic acid, blood	mEq/l	0–0.11	1,000	0–110	μmol/l
Quinidine, serum	μg/ml	0	3.082	0	μmol/l
Salicylate, plasma	mg/100 ml	0	0.07240	0	mmol/l
Sodium, serum	mEq/l	135–145	1.0	135–145	mmol/l
Sulfate, serum	mg/100 ml	0.5–1.5	104.1	50–150	μmol/l
Thyroxine, total, serum	μg/100 ml	4–11	12.87	50–140	nmol/l
Thyroxine, free, serum	ng/100 ml	0.8–2.4	0.01287	0.010–0.030	nmol/l
Transaminase (SGOT), serum	Karmen	10–40	0.008051	0.08–0.32	μmol.s^{-1}/l
Urea nitrogen, blood/serum	mg/100 ml	8–25	0.3569	2.9–8.9	mmol/l
Uric acid, serum	mg/100 ml	3.0–7.0	0.05948	0.18–0.42	mmol/l
Vitamin A, serum	μg/ml	0.15–0.6	3.491	0.5–2.1	μmol/l

Special Endocrine Tests

Test	Units	Reference range	Factor	Reference range (SI)	Units (SI)
Calcitonin, plasma	pg/ml	0	1.0	0	ng/l
Insulin, serum/plasma	μU/ml	6–26	1.0	6–26	10^{-2} int. unit/l
Parathyroid hormone, plasma	μl equiv.	<15	1.0	<15	arb. unit
Renin activity, plasma	ng/ml/hour	1.1 ± 0.8	0.2777	0.3 ± 0.2	ng.l^{-1}/s
Cortisol, plasma	μg/100 ml	5–25	0.02759	0.15–0.70	μmol/l
11-Deoxycortisol, plasma	μg/100 ml	>10	0.02903	>0.30	μmol/l
Triiodothyronine, serum	ng/100 ml	150–250	0.01538	2.3–3.9	nmol/l

Conversion of Traditional Units to SI Values for Normal Laboratory Tests (Continued)

Constituent	Traditional			SI[a]	
	Units[a]	Range	Multiplication Factor	Range	Units[a]
Hematologic Values					
Coagulation factor I (fibrinogen), plasma	g/100 ml	0.15–0.35	29.41	4.0–10.0	μmol/l
Coagulation factor II (prothrombin), plasma	%	70–130	0.01	0.70–1.30	*
Coagulation factor V, plasma	%	70–130	0.01	0.70–1.30	*
Coagulation factors VII–X, plasma	%	70–130	0.01	0.70–1.30	*
Coagulation factor X, plasma	%	70–130	0.01	0.70–1.30	*
Factor VIII, plasma	%	50–200	0.01	0.50–2.00	*
Factor IX, plasma	%	70–130	0.01	0.70–1.30	*
Factor XI, plasma	%	70–130	0.01	0.70–1.30	*
Factor XII (Hageman factor), plasma	%	70–130	0.01	0.70–1.30	*
Bleeding time, patient	min	3–8	0.06	0.18–0.48	ks
Clotting time, blood	min	<15	0.06	<0.90	ks
Prothrombin time, plasma	sec	control ± 2	1.0	control ± 2	arb. unit
Partial thromboplastin time (activated), plasma	sec	22–37	1.0	22–37	arb. unit
Blood clot lysis time, whole blood	lysis/no lysis	0	1.0	0	arb. unit
Euglobulin lysis time, plasma	lysis/no lysis	0	1.0	0	arb. unit
Fibrinogen split products (method 1), serum	dilution	neg. react. at > 1:2	1.0	2	arb. unit
Fibrinogen split products (method 2), serum	dilution	pos. react. at > 1:2	1.0	8	arb. unit
Plasminogen, plasma	casein units/ml	3–5	1.0	3–5	arb. unit

Test	Units	control ± 5		control ± 5	SI units
Thrombin time, plasma	sec		1.0		arb. unit
Hematocrit, blood	%	42–50	0.01	0.42–0.50	*
Hemoglobin (tetramer), blood	g/100 ml	13–16	0.1551	2.02–2.48	mmol/l
2,3-DPG, blood	—	—	—	4.2	μmol/l
			—	0.90	mol 2,3-DPG per mol Hb
Leukocyte count, blood	per mm³	4,800–10,800	10⁶	4.8–10.8	10⁹/l
Fetal hemoglobin, blood	%	<2	0.01	<0.02	*
Hemoglobin, methemoglobin, and sulfhemoglobin, blood	absent/present	0	1.0	0	arb. unit
Hemoglobin (monomer), serum	mg/100 ml	2–3	0.6205	1.2–1.9	μmol/l
Platelet count, blood	mm³	200,000–350,000	10⁶	200–350	10⁹/l
Clot retraction, plasma	%/2 hours	50–100	1.0	50–100	arb. unit
Platelet aggregation, plasma	—	Full response	1.0	1	arb. unit
Platelet factor 3, plasma	sec	33–57	1.0	33–57	sec
Reticulocyte count, blood	% red cells	0.5–1.5	0.01	0.005–0.015	*
Vitamin B12, serum	pg/ml	200–800	0.738	150–590	pmol/l
Cerebrospinal Fluid Values					
Bilirubin, cerebrospinal fluid	mg/100 ml	0	17.1	0	μmol/l
Cell count, cerebrospinal fluid	arb. unit	0–5	1.0	0–5	arb. unit
Chloride, cerebrospinal fluid	mEq/l	120–130	1.0	120–130	mmol/l
Albumin, cerebrospinal fluid	%	80	0.01	0.80	*
γ-Globulin, cerebrospinal fluid	%	10	0.01	0.10	*
Glucose, cerebrospinal fluid	mg/100 ml	50–75	0.05551	2.8–4.2	mmol/l
Pressure, cerebrospinal fluid	mm H₂O	70–180	1.0	70–180	arb. unit
Protein, cerebrospinal fluid	mg/100 ml	15–45	0.01	0.15–0.45	g/l

[a] SI = Système International. Units: *arb.* = arbitrary; *int.* = international. * = the relative amount of substance is expressed with a reference unit of 1. The retention should be defined in the test description. kPa = kilo Pascal. Mass measurements: *pg* = picogram; *ng* = nanogram; *μg* = microgram; *mg* = milligram; *g* = gram; *kg* = kilogram. Amounts of substance (molar) measurements: *pmol* = picomole; *nmol* = nanomole; *μmol* = micromole; *mmol* = millimole. Volume measurements: *μl* = microliter; *ml* = milliliter; *l* = liter. Time: *sec* = second; *ks* = kilosecond (1 kilosecond = 16.67 minutes). SOURCE: D. S. Young.[21,22] Reprinted and modified by permission from the *New England Journal of Medicine* 292:795–802, 1975.

References

1. Abel, F. L., Waldhausen, J. A., Daly, W. J., and Pearce, W. L.   Pulmonary blood volume in hemorrhagic shock in the dog and primate. *Am. J. Physiol.* 213:1072–1078, 1967.
2. Abel, R. M., Beck, C. H., Abbott, W. M., Ryan, J. A., Jr., Barnett, G. O., and Fischer, J. E.   Improved survival from acute renal failure after treatment with intravenous essential L-amino acids and glucose. *N. Engl. J. Med.* 288:695–699, 1973.
3. Abernathy, W. S.   Complete heart block caused by the Swan-Ganz catheter. *Chest* 65:349, 1974.
4. Abrams, J. S., Deane, R. S., and Davis, J. H.   Adverse effects of salt and water retention on pulmonary function in patients with multiple trauma. *J. Trauma* 13:788–798, 1973.
5. Abrams, L. D.   Physiotherapy in chest injuries. *Physiotherapy* 55:100–101, 1969.
6. Achauer, B. M., Allyn, P. A., Furnas, D. W., and Bartlett, R. H.   Pulmonary complications of burns: The major threat to the burn patient. *Ann. Surg.* 177:311–319, 1973.
7. Adamson, I. Y. R., Bowden, D. H., and Wyatt, J. P.   Oxygen poisoning in mice: Ultrastructural and surfactant studies during exposure and recovery. *Arch. Pathol.* 90:463–472, 1970.
8. Adar, R., Franklin, A., and Salzman, E. W.   Effect of furosemide on mesenteric blood flow in dogs. *Pharmacol. Res. Commun.* 6:485–491, 1974.
9. Adler, D. C., and Bryan-Brown, C. W.   Use of the axillary artery for intravascular monitoring. *Crit. Care Med.* 1:148–150, 1973.
10. Adler, J. L., and Finland, M.   Susceptibility of recent isolates of *Pseudomonas aeruginosa* to gentamicin, polymyxin, and five penicillins, with observations on the pyocin and immunotypes of the strains. *Appl. Microbiol.* 22:870–875, 1971.
11. Agress, C. M., Wegner, S., Forrester, J. S., Chatterjee, K., Parmley, W. W., and Swan, H. J. C.   An indirect method for evaluation of left ventricular function in acute myocardial infarction. *Circulation* 46:291–297, 1972.
12. Al Bazzaz, F. J., and Kazemi, H.   Arterial hypoxemia and distribution of pulmonary perfusion after uncomplicated myocardial infarction. *Am. Rev. Respir. Dis.* 106:721–728, 1972.
13. Albert, R. E., Alessandro, D., Lippmann, M., and Berger, J.   Long-term smoking in the donkey. Effect on tracheobronchial particle clearance. *Arch. Environ. Health* 22:12–19, 1971.
14. Albrecht, M., and Clowes, G. H. A., Jr.   The increase of circulatory requirements in the presence of inflammation. *Surgery* 56:158–171, 1964.
15. Albrecht, W. H., and Dryden, G. E.   Five-year experience with the develop-

ment of an individually clean anesthesia system. *Anesth. Analg.* (Cleve.) 53:24–28, 1974.

16. Alderete, J. F., Jeri, F. R., Richardson, E. P., Jr., Sament, S., Schwab, R. S., and Young, R. R. Irreversible coma: A clinical, electroencephalographic, and neuropathological study. *Trans. Am. Neurol. Assoc.* 93:16–20, 1968.

17. Alderman, E. L., Branzi, A., Sanders, W., Brown, B. W., and Harrison, D. C. Evaluation of pulse-contour method of determining stroke volume in man. *Circulation* 46:546–558, 1972.

18. Alexander, I. G. S. The ultrastructure of the pulmonary alveolar vessels in Mendelson's (acid pulmonary aspiration) syndrome. *Br. J. Anaesth.* 40:408–414, 1968.

19. Alexander, J. I., Horton, P. W., Millar, W. T., Parikh, R. K., and Spence, A. A. The effect of upper abdominal surgery on the relationship of airway closing point to end tidal position. *Clin. Sci.* 43:137–141, 1972.

20. Alexander, J. I., Horton, P. W., Millar, W. T., and Spence, A. A. Lung volume changes in relation to airways closure in the postoperative period: A possible mechanism of postoperative hypoxaemia. *Br. J. Anaesth.* 43:1196–1197, 1971.

21. Alexander, J. I., and Spence, A. A. Apparent improvement in postoperative lung volumes by using the Entonox apparatus. A preliminary report. *Br. J. Anaesth.* 45:90–92, 1973.

22. Alexander, J. I., Spence, A. A., Parikh, R. K., and Stuart, B. The role of airway closure in postoperative hypoxaemia. *Br. J. Anaesth.* 45:34–40, 1973.

23. Alexander, J. K., Amad, K. H., and Cole, V. W. Observations on some clinical features of extreme obesity, with particular reference to cardiorespiratory effects. *Am. J. Med.* 32:512–524, 1962.

24. Alexander, J. P., and Frazer, M. J. L. Meteorism during treatment of respiratory-distress syndrome by intermittent positive-pressure ventilation. *N. Engl. J. Med.* 288:1246, 1973.

25. Alexander, S. C., Marshall, B. E., and Agnoli, A. Cerebral blood flow in the goat with sustained hypocarbia. *Scand. J. Clin. Lab. Invest.* 22(Suppl. 102):VIIIC, 1968.

26. Allardyce, D. B., Yoshida, S. H., and Ashmore, P. G. The importance of microembolism in the pathogenesis of organ dysfunction caused by prolonged use of the pump oxygenator. *J. Thorac. Cardiovasc. Surg.* 52:706–715, 1966.

27. Allen, E. V. Thromboangiitis obliterans. Methods of diagnosis of chronic occlusive arterial lesions distal to the wrist with illustrative cases. *Am. J. Med. Sci.* 178:237–244, 1929.

28. Allen, J. E., Goodman, D. B. P., Besarab, A., and Rasmussen, H. Studies on the biochemical basis of oxygen toxicity. *Biochim. Biophys. Acta* 320:708–728, 1973.

29. Ambiavagar, M., Chalon, J., Sianghio, G., and Zargham, I. Diagnosis of Thermal Trauma to the Respiratory Tract. Scientific abstracts, First World Congress on Intensive Care, London, England, June 24–27, 1974. Pp. 80–81.

30. Ames, A., III, Wright, R. L., Kowada, M., Thurston, J. M., and Majno, G. Cerebral ischemia. II. The no-reflow phenomenon. *Am. J. Pathol.* 52:437–454, 1968.

31. Amplatz, K. Percutaneous arterial catheterization and its application. *Am. J. Roentgenol. Radium Ther. Nucl. Med.* 87:265–275, 1962.

32. Amplatz, K., and Harner, R. A new subclavian artery catheterization technic. Preliminary report. *Radiology* 78:963–966, 1962.

33. Andersen, E. W., and Navaratne, R. A. Tetanus: A review of 356 cases with special reference to treatment with mephenesin. *Acta Anaesthesiol. Scand.* 2:81–89, 1958.
34. Anderson, D. O., and Ferris, B. G., Jr. Role of tobacco smoking in the causation of chronic respiratory disease. *N. Engl. J. Med.* 267:787–794, 1962.
35. Anderson, S., Herbring, B. G., and Widman, B. Accidental profound hypothermia: Case report. *Br. J. Anaesth.* 42:653–655, 1970.
36. Anderson, W. H., Dossett, B. E., Jr., and Hamilton, G. L. Prevention of postoperative pulmonary complications: Use of isoproterenol and intermittent positive pressure breathing on inspiration. *J.A.M.A.* 186:763–766, 1963.
37. Andrus, C. H., and Morton, J. H. Rupture of the diaphragm after blunt trauma. *Am. J. Surg.* 119:686–693, 1970.
38. Anthonisen, N. R., Danson, J., Robertson, P. C., and Ross, W. R. D. Airway closure as a function of age. *Respir. Physiol.* 8:58–65, 1969.
39. Antkowiak, J. G., Cohen, M. L., and Kyllonen, A. S. Tracheoesophageal fistula following blunt trauma. *Arch. Surg.* 109:529–531, 1974.
40. Aranda, J. V., Saheb, N., Stern, L., and Avery, M. E. Arterial oxygen tension and retinal vasoconstriction in newborn infants. *Am. J. Dis. Child.* 122:189–194, 1971.
41. Archie, J. P., Jr., Fixler, D. E., Ullyot, D. J., Hoffman, J. I. E., Utley, J. R., and Carlson, E. L. Measurement of cardiac output with end organ trapping of radioactive microspheres. *J. Appl. Physiol.* 35:148–154, 1973.
42. Ardran, G. M., Kemp, F. H., and Wegelius, C. Swallowing defects after poliomyelitis. *Br. J. Radiol.* 30:169–189, 1957.
43. Arfors, K.-E., and Malmberg, P. Thermodilution measurement of cardiac output. A study in dogs comparing direct Fick with an automated thermodilution method (Fischer cardiac output computer). *Acta Chir. Scand.* 138:761–764, 1972.
44. Arieff, A. I., and Friedman, E. A. Coma following nonnarcotic drug overdosage: Management of 208 adult patients. *Am. J. Med. Sci.* 266:405–426, 1973.
45. Arms, R. A., Dines, D. E., and Tinstman, T. C. Aspiration pneumonia. *Chest* 65:136–139, 1974.
46. Aronow, W. S., Harris, C. N., Isbell, M. W., Rokaw, S. N., and Imparato, B. Effect of freeway travel on angina pectoris. *Ann. Intern. Med.* 77:669–676, 1972.
47. Artz, J. S., Vincour, B., and Sampliner, J. E. Application of a critical care monitoring program in the diagnosis and management of critically ill patients in a community hospital. *Crit. Care Med.* 2:42–43, 1974.
48. Asch, M. J., Feldman, R. J., Walker, H. L., Foley, F. D., Popp, R. L., Mason, A. D., and Pruitt, B. A. Systemic and pulmonary hemodynamic changes accompanying thermal injury. *Ann. Surg.* 178:218–221, 1973.
49. Asch, M. J., White, M. G., and Pruitt, B. A., Jr. Acid base changes associated with topical sulfamylon therapy. Retrospective study of 100 burn patients. *Ann. Surg.* 172:946–950, 1970.
50. Ashbaugh, D. G. Oxygen toxicity in normal and hypoxemic dogs. *J. Appl. Physiol.* 31:664–668, 1971.
51. Ashbaugh, D. G., Peters, G. N., Halgrimson, C. G., Owens, J. C., and Waddell, W. R. Chest trauma. Analysis of 685 patients. *Arch. Surg.* 95:546–555, 1967.
52. Ashbaugh, D. G., and Petty, T. L. The use of corticosteroids in the treatment of respiratory failure associated with massive fat embolism. *Surg. Gynecol. Obstet.* 123:493–500, 1966.

53. Ashbaugh, D. G., and Petty, T. L.   Sepsis complicating the acute respiratory distress syndrome. *Surg. Gynecol. Obstet.* 135:865–869, 1972.
54. Ashbaugh, D. G., and Petty, T. L.   Positive end-expiratory pressure. Physiology, indications, and contraindications. *J. Thorac. Cardiovasc. Surg.* 65:165–170, 1973.
55. Ashbaugh, D. G., Petty, T. L., Bigelow, D. B., Harris, T. M., and Waddell, W. R.   Continuous positive-pressure breathing (CPPB) in adult respiratory distress syndrome. *J. Thorac. Cardiovasc. Surg.* 57:31–41, 1969.
56. Ashbaugh, D. G., and Uzawa, T.   Respiratory and hemodynamic changes after injection of free fatty acids. *J. Surg. Res.* 8:417–423, 1968.
57. Ashcraft, K. W., and Leape, L. L.   *Candida* sepsis complicating parenteral feeding. *J.A.M.A.* 212:454–456, 1970.
58. Ashmore, P. G., Swank, R. L., Gallery, R., Ambrose, P., and Prichard, K. H.   Effect of Dacron wool filtration on the microembolic phenomenon in extracorporeal circulation. *J. Thorac. Cardiovasc. Surg.* 63:240–248, 1972.
59. Astrup, P., Hellung-Larsen, P., Kjeldsen, K., and Mellemgaard, K.   The effect of tobacco smoking on the dissociation curve of oxyhemoglobin. Investigations in patients with occlusive arterial diseases and in normal subjects. *Scand. J. Clin. Lab. Invest.* 18:450–457, 1966.
60. Atkinson, W. J.   Posture of the unconscious patient. *Lancet* 1:404–405, 1970.
61. Atsmon, A., and Blum, I.   Treatment of acute porphyria variegata with propranolol. *Lancet* 1:196–197, 1970.
62. Attar, S., Boyd, D., Layne, E., McLaughlin, J., Mansberger, A. R., and Cowley, R. A.   Alteration in coagulation and fibrinolytic mechanisms in acute trauma. *J. Trauma* 9:939–965, 1969.
63. Aub, J. C., Pittman, H., and Brues, A. M.   The pulmonary complications: A clinical description. *Ann. Surg.* 117:834–840, 1943.
64. Auchincloss, J. H., Jr., Cook, E., and Renzetti, A. D.   Clinical and physiological aspects of a case of obesity, polycythemia and alveolar hypoventilation. *J. Clin. Invest.* 34:1537–1545, 1955.
65. Auchincloss, J. H., Jr., Gilbert, R., and Mullison, E.   A new self-inflating tracheostomy cuff of silicone rubber for use in patients requiring mechanical aid to ventilation. *Am. Rev. Respir. Dis.* 97:706–709, 1968.
66. Auchincloss, J. H., Jr., Sipple, J., and Gilbert, R.   Effect of obesity on ventilatory adjustment to exercise. *J. Appl. Physiol.* 18:19–24, 1963.
67. Auerbach, O., Hammond, E. C., Garfinkel, L., and Benante, C.   Relation of smoking and age to emphysema. Whole-lung section study. *N. Engl. J. Med.* 286:853–857, 1972.
68. Auerbach, O., Stout, A. P., Hammond, E. C., and Garfinkel, L.   Changes in bronchial epithelium in relation to cigarette smoking and in relation to lung cancer. *N. Engl. J. Med.* 265:253–267, 1961.
69. Auerbach, O., Stout, A. P., Hammond, E. C., and Garfinkel, L.   Smoking habits and age in relation to pulmonary changes. Rupture of alveolar septums, fibrosis and thickening of walls of small arteries and arterioles. *N. Engl. J. Med.* 269:1045–1054, 1963.
70. Auld, P. A. M., Kevy, S. V., and Eley, R. C.   Poliomyelitis in children: Experiences with 956 cases in the 1955 Massachusetts epidemic. *N. Engl. J. Med.* 263:1093–1100, 1960.
71. Austen, W. G., Sanders, C. A., Averill, J. H., and Friedlich, A. L.   Ruptured papillary muscle. Report of a case with successful mitral valve replacement. *Circulation* 32:597–601, 1965.
72. Autor, A. P.   Reduction of paraquat toxicity by superoxide dismutase. *Life Sci.* 14:1309–1319, 1974.

73. Avery, E. E., Mörch, E. T., and Benson, D. W.   Critically crushed chests. A new method of treatment with continuous mechanical hyperventilation to produce alkalotic apnea and internal pneumatic stabilization. *J. Thorac. Surg.* 32:291–309, 1956.

74. Aviet, T. A., and Crawford, J. S.   Serum magnesium levels and magnesium trisilicate therapy in labour. *Br. J. Anaesth.* 43:183–184, 1971.

75. Awe, W. C., Fletcher, W. S., and Jacob, S. W.   The pathophysiology of aspiration pneumonitis. *Surgery* 60:232–238, 1966.

76. Ayers, L., and Tierney, D.   High Po_2 and the pentose pathway in rat lungs. *Clin. Res.* 19:190, 1971.

77. Ayres, S. M., and Mueller, H.   Hypoxemia, hypercapnia and cardiac arrhythmias: The importance of regional abnormalities of vascular distensibility. *Chest* 63:981–985, 1973.

78. Babington, P. C. B., Baker, A. B., and Johnston, H. H.   Retrograde spread of organisms from ventilator to patient via the expiratory limb. *Lancet* 1:61–62, 1971.

79. Bachmann, F.   Evidence for hypercoagulability in heat stroke. *J. Clin. Invest.* 46:1033, 1967.

80. Bachofen, H., Hobi, H. J., and Scherrer, M.   Alveolar-arterial N_2 gradients at rest and during exercise in healthy men of different ages. *J. Appl. Physiol.* 34:137–142, 1973.

81. Baek, S. M., Brown, R. S., and Shoemaker, W. C.   Early prediction of acute renal failure and recovery. II. Renal function response to furosemide. *Ann. Surg.* 178:605–608, 1973.

82. Baetjer, A. M.   Dehydration and recovery of free alveolar macrophages. *Arch. Environ. Health* 22:28–31, 1971.

83. Baker, L. E., and Denniston, J. C.   Noninvasive measurement of intrathoracic fluids. *Chest* 65(Suppl.):35S–37S, 1974.

84. Baker, N. H., and Messert, B.   Acute intermittent porphyria with central neurogenic hyperventilation. *Neurology* 17:559–566, 1967.

85. Baker, P. L., Pazell, J. A., and Peltier, L. F.   Free fatty acids, catecholamines and arterial hypoxia in patients with fat embolism. *J. Trauma* 11:1026–1030, 1971.

86. Bakhle, Y. S., and Vane, J. R.   Pharmacokinetic function of the pulmonary circulation. *Physiol. Rev.* 54:1007–1045, 1974.

87. Balentine, J. D.   Pathologic effects of exposure to high oxygen tensions. *N. Engl. J. Med.* 275:1038–1040, 1966.

88. Balint, J. A., Bondurant, S., and Kyriakides, E. C.   Lecithin biosynthesis in cigarette smoking dogs. *Arch. Intern. Med.* 127:740–747, 1971.

89. Balis, M. E., Gerber, L. I., Rappaport, E. S., and Neville, W. E.   Mechanisms of blood-vascular reactions of the primate lung to acute endotoxemia. *Exp. Mol. Pathol.* 21:123–137, 1974.

90. Bannister, W. K., and Sattilaro, A. J.   Vomiting and aspiration during anesthesia. *Anesthesiology* 23:251–264, 1962.

91. Bannister, W. K., Sattilaro, A. J., and Otis, R. D.   Therapeutic aspects of aspiration pneumonia in experimental animals. *Anesthesiology* 22:440–443, 1961.

92. Banyai, A. L.   Pulmonary disease due to endogenous aspiration. *Chest* 62:254, 1972.

93. Barach, A. L., Eckman, M., Oppenheimer, E. T., Rumsey, C., Jr., and Soroka, M.   Observations on methods of increasing resistance to oxygen poisoning and studies of accompanying physiological effects. *Am. J. Physiol.* 142:462–475, 1944.

94. Barakat, T., and MacPhee, I. W.   Bilirubin and alkaline phosphatase clearance from blood-plasma by perfusion through activated carbon. *Br. J. Surg.* 58:355–358, 1971.

95. Baratz, R. A., Philbin, D. M., and Patterson, R. W.   Plasma anti-diuretic hormone and urinary output during continuous positive-pressure breathing in dogs. *Anesthesiology* 34:510–513, 1971.

96. Barber, H.   The effects of trauma, direct and indirect, on the heart. *Q. J. Med.* 13:137–167, 1944.

97. Barber, R. E., Lee, J., and Hamilton, W. K.   Oxygen toxicity in man: A prospective study in patients with irreversible brain damage. *N. Engl. J. Med.* 283:1478–1484, 1970.

98. Barr, P.-O.   Percutaneous puncture of the radial artery with multi-purpose Teflon catheter for indwelling use. *Acta Physiol. Scand.* 51:343–347, 1961.

99. Barrera, F., Reidenberg, M. M., and Winters, W. L.   Pulmonary function in the obese patient. *Am. J. Med. Sci.* 254:785–796, 1967.

100. Barrera, F., Reidenberg, M. M., Winters, W. L., and Hungspreugs, S.   Ventilation-perfusion relationships in the obese patient. *J. Appl. Physiol.* 26:420–426, 1969.

101. Barry, D., Meyskens, F. L., and Becker, C. E.   Phenothiazine poisoning: A review of 48 cases. *Calif. Med.* 118:1–5, 1973.

102. Bartlett, G. R., and Barnet, H. N.   Changes in the phosphate compounds of the human red blood cell during blood bank storage. *J. Clin. Invest.* 39:56–61, 1960.

103. Bartlett, J. G., Gorbach, S. L., and Finegold, S. M.   The bacteriology of aspiration pneumonia. *Am. J. Med.* 56:202–207, 1974.

104. Bartlett, R. H., Gazzaniga, A. B., and Geraghty, T. R.   The yawn maneuver: Prevention and treatment of postoperative pulmonary complications. *Surg. Forum* 22:196–198, 1971.

105. Bartlett, R. H., Gazzaniga, A. B., and Geraghty, T. R.   Respiratory maneuvers to prevent postoperative pulmonary complications. A critical review. *J.A.M.A.* 224:1017–1021, 1973.

106. Bartlett, R. H., and Munster, A. M.   An improved technique for prolonged arterial cannulation. *N. Engl. J. Med.* 279:92–93, 1968.

107. Bartlett, R. H., and Yahia, C.   Management of septic chemical abortion with renal failure. Report of five consecutive cases with five survivors. *N. Engl. J. Med.* 281:747–753, 1969.

108. Basu, D., Gallus, A., Hirsh, J., and Cade, J.   A prospective study of the value of monitoring heparin treatment with the activated partial thromboplastin time. *N. Engl. J. Med.* 287:324–327, 1972.

109. Basu, H. K.   Fibrinolysis and abruptio placentae. *J. Obstet. Gynaecol. Br. Commonw.* 76:481–496, 1969.

110. Bates, D. V., and Christie, R. V.   Effects of Aging on Respiratory Function in Man. In G. E. W. Wolstenholme and M. P. Cameron (Eds.), *Ciba Foundation Colloquia on Aging.* Vol. I, *General Aspects.* Boston: Little, Brown, 1955. Pp. 58–65.

111. Bates, D. V., Macklem, P. T., and Christie, R. V.   *Respiratory Function in Disease.* Philadelphia: Saunders, 1971.

112. Baxter, C. R., Cook, W. A., and Shires, G. T.   Serum myocardial depressant factor of burn shock. *Surg. Forum* 17:1–2, 1966.

113. Baxter, W. D., and Levine, R. S.   An evaluation of intermittent positive pressure breathing in the prevention of postoperative pulmonary complications. *Arch. Surg.* 98:795–798, 1969.

114. Bay, J., Nunn, J. F., and Prys-Roberts, C. Factors influencing arterial Po_2 during recovery from anaesthesia. *Br. J. Anaesth.* 40:398–407, 1968.
115. Bayley, T., Clements, J. A., and Osbahr, A. J. Pulmonary and circulatory effects of fibrinopeptides. *Circ. Res.* 21:469–485, 1967.
116. Beach, T., Millen, E., and Grenvik, A. Hemodynamic response to discontinuance of mechanical ventilation. *Crit. Care Med.* 1:85–90, 1973.
117. Beal, D. D., Lambeth, J. T., and Conner, G. H. Follow-up studies on patients treated with steroids following pulmonary thermal and acrid smoke injury. *Laryngoscope* 78:396–403, 1968.
118. Beal, J. M., Payne, M. A., Gilder, H., Johnson, G., Jr., and Carver, W. L. Experience with administration of an intravenous fat emulsion to surgical patients. *Metabolism* 6:673–681, 1957.
119. Beall, A. C., Jr., Arbegast, N. R., Hallman, G. L., and Cooley, D. A. Complete transection of the thoracic aorta due to rapid deceleration. Report of successful repair in two cases. *Am. J. Surg.* 114:769–773, 1967.
120. Beall, A. C., Jr., Arbegast, N. R., Ripepi, A. C., Bricker, D. L., Diethrich, E. B., Hallman, G. L., Cooley, D. A., and De Bakey, M. E. Aortic laceration due to rapid deceleration: Surgical management. *Arch. Surg.* 98:595–601, 1969.
121. Beall, A. C., Jr., Diethrich, E. B., Crawford, W., Cooley, D. A., and DeBakey, M. E. Surgical management of penetrating cardiac injuries. *Am. J. Surg.* 112:686–692, 1966.
122. Beall, A. C., Jr., Ochsner, J. L., Morris, G. C., Cooley, D. A., and DeBakey, M. E. Penetrating wounds of the heart. *J. Trauma* 1:195–204, 1961.
123. Beall, A. C., Jr., Patrick, T. A., Okies, J. E., Bricker, D. L., and DeBakey, M. E. Penetrating wounds of the heart: Changing patterns of surgical management. *J. Trauma* 12:468–472, 1972.
124. Bean, J. W., and Beckman, D. L. Centrogenic pulmonary pathology in mechanical head injury. *J. Appl. Physiol.* 27:807–812, 1969.
125. Beard, R. R., and Grandstaff, N. Carbon monoxide and cerebral function. *Ann. N.Y. Acad. Sci.* 174:385–395, 1970.
126. Becker, A., Barak, S., Braun, E., and Meyers, M. P. The treatment of postoperative pulmonary atelectasis with intermittent positive pressure breathing. *Surg. Gynecol. Obstet.* 111:517–522, 1960.
127. Becker, D. P., Robert, C. M., Jr., Nelson, J. R., and Stern, W. E. An evaluation of the definition of cerebral death. *Neurology* 20:459–462, 1970.
128. Becker, J., and Schampi, B. The incidence of postoperative venous thrombosis of the legs: A comparative study on the prophylactic effect of dextran 70 and electric calf-muscle stimulation. *Acta Chir. Scand.* 139:357–367, 1973.
129. Becker, R. M., Smith, M. R., and Dobell, A. R. C. Effect of platelet inhibition on platelet phenomena in cardiopulmonary bypass in pigs. *Ann. Surg.* 179:52–57, 1974.
130. Beckman, D. L., and Bean, J. W. Pulmonary pressure-volume changes attending head injury. *J. Appl. Physiol.* 29:631–636, 1970.
131. Beckman, D. L., Bean, J. W., and Baslock, D. R. Sympathetic influence on lung compliance and surface forces in head injury. *J. Appl. Physiol.* 30:394–399, 1971.
132. Beckman, D. L., and Mason, K. F. Sympathetic influence on the dynamic lung compliance. *Life Sci.* [I] 12:42–48, 1973.
133. Beckman, D. L., Mason, K. F., and Bean, J. W. Sympathetic factors in acute pulmonary injury. *Chest* 65(Suppl.):38S–39S, 1974.
134. Bedell, G. N., Wilson, W. R., and Seebohm, P. M. Pulmonary function in obese persons. *J. Clin. Invest.* 37:1049–1060, 1958.

135. Bedford, R. F. Percutaneous radial-artery cannulation—Increased safety using Teflon catheters. *Anesthesiology* 42:219–222, 1975.
136. Bedford, R. F., and Wollman, H. Complications of percutaneous radial-artery cannulation: An objective prospective study. *Anesthesiology* 38:228–236, 1973.
137. Bedson, H. S. Coma due to meprobamate intoxication. Report of a case confirmed by chemical analysis. *Lancet* 1:288–290, 1959.
138. Beecher, H. K. Effect of laparotomy on lung volume. Demonstration of a new type of pulmonary collapse. *J. Clin. Invest.* 12:651–658, 1933.
139. Beecher, H. K. Resuscitation and sedation of patients with burns which include the airway. *Ann. Surg.* 117:825–833, 1943.
140. Beecher, H. K. A definition of irreversible coma: Report of the Ad Hoc Committee of the Harvard Medical School to examine the definition of brain death. *J.A.M.A.* 205:337–340, 1968.
141. Behrendt, D. M., and Austen, W. G. *Patient Care in Cardiac Surgery.* Boston: Little, Brown, 1972.
142. Bell, H., Stubbs, D., and Pugh, D. Reliability of central venous pressure as an indicator of left atrial pressure: Study in patients with mitral valve disease. *Chest* 59:169–173, 1971.
143. Bell, J. W. Treatment of post-catheterization arterial injuries: Use of survey plethysmography. *Ann. Surg.* 155:591–602, 1962.
144. Bell, M. L., Herman, A. H., Smith, E. E., Egdahl, R. H., and Rutenburg, A. M. Role of lysosomal instability in the development of refractory shock. *Surgery* 70:341–347, 1971.
145. Beller, F. K., and Douglas, G. W. Thrombocytopenia indicating gram-negative infection and endotoxemia. *Obstet. Gynecol.* 41:521–524, 1973.
146. Beller, F. K., Graeff, H., and Gorstein, F. Disseminated intravascular coagulation during the continuous infusion of endotoxin in rabbits: Morphologic and physiologic studies. *Am. J. Obstet. Gynecol.* 103:544–554, 1969.
147. Bellville, J. W. Gas Analysis. In J. W. Bellville and C. S. Weaver (Eds.), *Techniques in Clinical Physiology: A Survey of Measurements in Anesthesiology.* New York: Macmillan, 1969. Pp. 189–204.
148. Belsey, R. The pulmonary complications of oesophageal disease. *Br. J. Dis. Chest* 54:342–348, 1960.
149. Benchimol, A., Desser, K. B., and Wang, T. F. Doppler measurement of phasic continuous left ventricular blood flow velocity during ventricular arrhythmias. *Am. Heart J.* 88:742–747, 1974.
150. Bender, A. N., Ringel, S. P., Engel, W. K., Daniels, M. P., and Vogel, Z. Myasthenia gravis: A serum factor blocking acetylcholine receptors of the human neuromuscular junction. *Lancet* 1:607–608, 1975.
151. Bendixen, H. H., Bullwinkel, B., Hedley-Whyte, J., and Laver, M. B. Atelectasis and shunting during spontaneous ventilation in anesthetized patients. *Anesthesiology* 25:297–301, 1964.
152. Bendixen, H. H., Egbert, L. D., Hedley-Whyte, J., Laver, M. B., and Pontoppidan, H. *Respiratory Care.* St. Louis: Mosby, 1965.
153. Bendixen, H. H., Hedley-Whyte, J., and Laver, M. B. Impaired oxygenation in surgical patients during general anesthesia with controlled ventilation: A concept of atelectasis. *N. Engl. J. Med.* 269:991–996, 1963.
154. Bendixen, H. H., Osgood, P. F., Hall, K. V., and Laver, M. B. Dose-dependent differences in catecholamine action on heart and periphery. *J. Pharmacol. Exp. Ther.* 145:299–306, 1964.
155. Bendixen, H. H., Smith, G. M., and Mead, J. Pattern of ventilation in young adults. *J. Appl. Physiol.* 19:195–198, 1964.

156. Bennett, S. H., Geelhoed, G. W., Aaron, R̊. K., Solis, R. T., and Hoye, R. C.   Pulmonary injury resulting from perfusion with stored bank blood in the baboon and dog. *J. Surg. Res.* 13:295–306, 1972.

157. Bennett, S. H., Geelhoed, G. W., Gralnick, H. R., and Hoye, R. C.   Effects of autotransfusion on blood elements. *Am. J. Surg.* 125:273–279, 1973.

158. Bennett, S. H., Geelhoed, G. W., Terrill, R. E., and Hoye, R. C.   Pulmonary effects of autotransfused blood. A comparison of fresh autologous and stored blood with blood retrieved from the pleural cavity in an in situ lung perfusion model. *Am. J. Surg.* 125:696–702, 1973.

159. Benoit, P. R., Hampson, L. G., and Burgess, J. H.   Value of arterial hypoxemia in diagnosis of pulmonary fat embolism. *Ann. Surg.* 175:128–137, 1972.

160. Benzinger, M.   Tympanic thermometry in surgery and anesthesia. *J.A.M.A.* 209:1207–1211, 1969.

161. Bergentz, S.-E., Hansson, L. O., and Norbäck, B.   Surgical management of complications of arterial puncture. *Ann. Surg.* 164:1021–1026, 1966.

162. Bergofsky, E. H.   Pulmonary insufficiency after nonthoracic trauma: Shock lung. *Am. J. Med. Sci.* 264:92–101, 1972.

163. Berman, A., and Franklin, R. L.   Precipitation of acute intermittent porphyria by griseofulvin therapy. *J.A.M.A.* 192:1005–1007, 1965.

164. Bernatz, P. E., Burnside, A. F., Jr., and Clagett, O. T.   Problem of the ruptured diaphragm. *J.A.M.A.* 168:877–881, 1958.

165. Bernéus, B., Carlsten, A., Holmgren, A., and Seldinger, S. I.   Percutaneous catheterization of peripheral arteries as a method for blood sampling. *Scand. J. Clin. Lab. Invest.* 6:217–221, 1954.

166. Berry, P. R., and Pontoppidan, H.   Oxygen consumption and blood gas exchange during controlled and spontaneous ventilation in patients with respiratory failure. *Anesthesiology* 29:177–178, 1968.

167. Berson, W., and Adriani, J.   "Silent" regurgitation and aspiration during anesthesia. *Anesthesiology* 15:644–649, 1954.

168. Beth Israel Hospital.   *Manual of Applied Clinical Nutrition* (8th ed.). Boston, 1971. Pp. 40–45.

169. Beutler, E., Meul, A., and Wood, L. A.   Depletion and regeneration of 2,3-diphosphoglyceric acid in stored red blood cells. *Transfusion* 9:109–114, 1969.

170. Beutler, E., and Wood, L.   The in vivo regeneration of red cell 2,3 diphosphoglyceric acid (DPG) after transfusion of stored blood. *J. Lab. Clin. Med.* 74:300–304, 1969.

171. Bevan, P. G.   Post-operative pneumoperitoneum and pulmonary collapse. *Br. Med. J.* 2:609–613, 1961.

172. Biddle, T. L., Khanna, P. K., Yu, P. N., Hodges, M., and Shah, P. M.   Lung water in patients with acute myocardial infarction. *Circulation* 49:115–123, 1974.

173. Bieber, G. F.   Review of 353 cases of premature separation of the placenta. *Am. J. Obstet. Gynecol.* 65:257–268, 1953.

174. Binenbaum, S. Z., and Hochberg, H. M.   Non-invasive assessment of cardiovascular function by the QD index: Proven and potential uses. *Crit. Care Med.* 1:118, 1973.

175. Birmingham Eclampsia Study Group.   Intravascular coagulation and abnormal lung-scans in pre-eclampsia and eclampsia. *Lancet* 2:889–891, 1971.

176. Birtch, A. G., Zakheim, R. M., Jones, L. G., and Barger, A. C.   Redistribution of renal blood flow produced by furosemide and ethacrynic acid. *Circ. Res.* 21:869–878, 1967.

177. Bishop, J. M., and Cole, R. B. The effects of inspired oxygen concentration, age and body position upon the alveolar-arterial oxygen tension difference (A-aD) and physiological deadspace. *J. Physiol.* (Lond.) 162:60P–61P, 1962.

178. Bishop, L. H., Jr., Estes, E. H., Jr., and McIntosh, H. D. The electrocardiogram as a safeguard in pericardiocentesis. *J.A.M.A.* 162:264–265, 1956.

179. Björk, V. O., Grenvik, Å., Holmdahl, M.H:Son, and Westerholm, C.-J. Cardiac output and oxygen consumption during respirator treatment. *Acta Anaesthesiol. Scand.* [Suppl.] 15:158–160, 1964.

180. Blackburn, G. L., Flatt, J. P., Clowes, G. H. A., Jr., and O'Donnell, T. F. Peripheral intravenous feeding with isotonic amino acid solutions. *Am. J. Surg.* 125:447–454, 1973.

181. Blackburn, G. L., Flatt, J. P., Clowes, G. H. A., Jr., O'Donnell, T. F., and Hensle, T. E. Protein sparing therapy during periods of starvation with sepsis or trauma. *Ann. Surg.* 177:588–593, 1973.

182. Blackhall, M. I., Buckley, G. A., Roberts, D. V., Roberts, J. B., Thomas, B. H., and Wilson, A. Drug-induced neonatal myasthenia. *J. Obstet. Gynaecol. Br. Commonw.* 76:157–162, 1969.

183. Blair, E., Montgomery, A. V., and Swan, H. Posthypothermic circulatory failure. I. Physiologic observations on the circulation. *Circulation* 13:909–915, 1956.

184. Blair, E., Wise, A., and Mackay, A. G. Gram-negative bacteremic shock. Mechanisms and management. *J.A.M.A.* 207:333–336, 1969.

185. Blaisdell, F. W. Respiratory insufficiency syndrome: Clinical and pathological definition. *J. Trauma* 13:195–199, 1973.

186. Blaisdell, F. W., Lin, R. C., Jr., and Stallone, R. J. The mechanism of pulmonary damage following traumatic shock. *Surg. Gynecol. Obstet.* 130:15–22, 1970.

187. Blaisdell, F. W., and Schlobohm, R. M. The respiratory distress syndrome: A review. *Surgery* 74:251–262, 1973.

188. Blegvad, B. Caloric vestibular reaction in unconscious patients. *Arch. Otolaryngol.* 75:506–514, 1962.

189. Blitt, C. D., and Wright, W. A. An unusual complication of percutaneous internal jugular vein cannulation, puncture of an endotracheal tube cuff. *Anesthesiology* 40:306–307, 1974.

190. Blitt, C. D., Wright, W. A., Petty, W. C., and Webster, T. A. Central venous catheterization via the external jugular vein: A technique employing the J-wire. *J.A.M.A.* 229:817–818, 1974.

191. Bloch, M. Cerebral effects of rewarming following prolonged hypothermia: Significance for the management of severe cranio-cerebral injury and acute pyrexia. *Brain* 90:769–784, 1967.

192. Bloom, S., Zapol, W., Wonders, T., Berger, S., and Salzman, E. Platelet destruction during 24 hour membrane lung perfusion. *Trans. Am. Soc. Artif. Intern. Organs* 20:299–305, 1974.

193. Bluemle, L. W. Current status of chronic hemodialysis. *Am. J. Med.* 44:749–766, 1968.

194. Blumberg, A. G., Rosett, H. L., and Dobrow, A. Severe hypotensive reactions following meprobamate overdosage. *Ann. Intern. Med.* 51:607–612, 1959.

195. Bø, J., and Hognestad, J. Effects on the pulmonary circulation of suddenly induced intravascular aggregation of platelets. *Acta Physiol. Scand.* 85:523–531, 1972.

196. Bolton, P. M., Wood, C. B., Quartey-Papafio, J. B., and Blumgart, L. H. Blunt abdominal injury: A review of 59 consecutive cases undergoing surgery. *Br. J. Surg.* 60:657–663, 1973.

197. Bondurant, S. The alveolar lining: A method of extraction; The surface tension lowering effect of cigarette smoke. *J. Clin. Invest.* 39:973–974, 1960.

198. Bonnar, J. A review of obstetrical aspects of haemostasis. *Br. J. Haematol.* 25:274–275, 1973.

199. Bonnar, J., and Walsh, J. Prevention of thrombosis after pelvic surgery by British dextran 70. *Lancet* 1:614–616, 1972.

200. Booher, D., and Little, B. Current concepts: Vaginal hemorrhage in pregnancy. *N. Engl. J. Med.* 290:611–613, 1974.

201. Booth, D. J., Zuidema, G. D., and Cameron, J. L. Aspiration pneumonia: Pulmonary arteriography after experimental aspiration. *J. Surg. Res.* 12:48–52, 1972.

202. Bors, W., Saran, M., Lengfelder, E., Spöttl, R., and Michel, C. The relevance of the superoxide anion radical in biological systems. *Curr. Top. Radiat. Res.* 9:247–309, 1974.

203. Borst, H. G., Berglund, E., and McGregor, M. The effects of pharmacologic agents on the pulmonary circulation in the dog. Studies on epinephrine, nor-epinephrine, 5-hydroxytryptamine, acetylcholine, histamine, and aminophylline. *J. Clin. Invest.* 36:669–675, 1957.

204. Bosman, S. C. W., Terblanche, J., Saunders, S. J., Harrison, G. G., and Barnard, C. N. Cross-circulation between man and baboon. *Lancet* 2:583–585, 1968.

205. Bosomworth, P. P., and Hamelberg, W. Etiologic and therapeutic aspects of aspiration pneumonitis. *Surg. Forum* 13:158–159, 1962.

206. Boucher, J. K., Rudy, L. W., Jr., and Edmunds, L. H., Jr. Organ blood flow during pulsatile cardiopulmonary bypass. *J. Appl. Physiol.* 36:86–90, 1974.

207. Boutros, A. R. Effects of nitrous oxide–curare, ether and cyclopropane on postoperative respiratory adequacy. *Anesthesiology* 26:743–750, 1965.

208. Bove, A. A., and Lynch, P. R. Measurement of canine left ventricular performance by cineradiography of the heart. *J. Appl. Physiol.* 29:877–883, 1970.

209. Bowden, D. H., and Adamson, I. Y. R. Reparative changes following pulmonary cell injury: Ultrastructural, cytodynamic and surfactant studies in mice after oxygen exposure. *Arch. Pathol.* 92:279–283, 1971.

210. Bowden, D. H., Adamson, I. Y. R., and Wyatt, J. P. Reactions of the lung cells to a high concentration of oxygen. *Arch. Pathol.* 86:671–675, 1968.

211. Bowen, B. D. The relation of age and obesity to vital capacity. *Arch. Intern. Med.* 31:579–589, 1923.

212. Boyan, C. P. Cold or warmed blood for massive transfusions. *Ann. Surg.* 160:282–286, 1964.

213. Boyd, A. D., Engelman, R. M., Beaudet, R. L., Lackner, H., and Spencer, F. C. Disseminated intravascular coagulation following extracorporeal circulation. *J. Thorac. Cardiovasc. Surg.* 64:685–693, 1972.

214. Boyd, W. A. Blood pressure monitoring. *Int. Anesthesiol. Clin.* 3:417–433, 1965.

215. Boylan, J. W., and Antkowiak, D. E. Mechanism of diuresis during negative pressure breathing. *J. Appl. Physiol.* 14:116–120, 1959.

216. Brain, M. C. Microangiopathic hemolytic anemia. *N. Engl. J. Med.* 281:833–835, 1969.

217. Bramson, M. L., Osborn, J. J., Main, F. B., O'Brien, M. F., Wright, J. S., and Gerbode, F. A new disposable membrane oxygenator with integral heat exchange. *J. Thorac. Cardiovasc. Surg.* 50:391–400, 1965.

218. Brandenburg, R. O., McGoon, D. C., Campeau, L., and Giuliani, E. R. Traumatic rupture of the chordae tendineae of the tricuspid valve. Successful repair twenty-four years later. *Am. J. Cardiol.* 18:911–915, 1966.

219. Brandstater, B., and Muallem, M. Atelectasis following tracheal suctioning in infants. *Anesthesiology* 31:468–473, 1969.
220. Brantigan, J. W., Gott, V. L., Vestal, M. L., Fergusson, G. J., and Johnston, W. H. A nonthrombogenic diffusion membrane for continuous in vivo measurement of blood gases by mass spectrometry. *J. Appl. Physiol.* 28:375–377, 1970.
221. Brantley, W. M., Del Valle, R. A., and Schoenbucher, A. K. Pneumothorax, bilateral, spontaneous complicating pregnancy. *Am. J. Obstet. Gynecol.* 81:42–44, 1961.
222. Brashear, R. E., and Christian, J. C. Endobronchial lavage phospholipids and protein in rats protected from oxygen toxicity by hypoxia pretreatment. *Metabolism* 22:1345–1348, 1973.
223. Brashear, R. E., and DeAtley, R. E. Decreased pulmonary oxygen toxicity by pretreatment with hypoxia. *Arch. Environ. Health* 24:77–81, 1972.
224. Brashear, R. E., and Ross, J. C. Hemodynamic effects of elevated cerebrospinal fluid pressure: Alterations with adrenergic blockade. *J. Clin. Invest.* 49:1324–1333, 1970.
225. Brashear, R. E., Sharma, H. M., and DeAtley, R. E. Prolonged survival breathing oxygen at ambient pressure. *Am. Rev. Respir. Dis.* 108:701–704, 1973.
226. Brauer, R. W., Parrish, D. E., Way, R. O., Pratt, P. C., and Pessotti, R. L. Protection by altitude acclimatization against lung damage from exposure to oxygen at 825 mm Hg. *J. Appl. Physiol.* 28:474–481, 1970.
227. Braun, P., Weinstein, M., Farber, M., and Fineberg, H. An inventory of subjects for study by the Center for the Analysis of Health Practices. A working paper of the Harvard University Graduate School of Public Health, Boston, Mass., 1976.
228. Braunwald, E. Control of myocardial oxygen consumption. Physiologic and clinical considerations. *Am. J. Cardiol.* 27:416–432, 1971.
229. Braunwald, E., Covell, J. W., Maroko, P. R., and Ross, J., Jr. Effects of drugs and of counterpulsation on myocardial oxygen consumption. Observations on the ischemic heart. *Circulation* 39, 40(Suppl. IV):220–230, 1969.
230. Braunwald, E., and Swan, H. J. C. (Eds.). Cooperative study on cardiac catheterization. American Heart Association Monograph No. 20. *Circulation* 37, 38(Suppl. III):1–113, 1968.
231. Brennan, M. F., Goldman, M. H., O'Connell, R. C., Kundsin, R. B., and Moore, F. D. Prolonged parenteral alimentation: Candida growth and the prevention of candidemia by amphotericin instillation. *Ann. Surg.* 176:265–270, 1972.
232. Brewis, R. A. L. Oxygen toxicity during artificial ventilation. *Thorax* 24:656–666, 1969.
233. Brigham, K. L., and Snell, J. D., Jr. In vivo assessment of pulmonary vascular integrity in experimental pulmonary edema. *J. Clin. Invest.* 52:2041–2052, 1973.
234. Brigham, K. L., Woolverton, W. C., Blake, L. H., and Staub, N. C. Increased sheep lung vascular permeability caused by Pseudomonas bacteremia. *J. Clin. Invest.* 54:792–804, 1974.
235. Briscoe, C. E. A comparison of jugular and central venous pressure measurements during anaesthesia. *Br. J. Anaesth.* 45:173–177, 1973.
236. Brisman, R., Parks, L. C., and Benson, D. W. Pitfalls in the clinical use of central venous pressure. *Arch. Surg.* 95:902–907, 1967.
237. Bristow, G. K., and Kirk, B. W. Venous admixture and lung water in healthy subjects over 50 years of age. *J. Appl. Physiol.* 30:552–557, 1971.

238. Brochmann-Hanssen, E., and Svendsen, A. B. Separation and identification of barbiturates and some related compounds by means of gas-liquid chromatography. *J. Pharmaceut. Sci.* 51:318–321, 1962.

239. Broder, G., and Weil, M. H. Excess lactate: An index of reversibility of shock in human patients. *Science* 143:1457–1459, 1964.

240. Brodsky, J. B. A simple method to determine patency of the ulnar artery intraoperatively prior to radial-artery cannulation. *Anesthesiology* 42:626–627, 1975.

241. Brodsky, J. B., and Burgess, G. E., III. Pulmonary embolism with factor XI deficiency. *J.A.M.A.* 234:1156–1157, 1975.

242. Broennle, A. M., Tung, C. K., Buchman, B., and Laver, M. B. Oxyhemoglobin dissociation following massive transfusion in man. *Fed. Proc.* 29:329, 1970.

243. Bromage, P. R. Spirometry in assessment of analgesia after abdominal surgery: A method of comparing analgesic drugs. *Br. Med. J.* 2:589–593, 1955.

244. Brooks, D. K. Organ failure following surgery. *Adv. Surg.* 6:289–314, 1972.

245. Brown, A., Mohamed, S. D., Montgomery, R. D., Armitage, P., and Laurence, D. R. Value of a large dose of antitoxin in clinical tetanus. *Lancet* 2:227–230, 1960.

246. Brown, A. E., Sweeney, D. B., and Lumley, J. Percutaneous radial artery cannulation. *Anaesthesia* 24:532–536, 1969.

247. Brown, D. R., and Starek, P. Sodium nitroprusside–induced improvement in cardiac function in association with left ventricular dilatation. *Anesthesiology* 41:521–523, 1974.

248. Brown, H. I., Goldiner, P. L., and Turnbull, A. D. The reliability of the 25-gauge needle for arterial blood sampling. *Anesthesiology* 37:363, 1972.

249. Brown, H. W., and Plum, F. The neurologic basis of Cheyne-Stokes respiration. *Am. J. Med.* 30:849–860, 1961.

250. Browne, A. G. R., Pontoppidan, H., Chiang, H., Geffin, B., and Wilson, R. Physiological Criteria for Weaning Patients from Prolonged Artificial Ventilation. Abstracts of scientific papers, Annual Meeting of the American Society of Anesthesiologists, Boston, Mass., September 30–October 4, 1972. Pp. 69–70.

251. Browse, N. L., and Negus, D. Prevention of postoperative leg vein thrombosis by electrical muscle stimulation. An evaluation with 125 I-labelled fibrinogen. *Br. Med. J.* 3:615–618, 1970.

252. Brubaker, L. H., and Nolph, K. D. Mechanisms of recovery from neutropenia induced by hemodialysis. *Blood* 38:623–631, 1971.

253. Bruner, J. M. R. Hazards of electrical apparatus. *Anesthesiology* 28:396–425, 1967.

254. Bruner, J. M. R. Common abuses and failures of electrical equipment. *Anesth. Analg.* (Cleve.) 51:810–820, 1972.

255. Bruner, J. M. R., Aronow, S., and Cavicchi, R. V. Electrical incidents in a large hospital: A 42 month register. *J. Assoc. Adv. Med. Instrum.* 6:222–230, 1972.

256. Bryant, L. R. Intermittent positive-pressure breathing. *J. Thorac. Cardiovasc. Surg.* 59:303, 1970.

257. Bryant, L. R., Rams, J. J., Trinkle, J. K., and Malette, W. G. Present-day risk of thoracotomy in patients with compromised pulmonary function. *Arch. Surg.* 101:140–144, 1970.

258. Bryant, L. R., Trinkle, J. K., and Dubilier, L. Reappraisal of tracheal injury from cuffed tracheostomy tubes. Experiments in dogs. *J.A.M.A.* 215:625–628, 1971.

259. Bryant, L. R., Trinkle, J. K., Mobin-Uddin, K., Baker, J., and Griffen, W. O., Jr.   Bacterial colonization profile with tracheal intubation and mechanical ventilation. *Arch. Surg.* 104:647–651, 1972.

260. Buckberg, G., Cohn, J., and Darling, C.   *Escherichia coli* bacteremic shock in conscious baboons. *Ann. Surg.* 173:122–130, 1971.

261. Buckberg, G. D., Lipman, C. A., Hahn, J. A., Smith, M. J., and Hennessen, J. A.   Pulmonary changes following hemorrhagic shock and resuscitation in baboons. *J. Thorac. Cardiovasc. Surg.* 59:450–460, 1970.

262. Buckley, M. J., Craver, J. M., Gold, H. K., Mundth, E. D., Daggett, W. M., and Austen, W. G.   Intra-aortic balloon pump assist for cardiogenic shock after cardiopulmonary bypass. *Circulation* 47, 48(Suppl. III):90–94, 1973.

263. Buckley, M. J., Mundth, E. D., Daggett, W. M., DeSanctis, R. W., Sanders, C. A., and Austen, W. G.   Surgical therapy for early complications of myocardial infarction. *Surgery* 70:814–820, 1971.

264. Buist, A. S., and Ross, B. B.   Predicted values for closing volumes using a modified single breath nitrogen test. *Am. Rev. Respir. Dis.* 107:744–752, 1973.

265. Buist, A. S., Van Fleet, D. L., and Ross, B. B.   A comparison of conventional spirometric tests and the test of closing volume in an emphysema screening center. *Am. Rev. Respir. Dis.* 107:735–743, 1973.

266. Bunker, J. P.   Metabolic effects of blood transfusion. *Anesthesiology* 27:446–455, 1966.

267. Bunker, J. P., Bendixen, H. H., and Murphy, A. J.   Hemodynamic effects of intravenously administered sodium citrate. *N. Engl. J. Med.* 266:372–377, 1962.

268. Bunker, J. P., Bendixen, H. H., Sykes, M. K., Todd, D. P., and Surtees, A. D.   A comparison of ether anesthesia with thiopental–nitrous oxide–succinylcholine for upper abdominal surgery. *Anesthesiology* 20:745–752, 1959.

269. Bunn, H. F., May, M. H., Kocholaty, W. F., and Shields, C. E.   Hemoglobin function in stored blood. *J. Clin. Invest.* 48:311–321, 1969.

270. Burdon, D. W., and Whitby, J. L.   Contamination of hospital disinfectants with *Pseudomonas* species. *Br. Med. J.* 2:153–156, 1967.

271. Burger, E. J., Jr., and Macklem, P.   Airway closure: Demonstration by breathing 100% O_2 at low lung volumes and by N_2 washout. *J. Appl. Physiol.* 25:139–148, 1968.

272. Burger, E. J., Jr., and Mead, J.   Static properties of lungs after oxygen exposure. *J. Appl. Physiol.* 27:191–197, 1969.

273. Burgess, G. E., III.   Antacids for obstetric patients. *Am. J. Obstet. Gynecol.* 123:577–579, 1975.

274. Burke, J. F.   Early diagnosis of traumatic rupture of the bronchus. *J.A.M.A.* 181:682–686, 1962.

275. Burke, J. F., Pontoppidan, H., and Welch, C. E.   High output respiratory failure: An important cause of death ascribed to peritonitis or ileus. *Ann. Surg.* 158:581–592, 1963.

276. Burnham, S. C., Martin, W. E., and Cheney, F. W.   The effects of various tidal volumes on gas exchange in pulmonary edema. *Anesthesiology* 37:27–31, 1972.

277. Burton, J. D. K.   Effects of dry anaesthetic gases on the respiratory mucous membrane. *Lancet* 1:235–238, 1962.

278. Burwell, C. S., Robin, E. D., Whaley, R. D., and Bickelmann, A. G.   Extreme obesity associated with alveolar hypoventilation—A Pickwickian syndrome. *Am. J. Med.* 21:811–818, 1956.

279. Bushnell, L. S. An adverse effect of respiratory therapy. *Anesthesiology* 29:1085–1086, 1968.
280. Bushnell, L. S. Management of drug poisoning. *Clin. Trends Anesthesiol.* 1(4):1–4, 1971.
281. Bushnell, S. S. *Respiratory Intensive Care Nursing.* Boston: Little, Brown, 1973.
282. Cahill, J. M. Respiratory problems in surgical patients. *Am. J. Surg.* 116:362–368, 1968.
283. Cahill, J. M., and Byrne, J. J. Ventilatory mechanics in hypovolemic shock. *J. Appl. Physiol.* 19:679–682, 1964.
284. Cahill, J. M., Jouasset-Strieder, D., and Byrne, J. J. Lung function in shock. *Am. J. Surg.* 110:324–329, 1965.
285. Caldwell, P. R. B., Lee, W. L., Jr., Schildkraut, H. S., and Archibald, E. R. Changes in lung volume, diffusing capacity, and blood gases in men breathing oxygen. *J. Appl. Physiol.* 21:1477–1483, 1966.
286. Cameron, G. R., and De, S. N. Experimental pulmonary oedema of nervous origin. *J. Pathol. Bacteriol.* 61:375–387, 1949.
287. Cameron, J. L., Anderson, R. P., and Zuidema, G. D. Aspiration pneumonia. A clinical and experimental review. *J. Surg. Res.* 7:44–53, 1967.
288. Cameron, J. L., Caldini, P., Toung, J. K., and Zuidema, G. D. Aspiration pneumonia: Physiologic data following experimental aspiration. *Surgery* 72:238–245, 1972.
289. Cameron, J. L., Mitchell, W. H., and Zuidema, G. D. Aspiration pneumonia: Clinical outcome following documented aspiration. *Arch. Surg.* 106:49–52, 1973.
290. Cameron, J. L., Reynolds, J., and Zuidema, G. D. Aspiration in patients with tracheostomies. *Surg. Gynecol. Obstet.* 136:68–70, 1973.
291. Cameron, J. L., Sebor, J., Anderson, R. P., and Zuidema, G. D. Aspiration pneumonia. Results of treatment by positive-pressure ventilation in dogs. *J. Surg. Res.* 8:447–457, 1968.
292. Campbell, E. J. M., Nunn, J. F., and Peckett, B. U. A comparison of artificial ventilation and spontaneous respiration with particular reference to ventilation-bloodflow relationships. *Br. J. Anaesth.* 30:166–175, 1958.
293. Cantarovich, F., Galli, C., Benedetti, L., Chena, C., Castro, L., Correa, C., Loredo, J. P., Ferandez, J. C., Locatelli, A., and Tizado, J. High dose frusemide in established acute renal failure. *Br. Med. J.* 4:449–450, 1973.
294. Cara, M., Poisvert, M., Martinez-Almoyna, M., Caille, C., Cardinaud, J. P., Castaing, R., Winckler, C., Decreau, M., Echter, E., Milhaud, A., Nemitz, B., Franc, B., Haegel, A., Jolis, P., Hanote, P., Huguenard, P., Larcan, A., Lareng, L., Virenque, C., Menthonnex, P., Stieglitz, P., Rendoing, J., Seys, A., Serre, L., and Tonellot, J. L. Medical Emergency Mobile Services in France (S.A.M.U.). Scientific abstracts, First World Congress on Intensive Care, London, England, June 24–27, 1974. P. 2.
295. Carden, E., and Doll, W. A doppler flowmeter for detecting air and other emboli, incorporating a simple method of screening against interference. *Anesthesiology* 33:551–552, 1970.
296. Carey, J. S., Williamson, H., and Scott, C. R. Accuracy of cardiac output computers. *Ann. Surg.* 174:762–768, 1971.
297. Carlsson, C.-A., von Essen, C., and Löfgren, J. Factors affecting the clinical course of patients with severe head injuries. *J. Neurosurg.* 29:242–251, 1968.
298. Carr, D. J., and Crampton, R. F. Ethchlorvynol. *Br. Med. J.* 1:262, 1963.
299. Carrière, S., Thorburn, G. D., O'Morchoe, C. C. C., and Barger, A. C. Intra-

renal distribution of blood flow in dogs during hemorrhagic hypotension. *Circ. Res.* 19:167–179, 1966.

300. Carroll, R. G.   Evaluation of tracheal tube cuff designs. *Crit. Care Med.* 1:45–46, 1973.

301. Carroll, R. G., Hedden, M., and Safar, P.   Intratracheal cuffs: Performance characteristics. *Anesthesiology* 31:275–281, 1969.

302. Carroll, R. G., McGinnis, G. E., and Grenvik, A.   Performance characteristics of tracheal cuffs. *Int. Anesthesiol. Clin.* 12(3):111–141, 1974.

303. Carson, I. W., Moore, J., Balmer, J. P., Dundee, J. W., and McNabb, T. G.   Laryngeal competence with ketamine and other drugs. *Anesthesiology* 38:128–133, 1973.

304. Carter, A. E., and Eban, R.   The prevention of postoperative deep venous thrombosis with dextran 70. *Br. J. Surg.* 60:681–683, 1973.

305. Carter, J. H., Burdge, R., Powers, S. R., Jr., and Campbell, C. J.   An analysis of 17 fatal and 31 nonfatal injuries following an airplane crash. *J. Trauma* 13:346–353, 1973.

306. Case records of the Massachusetts General Hospital.   Barbiturate intoxication with progressive respiratory insufficiency. *N. Engl. J. Med.* 282:1087–1096, 1970.

307. Case records of the Massachusetts General Hospital.   Pneumonia treated by extracorporeal membrane oxygenation. *N. Engl. J. Med.* 292:1174–1181, 1975.

308. Cassell, E. J., Lebowitz, M., and McCarroll, J. R.   The relationship between air pollution, weather, and symptoms in an urban population. Clarification of conflicting findings. *Am. Rev. Respir. Dis.* 106:677–683, 1972.

309. Cavanagh, D., Rao, P. S., Sutton, D. M. C., Bhagat, B. D., and Bachmann, F.   Pathophysiology of endotoxin shock in the primate. *Am. J. Obstet. Gynecol.* 108:705–719, 1970.

310. Cawley, L. P., Douglass, R. C., and Schneider, C. L.   Nonfatal pulmonary amniotic embolism. *Obstet. Gynecol.* 14:615–620, 1959.

311. Chamberlain, D. A., Leinbach, R. C., Vassaux, C. E., Kastor, J. A., DeSanctis, R. W., and Sanders, C. A.   Sequential atrioventricular pacing in heart block complicating acute myocardial infarction. *N. Engl. J. Med.* 282:577–582, 1970.

312. Chan, J. C. M.   Acid-base problems after intravenous amino acids. *N. Engl. J. Med.* 288:420, 1973.

313. Chance, B., Jamieson, D., and Coles, H.   Energy-linked pyridine nucleotide reduction: Inhibitory effects of hyperbaric oxygen in vitro and in vivo. *Nature* 206:257–263, 1965.

314. Chaplin, H., Jr., Beutler, E., Collins, J. A., Giblett, E. R., and Polesky, H. F.   Current status of red-cell preservation and availability in relation to the developing national blood policy. *N. Engl. J. Med.* 291:68–75, 1974.

315. Chapman, R. L., Modell, J. H., Ruiz, B. C., Calderwood, H. W., Hood, C. I., and Graves, S. A.   Effect of continuous positive-pressure ventilation and steroids on aspiration of hydrochloric acid (pH 1.8) in dogs. *Anesth. Analg.* (Cleve.) 53:556–562, 1974.

316. Charytan, C., and Purtilo, D.   Glomerular capillary thrombosis and acute renal failure after epsilon amino-caproic acid therapy. *N. Engl. J. Med.* 280:1102–1104, 1969.

317. Chase, H. F.   The role of delayed gastric emptying time in the etiology of aspiration pneumonia. *Am. J. Obstet. Gynecol.* 56:673–679, 1948.

318. Chatterjee, K., Parmley, W. W., Ganz, W., Forrester, J., Walinsky, P., Crexells, C., and Swan, H. J. C.   Hemodynamic and metabolic responses to vasodilator therapy in acute myocardial infarction. *Circulation* 48:1183–1193, 1973.

319. Chatterjee, K., Parmley, W. W., Swan, H. J. C., Berman, G., Forrester, J., and Marcus, H. S. Beneficial effects of vasodilator agents in severe mitral regurgitation due to dysfunction of subvalvar apparatus. *Circulation* 48: 684–690, 1973.

320. Chazan, J. A., and Garella, S. Glutethimide intoxication. A prospective study of 70 patients treated conservatively without hemodialysis. *Arch. Intern. Med.* 128: 215–219, 1971.

321. Chen, H. I., and Chai, C. Y. Pulmonary edema and hemorrhage as a consequence of systemic vasoconstriction. *Am. J. Physiol.* 227: 144–151, 1974.

322. Chen, H. I., Sun, S. C., and Chai, C. Y. Pulmonary edema and hemorrhage resulting from cerebral compression. *Am. J. Physiol.* 224: 223–229, 1973.

323. Cheney, F. W., Jr., and Butler, J. The effects of ultrasonically-produced aerosols on airway resistance in man. *Anesthesiology* 29: 1099–1106, 1968.

324. Cheney, F. W., Jr., and Martin, W. E. Effects of continuous positive-pressure ventilation on gas exchange in acute pulmonary edema. *J. Appl. Physiol.* 30: 378–381, 1971.

325. Cherington, M. Botulism: Ten-year experience. *Arch. Neurol.* 30: 432–437, 1974.

326. Cherington, M., and Ginsberg, S. Type B botulism: Neurophysiologic studies. *Neurology* 21: 43–46, 1971.

327. Cherington, M., and Ryan, D. W. Botulism and guanidine. *N. Engl. J. Med.* 278: 931–933, 1968.

328. Cherniack, N. S., and Longobardo, G. S. Cheyne-Stokes breathing: An instability in physiologic control. *N. Engl. J. Med.* 288: 952–957, 1973.

329. Chester, E. H., Racz, I., Barlow, P. B., and Baum, G. L. Bronchodilator therapy: Comparison of acute response to three methods of administration. *Chest* 62: 394–399, 1972.

330. Chesterman, J. T., and Satsangi, P. N. Rupture of the trachea and bronchi by closed injury. *Thorax* 21: 21–27, 1966.

331. Chevalier, R. B., Krumholz, R. A., and Ross, J. C. Reaction of nonsmokers to carbon monoxide inhalation. Cardiopulmonary responses at rest and during exercise. *J.A.M.A.* 198: 1061–1064, 1966.

332. Chien, S., Chang, C., Dellenback, R. J., Vsami, S., and Gregorsen, M. I. Hemodynamic changes in endotoxin shock. *Am. J. Physiol.* 210: 1401–1410, 1966.

333. Chinard, F. P., and Enns, T. Transcapillary pulmonary exchange of water in the dog. *Am. J. Physiol.* 178: 197–202, 1954.

334. Chiodi, H., Dill, D. B., Consolazio, F., and Horvath, S. M. Respiratory and circulatory responses to acute carbon monoxide poisoning. *Am. J. Physiol.* 134: 683–693, 1941.

335. Chodoff, P., Margand, P. M. S., and Imbembo, A. L. Applied pulmonary physiology: Morbid obesity and pulmonary function. *Crit. Care Med.* 2: 123–128, 1974.

336. Chow, C. K., and Tappel, A. L. Activities of pentose shunt and glycolytic enzymes in lungs of ozone-exposed rats. *Arch. Environ. Health* 26: 205–208, 1973.

337. Christoforides, C., and Hedley-Whyte, J. Supersaturation of blood with O_2. *J. Appl. Physiol.* 26: 239–240, 1969.

338. Christoforides, C., and Hedley-Whyte, J. Effect of temperature and hemoglobin concentration on solubility of O_2 in blood. *J. Appl. Physiol.* 27: 592–596, 1969.

339. Christoforides, C., Laasberg, L. H., and Hedley-Whyte, J. Effect of temperature on solubility of O_2 in human plasma. *J. Appl. Physiol.* 26: 56–60, 1969.

340. Christy, J. H.   Treatment of gram-negative shock. *Am. J. Med.* 50: 77–88, 1971.

341. Chun, G. M. H., and Ellestad, M. H.   Perforation of the pulmonary artery by a Swan-Ganz catheter. *N. Engl. J. Med.* 284: 1041–1042, 1971.

342. Churchill, E. D., and McNeil, D.   The reduction in vital capacity following operation. *Surg. Gynecol. Obstet.* 44: 483–488, 1927.

343. Churchill-Davidson, H. C., and Richardson, A. T.   Myasthenic crisis. Therapeutic use of *d*-tubocurarine. *Lancet* 1: 1221–1224, 1957.

344. Civetta, J. M.   Pulmonary-artery-pressure determination: Electronic superior to manometric. *N. Engl. J. Med.* 285: 1145–1146, 1971.

345. Civetta, J. M.   The inverse relationship between cost and survival. *J. Surg. Res.* 14: 265–269, 1973.

346. Civetta, J. M.   Clinical Significance of Right-sided Venous and Arterial Pressure. Refresher course lectures, Annual Meeting of the American Society of Anesthesiologists, San Francisco, Calif., October 7–11, 1973. Lecture no. 106.

347. Civetta, J. M., and Gabel, J. C.   Flow directed–pulmonary artery catheterization in surgical patients: Indications and modifications of technic. *Ann. Surg.* 176: 753–756, 1972.

348. Civetta, J. M., Gabel, J. C., and Laver, M. B.   Disparate ventricular function in surgical patients. *Surg. Forum* 22: 136–139, 1971.

349. Claeys, D. W., Lockhart, C. H., and Hinckle, J. E.   The effects of translaryngeal block and Innovar on glottic competence. *Anesthesiology* 38: 485–486, 1973.

350. Clagett, G. P., and Salzman, E. W.   Prevention of venous thromboembolism in surgical patients. *N. Engl. J. Med.* 290: 93–96, 1974.

351. Clark, J. M.   Derivation of Pulmonary Oxygen Tolerance Curves Describing the Rate of Development of Pulmonary Oxygen Toxicity in Man. Ph.D. thesis, Graduate School of Arts and Sciences, University of Pennsylvania, 1970.

352. Clark, J. M., and Lambertsen, C. J.   Rate of development of pulmonary O_2 toxicity in man during O_2 breathing of 2.0 Ata. *J. Appl. Physiol.* 30: 739–752, 1971.

353. Clark, J. M., and Lambertsen, C. J.   Pulmonary oxygen toxicity: A review. *Pharmacol. Rev.* 23: 37–133, 1971.

354. Clark, J. S., Veasy, L. G., Jung, A. L., and Jenkins, J. L.   Automated Po_2, Pco_2, and pH monitoring of infants. *Comput. Biomed. Res.* 4: 262–274, 1971.

355. Clark, S. S., and Prudencio, R. F.   Lower urinary tract injuries associated with pelvic fractures. Diagnosis and treatment. *Surg. Clin. North Am.* 52: 183–201, 1972.

356. Clarke, G. M., Smith, G., Sandison, A. T., and Ledingham, I. McA.   Acute pulmonary oxygen toxicity in spontaneously breathing anesthetized dogs. *Am. J. Physiol.* 224: 248–255, 1973.

357. Clèdes, M. J., Bony, D., Emeriau, M., and Potaux, L.   Le poumon des péritonites. *Bordeaux Médical* 16: 1989–1998, 1972.

358. Clements, J. A.   Pulmonary surfactant. *Am. Rev. Respir. Dis.* 101: 984–990, 1970.

359. Clements, J. A.   Smoking and pulmonary surfactant. *N. Engl. J. Med.* 286: 261–262, 1972.

360. Clements, J. A.   Biochemical aspects of pulmonary function: Introductory remarks. *Fed. Proc.* 33: 2231, 1974.

361. Clements, J. A., and Fisher, H. K.   The oxygen dilemma. *N. Engl. J. Med.* 282: 976–977, 1970.

362. Clifton, J. S., and Parker, D.   Galvanic cell transducers for the in vivo measurement of oxygen tension. *Phys. Med. Biol.* 15: 183, 1970.

363. Cline, M. J., Melmon, K. L., Davis, W. C., and Williams, H. E. Mechanism of endotoxin interaction with human leukocytes. *Br. J. Haematol.* 15: 539–547, 1968.
364. Cloeron, S. E., and Lippert, T. H. Effect of plasma volume expanders in toxemia of pregnancy. *N. Engl. J. Med.* 287: 1356–1357, 1972.
365. Clowes, G. H. A., Jr. Pulmonary abnormalities in sepsis. *Surg. Clin. North Am.* 54: 993–1013, 1974.
366. Clowes, G. H. A., Jr., Farrington, G. H., Zuschneid, W., Cossette, G. R., and Saravis, C. Circulating factors in the etiology of pulmonary insufficiency and right heart failure accompanying severe sepsis (peritonitis). *Ann. Surg.* 171: 663–678, 1970.
367. Clowes, G. H. A., Jr., Hopkins, A. L., and Neville, W. E. An artificial lung dependent upon diffusion of oxygen and carbon dioxide through plastic membranes. *J. Thorac. Surg.* 32: 630–637, 1956.
368. Clowes, G. H. A., Jr., Vucinic, M., and Weidner, M. G. Circulatory and metabolic alterations associated with survival or death in peritonitis: Clinical analysis of 25 cases. *Ann. Surg.* 163: 866–885, 1966.
369. Clowes, G. H. A., Jr., Zuschneid, W., Turner, M., Blackburn, G., Rubin, J., Toala, P., and Green, G. Observations on the pathogenesis of the pneumonitis associated with severe infections in other parts of the body. *Ann. Surg.* 167: 630–650, 1968.
370. Coalson, J. J., Beller, J. J., and Greenfield, L. J. Effects of 100% oxygen ventilation on pulmonary ultrastructure and mechanics. *J. Pathol.* 104: 267–273, 1971.
371. Coalson, J. J., Hinshaw, L. B., and Guenter, C. A. The pulmonary ultrastructure in septic shock. *Exp. Mol. Pathol.* 12: 84–103, 1970.
372. Coates, E. O., Jr., Bower, G. C., and Reinstein, N. Chronic respiratory disease in postal employees. Epidemiological survey of a group employed in one building. *J.A.M.A.* 191: 161–166, 1965.
373. Cohen, G., and Heikkilar, R. E. The generation of hydrogen peroxide, superoxide radical and hydroxyl radical by 6-hydroxydopamine, dialuric acid, and related cytotoxic agents. *J. Biol. Chem.* 249: 2447–2452, 1974.
374. Cohen, M. M., and Silen, W. Effect of indomethacin on dog gastric mucosal permeability. *Surg. Forum* 22: 313–315, 1971.
375. Cohen, S. I., Deane, M., and Goldsmith, J. R. Carbon monoxide and survival from myocardial infarction. *Arch. Environ. Health* 19: 510–517, 1969.
376. Cohen, S. I., and Weintraub, R. M. A new application of counterpulsation. Safer laparotomy after recent myocardial infarction. *Arch. Surg.* 110: 116–117, 1975.
377. Cohn, H. E., Solit, R. W., Schatz, N. J., and Schlezinger, N. Surgical treatment in myasthenia gravis. A 27 year experience. *J. Thorac. Cardiovasc. Surg.* 68: 876–883, 1974.
378. Cohn, J. E., Carrol, D. G., Armstrong, B. W., Shepard, R. H., and Riley, R. L. Maximal diffusing capacity of the lung in normal male subjects of different ages. *J. Appl. Physiol.* 6: 588–597, 1954.
379. Cohn, J. E., and Donoso, H. D. Mechanical properties of lung in normal men over 60 years old. *J. Clin. Invest.* 42: 1406–1410, 1963.
380. Cohn, J. N. Blood pressure and cardiac performance. *Am. J. Med.* 55: 351–361, 1973.
381. Cohn, J. N. Vasodilator therapy for heart failure. The influence of impedance on left ventricular performance. *Circulation* 48: 5–8, 1973.
382. Cohn, J. N., Mathew, K. J., Franciosa, J. A., and Snow, J. A. Chronic

vasodilator therapy in the management of cardiogenic shock and intractable left ventricular failure. *Ann. Intern. Med.* 81: 777–780, 1974.

383. Cohn, J. N., Tristoni, F. E., and Khatri, I. M.   Studies in clinical shock and hypotension. VI. Relationship between left and right ventricular function. *J. Clin. Invest.* 48: 2008–2018, 1969.

384. Cohn, R.   Nonpenetrating wounds of the lungs and bronchi. *Surg. Clin. North Am.* 52: 585–595, 1972.

385. Cole, J. S., Martin, W. E., Cheung, P. W., and Johnson, C. C.   Clinical studies with a solid state fiberoptic oximeter. *Am. J. Cardiol.* 29: 383–388, 1972.

386. Cole, R. B., and Bishop, J. M.   Effect of varying inspired O_2 tension on alveolar-arterial O_2 tension difference in man. *J. Appl. Physiol.* 18: 1043–1048, 1963.

387. Colebatch, H. J. H., and Halmagyi, D. F. J.   Lung mechanics and resuscitation after fluid aspiration. *J. Appl. Physiol.* 16: 684–696, 1961.

388. Colebatch, H. J. H., and Halmagyi, D. F. J.   Reflex airway reaction to fluid aspiration. *J. Appl. Physiol.* 17: 787–794, 1962.

389. Colebatch, H. J. H., and Halmagyi, D. F. J.   Reflex pulmonary hypertension of fresh-water aspiration. *J. Appl. Physiol.* 18: 179–185, 1963.

390. Colebatch, H. J. H., Olsen, C. R., and Nadel, J. A.   Effect of histamine, serotonin, and acetylcholine on the peripheral airways. *J. Appl. Physiol.* 21: 217–226, 1966.

391. Coleman, B. D.   Septic shock in pregnancy. *Obstet. Gynecol.* 24: 895–902, 1964.

392. Coleman, S. S., and Anson, B. J.   Arterial patterns in the hand based upon a study of 650 specimens. *Surg. Gynecol. Obstet.* 113: 409–424, 1961.

393. Colgan, F. J., Barrow, R. E., and Fanning, G. L.   Constant positive-pressure breathing and cardiorespiratory function. *Anesthesiology* 34: 145–151, 1971.

394. Colgan, F. J., and Marocco, P. P.   The cardiorespiratory effects of constant and intermittent positive-pressure breathing. *Anesthesiology* 36: 444–448, 1972.

395. Collins, C. D., Drake, C. S., and Knowelden, J.   Chest complications after upper abdominal surgery: Their anticipation and prevention. *Br. Med. J.* 1: 401–406, 1968.

396. Collins, J. A., Braitberg, A., and Butcher, H. R., Jr.   Changes in lung and body weight and lung water content in rats treated for hemorrhage with various fluids. *Surgery* 73: 401–411, 1973.

397. Colman, R. W.   The effect of proteolytic enzymes on bovine factor V. I. Kinetics of activation and inactivation by bovine thrombin. *Biochemistry* 8: 1438–1445, 1969.

398. Colman, R. W.   Fragmentation of erythrocytes. *N. Engl. J. Med.* 280: 563, 1969.

399. Colman, R. W.   Hemorrhagic Disorders. IV. Intravascular Coagulation and Fibrinolysis. In W. S. Beck (Ed.), *Hematology.* Cambridge, Mass.: M.I.T. Press, 1973. Pp. 444–465.

400. Colman, R. W.   Formation of human plasma kinin. *N. Engl. J. Med.* 291: 509–515, 1974.

401. Colman, R. W., O'Donnell, T. F., Talamo, R. C., and Clowes, G. H. A., Jr.   Bradykinin formation in sepsis: Relation to hepatic dysfunction and hypotension. *Clin. Res.* 21: 596, 1973.

402. Colman, R. W., Robboy, S. J., and Minna, J. D.   Disseminated intravascular coagulation (DIC): An approach. *Am. J. Med.* 52: 679–689, 1972.

403. Comroe, J. H., Jr., Dripps, R. D., Dumke, P. R., and Deming, M.   Oxygen toxicity. The effect of inhalation of high concentrations of oxygen for 24 hours

on normal men at sea level and at a simulated altitude of 18,000 feet. *J.A.M.A.* 128: 710–717, 1945.

404. Comroe, J. H., Jr., Forster, R. E., II, Dubois, A. B., Briscoe, W. A., and Carlsen, E. *The Lung. Clinical Physiology and Pulmonary Function Tests* (2nd ed.). Chicago: Year Book, 1962.

405. Comstock, G. W., Brownlow, W. J., Stone, R. W., and Sartwell, P. E. Cigarette smoking and changes in respiratory findings. *Arch. Environ. Health* 21: 50–57, 1970.

406. Condon, R. E., Bomdeck, C. T., and Steigmann, F. Heterologous bovine liver perfusion therapy of acute hepatic failure. *Am. J. Surg.* 119: 147–153, 1970.

407. Congdon, J. E., Kardinal, C. G., and Wallin, J. D. Monitoring heparin therapy in hemodialysis. *J.A.M.A.* 226: 1529–1533, 1973.

408. Conn, J. H., Hardy, J. D., Fain, W. R., and Netterville, R. E. Thoracic trauma: Analysis of 1,022 cases. *J. Trauma* 3: 22–40, 1963.

409. Connell, R. S., Page, U. S., Bartley, T. D., Bigelow, J. C., and Webb, M. C. The effect on pulmonary ultrastructure of Dacron-wool filtration during cardiopulmonary bypass. *Ann. Thorac. Surg.* 15: 217–229, 1973.

410. Connell, R. S., and Swank, R. L. Pulmonary microembolism after blood transfusion: An electron microscopic study. *Ann. Surg.* 177: 40–50, 1973.

411. Conroy, J. P. Smoking and the anesthetic risk. *Anesth. Analg.* (Cleve.) 48: 388–400, 1969.

412. Cook, W. A. Experimental shock lung model. *J. Trauma* 8: 793–799, 1968.

413. Cooper, J. D., and Grillo, H. C. Experimental production and prevention of injury due to cuffed tracheal tubes. *Surg. Gynecol. Obstet.* 129: 1235–1241, 1969.

414. Cooper, J. D., and Grillo, H. C. Analysis of problems related to cuffs on intratracheal tubes. *Chest* 62(Suppl.): 21S–27S, 1972.

415. Cooper, J. D., and Malt, R. A. Meteorism produced by nasotracheal intubation and ventilatory assistance. *N. Engl. J. Med.* 287: 652–653, 1972.

416. Cooper, K. E., Hunter, A. R., and Keatinge, W. R. Accidental hypothermia. *Int. Anesthesiol. Clin.* 2: 999–1013, 1964.

417. Cooperman, L. H., and Price, H. L. Pulmonary edema in the operative and postoperative period: A review of 40 cases. *Ann. Surg.* 172: 883–891, 1970.

418. Cooperman, L. H., Warden, J. C., and Price, H. L. Splanchnic circulation during nitrous oxide anesthesia and hypocarbia in normal man. *Anesthesiology* 29: 254–258, 1968.

419. Cope, O. Management of the Cocoanut Grove burns at the Massachusetts General Hospital. *Ann. Surg.* 117: 801–802, 1943.

420. Cope, O., and Rhinelander, F. W. The problem of burn shock complicated by pulmonary damage. *Ann. Surg.* 117: 915–928, 1943.

421. Coppel, D. L., Balmer, H. G. R., and Dundee, J. W. Civil disturbance and anesthetic workload in the Royal Victoria Hospital, Belfast. II. The respiratory and intensive care unit. *Anesth. Analg.* (Cleve.) 52: 147–155, 1973.

422. Coppel, D. L., and Gray, R. C. Intensive Care and Disturbances. Scientific abstracts, First World Congress on Intensive Care, London, England, June 24–27, 1974. P. 4.

423. Corbett, J. L., Kerr, J. H., Prys-Roberts, C., Crampton Smith, A., and Spalding, J. M. K. Cardiovascular disturbances in severe tetanus due to overactivity of the sympathetic nervous system. *Anaesthesia* 24: 198–212, 1969.

424. Cornell, W. P., Braunwald, E., and Brockenbrough, E. C. Use of krypton[85] for the measurement of cardiac output by the single-injection indicator-dilution technique. *Circ. Res.* 9: 984–988, 1961.

425. Cornil, A., Thys, J. P., Ectors, M., and Degaute, J. P. Progress in the

Treatment of Tetanus. Scientific abstracts, First World Congress on Intensive Care, London, England, June 24–27, 1974. P. 115.

426. Corrigan, J. J., Jr., and Jordan, C. M. Heparin therapy in septicemia with disseminated intravascular coagulation. Effect on mortality and on correction of hemostatic defects. *N. Engl. J. Med.* 283:778–782, 1970.

427. Corrigan, J. J., Jr., Ray, W. L., and May, N. Changes in the blood coagulation system associated with septicemia. *N. Engl. J. Med.* 279:851–856, 1968.

428. Cotton, E. K., Abrams, G., Vanhoutte, J., and Burrington, J. Removal of aspirated foreign bodies by inhalation and postural drainage. A survey of 24 cases. *Clin. Pediatr.* (Phila.) 12:270–276, 1973.

429. Cottrell, J. E., and Siker, E. S. Preoperative intermittent positive pressure breathing therapy in patients with chronic obstructive lung disease: Effect on postoperative pulmonary complications. *Anesth. Analg.* (Cleve.) 52:258–262, 1973.

430. Cournand, A., Motley, H. L., Werko, L., and Richards, D. W. Physiological studies of the effects of intermittent positive pressure breathing on cardiac output in man. *Am. J. Physiol.* 152:162–174, 1948.

431. Cournand, A., and Ranges, H. A. Catheterization of the right auricle in man. *Proc. Soc. Exp. Biol. Med.* 46:462–466, 1941.

432. Couture, J., Picken, J., Trop, D., Ruff, F., Lousada, N., Houseley, E., and Bates, D. V. Airway closure in normal obese and anesthetized supine subjects. *Fed. Proc.* 29:269, 1970.

433. Cowger, M. L., and Labbe, R. F. Contraindications of biological-oxidation inhibitors in the treatment of porphyria. *Lancet* 1:88–89, 1965.

434. Craddock, P. R., Yawata, Y., VanSanten, L., Gilberstadt, S., Silvis, S., and Jacob, H. S. Acquired phagocyte dysfunction. A complication of the hypophosphatemia of parenteral hyperalimentation. *N. Engl. J. Med.* 290:1403–1407, 1974.

435. Craig, D. B., and McCarthy, D. S. Airway closure and lung volumes during breathing with maintained airway positive pressures. *Anesthesiology* 36:540–543, 1972.

436. Craig, R. G., Jones, R. A., Sproul, G. J., and Kinyon, G. E. The alternate methods of central venous system catheterization. *Am. Surg.* 34:131–134, 1968.

437. Crampton Smith, A., and Hahn, C. E. W. Electrodes for the measurement of oxygen and carbon dioxide tensions. *Br. J. Anaesth.* 41:731–741, 1969.

438. Crampton Smith, A., and Spalding, J. M. K. The treatment of severe tetanus. *Oxford Med. Sch. Gaz.* 22:21–26, 1970.

439. Crampton Smith, A., Spalding, J. M. K., and Watson, W. E. CO_2 as stimulus to spontaneous ventilation after prolonged artificial ventilation. *J. Physiol.* 160:32–39, 1962.

440. Crapo, J. D., and Tierney, D. F. Superoxide dismutase and pulmonary oxygen toxicity. *Am. J. Physiol.* 226:1401–1407, 1974.

441. Crawford, H., and Mollison, P. L. Reversal of electrolyte changes in stored red cells after transfusion. *J. Physiol.* 129:639–647, 1955.

442. Crawford, J. S. Some aspects of obstetric anaesthesia. *Br. J. Anaesth.* 28:201–208, 1956.

443. Crawford, J. S. The anaesthetist's contribution to maternal mortality. *Br. J. Anaesth.* 42:70–73, 1970.

444. Crawford, J. S. Maternal mortality associated with anaesthesia. *Lancet* 2:918–919, 1972.

445. Crawford, J. S. *Principles and Practice of Obstetric Anaesthesia.* Oxford: Blackwell, 1972. Pp. 193–197.

446. Credle, W. F., Jr., Smiddy, J. F., Shea, D. W., and Elliott, R. C. Fiberoptic bronchoscopy in acute respiratory failure in the adult. *N. Engl. J. Med.* 288: 49–50, 1973.

447. Creech, O., Jr., and Pearce, C. W. Stab and gunshot wounds of the chest. *Am. J. Surg.* 105: 469–483, 1963.

448. Crexells, C., Bourassa, M. G., and Biron, P. Effects of dopamine on myocardial metabolism in patients with ischaemic heart disease. *Cardiovasc. Res.* 7: 438–445, 1973.

449. Crexells, C., Chatterjee, K., Forrester, J. S., Dikshit, K., and Swan, H. J. C. Optimal level of filling pressure in the left side of the heart in acute myocardial infarction. *N. Engl. J. Med.* 289: 1263–1266, 1973.

450. Cross, C. E. The granular type II pneumonocyte and lung antioxidant defense. *Ann. Intern. Med.* 80: 409–411, 1974.

451. Cross, C. E., DeLucia, A. J., and Mustafa, M. G. Low-level ozone exposure enhances lung antioxidant defense systems in rodents and primates. *Clin. Res.* 22: 199A, 1974.

452. Cross, M. H., and Houlihan, R. T. Sympathoadrenomedullary response of the rat to high oxygen exposures. *J. Appl. Physiol.* 27: 523–527, 1969.

453. Cuello, L., Vazquez, E., Rios, R., and Raffucci, F. L. Autologous blood transfusion in thoracic and cardiovascular surgery. *Surgery* 62: 814–818, 1967.

454. Cuevas, P., de la Maza, L. M., Gilbert, J., and Fine, J. The lung lesion in four different types of shock in rabbits. *Arch. Surg.* 104: 319–322, 1972.

455. Cullen, D. J. Interpretation of blood-pressure measurements in anesthesia. *Anesthesiology* 40: 6–12, 1974.

456. Cullen, D. J. Care of the Critically Ill. Refresher course lectures, Annual Meeting of the American Society of Anesthesiologists, Washington, D.C., October 12–16, 1974. Lecture no. 107.

457. Cullen, D. J., and Ferrara, L. C. Comparative evaluation of blood filters: A study in vitro. *Anesthesiology* 41: 568–575, 1974.

458. Cullen, J. H., and Formel, P. F. The respiratory defects in extreme obesity. *Am. J. Med.* 32: 525–531, 1962.

459. Cullen, P., Modell, J. H., Kirby, R. R., Klein, E. F., Jr., and Long, W. Treatment of patients with flail chest by intermittent mandatory ventilation and PEEP. *Crit. Care Med.* 3: 45, 1975.

460. Culver, G. A., Makel, H. P., and Beecher, H. K. Frequency of aspiration of gastric contents by the lungs during anesthesia and surgery. *Ann. Surg.* 133: 289–292, 1951.

461. Currie, W. D., Pratt, P. C., and Sanders, A. P. Hyperoxia and lung metabolism. *Chest* 66 (Suppl., Pt. 2): 19S–21S, 1974.

462. Curry, C. R., and Quie, P. G. Fungal septicemia in patients receiving parenteral hyperalimentation. *N. Engl. J. Med.* 285: 1221–1225, 1971.

463. Curtin, J. W., Holinger, P. H., and Greeley, P. W. Blunt trauma to the larynx and upper trachea: Immediate treatment, complications and late reconstructive procedures. *J. Trauma* 6: 493–502, 1966.

464. Curtis, J. R., Eastwood, J. B., Smith, E. K. M., Storey, J. M., Verroust, P. J., De Wardener, H. E., Wing, A. J., and Wolfson, E. M. Maintenance haemodialysis. *Q. J. Med.* (N. S.) 38: 49–89, 1969.

465. Cushing, H. Concerning a definite regulatory mechanism of the vasomotor centre which controls blood pressure during cerebral compression. *Bull. Johns Hopkins Hosp.* 12: 290–292, 1901.

466. Cushing, H. Some experimental and clinical observations concerning states of increased intracranial tension. *Am. J. Med. Sci.* 124: 375–400, 1902.

467. Czapek, E. E.   Coagulation problems. *Int. Anesthesiol. Clin.* 11(2):175–201, 1973.
468. Daggett, W. M., Burwell, L. R., Lawson, D. W., and Austen, W. G.   Resection of acute ventricular aneurysm and ruptured interventricular septum after myocardial infarction. *N. Engl. J. Med.* 283:1507–1508, 1970.
469. Daily, P. O., Griepp, R. B., and Shumway, N. E.   Percutaneous internal jugular vein cannulation. *Arch. Surg.* 101:534–536, 1970.
470. Dalldorf, F. G., Pate, D. H., and Langdell, R. D.   Pulmonary capillary thrombosis in experimental pneumococcal septicemia. *Arch. Pathol.* 85:149–161, 1968.
471. Dalrymple, D. G., Parbrook, G. D., and Steel, D. F.   Factors predisposing to postoperative pain and pulmonary complications. A study of female patients undergoing elective cholecystectomy. *Br. J. Anaesth.* 45:589–597, 1973.
472. Dalton, B., and Laver, M. B.   Vasospasm with an indwelling radial artery cannula. *Anesthesiology* 34:194–197, 1971.
473. Dammann, J. F., Jr., Wright, D. J., Updike, O. L., and Bowers, D. L.   Assessment of continuous monitoring in the critically ill patient. *Dis. Chest* 55:240–244, 1969.
474. Damus, P. S., and Salzman, E. W.   Disseminated intravascular coagulation. *Arch. Surg.* 104:262–265, 1972.
475. Darling, R. C.   Ruptured arteriosclerotic abdominal aortic aneurysms. A pathologic and clinical study. *Am. J. Surg.* 119:397–401, 1970.
476. Da Silva, A. M. T., and Hamosh, P.   Effect of smoking a single cigarette on the "small airways." *J. Appl. Physiol.* 34:361–365, 1973.
477. Dave, K. S., Bekassy, S. M., Wooler, G. H., and Ionescu, M. I.   Spontaneous rupture of the diaphragm during delivery. *Br. J. Surg.* 60:666–668, 1973.
478. Davidson, C. S., and Gabuzda, G. J.   Hepatic Coma. In L. Schiff (Ed.), *Diseases of the Liver.* Philadelphia: Lippincott, 1969. Pp. 378–409.
479. Davidson, C. S., McDermott, W. V., Jr., and Trey, C.   Sustaining life during fulminant hepatic failure. *Ann. Intern. Med.* 71:415–418, 1969.
480. Davies, D. M., Millar, E. J., and Miller, I. A.   Accidental hypothermia treated by extracorporeal blood-warming. *Lancet* 1:1036–1037, 1967.
481. Davies, H. C., and Davies, R. E.   Biochemical Aspects of Oxygen Poisoning. In W. O. Fenn and H. Rahn (Eds.), *Handbook of Physiology.* Volume II, Section 3, *Respiration.* Washington, D.C.: American Physiological Society, 1965. Pp. 1047–1058.
482. Davis, A. G., and Spence, A. A.   Postoperative hypoxemia and age. *Anesthesiology* 37:663–664, 1972.
483. Davis, F. G., and Cullen, D. J.   Post-extubation Aspiration Following Prolonged Intubation. Abstracts of scientific papers, Annual Meeting of the American Society of Anesthesiologists, Washington, D.C., October 12–16, 1974. Pp. 181–182.
484. Davis, J. M., Bartlett, E., and Termini, B. A.   Overdosage of psychotropic drugs: A review. I. Major and minor tranquilizers. *Dis. Nerv. Syst.* 29:157–164, 1968.
485. Davis, J. T.   The influence of intrathoracic pressure on fluid and electrolyte balance. *Chest* 62(Suppl.):118S–125S, 1972.
486. Day, E. A., and Morgan, E. B.   Accidental hypothermia: Report of a case following alcohol and barbiturate overdose. *Anaesth. Intensive Care* 2:73–76, 1974.
487. Dean, H. R.   Twenty-five cases of tetanus. *Lancet* 1:673–680, 1917.
488. Deane, R. S., Mills, E. L., and Hamel, A. J.   Antibacterial action of copper in respiratory therapy apparatus. *Chest* 58:373–377, 1970.

489. Decker, W. J., Thompson, H. L., and Arneson, L. A. Glutethimide rebound. *Lancet* 1: 778–779, 1970.
490. Deeb, E. N., and Natsios, G. A. Contamination of "in-use" hyperalimentation solutions. *N. Engl. J. Med.* 286: 613, 1972.
491. Defalque, R. J. Percutaneous catheterization of the internal jugular vein. *Anesth. Analg.* (Cleve.) 53: 116–121, 1974.
492. Dehm, M. M., and Bruce, R. A. Longitudinal variations in maximal oxygen intake with age and activity. *J. Appl. Physiol.* 33: 805–807, 1972.
493. DeLemos, R., Wolfsdorf, J., Nachman, R., Block, A. J., Leiby, G., Wilkinson, H. A., Allen, T., Haller, J. A., Morgan, W., and Avery, M. E. Lung injury from oxygen in lambs: The role of artificial ventilation. *Anesthesiology* 30: 609–618, 1969.
494. deLeval, M. R., Hills, J. D., Mielke, H., Bramson, M. L., Smith, C., and Gerbode, F. Platelet kinetics during extracorporeal circulation. *Trans. Am. Soc. Artif. Intern. Organs* 18: 355–357, 1972.
495. Del Guercio, L. R. M., Cohn, J. D., Greenspan, M., Feins, N. R., and Kornitzer, G. Pulmonary and Systemic Arteriovenous Shunting in Clinical Septic Shock. In I. W. Brown, Jr. and B. G. Cox (Eds.), *Proceedings of the Third International Conference on Hyperbaric Medicine.* National Research Council Publication no. 1404. Washington, D. C.: National Academy of Sciences, 1966. Pp. 337–342.
496. Del Guercio, L. R. M., Commaraswamy, R. P., Feins, N. R., Wollman, S. B., and State, D. Pulmonary arteriovenous admixture and the hyperdynamic cardiovascular state in surgery for portal hypertension. *Surgery* 56: 57–74, 1964.
497. Dempsey, J. A., Reddan, W., Balke, B., and Rankin, J. Work capacity determinants and physiologic cost of weight-supported work in obesity. *J. Appl. Physiol.* 21: 1815–1820, 1966.
498. Dempsey, J. A., Reddan, W., Rankin, J., and Balke, B. Alveolar-arterial gas exchange during muscular work in obesity. *J. Appl. Physiol.* 21: 1807–1814, 1966.
499. DeMuth, W. E., Jr., and Zinsser, H. F., Jr. Myocardial contusion. *Arch. Intern. Med.* 115: 434–442, 1965.
500. DePalma, R. G., Coil, J., Davis, J. H., and Holden, W. D. Cellular and ultrastructural changes in endotoxemia: A light and electron microscopic study. *Surgery* 62: 505–515, 1967.
501. Dewar, K. M. S., Smith, G., Spence, A. A., and Ledingham, I. McA. Effect of hyperoxia on airways resistance in man. *J. Appl. Physiol.* 32: 486–490, 1972.
502. Deykin, D. The clinical challenge of disseminated intravascular coagulation. *N. Engl. J. Med.* 283: 636–644, 1970.
503. Deysine, M., Lieblich, N., and Aufses, A. H., Jr. Albumin changes during clinical septic shock. *Surg. Gynecol. Obstet.* 137: 475–478, 1973.
504. Diament, M. L., and Palmer, K. N. V. Postoperative changes in gas tensions of arterial blood and in ventilatory function. *Lancet* 2: 180–182, 1966.
505. Diament, M. L., and Palmer, K. N. V. Venous/arterial pulmonary shunting as the principal cause of postoperative hypoxaemia. *Lancet* 1: 15–17, 1967.
506. Diament, M. L., and Palmer, K. N. V. Spirometry for preoperative assessment of airways resistance. *Lancet* 1: 1251–1253, 1967.
507. Diamond, G., Marcus, H., McHugh, T., Swan, H. J. C., and Forrester, J. Catheterization of left ventricle in acutely ill patients. *Br. Heart J.* 33: 489–493, 1971.
508. Dick, W. Aspects of humidification: Requirements and techniques. *Int. Anesthesiol. Clin.* 12(4): 217–239, 1974.

509. Dickie, K. J., deGroot, W. J., Cooley, R. N., Bond, T. P., and Guest, M. M. Hemodynamic effects of bolus infusion of urokinase in pulmonary thromboembolism. *Am. Rev. Respir. Dis.* 109:48–56, 1974.

510. Dikshit, K., Vyden, J. K., Forrester, J. S., Chatterjee, K., Prakash, R., and Swan, H. J. C.   Renal and extrarenal hemodynamic effects of furosemide in congestive heart failure after acute myocardial infarction. *N. Engl. J. Med.* 288:1087–1090, 1973.

511. Dill, D. B., and Consolazio, C. F.   Responses to exercise as related to age and environmental temperature. *J. Appl. Physiol.* 17:645–648, 1962.

512. Dill, D. B., Graybiel, A., Hurtado, A., and Taquini, A. C.   Gaseous exchange in the lungs in old age. *J. Am. Geriatr. Soc.* 11:1063–1076, 1963.

513. Dilley, R. B., Ross, J., Jr., and Bernstein, E. F.   Serial hemodynamics during intra-aortic balloon counterpulsation for cardiogenic shock. *Circulation* 47, 48(Suppl. III):99–104, 1973.

514. Dimmick, J. E., Bove, K. E., McAdams, A. J., and Benzing, G., III.   Fiber embolization—A hazard of cardiac surgery and catheterization. *N. Engl. J. Med.* 292:685–687, 1975.

515. Dines, D. E., Linscheid, R. L., and Didier, E. P.   Fat embolism syndrome. *Mayo Clin. Proc.* 47:237–240, 1972.

516. Dinnick, O. P.   Discussions on anaesthesia for obstetrics: An evaluation of general and regional methods. *Proc. R. Soc. Med.* 50:547–552, 1957.

517. DiVincenti, F. C., Pruitt, B. A., Jr., and Reckler, J. M.   Inhalation injuries. *J. Trauma* 11:109–117, 1971.

518. Dobbie, A. K.   Electricity in hospitals. *Biomed. Eng.* 7:12–20, 1972.

519. Dodge, P. R., and Swartz, M. N.   Bacterial meningitis: A review of selected aspects. II. Special neurologic problems, postmeningitic complications and clinicopathologic correlations. *N. Engl. J. Med.* 272:954–960, 1965.

520. Dodsworth, J. M., James, J. H., Cummings, M. C., and Fischer, J. E.   Depletion of brain norepinephrine in acute hepatic coma. *Surgery* 75:811–820, 1974.

521. Doležal, V.   The effect of long lasting oxygen inhalation upon respiratory parameters in man. *Physiol. Bohemoslov.* 11:149–158, 1962.

522. Don, H. F., Wahba, W. M., and Craig, D. B.   Airway closure, gas trapping, and the functional residual capacity during anesthesia. *Anesthesiology* 36:533–539, 1972.

523. Donald, K. W.   Oxygen poisoning in man. *Br. Med. J.* 1:667–672, 712–717, 1947.

524. Donald, K. W., Renzetti, A., Riley, R. L., and Cournand, A.   Analysis of factors affecting concentrations of oxygen and carbon dioxide in gas and blood of lungs: Results. *J. Appl. Physiol.* 4:497–525, 1952.

525. Donnelly, W. A., Grossman, A. A., and Grem, F. M.   Local sequelae of endotracheal anesthesia as observed by examination of one hundred patients. *Anesthesiology* 9:490–497, 1948.

526. Donovan, A. J., Turrill, F. L., and Facey, F. L.   Hepatic trauma. *Surg. Clin. North Am.* 48:1313–1335, 1968.

527. Dornette, W. H. L.   Thermometry in clinical practice. *Int. Anesthesiol. Clin.* 3:473–488, 1965.

528. Dornette, W. H. L.   *Clinical Anesthesia: Monitoring in Anesthesia.* Philadelphia: Davis, 1973.

529. Dorricott, N. J., Eisenberg, H., and Silen, W.   Effect of intra-arterial vasopressin on canine gastric mucosal permeability. *Gastroenterology* 65:625–629, 1973.

530. Dotter, C. T., Rösch, J., and Bilbao, M. K.   Transluminal extraction of cathe-

ter and guide fragments from the heart and great vessels; 29 collected cases. *Am. J. Roentgenol. Radium Ther. Nucl. Med.* 111:467–472, 1971.

531. Douglas, C. G., Haldane, J. S., and Haldane, J. B. S. The laws of combination of haemoglobin with carbon monoxide and oxygen. *J. Physiol.* (Lond.) 44:275–304, 1912.

532. Douglas, F. G., and Chong, P. Y. Influence of obesity on peripheral airways patency. *J. Appl. Physiol.* 33:559–563, 1972.

533. Douglas, M. E., Downs, J. B., Dannemiller, F. J., and Hodges, M. R. Thrombocytopenia and the Adult Respiratory Distress Syndrome. Abstracts of scientific papers, Annual Meeting of the American Society of Anesthesiologists, Washington, D.C., October 12–16, 1974. Pp. 245–246.

534. Dowd, J., and Jenkins, L. C. The lung in shock: A review. *Can. Anaesth. Soc. J.* 19:309–318, 1972.

535. Downs, J. B., Chapman, R. L., Modell, J. H., and Hood, C. I. An evaluation of steroid therapy in aspiration pneumonitis. *Anesthesiology* 40:129–135, 1974.

536. Downs, J. B., Klein, E. F., Jr., Desautels, D., Modell, J. H., and Kirby, R. R. Intermittent mandatory ventilation: A new approach to weaning patients from mechanical ventilators. *Chest* 64:331–335, 1973.

537. Downs, J. B., Perkins, H. M., and Sutton, W. W. Successful weaning after five years of mechanical ventilation. *Anesthesiology* 40:602–603, 1974.

538. Downs, J. B., Rackstein, A. D., Klein, E. F., Jr., and Hawkins, I. F. Hazards of radial-artery catheterization. *Anesthesiology* 38:283–286, 1973.

539. Drachman, D. A., and Adams, R. D. Herpes simplex and acute inclusion-body encephalitis. *Arch. Neurol.* 7:45–63, 1962.

540. Drazen, E. C., and Wechsler, A. E. Review of Computer-based Patient Monitoring Systems in the United States. Scientific abstracts, First World Congress on Intensive Care, London, England, June 24–27, 1974. P. 139.

541. Drinker, C. K. *Carbon Monoxide Asphyxia.* New York: Oxford University Press, 1938.

542. Drinker, P. A. Prolonged extracorporeal respiratory support: Engineering view and progress report. *Transplant. Proc.* 3:1429–1436, 1971.

543. Dripps, R. D., and Deming, M. V. N. Postoperative atelectasis and pneumonia. Diagnosis, etiology and management based upon 1,240 cases of upper abdominal surgery. *Ann. Surg.* 124:94–110, 1946.

544. Drop, L. J. Interdependence Between Plasma Ionized Calcium and Hemodynamic Performance. Ph.D. dissertation, De Katholieke Universiteit te Nijmegen. Boston: Massachusetts General Hospital Printing Office, 1974.

545. Drop, L. J., and Cullen, D. J. Effect of Calcium Chloride and Calcium Gluceptate on Hemodynamic Function and Plasma Levels in Man. Abstracts of scientific papers, Annual Meeting of the American Society of Anesthesiologists, Washington, D.C., October 12–16, 1974. Pp. 337–338.

546. Drury, D. R., Henry, J. P., and Goodman, J. The effects of continuous pressure breathing on kidney function. *J. Clin. Invest.* 26:945–951, 1947.

547. DuBois, A. B., Hyde, R. W., and Hendler, E. Pulmonary mechanics and diffusing capacity following simulated space flight of 2 weeks duration. *J. Appl. Physiol.* 18:696–698, 1963.

548. DuBois, A. B., Turaids, T., Mammen, R. E., and Nobrega, F. T. Pulmonary atelectasis in subjects breathing oxygen at sea level or at simulated altitude. *J. Appl. Physiol.* 21:828–836, 1966.

549. DuBois, D., and DuBois, E. F. A formula to estimate the approximate surface area if height and weight be known. *Arch. Intern. Med.* 17:863–871, 1916.

550. DuBois, E. F. *Basal Metabolism in Health and Disease.* Philadelphia: Lea & Febiger, 1936. Pp. 410–442.
551. Ducker, T. B. Increased intracranial pressure and pulmonary edema. I. Clinical study of 11 patients. *J. Neurosurg.* 28:112–117, 1968.
552. Ducker, T. B., and Simmons, R. L. Increased intracranial pressure and pulmonary edema. II. The hemodynamic response of dogs and monkeys to increased intracranial pressure. *J. Neurosurg.* 28:118–123, 1968.
553. Ducker, T. B., Simmons, R. L., and Anderson, R. W. Increased intracranial pressure and pulmonary edema. III. The effect of increased intracranial pressure on the cardiovascular hemodynamics of chimpanzees. *J. Neurosurg.* 29:475–483, 1968.
554. Ducker, T. B., Simmons, R. L., and Martin, A. M., Jr. Pulmonary edema as a complication of intracranial disease. *Am. J. Dis. Child.* 118:638–641, 1969.
555. Dudley, W. R., and Marshall, B. E. Steroid treatment for acid-aspiration pneumonitis. *Anesthesiology* 40:136–141, 1974.
556. Dudrick, S. J., MacFadyen, B. V., Van Burren, C. T., Ruberg, R. L., and Maynard, A. T. Parenteral hyperalimentation. Metabolic problems and solution. *Ann. Surg.* 176:259–264, 1972.
557. Dudrick, S. J., Steiger, E., and Long, J. M. Renal failure in surgical patients. Treatment with intravenous essential amino acids and hypertonic glucose. *Surgery* 68:180–186, 1970.
558. Dudrick, S. J., Wilmore, D. W., Vars, H. M., and Rhoads, J. E. Long-term total parenteral nutrition with growth, development, and positive nitrogen balance. *Surgery* 64:134–142, 1968.
559. Dudrick, S. J., Wilmore, D. W., Vars, H. M., and Rhoads, J. E. Can intravenous feeding as a sole means of nutrition support growth in the child and restore weight loss in an adult? *Ann. Surg.* 169:974–984, 1969.
560. Duguid, H., Simpson, R. G., and Stowers, J. M. Accidental hypothermia. *Lancet* 2:1213–1219, 1961.
561. Dunkman, W. B., Leinbach, R. C., Buckley, M. J., Mundth, E. D., Kantrowitz, A. R., Austen, W. G., and Sanders, C. A. Clinical and hemodynamic results of intraaortic balloon pumping and surgery for cardiogenic shock. *Circulation* 46:465–477, 1972.
562. Dunn, J., Kirsch, M. M., Harness, J., Carroll, M., Straker, J., and Sloan, H. Hemodynamic, metabolic, and hematologic effects of pulsatile cardiopulmonary bypass. *J. Thorac. Cardiovasc. Surg.* 68:138–147, 1974.
563. Dupont, F. S., and Sphire, R. D. Pulmonary lavage. *Crit. Care Med.* 2:161–162, 1974.
564. Dupont, J. R., and Earle, K. M. Human rabies encephalitis. A study of 49 fatal cases with a review of the literature. *Neurology* 15:1023–1034, 1965.
565. Dyer, I., and Barclay, D. L. Accidental trauma complicating pregnancy and delivery. *Am. J. Obstet. Gynecol.* 83:907–929, 1962.
566. Dyer, I., and McCaughey, E. V. Abruptio placentae. A ten year survey. *Am. J. Obstet. Gynecol.* 77:1176–1186, 1959.
567. Eales, L. The acute porphyria attack. III. Acute porphyria: The precipitating and aggravating factors. *S. Afr. J. Lab. Clin. Med.* 17:120–125, 1971. (Suppl. to *S. Afr. Med. J.* 45:1971.)
568. Eastridge, C. E., Hughes, F. A., Jr., Pate, J. W., Cole, F., and Richardson, R. Tracheobronchial injury caused by blunt trauma. *Am. Rev. Respir. Dis.* 101:230–237, 1970.
569. Ebaugh, F. G., Barnacle, C. H., and Ewalt, J. R. Delirious episodes associated with artificial fever. A study of 200 cases. *Am. J. Psychiatry* 93:191–215, 1936.

570. Ebert, R. V., and Stead, E. A., Jr. Circulatory failure in acute infections. *J. Clin. Invest.* 20: 671–679, 1941.

571. Ebert, R. V., and Terracio, M. J. The bronchiolar epithelium in cigarette smokers. Observations with the scanning electron microscope. *Am. Rev. Respir. Dis.* 111: 4–11, 1975.

572. Eckenhoff, J. E., Enderby, G. E. H., Larson, A., Edridge, A., and Judevine, D. E. Pulmonary gas exchange during deliberate hypotension. *Br. J. Anaesth.* 35: 750–758, 1963.

573. Eckhauser, F. E., Billote, J., Burke, J. F., and Quinby, W. C. Tracheostomy complicating massive burn injury: A plea for conservatism. *Am. J. Surg.* 127: 418–422, 1974.

574. Edelman, N. H., Mittman, C., Norris, A. H., and Shock, N. W. Effects of respiratory pattern on age differences in ventilation uniformity. *J. Appl. Physiol.* 24: 49–53, 1968.

575. Editorial. Airport disasters. *Br. Med. J.* 3: 387, 1971.

576. Edwards, G., Morton, H. J. V., Pask, E. A., and Wylie, W. D. Deaths associated with anaesthesia: A report on 1,000 cases. *Anaesthesia* 11: 194–220, 1956.

577. Egbert, L. D., Battit, G. E., Turndorf, H., and Beecher, H. K. The value of the preoperative visit by an anesthetist. A study of doctor-patient rapport. *J.A.M.A.* 185: 553–555, 1963.

578. Egbert, L. D., Battit, G. E., Welch, C. E., and Bartlett, M. K. Reduction of postoperative pain by encouragement and instruction of patients; a study of doctor-patient rapport. *N. Engl. J. Med.* 270: 825–827, 1964.

579. Egbert, L. D., and Bendixen, H. H. Effect of morphine on breathing pattern: A possible factor in atelectasis. *J.A.M.A.* 188: 485–488, 1964.

580. Egbert, L. D., Laver, M. B., and Bendixen, H. H. The effect of site of operation and type of anesthesia upon the ability to cough in the postoperative period. *Surg. Gynecol. Obstet.* 115: 295–298, 1962.

581. Eichenholz, A., Mulhausen, R. O., Anderson, W. E., and MacDonald, F. M. Primary hypocapnia: A cause of metabolic acidosis. *J. Appl. Physiol.* 17: 283–288, 1962.

582. Eickhoff, T. C., Brachman, P. S., Bennett, J. V., and Brown, J. F. Surveillance of nosocomial infections in community hospitals. I. Surveillance methods, effectiveness, and initial results. *J. Infect. Dis.* 120: 305–317, 1969.

583. Eiseman, B., and Soyer, T. Prosthetics in hepatic assistance. *Transplant. Proc.* 3: 1519–1524, 1971.

584. Elkins, R. C., Peyton, M. D., Hinshaw, L. B., and Greenfield, L. J. Clinical hemodynamic and respiratory responses to graded positive end-expiratory pressure. *Surg. Forum* 25: 226–229, 1974.

585. Eller, W. C., and Haugen, R. K. Food asphyxiation—Restaurant rescue. *N. Engl. J. Med.* 289: 81–82, 1973.

586. Ellison, N., Beatty, C. P., Blake, D. R., Wurzel, H. A., and MacVaugh, H., III. Heparin rebound. Studies in patients and volunteers. *J. Thorac. Cardiovasc. Surg.* 67: 723–729, 1974.

587. Ellison, N., Ominsky, A. J., and Wollman, H. Is protamine a clinically important anticoagulant? A negative answer. *Anesthesiology* 35: 621–629, 1971.

588. Ellman, L., Carvalho, A., and Colman, R. W. The Thrombo-Wellcotest as a screening test for disseminated intravascular coagulation. *N. Engl. J. Med.* 288: 633–634, 1973.

589. El-Naggar, M. Weaning. *Mid. East J. Anaesth.* 3: 401–406, 1972.

590. Elsberry, D. D., Rhoda, D. A., and Beisel, W. R. Hemodynamics of

staphylococcal B enterotoxemia and other types of shock in monkeys. *J. Appl. Physiol.* 27:164–169, 1969.

591. Emirgil, C., Sobol, B. J., Campodonico, S., Herbert, W. H., and Mechkati, R. Pulmonary circulation in the aged. *J. Appl. Physiol.* 23:631–640, 1967.

592. English, I. C. W., Frew, R. M., Pigott, J. F., and Zaki, M. Percutaneous catheterization of the internal jugular vein. *Anaesthesia* 24:521–531, 1969.

593. Epstein, B. S., Hardy, D. L., Harrison, H. N., Teplitz, C., Villarreal, Y., and Mason, A. D. Hypoxemia in the burned patient: A clinical-pathologic study. *Ann. Surg.* 158:924–932, 1963.

594. Epstein, B. S., Rose, L. R., Teplitz, C., and Moncrief, J. A. Experiences with low tracheostomy in the burn patient. *J.A.M.A.* 183:966–968, 1963.

595. Epstein, F. H. Acute Renal Failure. In M. M. Wintrobe et al. (Eds.), *Harrison's Principles of Internal Medicine* (7th ed.). New York: McGraw-Hill, 1974. Pp. 1383–1388.

596. Erdmann, W., and Frey, R. Continuous blood-gas-controlled ventilation (CBC-ventilation): A step into the future of computer controlled therapy in intensive care units. *Crit. Care Med.* 1:120, 1973.

597. Erickson, D. R., Blair, E., Davis, J. H., and Dwyer, E. Pathodynamics of blunt chest trauma: A preliminary report. *Am. J. Surg.* 36:717–720, 1970.

598. Ersoz, C. J., Hedden, M., and Lain, L. Prolonged femoral arterial catheterization for intensive care. *Anesth. Analg.* (Cleve.) 49:160–164, 1970.

599. Estes, E. H., Jr., Sieker, H. O., McIntosh, H. D., and Welser, G. A. Reversible cardiopulmonary syndrome with extreme obesity. *Circulation* 16:179–187, 1957.

600. Eurenius, S., and Smith, R. M. Hemolysis in blood infused under pressure. *Anesthesiology* 39:650–651, 1973.

601. Evans, L. E. J., Roscoe, P., Swainson, C. P., and Prescott, L. F. Treatment of drug overdosage with naloxone, a specific narcotic antagonist. *Lancet* 1:452–455, 1973.

602. Evans, M. J., Stephens, R. J., and Freeman, G. Effects of nitrogen dioxide on cell renewal in the rat lung. *Arch. Intern. Med.* 128:57–60, 1971.

603. Evarts, C. M. Fat embolism syndrome: A review. *Surg. Clin. North Am.* 50:493–507, 1970.

604. Exton-Smith, A. N., Agate, J., Crockett, G. S., Irvine, R. E., and Wallis, M. G. Accidental hypothermia in the elderly. *Br. Med. J.* 2:1255–1258, 1964.

605. Faich, G. A., Graebner, R. W., and Sato, S. Failure of guanidine therapy in botulism A. *N. Engl. J. Med.* 285:773–776, 1971.

606. Faiman, M. D., Mehl, R. G., and Myers, M. B. Brain norepinephrine and serotonin in central oxygen toxicity. *Life Sci.* 10:21–34, 1971.

607. Fairley, H. B., and Blenkarn, G. D. Effect on pulmonary gas exchange of variations in inspiratory flow rate during intermittent positive-pressure ventilation. *Br. J. Anaesth.* 38:320–328, 1966.

608. Falke, K. J., Pontoppidan, H., Kumar, A., Leith, D. E., Geffin, B., and Laver, M. B. Ventilation with end-expiratory pressure in acute lung disease. *J. Clin. Invest.* 51:2315–2323, 1972.

609. Falla, S. T. Effect of explosion-blast on the lungs. Report of a case. *Br. Med. J.* 2:255–256, 1940.

610. Falsetti, H. L., Mates, R. E., Carroll, R. J., Gupta, R. L., and Bell, A. C. Analysis and correction of pressure wave distortion in fluid-filled catheter systems. *Circulation* 49:165–172, 1974.

611. Farber, M. O., Manfredi, F., Atkinson, K., and Passo, T. Oxygen transport during acute alkalosis and hyperphosphatemia in dogs. *Anesthesiology* 40:525–530, 1974.

612. Farhi, L. E., and Rahn, H. A theoretical analysis of the alveolar-arterial O_2 difference with special reference to the distribution effect. *J. Appl. Physiol.* 7:699–703, 1955.
613. Faridy, E. E. Effect of hydration and dehydration on elastic behavior of dogs' lungs. *J. Appl. Physiol.* 34:597–605, 1973.
614. Faridy, E. E., and Naimark, A. Effect of ventilation on lung metabolism. *Fed. Proc.* 29:661, 1970.
615. Faridy, E. E., and Naimark, A. Effect of distention on metabolism of excised dog lung. *J. Appl. Physiol.* 31:31–37, 1971.
616. Farrington, G. H., Saravis, C. A., Cossette, G. R., Miller, D. A., and Clowes, G. H. A., Jr. Blood-borne factors in the pulmonary response to sepsis (acute experimental peritonitis). *Surgery* 68:136–145, 1970.
617. Fassolt, A., Braun, U., and Graber, M. Gefahren des Katheters der oberen Hohlvene, mit besonderer Berücksichtigung des infraklavikulären Zugangs. *Helv. Chir. Acta* 37:18–22, 1970.
618. Favero, M. S., Carson, L. A., Bond, W. W., and Peterson, N. J. *Pseudomonas aeruginosa*: Growth in distilled water from hospitals. *Science* 173:836–838, 1971.
619. Fearon, D. T., Ruddy, S., McCabe, W. R., and Schur, P. H. Activation of the complement system by the properdin pathway in patients with gram-negative bacteremia. *J. Clin. Invest.* 53:23a, 1974.
620. Feeley, T. W., du Moulin, G. C., Hedley-Whyte, J., Bushnell, L. S., Gilbert, J. P., and Feingold, D. S. Aerosol polymyxin and pneumonia in seriously ill patients. *N. Engl. J. Med.* 293:471–475, 1975.
621. Feeley, T. W., and Hedley-Whyte, J. Weaning from controlled ventilation and supplemental oxygen. *N. Engl. J. Med.* 292:903–906, 1975.
622. Feeley, T. W., McClelland, K. J., and Malhotra, I. V. The hazards of bulk oxygen delivery systems. *Lancet* 1:1416–1418, 1975.
623. Feeley, T. W., Saumarez, R., Klick, J. M., McNabb, T. G., and Skillman, J. J. Positive end-expiratory pressure in weaning patients from controlled ventilation: A prospective randomised trial. *Lancet* 2:725–729, 1975.
624. Fegler, G. Measurement of cardiac output in anaesthetized animals by a thermo-dilution method. *Q. J. Exp. Physiol.* 39:153–164, 1954.
625. Feingold, D. S. Hospital-acquired infections. *N. Engl. J. Med.* 283:1384–1391, 1970.
626. Fell, R. H., Gunning, A. J., Bardhan, K. D., and Triger, D. R. Severe hypothermia as a result of barbiturate overdose complicated by cardiac arrest. *Lancet* 1:392–394, 1968.
627. Felner, J. M., and Dowell, V. R., Jr. "Bacteroides" bacteremia. *Am. J. Med.* 50:787–796, 1971.
628. Ferguson, R. K., and Reid, D. E. Rupture of the uterus: A twenty year report from the Boston Lying-In Hospital. *Am. J. Obstet. Gynecol.* 76:172–180, 1958.
629. Fernandez, J. P., O'Rourke, R. A., and Ewy, G. A. Rapid active external rewarming in accidental hypothermia. *J.A.M.A.* 212:153–156, 1970.
630. Ferris, B. G., Jr., and Pollard, D. S. Effect of deep and quiet breathing on pulmonary compliance in man. *J. Clin. Invest.* 39:143–149, 1960.
631. Figueras, J., Stein, L., Balda, V., Shubin, H., and Weil, M. H. The pulmonary diastolic gradient in 112 acutely ill patients: Difference between cardiac and non-cardiac cases. *Crit. Care Med.* 3:45–46, 1975.
632. Finley, T. N., and Ladman, A. J. Low yield of pulmonary surfactant in cigarette smokers. *N. Engl. J. Med.* 286:223–227, 1972.
633. Finnerty, F. A., Jr. Toxemia of pregnancy as seen by an internist: An analysis of 1,081 patients. *Ann. Intern. Med.* 44:358–375, 1956.

634. Fischer, E. G.   Impaired perfusion following cerebrovascular stasis. A review. *Arch. Neurol.* 29:361–364, 1973.
635. Fischer, J. E.   Hepatic coma in cirrhosis, portal hypertension, and following portacaval shunt. Its etiologies and the current status of its treatment. *Arch. Surg.* 108:325–336, 1974.
636. Fischer, J. E., and Baldessarini, R. J.   False neurotransmitters and hepatic failure. *Lancet* 2:75–80, 1971.
637. Fischer, J. E., Funovics, J. M., Aguirre, A., James, J. H., Keane, J. M., Wesdorp, R. I. C., Yoshimura, N., and Westman, T.   The role of plasma amino acids in hepatic encephalopathy. *Surgery* 78:276–288, 1975.
638. Fischer, J. E., and James, J. H.   Treatment of hepatic coma and hepatorenal syndrome. Mechanisms of action of L-dopa and aramine. *Am. J. Surg.* 123:222–230, 1972.
639. Fischer, J. E., Yoshimura, N., Aguirre, A., James, J. H., Cummings, M. G., Abel, R. M., and Deindoerfer, F.   Plasma amino acids in patients with hepatic encephalopathy. Effects of amino acid infusions. *Am. J. Surg.* 127:40–47, 1974.
640. Fish, J. S.   Marginal placental rupture. *Clin. Obstet. Gynecol.* 3:599–615, 1960.
641. Fisher, A. B., Diamond, S., and Mellen, S.   Effect of O_2 exposure on metabolism of the rabbit alveolar macrophage. *J. Appl. Physiol.* 37:341–345, 1974.
642. Fisher, A. B., Diamond, S., Mellen, S., and Zubrow, A.   Effect of 48- and 72-hour oxygen exposure on the rabbit alveolar macrophage. *Chest* 66(Suppl., Pt. 2):4S–6S, 1974.
643. Fisher, A. B., and Furia, L.   Redox changes of isolated perfused rat lung with metabolic inhibitors. *Physiologist* 17:222, 1974.
644. Fisher, A. B., Hyde, R. W., Puy, R. J. M., Clark, J. M., and Lambertsen, C. J.   Effect of oxygen at 2 atmospheres on the pulmonary mechanics of normal man. *J. Appl. Physiol.* 24:529–536, 1968.
645. Fisher, C. M.   The neurological examination of the comatose patient. *Acta Neurol. Scand.* 45(Suppl. 36):1–56, 1969.
646. Fishman, A. P., and Pietra, G. G.   Handling of bioactive materials by the lung. *N. Engl. J. Med.* 291:953–959, 1974.
647. Flacke, W.   Treatment of myasthenia gravis. *N. Engl. J. Med.* 288:27–31, 1973.
648. Flanagan, J. P., Gradisar, I. A., Gross, R. J., and Kelly, T. R.   Air embolus—A lethal complication of subclavian venipuncture. *N. Engl. J. Med.* 281:488–489, 1969.
649. Fleming, W. H., and Bowen, J. C.   Early complications of long-term respiratory support. *J. Thorac. Cardiovasc. Surg.* 64:729–737, 1972.
650. Fletcher, W. S.   Nonpenetrating trauma to the gallbladder and extrahepatic bile ducts. *Surg. Clin. North Am.* 52:711–717, 1972.
651. Flowers, C. E., Jr.   Magnesium sulfate in obstetrics. A study of magnesium in plasma, urine, and muscle. *Am. J. Obstet. Gynecol.* 91:763–772, 1965.
652. Foley, F. D., Moncrief, J. A., and Mason, A. D.   Pathology of the lung in fatally burned patients. *Ann. Surg.* 167:251–264, 1968.
653. Ford, P. J., and Weintraub, R. M.   *Intra-aortic Balloon Pumping Manual.* Boston: Beth Israel Hospital, 1974.
654. Forrester, J. S., Diamond, G., Ganz, W., Danzig, R., and Swan, H. J. C.   Right and left heart pressures in the acutely ill patient. *Clin. Res.* 18:306, 1970.
655. Forrester, J. S., Diamond, G., McHugh, T. J., and Swan, H. J. C.   Filling pressures in the right and left sides of the heart in acute myocardial infarction: A reappraisal of central-venous-pressure monitoring. *N. Engl. J. Med.* 285:190–193, 1971.

656. Forrester, J. S., Ganz, W., Diamond, G., McHugh, T., Chonette, D. W., and Swan, H. J. C. Thermodilution cardiac output determination with a single flow-directed catheter. *Am. Heart J.* 83:306–311, 1972.

657. Forssmann, W. Die Sondierung des rechten Herzens. *Klin. Wochenschr.* 8:2085–2087, 1929.

658. Forthman, H. J., and Shepard, A. Postoperative pulmonary complications. *South. Med. J.* 62:1198–1200, 1969.

659. Fox, C. L., Jr., and Stanford, J. W. Comparative efficacy of hypo-, iso-, and hypertonic sodium solutions in experimental burn shock. *Surgery* 75:71–79, 1974.

660. Franciosa, J. A., Guiha, N. H., Limas, C. J., Rodriguera, E., and Cohn, J. N. Improved left ventricular function during nitroprusside infusion in acute myocardial infarction. *Lancet* 1:650–654, 1972.

661. Francis, E. Laboratory studies on tetanus. *U.S. Hyg. Lab. Bull.* 95:7–73, 1914.

662. Frank, N. R., Mead, J., and Ferris, B. G., Jr. The mechanical behavior of the lungs in healthy elderly persons. *J. Clin. Invest.* 36:1680–1687, 1957.

663. Frazier, H. S., and Yager, H. The clinical use of diuretics. *N. Engl. J. Med.* 288:246–249, 455–457, 1973.

664. Freeark, R. J. Penetrating wounds of the abdomen. *N. Engl. J. Med.* 291:185–188, 1974.

665. Freeman, J., and Nunn, J. F. Ventilation-perfusion relationships after hemorrhage. *Clin. Sci.* 24:135–147, 1963.

666. Friedman, N. J., Hoag, M. S., Robinson, A. J., and Aggelar, P. M. Hemorrhagic syndrome following transurethral prostatic resection for benign adenoma. *Arch. Intern. Med.* 124:341–349, 1969.

667. Friedman, S. A. Prevalence of palpable wrist pulses. *Br. Heart J.* 32:316, 1970.

668. Froeb, H. F., and Kim, B. M. Tracheostomy and respiratory dead space in emphysema. *J. Appl. Physiol.* 19:92–96, 1964.

669. Froese, A. B., and Bryan, A. C. Effects of anesthesia and paralysis on diaphragmatic mechanics in man. *Anesthesiology* 41:242–255, 1974.

670. Fuchsig, P., Brücke, P., Blümel, G., and Gottlob, R. A new clinical and experimental concept on fat embolism. *N. Engl. J. Med.* 276:1192–1193, 1967.

671. Fuller, R. H. Drowning and the postimmersion syndrome. A clinicopathologic study. *Milit. Med.* 128:22–36, 1963.

672. Fuller, R. H. The clinical pathology of human near-drowning. *Proc. R. Soc. Med.* 56:33–38, 1963.

673. Fulton, R. L., and Peter, E. T. The progressive nature of pulmonary contusion. *Surgery* 67:499–506, 1970.

674. Fulton, R. L., and Peter, E. T. Physiologic effects of fluid therapy after pulmonary contusion. *Am. J. Surg.* 126:773–777, 1973.

675. Fuson, R. L., Saltzman, H. A., Smith, W. W., Whalen, R. E., Osterhout, S., and Parker, R. T. Clinical hyperbaric oxygenation with severe oxygen toxicity. Report of a case. *N. Engl. J. Med.* 273:415–419, 1965.

676. Gaar, K. A., Jr., Taylor, A. E., Owens, L. J., and Guyton, A. C. Effect of capillary pressure and plasma protein on development of pulmonary edema. *Am. J. Physiol.* 213:79–82, 1967.

677. Gacad, G., and Massaro, D. Hyperoxia: Influence on lung mechanics and protein synthesis. *J. Clin. Invest.* 52:559–565, 1973.

678. Gaensler, E. A. Analysis of the ventilatory defect by timed capacity measurements. *Am. Rev. Tuberc.* 64:256–278, 1951.

679. Gaisford, W. D., Pandey, N., and Jensen, C. G. Pulmonary changes in treated hemorrhagic shock. II. Ringer's lactate solution versus colloid infusion. *Am. J. Surg.* 124:738–743, 1972.

680. Galbo, H., and Paulev, P.-E.   Cardiac function during rest and supine cycling examined with a new noninvasive technique (CED). *J. Appl. Physiol.* 36:113–117, 1974.

681. Gallin, J. I., Kaye, D., and O'Leary, W. M.   Serum lipids in infection. *N. Engl. J. Med.* 281:1081–1086, 1969.

682. Gallitano, A. L., Kondi, E. S., and Deckers, P. J.   A safe approach to the subclavian vein. *Surg. Gynecol. Obstet.* 135:96–98, 1972.

683. Gallus, A. S., Hirsh, J., Tuttle, R. J., Trebilcock, R., O'Brien, S. E., Carroll, J. J., Minder, J. H., and Hudecki, S. M.   Small subcutaneous doses of heparin in prevention of venous thrombosis. *N. Engl. J. Med.* 288:545–551, 1973.

684. Ganz, W., Donoso, R., Marcus, H. S., Forrester, J. S., and Swan, H. J. C.   A new technique for measurement of cardiac output by thermodilution in man. *Am. J. Cardiol.* 27:392–396, 1971.

685. Garan, H., Smith, T. W., and Powell, W. J., Jr.   The central nervous system as a site of action for the coronary vasoconstrictor effect of digoxin. *J. Clin. Invest.* 54:1365–1372, 1974.

686. Gardner, P., Griffin, W. B., Swartz, M. N., and Kunz, L. J.   Nonfermentative gram-negative bacilli of nosocomial interest. *Am. J. Med.* 48:735–749, 1970.

687. Gardner, R. M., Schwartz, R., Wong, H. C., and Burke, J. P.   Percutaneous indwelling radial-artery catheters for monitoring cardiovascular function; Prospective study of the risk of thrombosis and infection. *N. Engl. J. Med.* 290:1227–1231, 1974.

688. Garella, S., Dana, C. L., and Chazan, J. A.   Severity of metabolic acidosis as a determinant of bicarbonate requirements. *N. Engl. J. Med.* 289:121–126, 1973.

689. Garzon, A. A., Gourin, A., Seltzer, B., Chiu, C.-J., and Karlson, K. E.   Severe blunt chest trauma. Studies of pulmonary mechanics and blood gases. *Ann. Thorac. Surg.* 2:629–639, 1966.

690. Garzon, A. A., Seltzer, B., Song, I. C., Bromberg, B. E., and Karlson, K. E.   Respiratory mechanics in patients with inhalation burns. *J. Trauma* 10:57–61, 1970.

691. Gauss, H.   The pathology of fat embolism. *Arch. Surg.* 9:593–605, 1924.

692. Geddes, L. A.   *The Direct and Indirect Measurement of Blood Pressure.* Chicago: Year Book, 1970.

693. Geer, R. T., Soma, L. R., Barnes, C., Leatherman, J., and Marshall, B. E.   Therapy of Pulmonary Edema: Albumin and/or Diuretic? Abstracts of scientific papers, Annual Meeting of the American Society of Anesthesiologists, Washington, D.C., October 12–16, 1974. Pp. 321–322.

694. Geffin, B., and Pontoppidan, H.   Reduction of tracheal damage by the pre-stretching of inflatable cuffs. *Anesthesiology* 31:462–463, 1969.

695. Geha, D. G., Davis, N. J., and Lappas, D. G.   Persistent atrial arrhythmias associated with placement of Swan-Ganz catheter. *Anesthesiology* 39:651–653, 1973.

696. Geiger, K., Gallagher, M. L., and Hedley-Whyte, J.   Cellular distribution and clearance of aerosolized dipalmitoyl lecithin. *J. Appl. Physiol.* 39:759–766, 1975.

697. Geiran, O., and Solheim, K.   Cardiac and aortic injuries. *Scand. J. Thorac. Cardiovasc. Surg.* 8:27–33, 1974.

698. Georg, J., Hornum, I., and Mellemgaard, K.   The mechanism of hypoxaemia after laparotomy. *Thorax* 22:382–386, 1967.

699. German, J. C., Allyn, P. A., and Bartlett, R. H.   Pulmonary artery pressure monitoring in acute burn management. *Arch. Surg.* 106:788–791, 1973.

700. Gerst, P. H., Rattenborg, C., and Holaday, D. A.   The effects of hemorrhage

on pulmonary circulation and respiratory gas exchange. *J. Clin. Invest.* 38:524–538, 1959.

701. Gett, P. M., Jones, E. S., and Shepherd, G. F.   Pulmonary oedema associated with sodium retention during ventilator treatment. *Br. J. Anaesth.* 43:460–470, 1971.

702. Giammona, S. T., and Modell, J. H.   Drowning by total immersion. Effects on pulmonary surfactant of distilled water, isotonic saline, and sea water. *Am. J. Dis. Child.* 114:612–616, 1967.

703. Giammona, S. T., Tocci, P., and Webb, W. R.   Effects of cigarette smoke on incorporation of radioisotopically labelled palmitic acid into pulmonary surfactant and on surface activity of canine lung extracts. *Am. Rev. Respir. Dis.* 104:358–367, 1971.

704. Giannella, R. A., Broitman, S. A., and Zamcheck, N.   Gastric acid barrier to ingested microorganisms in man: Studies in vivo and in vitro. *Gut* 13:251–256, 1972.

705. Gibbon, J. H.   Artificial maintenance of circulation during experimental occlusion of pulmonary artery. *Arch. Surg.* 34:1105–1131, 1937.

706. Gibbs, N. M.   Venous thrombosis of the lower limbs, with particular reference to bed-rest. *Br. J. Surg.* 45:209–236, 1957.

707. Gibson, J. G., Rees, S. B., and McManus, T. J.   Replacement of blood loss during surgical procedures with blood collected in citrate phosphate dextrose solution. *N. Engl. J. Med.* 262:595–597, 1960.

708. Giebisch, G., Berger, L., and Pitts, R. F.   The extrarenal response to acute acid-base disturbances of respiratory origin. *J. Clin. Invest.* 34:231–245, 1955.

709. Gilbert, R., and Mullison, E.   A new self-inflating tracheostomy cuff of silicone rubber for use in patients requiring mechanical aid to ventilation. *Am. Rev. Respir. Dis.* 97:706–709, 1968.

710. Gilbert, R., Sipple, J. H., and Auchincloss, J. H., Jr.   Respiratory control and work of breathing in obese subjects. *J. Appl. Physiol.* 16:21–26, 1961.

711. Gilbert, R. P.   Mechanisms of the hemodynamic effects of endotoxin. *Physiol. Rev.* 40:245–279, 1960.

712. Gilbert, R. P., Honig, K. P., Griffin, J. A., Becker, R. J., and Adelson, B. H.   Hemodynamics of shock due to infection. *Stanford Med. Bull.* 13:239–246, 1955.

713. Gilder, H., and McSherry, C. K.   Mechanisms of oxygen inhibition of pulmonary surfactant synthesis. *Surgery* 76:72–79, 1974.

714. Gillies, R. R., and Govah, J. R. W.   Typing of *Pseudomonas pyocyanea* by pyocine production. *J. Pathol. Bacteriol.* 91:339–345, 1966.

715. Gilston, A.   Clinical assessment versus scientific measurement. *Crit. Care Med.* 1:331, 1973.

716. Ginsberg, M. D., Hedley-Whyte, E. T., and Richardson, E. P., Jr.   Hypoxic-ischemic leukoencephalopathy in man. *Arch. Neurol.* 33:5–14, 1976.

717. Giordano, J. M., Campbell, D. A., and Joseph, W. L.   The effect of intravenously administered albumin on dogs with pulmonary interstitial edema. *Surg. Gynecol. Obstet.* 137:593–596, 1973.

718. Giordano, J. M., Joseph, W. L., Klingenmaier, C. H., and Adkins, P. C.   The management of interstitial pulmonary edema. Significance of hypoproteinemia. *J. Thorac. Cardiovasc. Surg.* 64:739–744, 1972.

719. Glancy, D. L., Yarnell, P., and Roberts, W. C.   Traumatic left ventricular aneurysm. Cardiac thrombosis following aneurysmectomy. *Am. J. Cardiol.* 20:428–433, 1967.

720. Glauser, F. L., Wilson, A. F., Hoshiko, M., Watanabe, M., and Davis,

J.   Pulmonary parenchymal tissue (Vt) changes in pulmonary edema. *J. Appl. Physiol.* 36:648–652, 1974.

721. Glen, W. W. L., Holcomb, W. G., McLaughlin, A. J., O'Hare, J. M., Hogan, J. F., and Yasuda, R.   Total ventilatory support in a quadriplegic patient with radiofrequency electrophrenic respiration. *N. Engl. J. Med.* 286:513–516, 1972.

722. Glenn, T. M., and Lefer, A. M.   Role of lysosomes in the pathogenesis of splanchnic ischemic shock in cats. *Circ. Res.* 27:783–797, 1970.

723. Gocke, D. J.   A prospective study of posttransfusion hepatitis. The role of Australia antigen. *J.A.M.A.* 219:1165–1170, 1972.

724. Golbert, T. M., Sanz, C. J., Rose, H. D., and Leitschuh, T. H.   Comparative evaluation of treatments of alcohol withdrawal syndromes. *J.A.M.A.* 201:99–102, 1967.

725. Gold, H. K., Leinbach, R. C., Sanders, C. A., Buckley, M. J., Mundth, E. D., and Austen, W. G.   Intraaortic balloon pumping for ventricular septal defect or mitral regurgitation complicating acute myocardial infarction. *Circulation* 47:1191–1196, 1973.

726. Goldberg, I., and Cherniack, R. M.   The effect of nebulized bronchodilator delivered with and without IPPB on ventilatory function in chronic obstructive emphysema. *Am. Rev. Respir. Dis.* 91:13–20, 1965.

727. Goldberg, I. S., and Lourenço, R. V.   Deposition of aerosols in pulmonary disease. *Arch. Intern. Med.* 131:88–91, 1973.

728. Goldberg, L. I.   Dopamine—Clinical uses of an endogenous catecholamine. *N. Engl. J. Med.* 291:707–710, 1974.

729. Goldberg, L. I., McDonald, R. H., Jr., and Zimmerman, A. M.   Sodium diuresis produced by dopamine in patients with congestive heart failure. *N. Engl. J. Med.* 269:1060–1064, 1963.

730. Golden, M. S., Pinder, T., Jr., Anderson, W. T., and Cheitlin, M. D.   Fatal pulmonary hemorrhage complicating use of flow-directed balloon-tipped catheter in patient receiving anticoagulant therapy. *Am. J. Cardiol.* 32:865–867, 1973.

731. Golding, M. R., Martinez, A., deJong, P., Mendosa, M., Fries, C. C., Sawyer, P. N., Hennigar, G. R., and Wesolowski, S. A.   The role of sympathectomy in frostbite, with a review of 68 cases. *Surgery* 57:774–777, 1965.

732. Goldman, D. A., Martin, W. T., and Worthington, J. W.   Growth of bacteria and fungi in total parenteral nutrition solutions. *Am. J. Surg.* 126:314–318, 1973.

733. Goldman, R. H., and Harrison, D. C.   The effects of hypoxia and hypercarbia on myocardial catecholamines. *J. Pharmacol. Exp. Ther.* 174:307–314, 1970.

734. Goldsmith, J. R.   Carbon monoxide and coronary heart disease: Compelling evidence in angina pectoris. *Ann. Intern. Med.* 77:808–810, 1972.

735. Goldstein, E., Lippert, W., and Warshaver, D.   Pulmonary alveolar macrophage: Defender against bacterial infection of the lung. *J. Clin. Invest.* 54:519–528, 1974.

736. Gomes, M. M. R., and McGoon, D. C.   Bleeding patterns after open-heart surgery. *J. Thorac. Cardiovasc. Surg.* 60:87–97, 1970.

737. Goodman, A. A., and Frey, C. F.   Massive upper gastrointestinal hemorrhage following surgical operations. *Ann. Surg.* 167:180–184, 1968.

738. Goodman, J. R., Lim, R. C., Jr., Blaisdell, F. W., Hall, A. D., and Thomas, A. N.   Pulmonary microembolism in experimental shock. An electron microscopic study. *Am. J. Pathol.* 52:391–400, 1968.

739. Goodman, L. S., and Gilman, A., (Eds.) *The Pharmacological Basis of Therapeutics* (5th ed.). New York: Macmillan, 1975. Pp. 787–791.

740. Goodnight, S. H., Kenoyer, G., Rapaport, S. I., Patch, M. J., Lee, J. A., and Kurze, T. Defibrination after brain-tissue destruction: A serious complication of head injury. *N. Engl. J. Med.* 290:1043–1047, 1974.

741. Gorbach, S. L., and Barlett, J. G. Anaerobic infections. *N. Engl. J. Med.* 290:1177–1184, 1237–1245, 1289–1294, 1974.

742. Gordon, M. J., Skillman, J. J., Zervas, N. T., and Silen, W. Divergent nature of gastric mucosal permeability and gastric acid secretion in sick patients with general surgical and neurosurgical disease. *Ann. Surg.* 178:285–294, 1973.

743. Gotsman, M. S., and Schrire, V. A pericardiocentesis electrode needle. *Br. Heart J.* 28:566–569, 1966.

744. Gottschalk, P. G., and Thomas, J. E. Heat stroke. *Proc. Mayo Clin.* 41:470–482, 1966.

745. Gottschall, J., Osgood, R. W., Stein, J. H., and Ferris, T. F. Mechanism of the oliguria in a model of nephrotoxic acute renal failure in the dog. *J. Clin. Invest.* 53:29a, 1974.

746. Gould, A. B., Jr. Effect of obesity on respiratory complications following general anesthesia. *Anesth. Analg.* (Cleve.) 41:448–452, 1962.

747. Gould, V. E., Tosco, R., Wheelis, R. F., Gould, N. S., and Kapanci, Y. Oxygen pneumonitis in man. Ultrastructural observations on the development of alveolar lesions. *Lab. Invest.* 26:499–508, 1972.

748. Gould, V. E., Wheelis, R. F., and Gould, N. S. Ultrastructural observations on human oxygen pneumonitis. *Am. J. Pathol.* 62:49a, 1971.

749. Goulon, M., Gajdos, Ph., Raphael, J. C., Barois, A., Nouailhat, F., Dequirot, A., and Babinet, P. Successful Respiratory Support with R.P. Membrane Oxygenator—Report of Two Cases. Scientific abstracts, First World Congress on Intensive Care, London, England, June 24–27, 1974. P. 74.

750. Govindaraj, M. The effect of dehydration on the ventilatory capacity in normal subjects. *Am. Rev. Respir. Dis.* 105:842–844, 1972.

751. Granholm, L., and Siesjö, B. K. The effects of hypercapnia and hypocapnia upon the cerebrospinal fluid lactate and pyruvate concentrations and upon the lactate pyruvate, ATP, ADP, phosphocreatin and creatine concentrations of cat brain tissue. *Acta Physiol. Scand.* 75:257–266, 1969.

752. Graves, C. L., Stauffer, W. M., Klein, R. L., and Underwood, P. S. Aortic pulse contour calculation of cardiac output. *Anesthesiology* 29:580–584, 1968.

753. Graystone, P., and Towell, M. E. Electric shock hazard associated with pressure transducers. *Anesthesiology* 34:79–80, 1971.

754. Green, D., Seeler, R. A., Allen, N., and Alavi, I. A. The role of heparin in the management of consumption coagulopathy. *Med. Clin. North Am.* 56:193–200, 1972.

755. Green, G. M., and Carolin, D. The depressant effect of cigarette smoke on the in vitro antibacterial activity of alveolar macrophages. *N. Engl. J. Med.* 276:421–427, 1967.

756. Green, G. M., and Kass, E. H. The role of alveolar macrophage in the clearance of bacteria from the lung. *J. Exp. Med.* 119:167–176, 1964.

757. Greenberg, M., and Childress, J. Vaccination against rabies with duck-embryo and Semple vaccines. *J.A.M.A.* 173:333–337, 1960.

758. Greene, H. L., and Nemir, P., Jr. Air embolism as a complication during parenteral alimentation. *Am. J. Surg.* 121:614–616, 1971.

759. Greene, J. F., Jr., and Cummings, K. C. Aseptic thrombotic endocardial vegetations. A complication of indwelling pulmonary artery catheters. *J.A.M.A.* 225:1525–1526, 1973.

760. Greene, N. M. Fatal cardiovascular and respiratory failure associated with tracheostomy. *N. Engl. J. Med.* 261:846–848, 1959.

761. Greene, R., Hoop, B., and Kazemi, H. Use of ^{13}N in studies of airway closure and regional ventilation. *J. Nucl. Med.* 12:719–723, 1971.

762. Greene, W. H., Moody, M., Schimpff, S., Young, V. M., and Wiernik, P. H. *Pseudomonas aeruginosa* resistant to carbenicillin and gentamicin. Epidemiologic and clinical aspects in a cancer center. *Ann. Intern. Med.* 79:684–689, 1973.

763. Greenfield, J. C., Jr., and Tindall, G. T. Effect of acute increase in intracranial pressure on blood flow in the internal carotid artery of man. *J. Clin. Invest.* 44:1343–1351, 1965.

764. Greenfield, L. J., Ebert, P. A., and Benson, D. W. Effect of positive pressure ventilation on surface tension properties of lung extracts. *Anesthesiology* 25:312–316, 1964.

765. Greenfield, L. J., Singleton, R. P., McCaffree, D. R., and Coalson, J. J. Pulmonary effects of experimental graded aspiration of hydrochloric acid. *Ann. Surg.* 170:74–86, 1969.

766. Greenfield, S., Teres, D., Bushnell, L. S., Hedley-Whyte, J., and Feingold, D. S. Prevention of gram-negative bacillary pneumonia using aerosol polymyxin as prophylaxis. I. Effect on the colonization pattern of the upper respiratory tract of seriously ill patients. *J. Clin. Invest.* 52:2935–2940, 1973.

767. Greenspan, M., and Del Guercio, L. R. M. Cardiorespiratory determinants of survival in cirrhotic patients requiring surgery for portal hypertension. *Am. J. Surg.* 115:43–56, 1968.

768. Gregory, E. M., and Fridovich, I. Oxygen toxicity and the superoxide dismutase. *J. Bacteriol.* 114:1193–1197, 1973.

769. Greifenstein, F. E., King, R. M., Latch, S. S., and Comroe, J. H., Jr. Pulmonary function studies in healthy men and women 50 years and older. *J. Appl. Physiol.* 4:641–648, 1951.

770. Grenvik, A. Respiratory, circulatory and metabolic effects of respirator treatment. A clinical study in postoperative thoracic surgical patients. *Acta Anaesthesiol. Scand.* [Suppl.] 19:1–122, 1966.

771. Grenvik, A., Orr, M., Smith, J., and Van Horn, G. Evaluation and Management of Brain Dead Patients. Scientific abstracts, First World Congress on Intensive Care, London, England, June 24–27, 1974. P. 100.

772. Grieble, H. G., Colton, F. R., Bird, T. J., Toigo, A., and Griffith, L. G. Fine-particle humidifiers: Source of *Pseudomonas aeruginosa* infections in a respiratory-disease unit. *N. Engl. J. Med.* 282:531–535, 1970.

773. Griffo, Z. J., and Roos, A. Effect of O_2 breathing on pulmonary compliance. *J. Appl. Physiol.* 17:233–238, 1962.

774. Grillo, H. C. Obstructive lesions of the trachea. *Ann. Otol. Rhinol. Laryngol.* 82:770–777, 1973.

775. Grillo, H. C., Cooper, J. D., Geffin, B., and Pontoppidan, H. A low-pressure cuff for tracheostomy tubes to minimize tracheal injury. A comparative clinical trial. *J. Thorac. Cardiovasc. Surg.* 62:898–907, 1971.

776. Groen, G. P. Uterine rupture in rural Nigeria. Review of 144 cases. *Obstet. Gynecol.* 44:682–687, 1974.

777. Grover, R. F., and Reeves, J. T. Loss of hypoxic pulmonary vasoconstriction in dogs given small amounts of endotoxin. *Chest* 65(Suppl.):50S–51S, 1974.

778. Guenter, C. A., Fiorica, V., and Hinshaw, L. B. Cardiorespiratory and metabolic responses to live *E. coli* and endotoxin in the monkey. *J. Appl. Physiol.* 26:780–786, 1969.

779. Guenter, C. A., and Hinshaw, L. B. Hemodynamic and respiratory effects of dopamine on septic shock in the monkey. *Am. J. Physiol.* 219:335–339, 1970.

780. Guenter, C. A., and Hinshaw, L. B. Comparison of septic shock due to gram-negative and gram-positive organisms. *Proc. Soc. Exp. Biol. Med.* 134:780–783, 1970.

781. Guiha, N. H., Cohn, J. N., Mikulic, E., Franciosa, J. A., and Limas, C. J. Treatment of refractory heart failure with infusion of nitroprusside. *N. Engl. J. Med.* 291:587–592, 1974.

782. Gump, F. E., Martin, P., and Kinney, J. M. Oxygen consumption and caloric expenditure in surgical patients. *Surg. Gynecol. Obstet.* 137:499–513, 1973.

783. Gump, F. E., Price, J. B., Jr., and Kinney, J. M. Whole body and splanchnic blood flow and oxygen consumption measurements in patients with intraperitoneal infection. *Ann. Surg.* 171:321–328, 1970.

784. Gunnar, R. M., Loeb, H. S., Winslow, E. J., Blain, C., and Robinson, J. Hemodynamic measurements in bacteremia and septic shock in man. *J. Infect. Dis.* 128(Suppl.):295S–298S, 1973.

785. Guyton, A. C., Farish, C. A., and Williams, J. W. An improved arteriovenous oxygen difference recorder. *J. Appl. Physiol.* 14:145–147, 1959.

786. Guyton, A. C., Jones, C. E., and Coleman, T. G. *Circulatory Physiology: Cardiac Output and Its Regulation.* Philadelphia: Saunders, 1973. Pp. 21–137.

787. Guyton, A. C., and Lindsey, A. W. Effect of elevated left atrial pressure and decreased plasma protein concentration on the development of pulmonary edema. *Circ. Res.* 7:649–657, 1959.

788. Haberman, P. B., Green, J. P., Archibald, C., Dunn, D. L., Hurwitz, S. R., Ashburn, W. L., and Moser, K. M. Determinants of successful selective tracheobronchial suctioning. *N. Engl. J. Med.* 289:1060–1063, 1973.

789. Hackney, J. D., Crane, M. G., Collier, C. C., Rokaw, S., and Griggs, D. E. Syndrome of extreme obesity and hypoventilation: Studies of etiology. *Ann. Intern. Med.* 51:541–552, 1959.

790. Hadden, J., Johnson, K., Smith, S., Price, L., and Giardina, E. Acute barbiturate intoxication: Concepts of management. *J.A.M.A.* 209:893–900, 1969.

791. Haldane, J. B. S. The dissociation of oxyhaemoglobin in human blood during partial CO poisoning. *J. Physiol.* (Lond.) 45:xxii–xxiv, 1912–1913.

792. Hales, C. A., and Kazemi, H. Small-airways function in myocardial infarction. *N. Engl. J. Med.* 290:761–765, 1974.

793. Hall, C. C. Aspiration pneumonitis: An obstetric hazard. *J.A.M.A.* 114:728–733, 1940.

794. Hall, R. J. C., Young, C., Sutton, G. C., and Cambell, S. Treatment of acute massive pulmonary embolism by streptokinase during labour and delivery. *Br. Med. J.* 4:647–649, 1972.

795. Hall, S. V., Johnson, E. E., and Hedley-Whyte, J. Renal hemodynamics and function with continous positive-pressure ventilation in dogs. *Anesthesiology* 41:452–461, 1974.

796. Hallberg, D., Holm, I., Obel, A. L., Schuberth, O., and Wretlind, A. Fat emulsions for complete intravenous nutrition. *Postgrad. Med. J.* 43:307–316, 1967.

797. Hallowell, P., Bland, J. H. L., Buckley, M. J., and Lowenstein, E. Transfusion of fresh autologous blood in open-heart surgery. A method for reducing bank blood requirements. *J. Thorac. Cardiovasc. Surg.* 64:941–948, 1972.

798. Halmagyi, D. F. J. Lung changes and incidence of respiratory arrest in rats after aspiration of sea and fresh water. *J. Appl. Physiol.* 16:41–44, 1961.

799. Halmagyi, D. F. J., and Colebatch, H. J. H. Ventilation and circulation after fluid aspiration. *J. Appl. Physiol.* 16:35–40, 1961.

800. Halmagyi, D. F. J., Colebatch, H. J. H., and Starzecki, B. Inhalation of blood, saliva, and alcohol: Consequences, mechanism and treatment. *Thorax* 17:244–250, 1962.

801. Halmagyi, D. F. J., Colebatch, H. J. H., Starzecki, B., and Horner, G. J.   Pulmonary alveolar-vascular reflex. *J. Appl. Physiol.* 19:105–112, 1964.

802. Hamelberg, W., and Bosomworth, P. P.   Aspiration pneumonitis: Experimental studies and clinical observations. *Anesth. Analg.* (Cleve.) 43:669–676, 1964.

803. Hamilton, W. K.   Atelectasis, pneumothorax, and aspiration as postoperative complications. *Anesthesiology* 22:708–722, 1961.

804. Hamilton, W. K., McDonald, J. S., Fischer, H. W., and Bethards, R.   Post operative respiratory complications: A comparison of arterial gas tensions, radiographs, and physical examination. *Anesthesiology* 25:607–612, 1964.

805. Hamilton, W. M., and Nemir, P., Jr.   The humoral factor in pulmonary embolism. *Arch. Surg.* 105:593–598, 1972.

806. Hammond, E. C.   Evidence on the effects of giving up cigarette smoking. *Am. J. Public Health* 55:682–691, 1965.

807. Hammond, E. C., Auerbach, O., Kirman, D., and Garfinkel, L.   Effects of cigarette smoking in dogs. *Arch. Environ. Health* 21:740–753, 1970.

808. Hansen, A. R., Kennedy, K. A., Ambre, J. J., and Fischer, L. J.   Glutethimide poisoning: A metabolite contributes to morbidity and mortality. *N. Engl. J. Med.* 292:250–252, 1975.

809. Hanson, J. S.   Exercise responses following production of experimental obesity. *J. Appl. Physiol.* 35:587–591, 1973.

810. Harbert, G. M., Jr., Claiborne, H. A., McGaughey, H. S., Wilson, L. A., and Thornton, W. N.   Convulsive toxemia. A report of 168 cases managed conservatively. *Am. J. Obstet. Gynecol.* 100:336–342, 1968.

811. Hardaker, W. T., Jr., and Wechsler, A. S.   Redistribution of renal intracortical blood flow during dopamine infusion in dogs. *Circ. Res.* 33:437–444, 1973.

812. Hardaway, R. M., III.   *Syndromes of Disseminated Intravascular Coagulation with Special Reference to Shock and Hemorrhage.* Springfield, Ill.: Thomas, 1966.

813. Hardaway, R. M., III.   Disseminated intravascular coagulation in experimental and clinical shock. *Am. J. Cardiol.* 20:161–173, 1967.

814. Hardaway, R. M., III.   Disseminated intravascular coagulation as a possible cause of acute respiratory failure. *Surg. Gynecol. Obstet.* 137:419–423, 1973.

815. Hardaway, R. M., III.   Acute respiratory failure and disseminated intravascular coagulation. *Crit. Care Med.* 2:40, 1974.

816. Harjola, P.-T., and Sivula, A.   Gastric ulceration following experimentally induced hypoxia and hemorrhagic shock: In vivo study of pathogenesis in rabbits. *Ann. Surg.* 163:21–28, 1966.

817. Harken, A. H., and Smith, R. M.   Aortic pressure versus Doppler-measured peripheral arterial pressure. *Anesthesiology* 38:184–186, 1973.

818. Harker, L. A., and Slichter, S. J.   Platelet and fibrinogen consumption in man. *N. Engl. J. Med.* 287:999–1005, 1972.

819. Harlan, W. R.   Gram-negative sepsis: Another piece of the mosaic. *N. Engl. J. Med.* 281:1127–1128, 1969.

820. Harp, J. R.   Criteria for the determination of death. *Anesthesiology* 40:391–397, 1974.

821. Harp, J. R., Wyche, M. Q., Marshall, B. E., and Wurzel, H. A.   Some factors determining rate of microaggregate formation in stored blood. *Anesthesiology* 40:398–400, 1974.

822. Harrington, R. B., and Olin, R.   Incomplete transverse myelitis following rabies duck embryo vaccination. *J.A.M.A.* 216:2137–2138, 1971.

823. Harris, J. O., Swenson, E. W., and Johnson, J. E., III.   Human alveolar

macrophages: Comparison of phagocytic ability, glucose utilization and ultrastructure in smokers and nonsmokers. *J. Clin. Invest.* 49:2086–2096, 1970.

824. Harrison, H. N. Respiratory tract injury, pathophysiology and response to therapy among burned patients. *Ann. N.Y. Acad. Sci.* 150:627–638, 1968.

825. Harrison, L. H., Beller, J. J., Hinshaw, L. B., Coalson, J. J., and Greenfield, L. J. Effects of endotoxin on pulmonary capillary permeability, ultrastructure, and surfactant. *Surg. Gynecol. Obstet.* 129:723–733, 1969.

826. Harrison, W. H., Jr., Gray, A. R., Couves, C. M., and Howard, J. M. Severe non-penetrating injuries to the chest. Clinical results in the management of 216 patients. *Am. J. Surg.* 100:715–722, 1960.

827. Hass, W. K., Siew, F. P., and Yee, D.-J. Progress in adaptation of mass spectrometer to study of human cerebral blood flow. *Circulation* 37, 38(Suppl. VI):96, 1968.

828. Hattwick, M. A. W., Weis, T. T., Stechschulte, C. J., Baer, G. M., and Gregg, M. B. Recovery from rabies: A case report. *Ann. Intern. Med.* 76:931–942, 1972.

829. Haugaard, N. Poisoning of cellular reactions by oxygen. *Ann. N.Y. Acad. Sci.* 117:736–744, 1965.

830. Haugaard, N. Cellular mechanics of oxygen toxicity. *Physiol. Rev.* 48:311–373, 1968.

831. Hausmann, W., and Lunt, R. L. The problem of the treatment of peptic aspiration pneumonia following obstetric anaesthesia (Mendelson's syndrome). *J. Obstet. Gynaecol. Br. Commonw.* 62:509–512, 1955.

832. Havard, C. W. H. Progress in myasthenia gravis. *Br. Med. J.* 3:437–440, 1973.

833. Hawiger, J., Niewiarowski, S., Gurewich, V., and Thomas, D. P. Measurement of fibrinogen and fibrin degradation products in serum by staphylococcal clumping test. *J. Lab. Clin. Med.* 75:93–108, 1970.

834. Hawker, R. E., and Celermajer, J. M. Comparison of pulmonary artery and pulmonary venous wedge pressure in congenital heart disease. *Br. Heart J.* 35:386–391, 1973.

835. Hayes, B., and Robinson, J. S. An assessment of methods of humidification of inspired gas. *Br. J. Anaesth.* 42:94–104, 1970.

836. Hayes, M. F., Jr., Morello, D. C., Rosenbaum, R. W., and Matsumoto, T. Radial artery catheterization by cutdown technique. *Crit. Care Med.* 1:151–152, 1973.

837. Hayes, M. F., Jr., Rosenbaum, R. W., Zibelman, M., and Matsumoto, T. Adult respiratory distress syndrome in association with acute pancreatitis. Evaluation of positive end expiratory pressure ventilation and pharmacologic doses of steroids. *Am. J. Surg.* 127:314–319, 1974.

838. Haymaker, W. R., and Kernohan, J. W. The Landry-Guillain-Barré syndrome. A clinicopathologic report of fifty fatal cases and a critique of the literature. *Medicine* 28:59–141, 1949.

839. Hayne, O. A., and Sherman, L. A. In vivo behavior of fibrinogen fragment D in experimental renal, hepatic and reticuloendothelial dysfunction. *Am. J. Pathol.* 71:219–237, 1973.

840. Hedden, M., Ersoz, C. J., Donnelly, W. H., and Safar, P. Laryngotracheal damage after prolonged use of orotracheal tubes in adults. *J.A.M.A.* 207:703–708, 1969.

841. Hedden, M., Ersoz, C. J., and Safar, P. Tracheoesophageal fistulas following prolonged artificial ventilation via cuffed tracheostomy tubes. *Anesthesiology* 31:281–289, 1969.

842. Hedden, M., and Miller, G. J. Mendelson's syndrome and its sequelae. *Can. Anaesth. Soc. J.* 19:351–359, 1972.

843. Hedley-Whyte, A. Acute cholecystitis. *Practitioner* 192:753–758, 1964.

844. Hedley-Whyte, E. T., and Craighead, J. E. Generalized cytomegalic inclusion disease after renal homotransplantation. Report of a case with isolation of virus. *N. Engl. J. Med.* 272:473–475, 1965.

845. Hedley-Whyte, J. Control of the uptake of oxygen. *N. Engl. J. Med.* 279:1152–1158, 1968.

846. Hedley-Whyte, J. Causes of pulmonary oxygen toxicity. *N. Engl. J. Med.* 283:1518–1519, 1970.

847. Hedley-Whyte, J., Berry, P., Bushnell, L. S., Darrah, H. K., and Morris, M. J. Effect of Posture on Respiratory Failure. In T. B. Boulton, R. Bryce-Smith, M. K. Sykes, G. B. Gillett, and A. L. Revell (Eds.), *Progress in Anaesthesiology, Proceedings of the Fourth World Congress of Anaesthesiologists, London, England, September 9–13, 1968*. International Congress Series No. 200. Amsterdam: Excerpta Medica, 1970. Pp. 1095–1103.

848. Hedley-Whyte, J., Corning, H., Laver, M. B., Austen, W. G., and Bendixen, H. H. Pulmonary ventilation-perfusion relations after heart valve replacement or repair in man. *J. Clin. Invest.* 44:406–416, 1965.

849. Hedley-Whyte, J., and Laasberg, L. H. Ethchlorvynol poisoning: Gas liquid chromatography in management. *Anesthesiology* 30:107–111, 1969.

850. Hedley-Whyte, J., and Laver, M. B. O_2 solubility in blood and temperature correction factors for P_{O_2}. *J. Appl. Physiol.* 19:901–906, 1964.

851. Hedley-Whyte, J., Laver, M. B., and Bendixen, H. H. Effect of changes in tidal ventilation on physiologic shunting. *Am. J. Physiol.* 206:891–897, 1964.

852. Hedley-Whyte, J., Morris, M. J., Darrah, H. K., Berry, P., Frank, N. R., and Woo, S. W. The effect of age on lung mechanics and ventilation-perfusion relations in respiratory failure. *Anesthesiology* 29:196–197, 1968.

853. Hedley-Whyte, J., Pontoppidan, H., Laver, M. B., Hallowell, P., and Bendixen, H. H. Arterial oxygenation during hypothermia. *Anesthesiology* 26:595–602, 1965.

854. Hedley-Whyte, J., Pontoppidan, H., and Morris, M. J. The relation of alveolar to tidal ventilation during respiratory failure in man. *Anesthesiology* 27:218–219, 1966.

855. Hedley-Whyte, J., Pontoppidan, H., and Morris, M. J. The response of patients with respiratory failure and cardiopulmonary disease to different levels of constant volume ventilation. *J. Clin. Invest.* 45:1543–1554, 1966.

856. Hedley-Whyte, J., Radford, E. P., Jr., and Laver, M. B. Nomogram for temperature correction or electrode calibration during P_{O_2} measurements. *J. Appl. Physiol.* 20:785–786, 1965.

857. Hedley-Whyte, J., and Winter, P. Oxygen therapy. *Clin. Pharmacol. Ther.* 8:696–737, 1967.

858. Heimbecker, R. O., Lemire, G., and Chen, C. Surgery for massive myocardial infarction. An experimental study of emergency infarctectomy with a preliminary report on the clinical application. *Circulation* 37, 38(Suppl. II):3–11, 1968.

859. Heinemann, H. O., and Fishman, A. P. Non-respiratory functions of the mammalian lung. *Physiol. Rev.* 49:1–47, 1969.

860. Heird, W. C., Dell, R. B., Driscoll, J. M., Jr., Grebin, B., and Winters, R. W. Metabolic acidosis resulting from intravenous alimentation mixtures containing synthetic amino acids. *N. Engl. J. Med.* 287:943–948, 1972.

861. Held, J. R., Tierkel, E. S., and Steele, J. H. Rabies in man and animals in the United States, 1946–1965. *Public Health Rep.* 82:1009–1018, 1967.

862. Helfant, R. H., Scherlag, B. J., and Damato, A. N. Diphenylhydantoin prevention of arrhythmias in the digitalis-sensitized dog after direct-current cardioversion. *Circulation* 37:424–428, 1968.

863. Hellman, E. S., Tschudy, D. P., and Bartter, F. C.   Abnormal electrolyte and water metabolism in acute intermittent porphyria. The transient inappropriate secretion of antidiuretic hormone. *Am. J. Med.* 32:734–746, 1962.

864. Helvey, W. M.   A problem of man and milieu: Prolonged exposure to pure oxygen. *Fed. Proc.* 22:1057–1059, 1963.

865. Henry, J. N., McArdle, A. H., Scott, H. J., and Gurd, F. N.   A study of the acute and chronic respiratory pathophysiology of hemorrhagic shock. *J. Thorac. Cardiovasc. Surg.* 54:666–678, 1967.

866. Hermreck, A. S., and Thal, A. P.   Mechanisms for the high circulatory requirements in sepsis and septic shock. *Ann. Surg.* 170:677–694, 1969.

867. Hershey, S. G., and Altura, B. M.   Function of the reticuloendothelial system in experimental shock and combined injury. *Anesthesiology* 30:138–143, 1969.

868. Hershey, S. G., Altura, B. M., and Altura, B. T.   Influence of Hydrocortisone and Methylprednisolone on Survival and Reticuloendothelial System Function after Induction of Hemorrhage and Bowel Ischemic Shock. Abstracts of scientific papers, Annual Meeting of the American Society of Anesthesiologists, Washington, D.C., October 12–16, 1974. P. 119.

869. Hershey, S. G., Del Guercio, L. R. M., and McConn, R. (Eds.).   *Septic Shock in Man.* Boston: Little, Brown, 1971.

870. Hewitt, R. L., Smith, A. D., Jr., Weichert, R. F., III, and Drapanas, T.   Penetrating cardiac injuries: Current trends in management. *Arch. Surg.* 101:683–688, 1970.

871. Hibbard, L. T.   Maternal mortality due to acute toxemia. *Obstet. Gynecol.* 42:263–270, 1973.

872. Higgs, B. E.   Factors influencing pulmonary gas exchange during the acute stages of myocardial infarction. *Clin. Sci.* 35:115–122, 1968.

873. Higgs, R. H., Smyth, R. D., and Castell, D. O.   Gastric alkalinization: Effect on lower-esophageal-sphincter pressure and serum gastrin. *N. Engl. J. Med.* 291:486–490, 1974.

874. Hilding, A. C.   Laryngotracheal damage during intratracheal anesthesia. Demonstration by staining the unfixed specimen with methylene blue. *Ann. Otol. Rhinol. Laryngol.* 80:565–581, 1971.

875. Hill, A. V.   *Living Machinery.* New York: Harcourt Brace Jovanovich, 1927.

876. Hill, D. W.   *Electronic Techniques in Anaesthesia and Surgery* (2nd ed.). London: Butterworth, 1973. Chaps. 1, 5.

877. Hill, J. D.   Blood filtration during extracorporeal circulation. *Ann. Thorac. Surg.* 15:313–316, 1973.

878. Hill, J. D., Aguilar, M. J., Baranco, A., de Lanerolle, P., and Gerbode, F.   Neuropathological manifestations of cardiac surgery. *Ann. Thorac. Surg.* 7:409–417, 1969.

879. Hill, J. D., deLeval, M. R., Dontigny, L., Bramson, M. L., Osborn, J. J., and Gerbode, F.   Clinical prolonged extracorporeal circulation for respiratory insufficiency. *Transplant. Proc.* 3:1437–1443, 1971.

880. Hill, J. D., deLeval, M. R., Fallat, R. J., Bramson, M. L., Eberhart, R. C., Schulte, H. D., Osborn, J. J., Barber, R., and Gerbode, F.   Acute respiratory insufficiency. Treatment with prolonged extracorporeal oxygenation. *J. Thorac. Cardiovasc. Surg.* 64:551–562, 1972.

881. Hill, J. D., deLeval, M. R., Mielke, C. H., Jr., Bramson, M. L., and Gerbode, F.   Clinical prolonged extracorporeal circulation for respiratory insufficiency: Hematological effects. *Trans. Am. Soc. Artif. Intern. Organs* 18:546–552, 1972.

882. Hill, J. D., Dontigny, L., deLeval, M. R., and Mielke, C. H., Jr.   A simple method of heparin management during prolonged extracorporeal circulation. *Ann. Thorac. Surg.* 17:129–134, 1974.

883. Hill, J. D., Fallat, R., Cohn, K., Eberhart, R., Dontigny, L., Bramson, M. L., Osborn, J. J., and Gerbode, F.   Clinical cardiopulmonary dynamics during prolonged extracorporeal circulation for acute respiratory insufficiency. *Trans. Am. Soc. Artif. Intern. Organs* 17:355–361, 1971.

884. Hill, J. D., O'Brien, T. G., Murray, J. J., Dontigny, L., Bramson, M. L., Osborn, J. J., and Gerbode, F.   Prolonged extracorporeal oxygenation for acute post-traumatic respiratory failure (shock-lung syndrome). *N. Engl. J. Med.* 286:629–634, 1972.

885. Hill, J. D., Osborn, J. J., Swank, R. L., Aguilar, M. J., deLanerolle, P., and Gerbode, F.   Experience using a new Dacron wool filter during extracorporeal circulation. *Arch. Surg.* 101:649–652, 1970.

886. Hill, L. B.   Injuries of the diaphragm following blunt trauma. *Surg. Clin. North Am.* 52:611–624, 1972.

887. Hill, R. B., Jr., Rowlands, D. T., Jr., and Rifkind, D.   Infectious pulmonary disease in patients receiving immunosuppressive therapy for organ transplantation. *N. Engl. J. Med.* 271:1021–1027, 1964.

888. Hillen, G. P., Gaisford, W. D., and Jensen, C. G.   Pulmonary changes in treated and untreated hemorrhagic shock. I. Early functional and ultrastructural alterations after moderate shock. *Am. J. Surg.* 122:639–649, 1971.

889. Hills, N. H., Pflug, J. J., Jeyasingh, K., Boardman, L., and Calnan, J. S.   Prevention of deep vein thrombosis by intermittent pneumatic compression of calf. *Br. Med. J.* 1:131–135, 1972.

890. Himmelhoch, S. R., Dekker, A., Gazzaniga, A. B., and Like, A. A.   Closed-chest cardiac resuscitation. A prospective clinical and pathological study. *N. Engl. J. Med.* 270:118–122, 1964.

891. Hinkle, J. E., and Cooperman, L. H.   Serum ionized calcium changes following citrated blood transfusion in anaesthetized man. *Br. J. Anaesth.* 43:1108–1112, 1971.

892. Hinkle, J. E., and Tantum, K. R.   A technique for measuring reactivity of the glottis. *Anesthesiology* 35:634–637, 1971.

893. Hinshaw, L. B., Emerson, T. E., Jr., and Reins, D. A.   Cardiovascular responses of the primate in endotoxin shock. *Am. J. Physiol.* 210:335–340, 1966.

894. Hinshaw, L. B., Greenfield, L. J., Owen, S. E., Archer, L. T., and Guenter, C. A.   Cardiac response to circulating factors in endotoxin shock. *Am. J. Physiol.* 222:1047–1053, 1972.

895. Hinshaw, L. B., Jordan, M. M., and Vick, J. A.   Histamine release and endotoxin shock in the primate. *J. Clin. Invest.* 40:1631–1637, 1961.

896. Hirshch, H., Swank, R. L., Breuer, M., and Hissen, W.   Screen filtration pressure of homologous and heterologous blood and electroencephalogram. *Am. J. Physiol.* 206:811–814, 1964.

897. Hirsch, J.   Jejunoileal shunt for obesity. *N. Engl. J. Med.* 290:962–963, 1974.

898. Hirsheimer, A., January, D. A., and Daversa, J. J.   An x-ray study of gastric function during labor. *Am. J. Obstet. Gynecol.* 36:671–673, 1938.

899. Hissen, W., and Swank, R. L.   Screen filtration pressure and pulmonary hypertension. *Am. J. Physiol.* 209:715–722, 1965.

900. Hites, R. A.   Computer Recording and Processing of Mass Spectra. Ph.D. thesis, Massachusetts Institute of Technology, Cambridge, Mass., 1968.

901. Hites, R. A., and Biemann, K.   Mass spectrometer-computer system particularly suited for gas chromatography of complex mixtures. *Anal. Chem.* 40:1217–1221, 1968.

902. Hlastala, M. P., Wranne, B., and Lenfant, C. J.   Cyclical variations in FRC and other respiratory variables in resting man. *J. Appl. Physiol.* 34:670–676, 1973.

903. Hobsley, M., and Silen, W. An Improved Procedure for the Continuous Sampling of Gastric Juice. Its Use to Study Effect of Arterial CO_2 Tension Changes on Gastric Secretory Activity. *Proceedings of the Third World Congress of Gastroenterology: Recent Advances in Gastroenterology, Tokyo, 1967.* Pp. 391–394.

904. Hodges, G. R., Fink, J. N., and Schlueter, D. P. Hypersensitivity pneumonitis caused by a contaminated cool-mist vaporizer. *Ann. Intern. Med.* 80:501–504, 1974.

905. Hodges, M., Downs, J. B., and Mitchell, L. A. Thermodilution and Fick cardiac index determinations following cardiac surgery. *Crit. Care Med.* 3:182–184, 1975.

906. Hodgkin, J. E., Bowser, M. A., and Burton, G. G. Respirator weaning. *Crit. Care Med.* 2:96–102, 1974.

907. Hodgkinson, C. P., and Nufeld, J. Premature separation of the normally implanted placenta. *Clin. Obstet. Gynecol.* 3:585–598, 1960.

908. Hogg, J. C., Agarawal, J. B., Gardiner, A. J. S., Palmer, W. H., and Macklem, P. T. Distribution of airway resistance with developing pulmonary edema in dogs. *J. Appl. Physiol.* 32:20–24, 1972.

909. Holcroft, J. W., and Trunkey, D. D. Extravascular lung water following hemorrhagic shock in the baboon: Comparison between resuscitation with Ringer's lactate and Plasmanate. *Ann. Surg.* 180:408–415, 1974.

910. Holden, W. D., Krieger, H., Levey, S., and Abbott, W. E. The effect of nutrition on nitrogen metabolism in the surgical patient. *Ann. Surg.* 146:563–577, 1957.

911. Holland, J., Milic-Emili, J., Macklem, P. T., and Bates, D. V. Regional distribution of pulmonary ventilation and perfusion in elderly subjects. *J. Clin. Invest.* 47:81–92, 1968.

912. Hollenberg, N. K., Epstein, M., Guttman, R. D., Conroy, M., Basch, R. I., and Merrill, J. P. Effect of sodium balance on intrarenal distribution of blood flow in normal man. *J. Appl. Physiol.* 28:312–317, 1970.

913. Holley, H. S., Milic-Emili, J., Becklake, M. R., and Bates, D. V. Regional distribution of pulmonary ventilation and perfusion in obesity. *J. Clin. Invest.* 46:475–481, 1967.

914. Hollmén, A., and Saukkonen, J. The effects of postoperative epidural analgesia versus centrally acting opiate on physiological shunt after upper abdominal operation. *Acta Anaesthesiol. Scand.* 16:147–154, 1972.

915. Holloway, R., Desai, S. D., Kelly, S. D., Thambiran, A. K., Strydom, S. E., and Adams, E. B. The effect of chest physiotherapy on the arterial oxygenation of neonates during treatment of tetanus by intermittent positive-pressure respiration. *S. Afr. Med. J.* 40:445–447, 1966.

916. Holt, J. H., and Branscomb, B. V. Hemodynamic responses to controlled 100% oxygen breathing in emphysema. *J. Appl. Physiol.* 20:215–220, 1965.

917. Holt, M. H. Central venous pressures via peripheral veins. *Anesthesiology* 28:1093–1095, 1967.

918. Holzbach, R. T., Wieland, R. G., Leiber, C. S., DeCarli, L. M., Koepke, K. R., and Green, S. G. Hepatic lipid in morbid obesity: Assessment at and subsequent to jejunoileal bypass. *N. Engl. J. Med.* 290:296–299, 1974.

919. Holzer, J., Karliner, J. S., O'Rourke, R. A., Pitt, W., and Ross, J., Jr. Effectiveness of dopamine in patients with cardiogenic shock. *Am. J. Cardiol.* 32:79–84, 1973.

920. Hood, R. M., and Sloan, H. E. Injuries of the trachea and major bronchi. *J. Thorac. Cardiovasc. Surg.* 38:458–477, 1959.

921. Hopkins, R. W., Pauly, R. P., Peters, T. E., and Simeone, F. A. Effects of levarterenol on blood flow in inflammation. *Arch. Surg.* 97:1032–1038, 1968.

922. Hopkins, R. W., Sabga, G., Penn, I., and Simeone, F. A. Hemodynamic aspects of hemorrhagic and septic shock. *J.A.M.A.* 191:731–735, 1965.

923. Horn, R. S., Haugaard, E. S., and Haugaard, N. The mechanism of the inhibition of glycolysis by oxygen in rat heart homogenate. *Biochim. Biophys. Acta* 99:549–552, 1965.

924. Horovitz, J. H., Carrico, C. J., and Shires, G. T. Pulmonary response to major injury. *Arch. Surg.* 108:349–355, 1974.

925. Horster, M., and Thurau, K. Micropuncture studies on the filtration rate of single superficial and juxtamedullary glomeruli in the rat kidney. *Pfluegers Arch.* 301:162–181, 1968.

926. Horton, J. M., and Lewin, W. S. Controlled Ventilation in the Management of Severe Head Injuries. In A. Arias, R. Llaurado, M. A. Nalda, and J. N. Lunn (Eds.), *Abstracts, Fourth European Congress of Anesthesiology, Madrid, Spain, September 5–11, 1974.* International Congress Series No. 330. Amsterdam: Excerpta Medica, 1974. P. 206.

927. Horton, J. M., and Lewin, W. S. Controlled Ventilation in the Management of Severe Head Injuries. Scientific abstracts, First World Congress on Intensive Care, London, England, June 24–27, 1974. P. 82.

928. Horwitz, D. L., Ballantine, T. V. N., and Herman, C. M. Acute effects of septic shock on plasma and red cell volumes in baboons. *J. Appl. Physiol.* 33:320–324, 1972.

929. Housley, E., Louzada, N., and Becklake, M. R. To sigh or not to sigh. *Am. Rev. Respir. Dis.* 101:611–614, 1970.

930. Howland, W. S., Schweizer, O., and Gould, P. A comparison of intraoperative measurements of coagulation. *Anesth. Analg.* (Cleve.) 53:657–663, 1974.

931. Hoye, R. C., Bennett, S. H., Geelhoed, G. W., and Gorschboth, C. Fluid volume and albumin kinetics occurring with major surgery. *J.A.M.A.* 222:1255–1261, 1972.

932. Hoye, R. C., and Ketcham, A. S. Shifts in body fluids during radical surgery. *Cancer* 20:1827–1831, 1967.

933. Hoye, R. C., Paulson, D. F., and Ketcham, A. S. Total circulating albumin deficits occurring with extensive surgical procedures. *Surg. Gynecol. Obstet.* 131:943–952, 1970.

934. Hsu, C.-T., Huang, P.-W., and Lin, C.-T. A term delivery complicated by spontaneous pneumothorax. Report of a case. *Obstet. Gynecol.* 14:527–529, 1959.

935. Huang, C. T., Cook, A. W., and Lyons, H. A. Severe craniocerebral trauma and respiratory abnormalities. I. Physiological studies with specific reference to effect of tracheostomy on survival. *Arch. Neurol.* 9:545–554, 1963.

936. Huber, G., LaForce, M., and Mason, R. Impairment and recovery of pulmonary antibacterial defense mechanisms after oxygen administration. *J. Clin. Invest.* 49:47a, 1970.

937. Huber, G., Mason, R., Pegg, C., and Norman, J. Production, reversal, and prevention of experimental hyaline membrane disease following disseminated intravascular coagulation. *Clin. Res.* 17:415, 1969.

938. Hudson, H. E., Harber, P. I., and Smith, T. C. Respiratory depression from alkalosis and opioid interaction in man. *Anesthesiology* 40:543–552, 1974.

939. Hughes, R. E., and Magovern, G. J. The relationship between right atrial pressure and blood volume. *Arch. Surg.* 79:238–243, 1959.

940. Hume, D. M., Mendez, G., Gayle, W. E., Smith, D. H., Abouna, G. M., and

Lee, H. M.   Current methods for support of patients in hepatic failure. *Transplant. Proc.* 3:1525–1535, 1971.

941. Hyde, R. W., and Rawson, A. J.   Unintentional iatrogenic oxygen pneumonitis—Response to therapy. *Ann. Intern. Med.* 71:517–531, 1969.

942. Iliff, L. D., Greene, R. E., and Hughes, J. M. B.   Effect of interstitial edema on distribution of ventilation and perfusion in isolated lung. *J. Appl. Physiol.* 33:462–467, 1972.

943. Inamdar, A. R., Wittner, M., and Rosenbaum, R. M.   Control of rate—limiting enzymes in tryptophan metabolism during O_2 toxicity. *J. Appl. Physiol.* 33:234–237, 1972.

944. Interiano, B., Hyde, R. W., Hodges, M., and Yu, P. N.   Interrelation between alterations in pulmonary mechanics and hemodynamics in acute myocardial infarction. *J. Clin. Invest.* 52:1994–2006, 1973.

945. Interiano, B., Stuard, I. D., and Hyde, R. W.   Acute respiratory distress syndrome in pancreatitis. *Ann. Intern. Med.* 77:923–926, 1972.

946. Irving, M.   Intravenous nutrition: The materials available. *Proc. R. Soc. Med.* 66:767–770, 1973.

947. Isern-Amaral, J., Stanley, T. H., Oster, H., and Liu, W.-S.   The Effects of Isolated Changes in Right and Left Ventricular Contractility on Pulmonary Shunting and Dead Space Ventilation after Orthotopic Cardiac Transplantation. Abstracts of scientific papers, Annual Meeting of the American Society of Anesthesiologists, Washington, D.C., October 12–16, 1974. P. 311.

948. Jackson, D. C.   Hypoxaemia in the immediate postoperative period. *Med. J. Aust.* 1:1044–1046, 1968.

949. Jackson, R., Greenfield, L. J., Coalson, J. J., and Hinshaw, L. B.   Evaluation of myocardial performance in subhuman primates subjected to endotoxin. *Crit. Care Med.* 2:48–49, 1974.

950. Jackson, R. R., and Davis, S. D.   Hydrostatic inflation for low-pressure tracheal cuffs. *J.A.M.A.* 212:1215–1216, 1970.

951. Jacobey, J. A., Taylor, W. J., Smith, G. T., Gorlin, R., and Harken, D. E.   A new therapeutic approach to acute coronary occlusion. II. Opening dormant coronary collateral channels by counterpulsation. *Am. J. Cardiol.* 11:218–227, 1963.

952. Jakschik, B. A., Marshall, G. R., Kourik, J. L., and Needleman, P.   Profile of circulating vasoactive substances in hemorrhagic shock and their pharmacologic manipulation. *J. Clin. Invest.* 54:842–852, 1974.

953. James, A. E., MacMillan, A. S., Jr., Eaton, S. B., and Grillo, H. C.   Roentgenology of tracheal stenosis resulting from cuffed tracheostomy. *Am. J. Roentgenol. Radium Ther. Nucl. Med.* 109:455–466, 1970.

954. James, P. M., Jr., Bevis, A., and Myers, R. T.   Experiences with central venous and pulmonary artery pressure in a series of 3,500 patients. *South. Med. J.* 65:1299–1307, 1972.

955. Janis, K. M., Kemmerer, W. T., and Kirby, R. R.   Intraoperative Doppler blood pressure measurements in infants. *Anesthesiology* 33:361–363, 1970.

956. Jenevin, E. P., Jr., and Weiss, D. L.   Platelet microemboli associated with massive blood transfusion. *Am. J. Pathol.* 45:313–334, 1964.

957. Jenkins, M. T., and Luhn, N. R.   Active management of tetanus based on experiences of an anesthesiology department. *Anesthesiology* 23:690–709, 1962.

958. Jenny, W. L.   Tracheostomy. *Int. Anesthesiol. Clin.* 9(4):139–149, 1971.

959. Jensen, N. K.   Recovery of pulmonary function after crushing injuries of the chest. *Dis. Chest* 22:319–346, 1952.

960. Jernigan, W. R., Gardner, W. C., Mahr, M. M., and Milburn, J. L.   Use of the internal jugular vein for placement of central venous catheter. *Surg. Gynecol. Obstet.* 130:520–524, 1970.

961. Jewett, J. F.   Spontaneous rupture of the uterus. *N. Engl. J. Med.* 287:930, 1972.

962. Jewitt, D., Birkhead, J., Mitchell, A., and Dollery, C.   Clinical cardiovascular pharmacology of dobutamine. A selective inotropic catecholamine. *Lancet* 2:363–367, 1974.

963. Jeyasingham, K., Althaus, U., Berg, E., and Albrechtsen, O.   Alterations in the plasma proteins and lipids of human and canine blood in bubble and disc oxygenators. *Scand. J. Thorac. Cardiovasc. Surg.* 6:172–177, 1972.

964. Johansen, S. H., Bech-Jansen, P., and Beck, O.   Alveolar-arterial oxygen tension gradients during perioperative replacement of fluid loss by physiologic saline. *Acta Anaesthesiol. Scand.* 16:127–131, 1972.

965. Johanson, W. G., Pierce, A. K., and Sanford, J. P.   Changing pharyngeal bacterial flora of hospitalized patients: Emergence of gram-negative bacilli. *N. Engl. J. Med.* 281:1137–1140, 1969.

966. Johanson, W. G., Pierce, A. K., Sanford, J. P., and Thomas, G. D.   Nosocomial respiratory infections with gram-negative bacilli: The significance of colonization of the respiratory tract. *Ann. Intern. Med.* 77:701–706, 1972.

967. John, R., and Thomas, J.   Chemical compositions of elastins isolated from aortas and pulmonary tissues of humans of different ages. *Biochem. J.* 127:261–269, 1972.

968. Johnson, E. E.   Splanchnic hemodynamic response to passive hyperventilation. *J. Appl. Physiol.* 38:156–162, 1975.

969. Johnson, E. E., and Hedley-Whyte, J.   Continuous positive-pressure ventilation and portal flow in dogs with pulmonary edema. *J. Appl. Physiol.* 33:385–389, 1972.

970. Johnson, E. E., and Hedley-Whyte, J.   Continuous positive-pressure ventilation and choledochoduodenal flow resistance. *J. Appl. Physiol.* 39:937–942, 1975.

971. Johnson, R. L., Jr., Spicer, W. S., Bishop, J. M., and Forster, R. E.   Pulmonary capillary blood volume, flow and diffusing capacity during exercise. *J. Appl. Physiol.* 15:893–902, 1960.

972. Johnson, R. W.   A complication of radial-artery cannulation. *Anesthesiology* 40:598–600, 1974.

973. Johnson, W. P., Jefferson, D., and Mengel, C. E.   In vivo hemolysis due to hyperoxia: Role in H_2O_2 accumulation. *Aerosp. Med.* 43:943–945, 1972.

974. Johnson, W. R., Jefferson, D., and Mengel, C. E.   In vivo formation of H_2O_2 in red cells during exposure to hyperoxia. *J. Clin. Invest.* 51:2211–2213, 1972.

975. Johnston, A. O. B., and Clark, R. G.   Malpositioning of central venous catheters. *Lancet* 2:1395–1397, 1972.

976. Johnston, D. A., and Bodey, G. P.   Oropharyngeal cultures of patients in protected environment units: Evaluation of semiquantitative technique during antibiotic prophylaxis. *Appl. Microbiol.* 23:846–851, 1972.

977. Johnston, I. H., Johnston, J. A., and Jennett, B.   Intracranial-pressure changes following head injury. *Lancet* 2:433–436, 1970.

978. Johnstone, R. E., and Greenhow, D. E.   Catheterization of dorsalis pedis artery. *Anesthesiology* 39:654–655, 1973.

979. Jones, E. A., Clain, D., Clink, H. M., MacGillivray, M., and Sherlock, S.   Hepatic coma due to acute hepatic necrosis treated by exchange blood-transfusion. *Lancet* 2:169–172, 1967.

980. Jones, R. B., Nelson, D. P., Shapiro, S., and Kiesow, L. A.   Synergism in the toxicities of lead and oxygen. *Experientia* 30:327–328, 1974.

981. Jordan, P. H., Jr., Boulafendis, D., and Guinn, G. A. Factors other than major vascular occlusion that contribute to intestinal infarction. *Ann. Surg.* 171:189–194, 1970.

982. Joyeuse, R., Ivanisevic, B., Longmire, W. P., Jr., and Maloney, J. V., Jr. The treatment of experimental hepatic coma by parabiotic cross circulation. *Surg. Forum* 13:334–336, 1962.

983. Jurado, R. A., Matucha, D., and Osborn, J. J. Cardiac output estimation by pulse contour methods: Validity of their use for monitoring the critically ill patient. *Surgery* 74:358–369, 1973.

984. Kafer, E. R. Respiratory function in pulmonary thromboembolic disease. *Am. J. Med.* 47:904–915, 1969.

985. Kafer, E. R. Pulmonary oxygen toxicity. A review of the evidence for acute and chronic oxygen toxicity in man. *Br. J. Anaesth.* 43:687–695, 1971.

986. Kakkar, V. V., Corrigan, T. P., and Fossard, D. P. Prevention of fatal postoperative pulmonary embolism by low doses of heparin. An international multicentre trial. *Lancet* 2:45–51, 1975.

987. Kakkar, V. V., Field, E. S., Nicolaides, A. N., Flute, P. T., Wessler, S., and Yin, E. T. Low doses of heparin in prevention of deep-vein thrombosis. *Lancet* 2:669–671, 1971.

988. Kallos, T., Wyche, M. Q., and Garman, J. K. The effects of Innovar on the functional residual capacity and total chest compliance. *Anesthesiology* 39:558–561, 1973.

989. Kaltreider, N. L., Fray, W. W., and Hyde, H. V. Z. The effect of age on the total pulmonary capacity and its subdivisions. *Am. Rev. Tuberc.* 37:662–689, 1938.

990. Kamen, J. M., and Wilkinson, C. J. A new low pressure cuff for endotracheal tubes. *Anesthesiology* 34:482–485, 1971.

991. Kampine, J. P., and Newmark, J. Miniature CO_2 sensors for continuous intravascular monitoring of blood P_{CO_2}. *Crit. Care Med.* 2:44–45, 1974.

992. Kane, R. C., Cohen, M. H., Fossieck, B. E., Jr., and Tvardzik, A. V. Absence of bacteremia after fiberoptic bronchoscopy. *Am. Rev. Respir. Dis.* 111:102–104, 1975.

993. Kapanci, Y., Tosco, R., Eggermann, J., and Gould, V. E. Oxygen pneumonitis in man. Light and electron microscopic morphometric studies. *Chest* 62:162–169, 1972.

994. Kapanci, Y., Weibel, E. R., Kaplan, H. P., and Robinson, F. R. Pathogenesis and reversibility of the pulmonary lesions of oxygen toxicity in monkeys. II. Ultrastructural and morphometric studies. *Lab. Invest.* 20:101–118, 1969.

995. Kaplan, A. L., Jacobs, W. M., and Ehresman, J. B. Aggressive management of pelvic abscess. *Am. J. Obstet. Gynecol.* 98:482–486, 1967.

996. Kaplan, H. P., Robinson, F. R., Kapanci, Y., and Weibel, E. R. Pathogenesis and reversibility of the pulmonary lesions of oxygen toxicity in monkeys. I. Clinical and light microscopic studies. *Lab. Invest.* 20:94–100, 1969.

997. Kaplan, P. M., and Gerin, J. L. Hepatitis B-specific DNA polymerase activity during post-transfusion hepatitis. *Nature* 249:762–764, 1974.

998. Kardos, G. G. Isoproterenol in the treatment of shock due to bacteremia with gram-negative pathogens. *N. Engl. J. Med.* 274:868–873, 1966.

999. Karim, F., and Reza, H. Effect of induced hypothermia and rewarming on renal hemodynamics in anesthetized dogs. *Life Sci.* 9:1153–1163, 1970.

1000. Karnovsky, M. J. The ultrastructural basis of capillary permeability studied with peroxidase as a tracer. *J. Cell Biol.* 35:213–236, 1967.

1001. Kassirer, J. P., Berkman, P. M., Lawrenz, D. R., and Schwartz, W. B. The critical rate of chloride in the correction of hypokalemic alkalosis in man. *Am. J. Med.* 38:172–189, 1965.

1002. Kastor, J. A., DeSanctis, R. W., Harthorne, J. W., and Schwartz, G. H. Transvenous atrial pacing in the treatment of refractory ventricular irritability. *Ann. Intern. Med.* 66:939–945, 1967.

1003. Katz, A. M., Birnbaum, M., Moylan, J., and Pellett, J. Gangrene of the hand and forearm: A complication of radial artery cannulation. *Crit. Care Med.* 2:270–272, 1974.

1004. Kaufman, B. J., Ferguson, M. H., and Cherniack, R. M. Hypoventilation in obesity. *J. Clin. Invest.* 38:500–507, 1959.

1005. Kaufman, J. J., and Brosman, S. A. Blunt injuries of the genitourinary tract. *Surg. Clin. North Am.* 52:747–760, 1972.

1006. Kazamias, T. M., Gander, M. P., Franklin, D. L., and Ross, J. Blood pressure measurement with Doppler ultrasonic flowmeter. *J. Appl. Physiol.* 30:585–588, 1971.

1007. Kazemi, H., Parsons, E. F., Valencia, L. M., and Strieder, D. J. Distribution of pulmonary blood flow after myocardial ischemia and infarction. *Circulation* 41:1025–1030, 1970.

1008. Kazyak, L., and Knoblock, E. C. Application of gas chromatography to analytical toxicology. *Anal. Chem.* 35:1448–1452, 1963.

1009. Keberle, H., Hoffmann, K., and Bernhard, K. The metabolism of glutethimide (Doriden). *Experientia* 18:105–111, 1962.

1010. Kellner, G. A., and Smart, J. F. Percutaneous placement of catheters to monitor "central venous pressure." *Anesthesiology* 36:515–516, 1972.

1011. Kellum, J. M., Jr., DeMeester, T. R., Elkins, R. C., and Zuidema, G. D. Respiratory insufficiency secondary to acute pancreatitis. *Ann. Surg.* 175:657–662, 1972.

1012. Kelly, R. E., and Laurence, D. R. Effect of chlorpromazine on convulsions of experimental and clinical tetanus. *Lancet* 1:118–121, 1956.

1013. Kelman, G. R. *Applied Cardiovascular Physiology.* New York: Appleton-Century-Crofts, 1971. Pp. 210–243.

1014. Kelman, G. R., and Nunn, J. F. *Computer Produced Physiological Tables for Calculations Involving the Relationships Between Blood Oxygen Tension and Content.* London: Butterworth, 1968.

1015. Kemmerer, W. T., Ware, R. W., Stegall, H. F., Morgan, J. L., and Kirby, R. Blood pressure measurement by Doppler ultrasonic detection of arterial wall motion. *Surg. Gynecol. Obstet.* 131:1141–1147, 1970.

1016. Kent, J. R., and Finegold, S. M. Human rabies transmitted by the bite of a bat with comments on the duck embryo vaccine. *N. Engl. J. Med.* 263:1058–1065, 1960.

1017. Kerber, R. E., Ridges, J. D., and Harrison, D. C. Electrocardiographic indications of atrial puncture during pericardiocentesis. *N. Engl. J. Med.* 282:1142–1143, 1970.

1018. Kerr, J. H., Corbett, J. L., Prys-Roberts, C., Crampton Smith, A., and Spalding, J. M. K. Involvement of the sympathetic nervous system in tetanus. Studies on 82 cases. *Lancet* 2:236–241, 1968.

1019. Kerstell, J. Pathogenesis of post-traumatic fat embolism. *Am. J. Surg.* 121:712–715, 1971.

1020. Kety, S. S. The theory and applications of the exchange of inert gases at the lungs and tissues. *Pharmacol. Rev.* 3:1–41, 1951.

1021. Kety, S. S., Shenkin, H. A., and Schmidt, C. F. The effects of increased intracranial pressure on cerebral circulatory functions in man. *J. Clin. Invest.* 27:493–499, 1948.

1022. Key, A., Parker, D., and Davies, R. Use of epoxy resin in oxygen electrodes. *Phys. Med. Biol.* 15:569–572, 1970.

1023. Khalil, K. G., Parker, F. B., Jr., Mukherjee, N., and Webb, W. R.   Thoracic duct injury: A complication of jugular vein catheterization. *J.A.M.A.* 221:908–909, 1972.

1024. Kilburn, K. H., and Dowell, A. R.   Renal function in respiratory failure. Effects of hypoxia, hyperoxia, and hypercapnia. *Arch. Intern. Med.* 127:754–762, 1971.

1025. Kilcoyne, M. M., and Cannon, P. J.   Influence of thoracic caval occlusion on intrarenal blood flow distribution and sodium excretion. *Am. J. Physiol.* 220:1220–1230, 1971.

1026. Kim, K. E., Onesti, G., Moyer, J. H., and Swartz, C.   Ethacrynic acid and furosemide. Diuretic and hemodynamic effects and clinical uses. *Am. J. Cardiol.* 27:407–415, 1971.

1027. Kimball, H. R., Melmon, M. L., and Wolff, S. M.   Endotoxin-induced kinin production in man. *Proc. Soc. Exp. Biol. Med.* 139:1078–1082, 1972.

1028. King, D. S.   Postoperative pulmonary complications. I. A statistical study based on two years' personal observation. *Surg. Gynecol. Obstet.* 56:43–50, 1933.

1029. King, E. G., Weily, H. S., Genton, E., and Ashbaugh, D. G.   Consumption coagulopathy in the canine oleic acid model of fat embolism. *Surgery* 69:533–541, 1971.

1030. Kinney, J. M.   Ventilatory failure in the postoperative patient. *Surg. Clin. North Am.* 43:619–630, 1963.

1031. Kinney, J. M.   Energy Demands in the Septic Patient. In S. G. Hershey, L. R. M. Del Guercio, and R. McConn (Eds.), *Septic Shock in Man.* Boston: Little, Brown, 1971. Pp. 119–130.

1032. Kinney, J. M., and Roe, C. F.   Caloric equivalent of fever. I. Patterns of postoperative response. *Ann. Surg.* 156:610–622, 1962.

1033. Kirby, R. R., Downs, J. B., Civetta, J. M., Modell, J. H., Dannemiller, F. J., Klein, E. F., and Hodges, M.   High level positive end expiratory pressure (PEEP) in acute respiratory insufficiency. *Chest* 67:156–163, 1975.

1034. Kirby, R. R., Kemmerer, W. T., and Morgan, J. L.   Transcutaneous Doppler measurement of blood pressure. *Anesthesiology* 31:86–89, 1969.

1035. Kirby, R. R., Robison, E. J., and Schulz, J.   Intermittent cuff inflation during prolonged positive-pressure ventilation. *Anesthesiology* 32:364–366, 1970.

1036. Kirkland, K., Edwards, D. G., and Whyte, H. M.   Oliguric renal failure: A report of 400 cases including classification, survival, and response to dialysis. *Aust. Ann. Med.* 14:275–281, 1965.

1037. Kirklin, J. W., Patrick, R. T., and Theye, R. A.   Theory and practice in the use of a pump-oxygenator for open intracardiac surgery. *Thorax* 12:93–98, 1957.

1038. Kisker, C. T., and Rush, R.   Detection of intravascular coagulation. *J. Clin. Invest.* 50:2235–2241, 1971.

1039. Kitamura, H., Sawa, T., and Ikezono, E.   Postoperative hypoxemia: The contribution of age to the maldistribution of ventilation. *Anesthesiology* 36:244–252, 1972.

1040. Kitamura, S., Echevarria, M., Kay, J. H., Krohn, B. G., Redington, J. V., Mendez, A., Zubiate, P., and Dunne, E. F.   Left ventricular performance before and after removal of the noncontractile area of the left ventricle and revascularization of the myocardium. *Circulation* 45:1005–1017, 1972.

1041. Klastersky, J., Geuning, C., Mouawad, E., and Daneau, D.   Endotracheal gentamicin in bronchial infections in patients with tracheostomy. *Chest* 61:117–120, 1972.

1042. Klastersky, J., Huysmans, E., Weerts, D., Hensgens, C., and Daneau, D.   Endotracheally administered gentamicin for the prevention of infections of the respiratory tract in patients with tracheostomy: A double-blind study. *Chest* 65:650–654, 1974.

1043. Klebanoff, G.   Early clinical experience with a disposable unit for the intraoperative salvage and reinfusion of blood loss (intraoperative autotransfusion). *Am. J. Surg.* 120:718–722, 1970.

1044. Klebanoff, G., Armstrong, R. G., Cline, R. E., Powell, J. R., and Bedingfield, J. R.   Resuscitation of a patient in stage IV hepatic coma using total body washout. *J. Surg. Res.* 13:159–165, 1972.

1045. Klebanoff, G., Phillips, J., and Evans, W.   Use of a disposable autotransfusion unit under varying conditions of contamination. *Am. J. Surg.* 120:351–354, 1970.

1046. Klein, R. L., Safar, P., and Grenvik, A.   Respiratory Care in Blunt Chest Injury—A Retrospective Review of 43 Cases. Abstracts of scientific papers, Annual Meeting of the American Society of Anesthesiologists, New York, October 19–21, 1970. Pp. 145–146.

1047. Kleiner, G. J., Merskey, C., Johnson, A. J., and Markus, W. B.   Defibrination in normal and abnormal parturition. *Br. J. Haematol.* 19:159–178, 1970.

1048. Klick, J. M., du Moulin, G. C., Hedley-Whyte, J., Teres, D., Bushnell, L. S., and Feingold, D. S.   Prevention of gram-negative bacillary pneumonia using polymyxin aerosol as prophylaxis. II. Effect on the incidence of pneumonia in seriously ill patients. *J. Clin. Invest.* 55:514–519, 1975.

1049. Klotz, U., Avant, G. R., Hoyumpa, A., Schenker, S., and Wilkinson, G. R.   The effects of age and liver disease on the disposition and elimination of diazepam in adult man. *J. Clin. Invest.* 55:347–359, 1975.

1050. Klug, T. J., and McPherson, R. C.   Postoperative complications in the elderly surgical patient. *Am. J. Surg.* 97:713–717, 1959.

1051. Kluge, R. M., and DuPont, H. L.   Factors affecting mortality of patients with bacteremia. *Surg. Gynecol. Obstet.* 137:267–269, 1973.

1052. Knott, P. J., and Curzon, G.   Effect of increased rat brain tryptophan on 5-hydroxytryptamine and 5-hydroxyindolyl acetic acid in the hypothalamus and other brain regions. *J. Neurochem.* 22:1065–1071, 1974.

1053. Knowlson, G. T. G., and Bassett, H. F. M.   The pressures exerted on the trachea by endotracheal inflatable cuffs. *Br. J. Anaesth.* 42:834–837, 1970.

1054. Knudson, J.   Duration of hypoxaemia after uncomplicated upper abdominal and thoraco-abdominal operations. *Anaesthesia* 25:372–377, 1970.

1055. Kogure, K., Scheinberg, P., Reinmuth, O. M., Fujishima, M., and Busto, R.   Mechanisms of cerebral vasodilatation in hypoxia. *J. Appl. Physiol.* 29:223–229, 1970.

1056. Kolobow, T., Spragg, R. G., Pierce, J. E., and Zapol, W. M.   Extended term (to 16 days) partial extracorporeal blood gas exchange with the spiral membrane lung in unanesthetized lambs. *Trans. Am. Soc. Artif. Intern. Organs* 17:350–354, 1971.

1057. Kolobow, T., and Zapol, W. M.   A new thin-walled nonkinking catheter for peripheral vascular cannulation. *Surgery* 68:625–629, 1970.

1058. Kolobow, T., and Zapol, W. M.   Partial and total extracorporeal respiratory gas exchange with the spiral membrane lung. *Adv. Cardiol.* 6:112–132, 1971.

1059. Kominos, S. D., Copeland, C. E., Grosiak, B., and Postic, B.   Introduction of *Pseudomonas aeruginosa* into a hospital via vegetables. *Appl. Microbiol.* 24:567–570, 1972.

1060. Kontos, H. A., Richardson, D. W., and Patterson, J. L., Jr.   Roles of hypercapnia and acidosis in the vasodilator response to hypercapnic acidosis. *Am. J. Physiol.* 215:1406–1408, 1968.

1061. Kopriva, C. J., Eltringham, R. J., and Siebert, P. E.   A comparison of the effects of intravenous Innovar and topical spray on the laryngeal closure reflex. *Anesthesiology* 40:596–598, 1974.

1062. Kopriva, C. J., Ratliff, J. L., Fletcher, J. R., Fortier, N. L., and Valeri, C. R. Biochemical and hematological changes associated with massive transfusion of ACD-stored blood in severely injured combat casualties. *Ann. Surg.* 176:585–589, 1972.

1063. Kowalski, E. Fibrinogen derivatives and their biologic activities. *Semin. Hematol.* 5:45–59, 1968.

1064. Krantz, M. L., and Edwards, W. L. The incidence of nonfatal aspiration in obstetric patients. *Anesthesiology* 39:359, 1973.

1065. Kreuzer, F., Rogeness, G. A., and Bornstein, P. Continuous recording in vivo of respiratory air oxygen tension. *J. Appl. Physiol.* 15:1157–1158, 1960.

1066. Krevans, J. R., Jackson, D. P., Conley, C. L., and Hartman, R. C. The nature of hemorrhagic disorder accompanying hemolytic transfusion reactions in man. *Blood* 12:834–843, 1957.

1067. Krieger, A. J., and Rosomoff, H. L. Sleep-induced apnea. 1. A respiratory and autonomic dysfunction syndrome following bilateral percutaneous cervical cordotomy. *J. Neurosurg.* 40:168–180, 1974.

1068. Krieger, A. J., and Rosomoff, H. L. Sleep induced apnea. 2. Respiratory failure after anterior spinal surgery. *J. Neurosurg.* 40:181–185, 1974.

1069. Kronenberg, R. S., and Drage, C. W. Attenuation of the ventilatory and heart rate responses to hypoxia and hypercapnia with aging in normal men. *J. Clin. Invest.* 52:1812–1819, 1973.

1070. Krumholz, R. A., and Hedrick, E. C. Pulmonary function differences in normal smoking and nonsmoking, middle-aged white-collar workers. *Am. Rev. Respir. Dis.* 107:225–230, 1973.

1071. Krumholz, R. A., Chevalier, R. B., and Ross, J. C. Changes in cardiopulmonary functions related to abstinence from smoking. Studies in young cigarette smokers at rest and exercise at three and six weeks of abstinence. *Ann. Intern. Med.* 62:197–207, 1965.

1072. Kugelberg, J., Schüller, H., Berg, B., and Kallum, B. Treatment of accidental hypothermia. *Scand. J. Thorac. Cardiovasc. Surg.* 1:142–146, 1967.

1073. Kuida, H., Hinshaw, L. B., Gilbert, R. P., and Visscher, M. B. Effect of gram-negative endotoxin on pulmonary circulation. *Am. J. Physiol.* 192:335–344, 1958.

1074. Kumar, A., Falke, K. J., Geffin, B., Aldredge, C. F., Laver, M. B., Lowenstein, E., and Pontoppidan, H. Continuous positive-pressure ventilation in acute respiratory failure. Effects on hemodynamics and lung function. *N. Engl. J. Med.* 283:1430–1436, 1970.

1075. Kumar, R., Hill, C. M., and McGeown, M. G. Acute renal failure in the elderly. *Lancet* 1:90–91, 1973.

1076. Kunin, C. M., and Bugg, A. Binding of polymyxin antibiotics to tissue: The major determinant of distribution and persistence in the body. *J. Infect. Dis.* 124:394–400, 1971.

1077. Kuperman, A. S., and Riker, J. B. The variable effect of smoking on pulmonary function. *Chest* 63:655–660, 1973.

1078. Kux, M., Coalson, J. J., Massion, W. H., and Guenter, C. A. Pulmonary effects of *E. coli* endotoxin: Role of leukocytes and platelets. *Ann. Surg.* 175:26–34, 1972.

1079. Kuzucu, E. Y. Measurement of temperature. *Int. Anesthesiol. Clin.* 3:435–449, 1965.

1080. Kvittingen, T. D., and Naess, A. Recovery from drowning in fresh water. *Br. Med. J.* 1:1315–1317, 1963.

1081. Kwaan, H. M., and Weil, M. H.   Differences in the mechanism of shock caused by bacterial infections. *Surg. Gynecol. Obstet.* 128:37–45, 1969.

1082. Kyle, J. L., and Riesen, W. H.   Stress and cigarette smoke effects on lung mitochondrial phosphorylation. *Arch. Environ. Health* 21:492–497, 1970.

1083. Ladegaard-Pederson, H. J.   Postoperative changes in blood volume and colloid osmotic pressure. *Acta Chir. Scand.* 135:95–104, 1969.

1084. LaForce, F. M., Kelly, W. J., and Huber, G. L.   Inactivation of staphylococci by alveolar macrophages with preliminary observations on the importance of alveolar lining material. *Am. Rev. Respir. Dis.* 108:784–790, 1974.

1085. Lahiri, S. K., Thomas, T. A., and Hodgson, R. M. H.   Single-dose antacid therapy for the prevention of Mendelson's syndrome. *Br. J. Anaesth.* 45:1143–1146, 1973.

1086. Lai, N. C. J., Coon, R. L., Macur, R. A., and Kampine, J. P.   A Combination Intravascular Sensor for Continuous On Line Measurement of Pco_2, pH, and HCO_3. Abstracts of scientific papers, Annual Meeting of American Society of Anesthesiologists, Washington, D.C., October 15–17, 1974. P. 369.

1087. Lal, S., Murtagh, J. G., Pollock, A. M., Fletcher, E., and Binnion, P. F.   Acute haemodynamic effects of frusemide in patients with normal and raised left atrial pressures. *Br. Heart J.* 31:711–717, 1969.

1088. Lambert, E. H., Rooke, E. D., Eaton, L. M., and Hodgson, C. H.   Myasthenic Syndrome Occasionally Associated with Bronchial Neoplasm: Neurophysiologic Studies. In H. R. Viets (Ed.), *Myasthenia Gravis.* Springfield, Ill.: Thomas, 1961. Pp. 362–410.

1089. Lambert, R. K., and Gremels, H.   On the factors concerned in the production of pulmonary oedema. *J. Physiol.* 61:98–112, 1926.

1090. Lamberti, J. J., Jr.   Catheter perforations of heart wall. *N. Engl. J. Med.* 291:679, 1974.

1091. Lamberti, J. J., Jr., Cohn, L. H., Lesch, M., and Collins, J. J., Jr.   Intra-aortic balloon counterpulsation. Indications and long-term results in postoperative left ventricular power failure. *Arch. Surg.* 109:766–771, 1974.

1092. Lambertsen, C. J.   Oxygen Toxicity. In *Fundamentals of Hyperbaric Medicine.* National Research Council Publication no. 1298. Washington, D.C.: National Academy of Sciences, 1966. Pp. 21–32.

1093. Lambie, J. M., Mahaffy, R. G., Barber, D. C., Karmody, A. M., Scott, M. M., and Matheson, N. A.   Diagnostic accuracy in venous thrombosis. *Br. Med. J.* 2:142–143, 1970.

1094. Landé, A. J.   Assisted circulation with membrane oxygenators. *Transplant. Proc.* 3:1479–1482, 1971.

1095. Landing, B. H.   The pathogenesis of amniotic fluid embolism. II. Uterine factors. *N. Engl. J. Med.* 243:590–596, 1950.

1096. Lane, R. E., and Andelman, S. L.   Maternal mortality in Chicago, 1956 through 1960. I. General analysis. *Am. J. Obstet. Gynecol.* 85:52–60, 1963.

1097. Lane, R. E., and Andelman, S. L.   Maternal mortality in Chicago, 1956 through 1960. II. Preventable factors in causes of death. *Am. J. Obstet. Gynecol.* 85:61–67, 1963.

1098. Langston, H. T., Milles, G., and Dalessandro, W.   Further experiences with autogenous blood transfusions. *Ann. Surg.* 158:333–336, 1963.

1099. Lapin, E. S., and Murray, J. A.   Hemoptysis with flow-directed cardiac catheterization. *J.A.M.A.* 220:1246, 1972.

1100. Lappas, D. G., Geha, D., Fischer, J. E., Laver, M. B., and Lowenstein, E.   Filling pressures of the heart and pulmonary circulation of the patient with coronary-artery disease after large intravenous doses of morphine. *Anesthesiology* 42:153–159, 1975.

1101. Lappas, D. G., Lell, W. A., Gabel, J. C., Civetta, J. M., and Lowenstein, E. Indirect measurement of left-atrial pressure in surgical patients—Pulmonary-capillary wedge and pulmonary-artery diastolic pressures compared with left-atrial pressure. *Anesthesiology* 38:394–397, 1973.
1102. Larkin, E. C., Williams, W. T., and Ulvedal, F. Human hematologic responses to 4 hrs. of isobaric hyperoxic exposure (100% oxygen at 760 mm Hg). *J. Appl. Physiol.* 34:417–421, 1973.
1103. Larmi, T. K. I., and Kärkölä, P. Plasma protein electrophoresis during a three-hour cardiopulmonary bypass in dogs. *Scand. J. Thorac. Cardiovasc. Surg.* 8:152–160, 1974.
1104. Larochelle, P., Mikulic, E., and Ogilvie, R. I. Effects of isoproterenol, diazoxide, ethacrynic acid, and furosemide on skeletal muscle vascular resistance. *Can. J. Physiol. Pharmacol.* 51:183–189, 1973.
1105. LaSalvia, L. A., and Steffen, E. A. Delayed gastric emptying time in labor. *Am. J. Obstet. Gynecol.* 59:1075–1081, 1950.
1106. Lash, R. F., Burdette, J. A., and Ozdil, T. Accidental profound hypothermia and barbiturate intoxication: A report of rapid "core" rewarming by peritoneal dialysis. *J.A.M.A.* 201:269–270, 1967.
1107. Lassen, N. A. Treatment of severe acute barbiturate poisoning by forced diuresis and alkalinisation of the urine. *Lancet* 2:338–342, 1960.
1108. Lassen, N. A. The luxury-perfusion syndrome and its possible relation to acute metabolic acidosis localised within the brain. *Lancet* 2:1113–1115, 1966.
1109. Lassen, N. A., and Pálvölgyi, R. Cerebral steal during hypercapnia and the inverse reaction during hypocapnia observed by the [133]xenon technique in man. *Scand. J. Clin. Lab. Invest.* 22(Suppl. 102):XIII–D, 1968.
1110. Laszlo, G., Archer, G. G., Darrell, J. H., Dawson, J. M., and Fletcher, C. M. The diagnosis and prophylaxis of pulmonary complications of surgical operation. *Br. J. Surg.* 60:129–134, 1973.
1111. Latimer, L. D., and Latimer, K. E. Continuous flushing systems: A critical review. *Anaesthesia* 29:307–317, 1974.
1112. Latimer, R. G., Dickman, M., Day, W. C., Gunn, M. L., and Schmidt, C. duW. Ventilatory patterns and pulmonary complications after upper abdominal surgery determined by preoperative and postoperative computerized spirometry and blood gas analysis. *Am. J. Surg.* 122:622–632, 1971.
1113. Laurenzi, G. A., Yin, S., and Guarneri, J. J. Adverse effect of oxygen on tracheal mucus flow. *N. Engl. J. Med.* 279:333–399, 1968.
1114. Lauria, J. I., and Anderson, M. N. Automatically inflated cuffed tube for ventilatory support. *Rev. Surg.* 26:75–76, 1969.
1115. Laver, M. B. Prevention of Postoperative Respiratory Complications. In L. J. Saidman and F. Moya (Eds.), *Complications of Anesthesia*. Springfield, Ill.: Thomas, 1970. Pp. 31–39.
1116. Laver, M. B. A fable of our time: Oxygen transport, or does the emperor have new clothes? *Anesthesiology* 36:105–106, 1972.
1117. Laver, M. B. Vasodilator Therapy. Presented at American Society of Anesthesiologists' Workshop: Anesthesia for Cardiovascular Surgery, Boston, Mass., November 2–3, 1974.
1118. Laver, M. B., and Bendixen, H. H. Atelectasis in the surgical patient: Recent conceptual advances. *Prog. Surg.* 5:1–37, 1966.
1119. Laver, M. B., Broennle, M., Trichet, B., Tung, C., and Jackson, E. Do Hormonal Factors Affect Oxygen Transport in Critically Ill Patients? In H. Chaplin, Jr., E. R. Jaffé, C. Lenfant, and C. R. Valeri (Eds.), *Preservation of Red Blood Cells*. Washington, D.C.: Division of Medical Sciences, National Academy of Sciences, National Research Council, 1973. Pp. 119–135.

1120. Laver, M. B., Morgan, J., Bendixen, H. H., and Radford, E. P., Jr.   Lung volume, compliance, and arterial oxygen tensions during controlled ventilation. *J. Appl. Physiol.* 19:725–733, 1964.

1121. Lawrence, R. M.   Postoperative hypoxia: Causes, limits, and prevention. *Int. Anesthesiol. Clin.* 9(4):31–82, 1971.

1122. Laws, A. K., and McIntyre, R. W.   Chest physiotherapy: A physiological assessment during intermittent positive pressure ventilation in respiratory failure. *Can. Anaesth. Soc. J.* 16:487–493, 1969.

1123. Lawson, D. R.   Pre-stretched cuffs on tracheostomy tubes. *Br. J. Anaesth.* 45:234, 1973.

1124. Lawson, D. W., Defalco, A. J., Phelps, J. A., Bradley, B. E., and McClenathan, J. E.   Corticosteroids as treatment for aspiration of gastric contents: An experimental study. *Surgery* 59:845–852, 1966.

1125. Lawson, D. W., and Grillo, H. C.   Closure of persistent tracheal stomas. *Surg. Gynecol. Obstet.* 130:995–996, 1970.

1126. Lawson, N. W., Ochsner, J. L., Mills, N. L., and Leonard, G. L.   Use of hemodilution and fresh autologous blood in open-heart surgery. *Anesth. Analg.* (Cleve.) 53:672–683, 1974.

1127. Leape, L. L.   Bronchial avulsion. Successful repair after bilateral pneumothorax. *J. Thorac. Cardiovasc. Surg.* 62:470–472, 1971.

1128. Leary, O. C., Jr., and Hertig, A. T.   The pathogenesis of amniotic fluid embolism. I. Possible placental factors—Aberrant squamous cells in placentas. *N. Engl. J. Med.* 243:588–590, 1950.

1129. Leblanc, P., Ruff, F., and Milic-Emili, J.   Effects of age and body position on "airway closure" in man. *J. Appl. Physiol.* 28:448–451, 1970.

1130. Lecky, J. H., and Ominsky, A. J.   Postoperative respiratory management. *Chest* 62(Suppl.):50S–57S, 1972.

1131. Ledingham, I. McA., and Mone, J. G.   Management of Severe Accidental Hypothermia. Scientific abstracts, First World Congress on Intensive Care, London, England, June 24–27, 1974. P. 111.

1132. Lee, A. B., Jr., and Kinney, J. M.   Ventilatory management of the pulmonary burn. *Ann. N.Y. Acad. Sci.* 150:738–754, 1968.

1133. Lee, C.-J., Lyons, J. H., and Moore, F. D.   Cardiovascular and metabolic responses to spontaneous and positive-pressure breathing of 100 per cent oxygen at one atmosphere pressure. *J. Thorac. Cardiovasc. Surg.* 53:770–780, 1967.

1134. Lee, J. A., and Atkinson, R. S.   *A Synopsis of Anaesthesia* (7th ed.). Baltimore: Williams & Wilkins, 1973. P. 111.

1135. Lee, Y.-H., and Kerstein, M. D.   Osteomyelitis and septic arthritis: A complication of subclavian venous catheterization. *N. Engl. J. Med.* 285:1179–1180, 1971.

1136. Lefer, A. M.   Role of a myocardial depressant factor in the pathogenesis of circulatory shock. *Fed. Proc.* 29:1836–1847, 1970.

1137. Lefer, A. M., Glenn, T. M., O'Neill, T. J., Lovett, W. L., Geissinger, W. T., and Wangensteen, S. L.   Inotropic influence of endogenous peptides in experimental hemorrhagic pancreatitis. *Surgery* 69:220–228, 1971.

1138. Lefrak, E. A., Stevens, P. M., Pitha, J., Balsinger, E., Noon, G. P., and Mayor, H. D.   Extracorporeal membrane oxygenation for fulminant influenza pneumonia. *Chest* 66:385–388, 1974.

1139. Leftwich, E. I., Witorsch, R. J., and Witorsch, P.   Positive end-expiratory pressure in refractory hypoxemia. A critical evaluation. *Ann. Intern. Med.* 79:187–193, 1973.

1140. Leinbach, R. C., Buckley, M. J., Austen, W. G., Petschek, H. E., Kantrowitz,

A. R., and Sanders, C. A. Effects of intra-aortic balloon pumping on coronary flow and metabolism in man. *Circulation* 43, 44(Suppl. I):77–81, 1971.

1141. Leinbach, R. C., Dinsmore, R. E., Mundth, E. D., Buckley, M. J., Dunkman, W. B., Austen, W. G., and Sanders, C. A. Selective coronary and left ventricular cineangiography during intraaortic balloon pumping for cardiogenic shock. *Circulation* 45:845–852, 1972.

1142. Leinbach, R. C., Gold, H. K., Dinsmore, R. E., Mundth, E. D., Buckley, M. J., Austen, W. G., and Sanders, C. A. The role of angiography in cardiogenic shock. *Circulation* 47, 48(Suppl. III):95–98, 1973.

1143. Leist, E. R., and Banwell, J. G. Products containing aspirin. *N. Engl. J. Med.* 291:710–712, 1974.

1144. Lemen, R., Jones, J. G., and Cowan, G. A mechanism of pulmonary-artery perforation by Swan-Ganz catheters. *N. Engl. J. Med.* 292:211–212, 1975.

1145. Lenfant, C. Effect of high $F_{I_{O_2}}$ on measurement of ventilation/perfusion distribution in man at sea level. *Ann. N.Y. Acad. Sci.* 121:797–808, 1965.

1146. Leonard, P. F. Medical Engineering in Anesthesiology. In C. D. Ray (Ed.), *Medical Engineering.* Chicago: Year Book, 1974. Pp. 345–369.

1147. Lepper, M. H., Kofman, S., Blatt, N., Dowling, H. F., and Jackson, G. G. Effect of eight antibiotics used singly and in combination on the tracheal flora following tracheotomy in poliomyelitis. *Antibiot. Chemother.* 4:829–843, 1954.

1148. Lepore, M. J., and Martel, A. J. Plasmapheresis with plasma exchange in hepatic coma. Methods and results in five patients with acute fulminant hepatic necrosis. *Ann. Intern. Med.* 72:165–174, 1970.

1149. LeQuesne, L. P. Relation between deep vein thrombosis and pulmonary embolism in surgical patients. *N. Engl. J. Med.* 291:1292–1294, 1974.

1150. Lerner, A. M., and Federman, M. J. Gram-negative bacillary pneumonia. *J. Infect. Dis.* 124:425–427, 1971.

1151. Levine, B. W., Talamo, R. C., and Kazemi, H. Action and metabolism of bradykinin in dog lung. *J. Appl. Physiol.* 34:821–826, 1973.

1152. Levine, O. R., Mellins, R. B., Senior, R. M., and Fishman, A. P. The application of Starling's law of capillary exchange to the lungs. *J. Clin. Invest.* 46:934–944, 1967.

1153. Levy, M. Renal function in dogs with acute selective hepatic venous outflow block. *Am. J. Physiol.* 227:1074–1083, 1974.

1154. Levy, M. Renal function during acute graded elevation of portal venous pressure. *Am. J. Physiol.* 227:1084–1087, 1974.

1155. Levy, S. E., and Simmons, D. H. Redistribution of alveolar ventilation following pulmonary thromboembolism in the dog. *J. Appl. Physiol.* 36:60–68, 1974.

1156. Lewinski, A. Evaluation of methods employed in the treatment of the chemical pneumonitis of aspiration. *Anesthesiology* 26:37–44, 1965.

1157. Lewis, B. M., and Gorlin, R. Effects of hypoxia on pulmonary circulation of the dog. *Am. J. Physiol.* 170:574–587, 1952.

1158. Lewis, F. J. Monitoring of patients in intensive care units. *Surg. Clin. North Am.* 51:15–23, 1971.

1159. Lewis, R. T., Burgess, J. H., and Hampson, L. G. Cardiorespiratory studies in critical illness. *Arch. Surg.* 103:335–340, 1971.

1160. Lichtman, M. A. Hypoalimentation during hyperalimentation. *N. Engl. J. Med.* 290:1432–1433, 1974.

1161. Liddle, E. B., Moore, G. H., and Corley, W. D. Acute respiratory insufficiency. Treated with extracorporeal oxygenation. *Rocky Mt. Med. J.* 71:691–693, 1974.

1162. Lifschitz, M. D., Brasch, R., Cuomo, A. J., and Menn, S. J. Marked hypercapnia secondary to severe metabolic alkalosis. *Ann. Intern. Med.* 77:405–409, 1972.

1163. Lillington, G. A., Anderson, M. W., and Brandenburg, R. O. The cardiorespiratory syndrome of obesity. *Dis. Chest* 32:1–20, 1957.

1164. Lim, R. C., Jr., Trunkey, D. D., and Blaisdell, F. W. Acute abdominal aortic injury. An analysis of operative and postoperative management. *Arch. Surg.* 109:706–711, 1974.

1165. Lindholm, .C.-E. Prolonged endotracheal intubation. *Acta Anaesthesiol. Scand.* [Suppl.] 33:1–131, 1969.

1166. Lindholm, C.-E., and Carroll, R. G. Influence of Translaryngeal Intubation on Mucus Clearance of the Airway. Abstracts of scientific papers, Annual Meeting of American Society of Anesthesiologists, Washington, D.C., October 12–16, 1974. Pp. 375–376.

1167. Lindholm, C.-E., Ollman, B., Snyder, J., Millen, E., and Grenvik, A. Cardiovascular effects of flexible fiberoptic bronchoscopy (FFB). *Crit. Care Med.* 3:49–50, 1975.

1168. Linton, A. L., and Ledingham, I. McA. Severe hypothermia with barbiturate intoxication. *Lancet* 1:24–26, 1966.

1169. Lipp, H., O'Donoghue, K., and Resnekov, L. Intracardiac knotting of a flow-directed balloon catheter. *N. Engl. J. Med.* 284:220, 1971.

1170. List, W. F., and Hiotakis, K. Respiratory Distress in Severe Eclampsia. Scientific abstracts, First World Congress on Intensive Care, London, England, June 24–27, 1974. P. 77.

1171. Little, J. M., Zylstra, P. L., West, J., and May, J. Circulatory patterns in the normal hand. *Br. J. Surg.* 60:652–655, 1973.

1172. Litwin, M. S., Smith, L. L., and Moore, F. D. Metabolic alkalosis following massive transfusion. *Surgery* 45:805–813, 1959.

1173. Llamas, R., Gupta, S. K., and Baum, G. L. A simple technique for prolonged arterial cannulation. *Anesthesiology* 31:289, 1969.

1174. Lloyd, T. C., Jr. Effect of increased intracranial pressure on pulmonary vascular resistance. *J. Appl. Physiol.* 35:332–335, 1973.

1175. Lockwood, P. The relationship between pre-operative lung function test results and post-operative complications in carcinoma of the bronchus. *Respiration* 30:105–106, 1973.

1176. Loeb, H. S., Cruz, A., Cheng, Y. T., Boswell, J., Pietras, R. J., Tobin, J. R., Jr., and Gunnar, R. M. Haemodynamic studies in shock associated with infection. *Br. Heart J.* 29:883–894, 1967.

1177. Loeb, H. S., Winslow, E. B. J., Rahimtoola, S. H., Rosen, K. M., and Gunnar, R. M. Acute hemodynamic effects of dopamine in patients with shock. *Circulation* 44:163–173, 1971.

1178. Lomholt, N. A. A new tracheostomy tube. I. Cuff with controlled pressure on the tracheal mucous membrane. *Acta Anaesthesiol. Scand.* 11:311–318, 1967.

1179. Lomholt, N. A. A new tracheostomy tube. II. Cuff with self-adjusting minimum pressure on the tracheal mucosa during inspiration and expiration. *Acta Anaesthesiol. Scand.* [Suppl.] 44:5–39, 1971.

1180. Longerbeam, J. K., Vannix, R., Wagner, W., and Joergenson, E. Central venous pressure monitoring. A useful guide to fluid therapy during shock and other forms of cardiovascular stress. *Am. J. Surg.* 110:220–229, 1965.

1181. Lopas, H., Birndorf, N. I., Bell, C. E., Jr., Robboy, S. J., and Colman, R. W. Immune hemolytic transfusion reaction in monkeys: Activation of the kallikrein system. *Am. J. Physiol.* 225:372–379, 1973.

1182. Lopas, H., Birndorf, N. I., and Robboy, S. J. Experimental transfusion reactions and disseminated intravascular coagulation produced by incompatible plasma in monkeys. *Transfusion* 11:196–204, 1971.

1183. Lorber, B., and Swenson, R. M.   Bacteriology of aspiration pneumonia. A prospective study of community- and hospital-acquired cases. *Ann. Intern. Med.* 81:329–331, 1974.

1184. Lourenço, R. V.   Diaphragm activity in obesity. *J. Clin. Invest.* 48:1609–1614, 1969.

1185. Lourenço, R. V., Klimek, M. F., and Borowski, C. J.   Deposition and clearance of 2μ particles in the tracheobronchial tree of normal subjects—Smokers and nonsmokers. *J. Clin. Invest.* 50:1411–1420, 1971.

1186. Louria, D. B., Hensle, T., and Rose, J.   The major medical complications of heroin addiction. *Ann. Intern. Med.* 67:1–22, 1967.

1187. Low, R. B.   Protein biosynthesis by the pulmonary alveolar macrophage: Conditions of assay and the effects of cigarette smoke extracts. *Am. Rev. Respir. Dis.* 110:466–477, 1974.

1188. Lowbury, E. J., Thom, B. T., Lilly, A., Babb, J. R., and Whitfall, K.   Sources of infection with *Pseudomonas aeruginosa* in patients with tracheostomy. *J. Med. Microbiol.* 3:39–56, 1970.

1189. Lowenstein, E., Little, J. W., III, and Lo, H. H.   Prevention of cerebral embolization from flushing radial-artery cannulas. *N. Engl. J. Med.* 285:1414–1415, 1971.

1190. Lown, B., Black, H., and Moore, F. D.   Digitalis, electrolytes and the surgical patient. *Am. J. Cardiol.* 6:309–337, 1960.

1191. Lown, B., Neuman, J., Amarasingham, R., and Berkovits, B. V.   Comparison of alternating current with direct current electroshock across the closed chest. *Am. J. Cardiol.* 10:223–233, 1962.

1192. Lozman, J., Powers, S. R., Jr., Older, T., Dutton, R. E., Roy, R. J., English, M., Marco, D., and Eckert, C.   Correlation of pulmonary wedge and left atrial pressures. A study in the patient receiving positive end expiratory pressure ventilation. *Arch. Surg.* 109:270–276, 1974.

1193. Lucas, C. E., Rector, F. E., Werner, M., and Rosenberg, I. K.   Altered renal homeostasis with acute sepsis: Clinical significance. *Arch. Surg.* 106:444–449, 1973.

1194. Lucas, C. E., Sugawa, C., Riddle, J., Rector, F., Rosenberg, B., and Walt, A. J.   Natural history and surgical dilemma of "stress" gastric bleeding. *Arch. Surg.* 102:266–272, 1971.

1195. Lucas, C. E., and Walt, A. J.   Critical decisions in liver trauma. Experience based on 604 cases. *Arch. Surg.* 101:277–283, 1970.

1196. Luchsinger, P. C., LaGarde, B., and Kilfeather, J. E.   Particle clearance from the human tracheobronchial tree. *Am. Rev. Respir. Dis.* 97:1046–1050, 1968.

1197. Ludwig, C. F. W.   *Die physiologischen Leistungen des Blutdrucks.* Leipzig: Hirzel, 1865.

1198. Ludwin, S. K., Northway, W. H., Jr., and Bensch, K. G.   Oxygen toxicity in the newborn. Necrotizing bronchiolitis in mice exposed to 100 per cent oxygen. *Lab. Invest.* 31:425–435, 1974.

1199. Lundberg, N., Troupp, H., and Lorin, H.   Continuous recording of the ventricular-fluid pressure in patients with severe acute traumatic brain injury. *J. Neurosurg.* 22:581–590, 1965.

1200. Lutch, J. S., and Murray, J. F.   Continuous positive-pressure ventilation: Effects on systemic oxygen transport and tissue oxygenation. *Ann. Intern. Med.* 76:193–202, 1972.

1201. Lynch, H. F., and Adolph, E. F.   Blood flow in small blood vessels during deep hypothermia. *J. Appl. Physiol.* 11:192–196, 1957.

1202. Macbeth, W. A. A. G., and Pope, G. R.   Effect of abdominal operation upon protein excretion in man. *Lancet* 1:215–217, 1968.

1203. MacCannell, K. L., McNay, J. L., Meyer, M. B., and Goldberg, L. I. Dopamine in the treatment of hypotension and shock. *N. Engl. J. Med.* 275:1389–1398, 1966.

1204. MacGregor, D. C., Armour, J. A., Goldman, B. S., and Bigelow, W. G.   The effects of ether, ethanol, propanol and butanol on tolerance to deep hypothermia. Experimental and clinical observations. *Dis. Chest* 50:523–529, 1966.

1205. MacGregor, R. R., Spagnuolo, P. J., and Lentnek, A. L.   Inhibition of granulocyte adherence by ethanol, prednisone, and aspirin, measured with an assay system. *N. Engl. J. Med.* 291:642–646, 1974.

1206. MacLean, L. D., McLean, A. P. H., and Duff, J. H.   Hemodynamic and metabolic abnormalities in septic shock. *Postgrad. Med.* 48:114–122, 1970.

1207. MacLean, L. D., Mulligan, W. G., McLean, A. P. H., and Duff, J. H.   Patterns of septic shock in man—A detailed study of 56 patients. *Ann. Surg.* 166:543–558, 1967.

1208. Macmillan, A. L., Corbett, J. L., Johnson, R. H., Crampton Smith, A., Spalding, J. M. K., and Wollner, L.   Temperature regulation in survivors of accidental hypothermia of the elderly. *Lancet* 2:165–169, 1967.

1209. Madding, G. F., and Kennedy, P. A.   *Trauma to the Liver* (2nd ed.). Philadelphia: Saunders, 1971.

1210. Maddock, R. K., Jr., and Bloomer, H. A.   Meprobamate overdosage: Evaluation of its severity and methods of treatment. *J.A.M.A.* 201:999–1003, 1967.

1211. Madras, P. N., Laird, J. D., Iatridis, E., Kantrowitz, A. R., Buckley, M. J., and Austen, W. G.   Effects of prolonged intraaortic balloon pumping. *Trans. Am. Soc. Artif. Intern. Organs* 15:400–405, 1969.

1212. Maier, H. C., and Cournand, A.   Studies of arterial oxygen saturation in the postoperative period after pulmonary resection. *Surgery* 13:199–213, 1943.

1213. Majid, P. A., Sharma, B., and Taylor, S. H.   Phentolamine for vasodilator treatment of severe heart-failure. *Lancet* 2:719–723, 1971.

1214. Malcolm-Smith, N. A., Grenvik, Å., and Westerholm, C. J.   A Comparison of Some Physiological Effects of Controlled and Assisted Ventilation. In T. B. Boulton, R. Bryce-Smith, M. K. Sykes, G. B. Gillett, and A. L. Revell (Eds.), *Progress in Anesthesiology, Proceedings of the Fourth World Congress of Anesthesiologists, London, England, September 9–13, 1968.* International Congress Series No. 200. Amsterdam: Excerpta Medica, 1970. Pp. 573–577.

1215. Malik, S. K., and Jenkens, D. E.   Alterations in airway dynamics following inhalation of ultrasonic mist. *Chest* 62:660–664, 1972.

1216. Mallory, G. K., Blackburn, N., Sparling, H. J., and Nickerson, D. A.   Maternal pulmonary embolism of amniotic fluid. Report of three cases and discussion of the literature. *N. Engl. J. Med.* 243:583–587, 1950.

1217. Mallory, T. B., and Brickley, W. J.   Pathology: With special reference to the pulmonary lesions. *Ann. Surg.* 117:865–884, 1943.

1218. Mann, G. V.   The influence of obesity on health. *N. Engl. J. Med.* 291:178–185, 226–232, 1974.

1219. Mann, P. E. G., Cohen, A. B., Finley, T. N., and Ladman, A. J.   Alveolar macrophages. Structural and functional differences between nonsmokers and smokers of marijuana and tobacco. *Lab. Invest.* 25:111–120, 1971.

1220. Mant, M. J., Hirsh, J., Pineo, G. F., and Luke, K. H.   Prolonged prothrombin time and partial thromboplastin time in disseminated intravascular coagulation not due to deficiency of factors V and VIII. *Br. J. Haematol.* 24:725–734, 1973.

1221. Mantle, J. A., Strand, E. M., Breinig, J. B., Russell, R. O., Jr., and Rackley, C. E. Quantitative continuous automated electrocardiographic and hemodynamic monitoring. *J. Clin. Invest.* 53:50a, 1974.

1222. Maran, A. G. D., and Stell, P. M. Acute laryngeal trauma. *Lancet* 2:1107–1110, 1970.

1223. Marcus, A. J. Perspective: Heparin therapy for disseminated intravascular coagulation. *Am. J. Med. Sci.* 264:365–366, 1972.

1224. Marder, V. J., Matchett, M. O., and Sherry, S. Detection of serum fibrinogen and fibrin degradation products. *Am. J. Med.* 51:71–82, 1971.

1225. Marder, V. J., and Shulman, N. R. High molecular weight derivatives of human fibrinogen produced by plasmin. II. Mechanism of their anticoagulant activity. *J. Biol. Chem.* 244:2120–2124, 1969.

1226. Marder, V. J., Shulman, N. R., and Carroll, W. R. High molecular weight derivatives of human fibrinogen produced by plasma. I. Physicochemical and immunological characterization. *J. Biol. Chem.* 244:2111–2119, 1969.

1227. Margaretten, W., McKay, D. G., and Phillips, L. L. The effect of heparin on endotoxin shock in the rat. *Am. J. Pathol.* 51:61–68, 1967.

1228. Marin, M. G., and Morrow, P. E. Effect of changing inspired O_2 and CO_2 levels on tracheal mucociliary transport rate. *J. Appl. Physiol.* 27:385–388, 1969.

1229. Marks, H. H. Influence of obesity on morbidity and mortality. *Bull. N.Y. Acad. Med.* 36:296–312, 1960.

1230. Maroko, P. R., Bernstein, E. F., Libby, P., DeLaria, G. A., Covell, J. W., Ross, J., Jr., and Braunwald, E. Effects of intraaortic balloon counterpulsation on the severity of myocardial ischemic injury following acute coronary occlusion. Counterpulsation and myocardial injury. *Circulation* 45:1150–1159, 1972.

1231. Maroko, P. R., Kjekshus, J. K., Sobel, B. E., Watanabe, T., Covell, J. W., Ross, J., Jr., and Braunwald, E. Factors influencing infarct size following experimental coronary artery occlusions. *Circulation* 43:67–82, 1971.

1232. Maroko, P. R., Libby, P., and Braunwald, E. Effect of pharmacologic agents on the function of the ischemic heart. *Am. J. Cardiol.* 32:930–936, 1973.

1233. Maroon, J. C., and Albin, M. S. Air embolism diagnosed by Doppler ultrasound. *Anesth. Analg.* (Cleve.) 53:399–402, 1974.

1234. Marschke, G., and Sarauw, A. Danger of polymyxin B inhalation. *Ann. Intern, Med.* 74:296–297, 1971.

1235. Marsden, E. How war wounds now. *The Sunday Times* (Lond.) Jan. 19, 1975.

1236. Marsh, H. M., Rehder, K., Sessler, A. D., and Fowler, W. S. Effects of mechanical ventilation, muscle paralysis, and posture on ventilation-perfusion relationships in anesthetized man. *Anesthesiology* 38:59–67, 1973.

1237. Marshall, B. E., and Millar, R. A. Some factors influencing post-operative hypoxaemia. *Anaesthesia* 20:408–428, 1965.

1238. Marshall, B. E., and Wyche, M. Q., Jr. Hypoxemia during and after anesthesia. *Anesthesiology* 37:178–209, 1972.

1239. Marshall, J. P., Chadwick, S. J., and Meyers, D. S. Catheter perforation of the right ventricle. A complication of endoscopy. *N. Engl. J. Med.* 290:890–891, 1974.

1240. Marshall, M. Adjusting Nutrition to Patient's Metabolic Capacity. Scientific abstracts, First World Congress on Intensive Care, London, England, June 24–27, 1974. P. 94.

1241. Marshall, W. J. S., Jackson, J. L. F., and Langfitt, T. W. Brain swelling caused by trauma and arterial hypertension. Hemodynamic effects. *Arch. Neurol.* 21:545–553, 1969.

1242. Martin, A. M., Jr., Simmons, R. L., and Heisterkamp, C. A., III. Respiratory insufficiency in combat casualties. I. Pathologic changes in the lungs of patients dying of wounds. *Ann. Surg.* 170:30–38, 1969.

1243. Martin, C. M., Cuomo, A. J., Geraghty, M. J., Zager, J. R., and Mandes, T. C. Gram-negative rod bacteremia. *J. Infect. Dis.* 119:506–517, 1969.

1244. Martin, W. E., Cheung, P. W., Johnson, C. C., and Wong, K. C. Continuous monitoring of mixed venous oxygen saturation in man. *Anesth. Analg.* (Cleve.) 52:784–793, 1973.

1245. Martinez, L. E., and Kalter, R. D. Extensive tracheal necrosis associated with a prestretched tracheostomy tube cuff. *Anesthesiology* 34:488–489, 1971.

1246. Marty, A. T. Hyperoncotic albumin therapy. *Surg. Gynecol. Obstet.* 139:105–109, 1974.

1247. Marty, A. T., Miyamoto, A. M., Weil, M. H., and Philips, P. A. Oncotic normalization after dilutional bypass and hypothermia. *Arch. Surg.* 109:61–64, 1974.

1248. Mason, J. W., Kleeberg, U., Dolan, P., and Colman, R. W. Plasma kallikrein and Hageman factor in gram-negative bacteremia. *Ann. Intern. Med.* 73:545–551, 1970.

1249. Massaro, G. D., and Massaro, D. Pulmonary granular pneumocytes: Loss of mitochondrial granules during hyperoxia. *J. Cell Biol.* 59:246–250, 1973.

1250. Massaro, G. D., and Massaro, D. Hyperoxia: A stereologic ultrastructural examination of its influence on cytoplasmic components of the pulmonary granular pneumocyte. *J. Clin. Invest.* 52:566–570, 1973.

1251. Massaro, G. D., and Massaro, D. Adaptation to hyperoxia: Influence on protein synthesis by lung and on granular pneumocyte ultrastructure. *J. Clin. Invest.* 53:705–709, 1974.

1252. Massumi, R. A., and Ross, A. M. Atraumatic, nonsurgical technic for removal of broken catheters from cardiac cavities. *N. Engl. J. Med.* 277:195–196, 1967.

1253. Mathews, J. I., and Gibbons, R. B. Embolization complicating radial artery puncture. *Ann. Intern. Med.* 75:87–88, 1971.

1254. Mathieu, A., Dalton, B., Fischer, J. E., and Kumar, A. Expanding aneurysm of the radial artery after frequent puncture. *Anesthesiology* 38:401–403, 1973.

1255. Matloff, J. M., Wolfson, S., Gorlin, R., and Harken, D. E. Control of postcardiac surgical tachycardias with propranolol. *Circulation* 37, 38(Suppl. II):133–138, 1968.

1256. Matsuura, Y., Najib, A., and Lee, W. H., Jr. Pulmonary compliance and surfactant activity in thermal burn. *Surg. Forum* 17:86–88, 1966.

1257. Matz, R. Complications of determining central venous pressure. *N. Engl. J. Med.* 273:703, 1965.

1258. Maynard, A. de L., Brooks, H. A., and Froix, C. J. L. Penetrating wounds of the heart: Report on a new series. *Arch. Surg.* 90:680–686, 1965.

1259. McCabe, W. R. Serum complement levels in bacteremia due to gram-negative organisms. *N. Engl. J. Med.* 288:21–23, 1973.

1260. McCabe, W. R., Kreger, B. E., and Johns, M. Type-specific and cross-reactive antibodies in gram-negative bacteremia. *N. Engl. J. Med.* 287:261–267, 1972.

1261. McCarthy, D. S., Spencer, R., Greene, R., and Milic-Emili, J. Measurement of "closing volume" as a simple and sensitive test for early detection of small airway disease. *Am. J. Med.* 52:747–753, 1972.

1262. McClenahan, J. B., and Urtnowski, A. Effect of ventilation on surfactant, and its turnover rate. *J. Appl. Physiol.* 23:215–220, 1967.

1263. McConn, R., and Del Guercio, L. R. M.   Respiratory function of blood in the acutely ill patient and the effect of steroids. *Ann. Surg.* 174:436–448, 1971.

1264. McConnell, R. Y., and Fox, R. T.   Experience with percutaneous internal jugular-innominate vein catheterization. *Calif. Med.* 117:1–6, 1972.

1265. McCord, J. M.   Free radicals and inflammation: Protection of synovial fluid by superoxide dismutase. *Science* 185:529–531, 1974.

1266. McCord, J. M., and Fridovich, I.   Superoxide dismutase: An enzymic function for erythrocuprein (hemocuprein). *J. Biol. Chem.* 244:6049–6055, 1969.

1267. McCredie, R. M., and Chia, B. L.   Measurement of pulmonary oedema in ischaemic heart disease. *Br. Heart J.* 35:1136–1140, 1973.

1268. McCutcheon, E. P., Evans, J. M., and Stanifer, R. R.   Direct blood-pressure measurement: Gadgets versus progress. *Anesth. Analg.* (Cleve.) 51:746–756, 1972.

1269. McDonald, R. H., Jr., Goldberg, L. I., McNay, J. L., and Tuttle, E. P., Jr.   Effects of dopamine in man: Augmentation of sodium excretion, glomerular filtration rate, and renal plasma flow. *J. Clin. Invest.* 43:1116–1124, 1964.

1270. McDonough, J. J., and Altemeier, W. A.   Subclavian venous thrombosis secondary to indwelling catheters. *Surg. Gynecol. Obstet.* 133:397–400, 1971.

1271. McDowall, R. A. W.   Pulmonary embolism and deep venous thrombosis in burned patients. *Br. J. Plast. Surg.* 26:176–177, 1973.

1272. McGinnis, G. E., Shively, J. G., Patterson, R. L., and Magovern, G. J.   An engineering analysis of intratracheal tube cuffs. *Anesth. Analg.* (Cleve.) 50:557–564, 1971.

1273. McHenry, A. G., Jr.   Management of acute inversion of the uterus. *Obstet. Gynecol.* 16:671–673, 1960.

1274. McHugh, T. J., Forrester, J. S., Adler, L., Zion, D., and Swan, H. J. C.   Pulmonary vascular congestion in acute myocardial infarction: Hemodynamic and radiologic correlations. *Ann. Intern. Med.* 76:29–33, 1972.

1275. McIntosh, H. D.   Arrhythmias. Cooperative study on cardiac catheterization. *Circulation* 37, 38(Suppl. III):27–35, 1968.

1276. McKay, D. G.   Trauma and disseminated intravascular coagulation. *J. Trauma* 9:646–660, 1969.

1277. McKay, D. G., Margaretten, W., and Csavossy, I.   An electron microscope study of endotoxin shock in rhesus monkeys. *Surg. Gynecol. Obstet.* 125:825–832, 1967.

1278. McKay, D. G., Müller-Berghaus, G., and Cruse, V.   Activation of Hageman factor by ellagic acid and the generalized Shwartzman reaction. *Am. J. Pathol.* 54:393–420, 1969.

1279. McLachlin, J., and Paterson, J. C.   Some basic observations on venous thrombosis and pulmonary embolism. *Surg. Gynecol. Obstet.* 93:1–8, 1951.

1280. McLean, A. P. H., Duff, J. H., Groves, A. C., Lapointe, R., and MacLean, L. D.   Oxygen Uptake in Septic Shock. In S. G. Hershey, L. R. M. Del Guercio, and R. McConn (Eds.), *Septic Shock in Man.* Boston: Little, Brown, 1971. Pp. 107–115.

1281. McLean, A. P. H., Duff, J. H., and MacLean, L. D.   Lung lesions associated with septic shock. *J. Trauma* 8:891–898, 1968.

1282. McManus, W. F., Eurenius, K., and Pruitt, B. A., Jr.   Disseminated intravascular coagulation in burned patients. *J. Trauma* 13:416–421, 1973.

1283. McNamara, J. J.   Microaggregates in Stored Blood: Physiologic Significance. In H. R. Chaplin, Jr., E. R. Jaffé, C. Lenfant, and C. R. Valeri (Eds.), *Preservation of Red Blood Cells.* Washington, D.C.: Division of Medical Sciences, National Academy of Sciences, National Research Council, 1973. Pp. 315–320.

1284. McNamara, J. J., Boatright, D., Burran, E. L., Molot, M. D., Summers, E., and Stremple, J. F.   Changes in some physical properties of stored blood. *Ann. Surg.* 174:58–60, 1971.

1285. McNamara, J. J., Burran, E. L., Larson, E., Omiya, G., Suehiro, G., and Yamase, H.   Effect of debris in stored blood on pulmonary microvasculature. *Ann. Thorac. Surg.* 14:133–138, 1972.

1286. McNamara, J. J., Burran, E. L., and Suehiro, G.   Effective filtration of banked blood. *Surgery* 71:594–597, 1972.

1287. McNamara, J. J., Molot, M. D., and Stremple, J. F.   Screen filtration pressure in combat casualties. *Ann. Surg.* 172:334–341, 1970.

1288. McNay, J. L., and Goldberg, L. I.   Comparison of the effects of dopamine, isoproterenol, norepinephrine and bradykinin on canine renal and femoral blood flow. *J. Pharmacol. Exp. Ther.* 151:23–31, 1966.

1289. McNicol, M. W., Kirby, B. J., Bhoola, K. D., Everest, M. E., Price, H. V., and Freedman, S. F.   Pulmonary function in acute myocardial infarction. *Br. Med. J.* 2:1270–1273, 1965.

1290. McNicol, M. W., and Smith, R.   Accidental hypothermia. *Br. Med. J.* 1:19–21, 1964.

1291. Mead, J.   Mechanical properties of lungs. *Physiol. Rev.* 41:281–330, 1961.

1292. Meathe, E. A., Uhl, R. R., Ozaki, G. T., and Saidman, L. J.   On-line Rate Spectral Analysis of the Electrocardiogram During Anesthesia. Abstracts of scientific papers, Annual Meeting of the American Society of Anesthesiologists, Washington, D.C., October 12–16, 1974. Pp. 385–386.

1293. Mehmel, H. C., Duvelleroy, M. A., and Laver, M. B.   Response of coronary blood flow to pH-induced changes in hemoglobin-O_2 affinity. *J. Appl. Physiol.* 35:485–489, 1973.

1294. Mehta, B., Briggs, D. K., Sommers, S. C., and Karpatkin, M.   Disseminated intravascular coagulation following cardiac arrest: A study of 15 patients. *Am. J. Med. Sci.* 264:353–363, 1972.

1295. Mela, L., Bacalzo, L. V., Jr., and Miller, L. D.   Defective oxidative metabolism of rat liver mitochondria in hemorrhagic and endotoxin shock. *Am. J. Physiol.* 220:571–577, 1971.

1296. Mellins, R. B., Levine, O. R., Wigger, H. J., Leidy, G., and Curnen, E. C.   Experimental meningococcemia: Model of overwhelming infection in unanesthetized monkeys. *J. Appl. Physiol.* 32:309–314, 1972.

1297. Mendelson, C. L.   The aspiration of stomach contents into the lungs during obstetric anesthesia. *Am. J. Obstet. Gynecol.* 52:191–203, 1946.

1298. Mengert, W. F., Goodson, J. H., Campbell, R. G., and Haynes, D. M.   Observations on the pathogenesis of premature separation of the normally implanted placenta. *Am. J. Obstet. Gynecol.* 66:1104–1112, 1953.

1299. Menzel, D. B.   Toxicity of ozone, oxygen, and radiation. *Annu. Rev. Pharmacol.* 10:379–391, 1970.

1300. Merrill, E. W.   Rheology of blood. *Physiol. Rev.* 49:863–888, 1969.

1301. Merrill, R. B., and Hingson, R. A.   Study of incidence of maternal mortality from aspiration of vomitus during anesthesia occurring in major obstetric hospitals in the United States. *Anesth. Analg.* (Cleve.) 39:121–135, 1951.

1302. Merskey, C.   Diagnosis and treatment of intravascular coagulation. *Br. J. Haematol.* 15:523–526, 1968.

1303. Merskey, C.   Defibrination syndrome or. . . ? *Blood* 41:599–603, 1973.

1304. Merskey, C., Johnson, A. J., and Lalezari, P.   Increase in fibrinogen and fibrin-related antigen in human serum due to in vitro lysis of fibrin by thrombin. *J. Clin. Invest.* 51:903–911, 1972.

1305. Meyer, J. A. Safety in the Use of Monitoring Equipment. In W. H. L. Dornette (Ed.), *Clinical Anesthesia: Monitoring in Anesthesia.* Philadelphia: Davis, 1973. Pp. 47–68.

1306. Michaelson, E. D., and Walsh, R. E. Osler's node—A complication of prolonged arterial cannulation. *N. Engl. J. Med.* 283:472–473, 1970.

1307. Michenfelder, J. D., Martin, J. T., Altenburg, B. M., and Rehder, K. Air embolism during neurosurgery: An evaluation of right-atrial catheters for diagnosis and treatment. *J.A.M.A.* 208:1353–1358, 1969.

1308. Michenfelder, J. D., Miller, R. H., and Gronert, G. A. Evaluation of an ultrasonic device (Doppler) for the diagnosis of venous air embolism. *Anesthesiology* 36:164–167, 1972.

1309. Mickal, A., Sellman, A. H., and Beebe, J. L. Ruptured tubo-ovarian abscess. *Am. J. Obstet. Gynecol.* 100:432–436, 1968.

1310. Miletich, D. J., Ivankovich, A. D., Albrecht, R. F., and Bonnet, R. Effect of Doxapram on Cerebral Blood Flow, Cardiac Output, and Arterial Blood Pressure in the Unanesthetized and Anesthetized Goat. Abstracts of scientific papers, Annual Meeting of the American Society of Anesthesiologists, Washington, D.C., October 12–16, 1974. Pp. 69–70.

1311. Milic-Emili, J., Henderson, J. A. M., Dolovich, M. B., Trop, D., and Kaneko, K. Regional distribution of inspired gas in the lung. *J. Appl. Physiol.* 21:749–759, 1966.

1312. Millar, R. A., and Gregory, I. C. Reduced oxygen content in equilibrated fresh heparinized and ACD-stored blood from cigarette smokers. *Br. J. Anaesth.* 44:1015–1019, 1972.

1313. Miller, D. R., and Sethi, G. Tracheal stenosis following prolonged cuffed intubation: Cause and prevention. *Ann. Surg.* 171:283–293, 1970.

1314. Miller, G. G., Witwer, M. W., Braude, A. I., and Davis, C. E. Rapid identification of *Candida albicans* septicemia in man by gas-liquid chromatography. *J. Clin. Invest.* 54:1235–1240, 1974.

1315. Miller, J. D., Stanek, A., and Langfitt, T. W. Concepts of cerebral perfusion pressure and vascular compression during intracranial hypertension. *Prog. Brain Res.* 35:411–432, 1972.

1316. Miller, J. M., and Sproule, B. J. Acute effects of inhalation of cigarette smoke on mechanical properties of the lungs. *Am. Rev. Respir. Dis.* 94:721–726, 1966.

1317. Miller, M. G., and Hall, S. V. Intra-aortic balloon counterpulsation in a high-risk cardiac patient undergoing emergency gastrectomy. *Anesthesiology* 42:103–105, 1975.

1318. Miller, M. G., Weintraub, R. M., Hedley-Whyte, J., Restall, D. S., and Alexander, M. Surgery for cardiogenic shock. *Lancet* 2:1342–1345, 1974.

1319. Miller, R. D. Complications of massive blood transfusions. *Anesthesiology* 39:82–93, 1973.

1320. Miller, R. D., Robbins, T. O., Tong, M. J., and Barton, S. L. Coagulation defects associated with massive blood transfusions. *Ann. Surg.* 174:794–801, 1971.

1321. Miller, R. D., Tong, M. J., and Robbins, T. O. Effects of massive transfusion of blood on acid-base balance. *J.A.M.A.* 216:1762–1765, 1971.

1322. Miller, R. L., Forsyth, R. P., Hoffbrand, B. I., and Melmon, K. L. Cardiovascular effects of hemorrhage during endotoxemia in unanesthetized monkeys. *Am. J. Physiol.* 224:1087–1091, 1973.

1323. Miller, W. F., Cade, J. R., and Cushing, I. E. Preoperative recognition and treatment of bronchopulmonary disease. *Anesthesiology* 18:483–497, 1957.

1324. Miller, W. W., Waldhausen, J. A., and Rashkind, W. J. Comparison of oxygen poisoning of the lung in cyanotic and acyanotic dogs. *N. Engl. J. Med.* 282:943–947, 1970.

1325. Milne, R. M., Griffiths, J. M. T., Gunn, A. A., and Ruckley, C. V.   Postoperative deep venous thrombosis: A comparison of diagnostic techniques. *Lancet* 2:445–447, 1971.

1326. Miranda, J. M., and Lourenço, R. V.   Influence of diaphragm activity on the measurement of total chest compliance. *J. Appl. Physiol.* 24:741–746, 1968.

1327. Mirowski, M., Mower, M. M., Gott, V. L., and Brawley, R. K.   Low energy ventricular defibrillation in man using a catheter electrode system. *Circulation* 45, 46(Suppl. II):108, 1972.

1328. Mittman, C., Edelman, N. H., Noggs, A. H., and Shock, N. W.   Relationship between chest wall and pulmonary compliance and age. *J. Appl. Physiol.* 20:1211–1216, 1965.

1329. Modell, J. H.   Resuscitation after aspiration of chlorinated fresh water. *J.A.M.A.* 185:651–655, 1963.

1330. Modell, J. H.   *The Pathophysiology and Treatment of Drowning and Near-Drowning.* Springfield, Ill.: Thomas, 1971.

1331. Modell, J. H., and Davis, J. H.   Electrolyte changes in human drowning victims. *Anesthesiology* 30:414–420, 1969.

1332. Modell, J. H., Davis, J. H., Giammona, S. T., Moya, F., and Mann, J. B.   Blood gas and electrolyte changes in human near-drowning victims. *J.A.M.A.* 203:337–343, 1968.

1333. Modell, J. H., Gaub, M., Moya, F., Vestal, B., and Swarz, H.   Physiologic effects of near-drowning with chlorinated fresh water, distilled water and isotonic saline. *Anesthesiology* 27:33–41, 1966.

1334. Modell, J. H., Giammona, S. T., and Davis, J. H.   Effect of chronic exposure to ultrasonic aerosols on the lung. *Anesthesiology* 28:680–688, 1967.

1335. Modell, J. H., and Moya, F.   Postoperative pulmonary complications. Incidence and management. *Anesth. Analg.* (Cleve.) 45:432–439, 1966.

1336. Modell, J. H., and Moya, F.   Effects of volume of aspirated fluid during chlorinated fresh water drowning. *Anesthesiology* 27:662–672, 1966.

1337. Modell, J. H., Moya, F., Newby, E. J., Ruiz, B. C., and Showers, A. V.   The effects of fluid volume in seawater drowning. *Ann. Intern. Med.* 67:68–80, 1967.

1338. Modell, J. H., Moya, F., Williams, H. D., and Weibley, T. C.   Changes in blood gases and A-aD$_{O_2}$ during near-drowning. *Anesthesiology* 29:456–465, 1968.

1339. Molinoff, P. B., Landsberg, L., and Axelrod, J.   An enzymatic assay for octopamine and other β–hydroxylated phenylethylamines. *J. Pharmacol. Exp. Ther.* 170:253–261, 1969.

1340. Monaco, R. N., Leeper, R. D., Robbins, J. J., and Calvy, G. L.   Intermittent acute porphyria treated with chlorpromazine. *N. Engl. J. Med.* 256:309–311, 1957.

1341. Monato, W. W., Chuntrasakul, C., and Ayvazian, V. H.   Hypertonic sodium solutions in the treatment of burn shock. *Am. J. Surg.* 126:778–783, 1973.

1342. Moncrief, J. A.   Burns. *N. Engl. J. Med.* 288:444–454, 1973.

1343. Monroe, P. W., Muchmore, H. G., Felton, F. G., and Pirtle, J. K.   Quantitation of microorganisms in sputum. *Appl. Microbiol.* 18:214–220, 1969.

1344. Monsees, L. R., and McQuarrie, D. G.   Can catheters be an electrical safety hazard? *Chest* 61:692, 1972.

1345. Moody, F. G., and Aldrete, J. S.   Hydrogen permeability of canine gastric secretory epithelium during formation of acute superficial erosions. *Surgery* 70:154–160, 1971.

1346. Moody, M. R., Young, V. M., Kenton, D. M., and Vermeulen, G. D. *Pseudomonas aeruginosa* in a center for cancer research. I. Distribution of intraspecies types from human and environmental sources. *J. Infect. Dis.* 125:95–101, 1972.

1347. Moore, F. D., and Brennan, M. F. Intravenous feeding. *N. Engl. J. Med.* 287:862–864, 1972.

1348. Moore, F. D., Lyons, J. H., Jr., Pierce, E. C., Jr., Morgan, A. P., Jr., Drinker, P. A., MacArthur, J. D., and Dammin, G. J. *Post-traumatic Pulmonary Insufficiency.* Philadelphia: Saunders, 1969.

1349. Moore, M., Jr. On surviving aircraft disaster. *J. Trauma* 11:190–191, 1971.

1350. Moorthy, S. S., and Losasso, A. M. Patency of the foramen ovale in the critically ill patient. *Anesthesiology* 41:405–407, 1974.

1351. Morgan, A. P. The pulmonary toxicity of oxygen. *Anesthesiology* 29:570–579, 1968.

1352. Morgan, A. P., Jenny, M. E., and Haessler, H. Phospholipids, acute pancreatitis, and the lungs: Effect of lecithinase infusion on pulmonary surface activity in dogs. *Ann. Surg.* 167:329–335, 1968.

1353. Morgan, B. C., Crawford, E. W., Hornbein, T. F., Martin, W. E., and Guntheroth, W. G. Hemodynamic effects of changes in arterial carbon dioxide tension during intermittent positive pressure ventilation. *Anesthesiology* 28:866–873, 1967.

1354. Morgan, B. C., Martin, W. E., Hornbein, T. F., Crawford, E. W., and Guntheroth, W. G. Hemodynamic effects of intermittent positive pressure respiration. *Anesthesiology* 27:584–590, 1966.

1355. Morgan, J. L., Kemmerer, W. T., and Halber, M. D. Doppler shifted ultrasound: History and applications in clinical medicine. *Minn. Med.* 52:503–506, 1969.

1356. Morgan, T. E. Biosynthesis of pulmonary surface-active lipid. *Arch. Intern. Med.* 127:401–407, 1971.

1357. Morgan, T. E., Finley, T. N., Huber, G. L., and Fialkow, H. Alterations in pulmonary surface active lipids during exposure to increased oxygen tension. *J. Clin. Invest.* 44:1737–1744, 1965.

1358. Moritz, A. R. Chemical methods for the determination of death by drowning. *Physiol. Rev.* 24:70–88, 1944.

1359. Moritz, A. R., Henriques, F. C., Jr., and McLean, R. The effects of inhaled heat on the air passages and lungs. An experimental investigation. *Am. J. Pathol.* 21:311–331, 1945.

1360. Moro, M., and Andrews, M. Prophylactic antibiotics in cesarean section. *Obstet. Gynecol.* 44:688–692, 1974.

1361. Morrell, M. T., and Dunnill, M. S. The post-mortem incidence of pulmonary embolism in a hospital population. *Br. J. Surg.* 55:347–352, 1968.

1362. Morris, M. J., Cade, D., and Clarke, B. Oxygen administration during artificial ventilation with pressure cycled respirators. *Anaesth. Intensive Care* 1:125–131, 1972.

1363. Mortensen, J. D. Clinical sequelae from arterial needle puncture, cannulation, and incision. *Circulation* 35:1118–1123, 1967.

1364. Morton, H. J. V. Tobacco smoking and pulmonary complications after operation. *Lancet* 1:368–370, 1944.

1365. Moseley, R. V., and Doty, D. B. Changes in the filtration characteristics of stored blood. *Ann. Surg.* 171:329–335, 1970.

1366. Moseley, R. V., and Doty, D. B. Death associated with multiple pulmonary emboli soon after battle injury. *Ann. Surg.* 171:336–346, 1970.

1367. Moser, K. M., Luchsinger, P. C., Adamson, J. S., McMahon, S. M., Schlueter,

D. P., Spivack, M., and Weg, J. G.   Respiratory stimulation with intravenous doxapram in respiratory failure: A double-blind co-operative study. *N. Engl. J. Med.* 288:427–431, 1973.

1368. Moser, K. M., and Stein, M. (Eds.).   *Pulmonary Thromboembolism.* Chicago: Year Book, 1973.

1369. Moses, D. C., Silver, T. M., and Bookstein, J. J.   The complementary roles of chest radiography, lung scanning, and selective pulmonary angiography in the diagnosis of pulmonary embolism. *Circulation* 49:179–188, 1974.

1370. Moskowitz, M. A., and Wurtman, R. J.   Catecholamines and neurologic diseases. *N. Engl. J. Med.* 293:274–280, 332–338, 1975.

1371. Moss, G.   The role of the central nervous system in shock: The centrineurogenic etiology of the respiratory distress syndrome. *Crit. Care Med.* 2:181–185, 1974.

1372. Moss, G., and Staunton, C.   Blood flow, needle size and hemolysis— Examining an old wives' tale. *N. Engl. J. Med.* 282:967, 1970.

1373. Moss, G., Staunton, C., and Stein, A. A.   The centrineurogenic etiology of the acute respiratory distress syndromes: Universal, species-independent phenomenon. *Am. J. Surg.* 126:37–41, 1973.

1374. Moss, G., Staunton, C., and Stein, A. A.   Cerebral etiology of the "shock lung syndrome." *J. Trauma* 12:885–890, 1972.

1375. Moss, G. S.   Pulmonary involvement in hypovolemic shock. *Annu. Rev. Med.* 23:201–228, 1972.

1376. Moss, G. S., Das Gupta, T. K., Newson, B., and Nyhus, L. M.   Effect of hemorrhagic shock on pulmonary interstitial sodium distribution in the primate lung. *Ann. Surg.* 177:211–221, 1973.

1377. Moss, G. S., Das Gupta, T. K., Newson, B., and Nyhus, L. M.   The effect of saline solution resuscitation on pulmonary sodium and water distribution. *Surg. Gynecol. Obstet.* 136:934–940, 1973.

1378. Moss, G. S., Proctor, H. J., Herman, C. M., Horner, L. D., and Litt, B. D.   Hemorrhagic shock in the baboon. I. Circulatory and metabolic effects of dilutional therapy: Preliminary report. *J. Trauma* 8:837–841, 1968.

1379. Moss, G. S., Siegel, D. C., Cochin, A., and Fresquez, V.   Effects of saline and colloid solutions on pulmonary function in hemorrhagic shock. *Surg. Gynecol. Obstet.* 133:53–58, 1971.

1380. Mostert, J. W., Kenny, G. M., and Murphy, G. P.   Safe placement of central venous catheter into internal jugular veins. *Arch. Surg.* 101:431–432, 1970.

1381. Moulopoulos, S. D., Topaz, S., and Kolff, W. J.   Diastolic balloon pumping (with carbon dioxide) in the aorta—A mechanical assistance to the failing circulation. *Am. Heart J.* 63:669–675, 1962.

1382. Mouridsen, H. T., and Faber, M.   Accumulation of serum-albumin at the operative wound site as a cause of postoperative hypoalbuminaemia. *Lancet* 2:723–725, 1966.

1383. Moxley, R. T., III, Pozefsky, T., and Lockwood, D. H.   Protein nutrition and liver disease after jejunoileal bypass for morbid obesity. *N. Engl. J. Med.* 290:921–926, 1974.

1384. Moylan, J. A., Jr., Wilmore, D. W., Mouton, D. E., and Pruitt, B. A., Jr.   Early diagnosis of inhalation injury using [133]xenon lung scan. *Ann. Surg.* 176:477–484, 1972.

1385. Mozersky, D. J., Buckley, C. J., Hagood, C. O., Jr., Capps, W. F., Jr., and Dannemiller, F. J., Jr.   Ultrasonic evaluation of the palmar circulation: A useful adjunct to radial artery cannulation. *Am. J. Surg.* 126:810–812, 1973.

1386. Mucklow, R. G., and Larard, D. G.   The effects of the inhalation of vomitus on the lungs: Clinical considerations. *Br. J. Anaesth.* 35:153–159, 1963.

1387. Mueller, H., Ayres, S. M., Conklin, E. F., Giannelli, S., Jr., Mazzara, J. T., Grace, W. T., and Nealon, T. F., Jr. The effects of intra-aortic counterpulsation on cardiac performance and metabolism in shock associated with acute myocardial infarction. *J. Clin. Invest.* 50:1885–1900, 1971.

1388. Mueller, H., Ayres, S. M., Giannelli, S., Jr., Conklin, E. F., Mazzara, J. T., and Grace, W. J. Effect of isoproterenol, l-norepinephrine, and intraaortic counterpulsation on hemodynamics and myocardial metabolism in shock following acute myocardial infarction. *Circulation* 45:335–351, 1972.

1389. Muldoon, S. M., Rehder, K., Didier, E. P., Divertie, M. B., Douglas, W. W., and Sessler, A. D. Respiratory care of patients undergoing intrathoracic operations. *Surg. Clin. North Am.* 53:843–857, 1973.

1390. Muller, D. J. A comparison of three approaches to alcohol-withdrawal states. *South. Med. J.* 62:495–496, 1969.

1391. Mundth, E. D., Buckley, M. J., and Austen, W. G. Myocardial revascularization during postinfarction shock. *Hosp. Practice* 8(1):113–123, 1973.

1392. Mundth, E. D., Buckley, M. J., Daggett, W. M., Sanders, C. A., and Austen, W. G. Surgery for complications of acute myocardial infarction. *Circulation* 45:1279–1291, 1972.

1393. Mundth, E. D., Buckley, M. J., Leinbach, R. C., DeSanctis, R. W., Sanders, C. A., Kantrowitz, A., and Austen, W. G. Myocardial revascularization for the treatment of cardiogenic shock complicating acute myocardial infarction. *Surgery* 70:78–87, 1971.

1394. Mundth, E. D., Buckley, M. J., Leinbach, R. C., Gold, H. K., Daggett, W. M., and Austen, W. G. Surgical intervention for the complications of acute myocardial ischemia. *Ann. Surg.* 178:379–388, 1973.

1395. Mundth, E. D., Yurchak, P. M., Buckley, M. J., Leinbach, R. C., Kantrowitz, A., and Austen, W. G. Circulatory assistance and emergency direct coronary-artery surgery for shock complicating acute myocardial infarction. *N. Engl. J. Med.* 283:1382–1384, 1970.

1396. Muneyuki, M., Ueda, Y., Urabe, N., Takeshita, H., and Inamoto, A. Postoperative pain relief and respiratory function in man: Comparison between intermittent intravenous injections of meperidine and continuous lumbar epidural analgesia. *Anesthesiology* 29:304–313, 1968.

1397. Munro, H. N., Fernstrom, J. D., and Wurtman, R. J. Insulin, plasma aminoacid imbalance, and hepatic coma. *Lancet* 1:722–724, 1975.

1398. Murakami, T., Wax, S. D., and Webb, W. R. Pulmonary microcirculation in hemorrhagic shock. *Surg. Forum* 21:25–27, 1970.

1399. Mushin, R., and Ziv, G. Epidemiological aspects of *Pseudomonas aeruginosa* in man, animals, and the environment. Application of pyocin typing. *Isr. J. Med. Sci.* 9:155–161, 1973.

1400. Mushin, W. W., Rendell-Baker, L., Thompson, P. W., and Mapleson, W. W. *Automatic Ventilation of the Lungs* (2nd ed.). Oxford: Blackwell, 1969.

1401. Muysers, K., Smidt, U., and Worth, G. Experiences with the MAT Respiration Mass Spectrometer. *Bull. Physiopathol. Respir.* (Nancy) 3:527–535, 1967.

1402. Myerowitz, R. L., Medeiros, A. A., and O'Brien, T. F. Recent experience with bacillemia due to gram-negative organisms. *J. Infect. Dis.* 124:239–246, 1971.

1403. Myschetsky, A., and Lassen, N. A. Urea-induced, osmotic diuresis and alkalinization of urine in acute barbiturate intoxication. *J.A.M.A.* 185:936–942, 1963.

1404. Nadel, J. A., and Comroe, J. H., Jr. Acute effects of inhalation of cigarette smoke on airway conductance. *J. Appl. Physiol.* 16:713–716, 1961.

1405. Nahrwold, M. L. Thermistor temperature monitor. *Anesth. Analg.* (Cleve.) 53:476–477, 1974.

494 *References*

1406. Naimark, A., and Cherniack, R. M.   Compliance of the respiratory system and its components in health and obesity. *J. Appl. Physiol.* 15:377–382, 1960.

1407. Naimark, A., Dugard, A., and Rangno, R. E.   Regional pulmonary blood flow and gas exchange in haemorrhagic shock. *J. Appl. Physiol.* 25:301–309, 1968.

1408. Nakata, K., Leong, G. F., and Brauer, R. W.   Direct measurement of blood pressures in minute vessels of the liver. *Am. J. Physiol.* 199:1181–1188, 1960.

1409. Namba, T., Brown, S. B., and Grob, D.   Neonatal myasthenia gravis: Report of two cases and review of the literature. *Pediatrics* 45:488–504, 1970.

1410. Nash, G., Blennerhassett, J. B., and Pontoppidan, H.   Pulmonary lesions associated with oxygen therapy and artificial ventilation. *N. Engl. J. Med.* 276:368–374, 1967.

1411. Naylor, B. A., Welch, M. H., Shafer, A. W., and Guenter, C. A.   Blood affinity for oxygen in hemorrhagic and endotoxic shock. *J. Appl. Physiol.* 32:829–833, 1972.

1412. Needleman, H. L., and Scanlon, J.   Getting the lead out. *N. Engl. J. Med.* 288:466–467, 1973.

1413. Neely, W. A., Robinson, W. T., McMullan, M. H., Bobo, W. O., Meadows, D. L., and Hardy, J. D.   Postoperative respiratory insufficiency: Physiological studies with therapeutic implications. *Ann. Surg.* 171:679–685, 1970.

1414. Nelson, J. H., Jr., Bernstein, R. L., Huston, J. W., Garcia, N. A., and Gartenlaub, C.   Percutaneous retrograde femoral arteriography in obstetrics and gynecology. *Obstet. Gynecol. Surg.* 16:1–19, 1961.

1415. Nemoto, E. M., and Frankel, H. M.   Cerebral oxygenation and metabolism during progressive hyperthermia. *Am. J. Physiol.* 219:1784–1788, 1970.

1416. Nesbitt, R. E. L., Jr.   Placenta previa and the low-lying placenta. *Clin. Obstet. Gynecol.* 3:569–584, 1960.

1417. Nesbitt, R. E. L., Jr., Powers, S. R., Jr., Boba, A., and Stein, A.   Experimental abruptio placentae. Histologic and physiologic studies. *Obstet. Gynecol.* 12:359–368, 1958.

1418. Neufeld, O., Smith, J. R., and Goldman, S. L.   Arterial oxygen tension in relation to age in hospital subjects. *J. Am. Geriatr. Soc.* 21:4–9, 1973.

1419. Neuschatz, J., and Crosby, W. H.   The prevention of postoperative thrombosis—A simple, safe approach. *Arch. Intern. Med.* 130:966–967, 1972.

1420. Newball, H. H., and Keiser, H. R.   Relative effects of bradykinin and histamine on the respiratory system of man. *J. Appl. Physiol.* 35:552–556, 1973.

1421. Newbower, R. S., Cooper, J. B., Ryan, J. F., and Maier, W. R.   Monitoring Temperature in Anesthesia: A New Method. Abstracts of scientific papers, Annual Meeting of the American Society of Anesthesiologists, Washington, D.C., October 12–16, 1974. Pp. 391–392.

1422. Newell, J. C., Levitzky, M. G., Krasney, J. A., and Dutton, R. E.   The influence of arterial Po_2 on the attenuation of blood flow to atelectatic lung. *Fed. Proc.* 33:447, 1974.

1423. Ng, W. S., and Rosen, M.   Positioning central venous catheters through the basilic vein. A comparison of catheters. *Br. J. Anaesth.* 45:1211–1214, 1973.

1424. Nichols, C. W., and Lambertsen, C. J.   Effects of high oxygen pressure on the eye. *N. Engl. J. Med.* 281:25–30, 1969.

1425. Nicholson, M. J.   Management of respiratory failure in acute pancreatitis. *Anesth. Analg.* (Cleve.) 53:84–88, 1974.

1426. Nicolaides, A. N., Dupont, P. A., Desai, S., Lewis, J. D., Douglas, J. N., Dodsworth, H., Fourides, G., Luck, R. J., and Jamieson, C. W.   Small doses of subcutaneous sodium heparin in preventing deep vein thrombosis after major surgery. *Lancet* 2:890–893, 1972.

1427. Niedrach, L. W., and Stoddard, W. H. A new approach to sensors for in vivo monitoring. I. Oxygen. *J. Assoc. Adv. Med. Instrum.* 6:121–125, 1972.

1428. Nielsen, B., and Thorn, N. A. Transient excess urinary excretion of antidiuretic material in acute intermittent porphyria with hyponatremia and hypomagnesemia. *Am. J. Med.* 38:345–358, 1965.

1429. Niemetz, J., and Marcus, A. J. Stimulation of leukocyte-derived procoagulant activity by platelets and platelet membranes. *J. Clin. Invest.* 53:56a, 1974.

1430. Niewoehner, D. E., and Kleinerman, J. Morphologic basis of pulmonary resistance in the human lung and effects of aging. *J. Appl. Physiol.* 36:412–418, 1974.

1431. Niewoehner, D. E., Kleinerman, J., and Rice, D. B. Pathologic changes in the peripheral airways of young cigarette smokers. *N. Engl. J. Med.* 291:755–758, 1974.

1432. Niinikoski, J., Goldstein, R., Linsey, M., and Hunt, T. K. Effect of oxygen-induced lung damage on tissue oxygen supply. *Acta Chir. Scand.* 139:591–595, 1973.

1433. Niinikoski, J., Nikkari, T., and Kulonen, E. Pulmonary oxygen toxicity: Composition of endobronchial saline extracts of rats during exposure to oxygen. *Aerosp. Med.* 42:525–529, 1971.

1434. Nilsson, E. On treatment of barbiturate poisoning. A modified clinical aspect. *Acta Med. Scand.* [Suppl.] 253:1–127, 1951.

1435. Nishijima, H., Shubin, H., Cavanilles, J., and Weil, M. H. Shock associated with gram-negative bacteremia. *Crit. Care Med.* 2:41–42, 1974.

1436. Nobel, J. J. A new portable clinical suction device. *Anesthesiology* 29:1217–1219, 1968.

1437. Noble, J., and Matthew, H. Acute poisoning by tricyclic antidepressants: Clinical features and management of 100 patients. *Clin. Toxicol.* 2:403–421, 1969.

1438. Nobles, E. R., Jr. Bacteroides infections. *Ann. Surg.* 177:601–606, 1973.

1439. Noehren, T. H. Is positive pressure breathing over-rated? *Chest* 57:507–509, 1970.

1440. Noehren, T. H., Lasry, J. E., and Legters, L. J. Intermittent positive pressure breathing (IPPB/I) for the prevention and management of postoperative pulmonary complications. *Surgery* 43:658–665, 1958.

1441. Noone, R. B., Graham, W. P., III, and Royster, H. P. Autotransfusion for blood loss in some major esthetic operations. *Plast. Reconstr. Surg.* 51:559–561, 1973.

1442. Norlander, O. P. The use of respirators in anaesthesia and surgery. *Acta Anaesthesiol. Scand.* [Suppl.] 30:1–74, 1968.

1443. Norlander, O. P. Preoperative and postoperative care and monitoring of patients undergoing cardiac surgery. *Int. Anesthesiol. Clin.* 10(4):153–172, 1972.

1444. Northway, W. H., Jr., Petriceks, R., and Shahinian, L. Quantitative aspects of oxygen toxicity in the newborn: Inhibition of lung DNA synthesis in the mouse. *Pediatrics* 50:67–72, 1972.

1445. Nossel, H. L., Yudelman, I., Canfield, R. E., Butler, V. P., Jr., Spanondis, K., Wilner, G. D., and Qureshi, G. D. Measurement of fibrinopeptide A in human blood. *J. Clin. Invest.* 54:43–53, 1974.

1446. Nunn, J. F. Influence of age and other factors on hypoxaemia in the postoperative period. *Lancet* 2:466–468, 1965.

1447. Nunn, J. F., Bergman, N. A., and Coleman, A. J. Factors influencing the arterial oxygen tension during anaesthesia with artificial ventilation. *Br. J. Anaesth.* 37:898–914, 1965.

1448. O'Brien, P., and Silen, W. Effect of bile salts and aspirin on the gastric mucosal blood flow. *Gastroenterology* 64:246–253, 1973.

1449. O'Brien, T. G., and Watkins, E., Jr. Gas-exchange dynamics of glycerolized frozen blood. *J. Thorac. Cardiovasc. Surg.* 40:611–624, 1960.

1450. O'Higgins, J. W. Fat embolism. *Br. J. Anaesth.* 42:163–168, 1970.

1451. Ollodart, R., and Mansberger, A. R. The effect of hypovolemic shock on bacterial defense. *Am. J. Surg.* 110:302–307, 1965.

1452. Olsson, P., Rådegran, K., and Swedenborg, J. Effects of disseminated intravascular coagulation on pulmonary circulation and respiration. *Int. Anesthesiol. Clin.* 10(4):173–179, 1972.

1453. Olsson, S. B., Wassen, R., Varnauskas, E., and Wallman, H. A simple analogue computer for cardiac output determination by thermodilution. *Cardiovasc. Res.* 6:303–308, 1972.

1454. Opie, L. H., and Spalding, J. M. K. Chest physiotherapy during intermittent positive-pressure respiration. *Lancet* 2:671–673, 1958.

1455. Orloff, M. J., and Charters, A. C. Injuries of the small bowel and mesentery and retroperitoneal hematoma. *Surg. Clin. North Am.* 52:729–734, 1972.

1456. Orr, R., Krous, H. F., and Hodson, W. A. Meconium Aspiration Syndrome: The Relationship of Clinical and Pathological Findings to Treatment. Abstracts of scientific papers, Annual Meeting of the American Society of Anesthesiologists, Washington, D. C., October 12–16, 1974. Pp. 297–298.

1457. Osborn, J. J. Experimental hypothermia: Respiratory and blood pH changes in relation to cardiac function. *Am. J. Physiol.* 175:389–398, 1953.

1458. Osborn, J. J. Monitoring respiratory function. *Crit. Care Med.* 2:217–220, 1974.

1459. Osborn, J. J., Beaumont, J. O., Raison, J. C. A., and Abbott, R. P. Computation for Quantitative On-line Measurements in an Intensive Care Ward. In R. W. Stacy and B. Waxman (Eds.), *Computers in Biomedical Research.* New York: Academic, 1969.

1460. Osborn, J. J., Beaumont, J. O., Raison, J. C. A., Russell, J., and Gerbode, F. Measurement and monitoring of acutely ill patients by digital computer. *Surgery* 64:1057–1070, 1968.

1461. Osborn, J. J., Gerbode, F., Johnston, J. B., Ross, J. K., Ogata, T., and Kerth, W. J. Blood chemical changes in perfusion hypothermia for cardiac surgery. *J. Thorac. Cardiovasc. Surg.* 42:462–474, 1961.

1462. Osborn, J. J., Swank, R. L., Hill, J. D., Aguilar, M. J., and Gerbode, F. Clinical use of a Dacron wool filter during perfusion for open-heart surgery. *J. Thorac. Cardiovasc. Surg.* 60:575–581, 1970.

1463. Osborn, J. R., Jones, R. C., and Jahnke, E. J., Jr. Traumatic tricuspid insufficiency. Hemodynamic data and surgical treatment. *Circulation* 30:217–222, 1964.

1464. Oski, F. A., Travis, S. F., Miller, L. D., Delivoria-Papadopoulos, M., and Cannon, E. The in vitro restoration of red cells 2,3-diphosphoglycerate levels in banked blood. *Blood* 37:52–58, 1971.

1465. Overholt, R. H. Postoperative pulmonary hypoventilation. *J.A.M.A.* 95:1484–1489, 1930.

1466. Overholt, R. H., and Veal, J. R. The incidence, character and significance of abnormal physical signs in the chest occurring after major surgical operations. *N. Engl. J. Med.* 208:242–247, 1933.

1467. Owings, J. M., Bomar, W. E., Jr., and Ramage, R. C. Parenteral hyperalimentation and its practical implications. *Ann. Surg.* 175:712–719, 1972.

1468. Oxorn, H. Maternal mortality: A 40 year survey. *Obstet. Gynecol.* 29:744–749, 1967.

1469. Paegle, R. D., Spain, D., and Davis, S.   Pulmonary morphology of chronic phase of oxygen toxicity in adult rats. *Chest* 66(Suppl.): 7S–8S, 1974.
1470. Page, D. W., Teres, D., and Hartshorn, J. W.   Fatal hemorrhage from Swan-Ganz catheter. *N. Engl. J. Med.* 291:260, 1974.
1471. Pain, M. C. F., Stannard, M., and Sloman, G.   Disturbances of pulmonary function after acute myocardial infarction. *Br. Med. J.* 2:591–594, 1967.
1472. Palmer, K. N. V., and Diament, M. L.   Relative contributions of obstructive and restrictive ventilatory impairment in the production of hypoxaemia and hypercapnia in chronic bronchitis. *Lancet* 1:1233–1234, 1968.
1473. Palmer, K. N. V., and Gardiner, A. J. S.   Effect of partial gastrectomy on pulmonary physiology. *Br. Med. J.* 1:347–349, 1964.
1474. Palmer, K. N. V., Gardiner, A. J. S., and McGregor, M. H.   Hypoxaemia after partial gastrectomy. *Thorax* 20:73–75, 1965.
1475. Palmer, K. N. V., and Sellick, B. A.   The prevention of postoperative pulmonary atelectasis. *Lancet* 1:164–168, 1953.
1476. Palmer, R. F., and Lasseter, K. C.   Sodium nitroprusside. *N. Engl. J. Med.* 292:294–297, 1975.
1477. Pamintuan, R. L., Brashear, R. E., Ross, J. C., and DeAtley, R. E.   Cardiovascular effects of experimental aspiration pneumonia in dogs. *Am. Rev. Respir. Dis.* 103:516–523, 1971.
1478. Parad, R., Simmons, G., Feldman, N., and Huber, G.   Impairment of adaptive tolerance to oxygen toxicity by systemic immunosuppression. *Chest* 67(Suppl.): 42S–43S, 1975.
1479. Paraskos, J. A., Adelstein, S. J., Smith, R. E., Rickman, F. D., Grossman, W., Dexter, L., and Dalen, J. E.   Late prognosis of acute pulmonary embolism. *N. Engl. J. Med.* 289:55–58, 1973.
1480. Parbrook, G. D., Steel, D. F., and Dalrymple, D. G.   Factors predisposing to postoperative pain and pulmonary complications. A study of male patients undergoing gastric surgery. *Br. J. Anaesth.* 45:21–33, 1973.
1481. Pareira, M. D.   *Therapeutic Nutrition with Tube Feeding.* Springfield, Ill.: Thomas, 1959.
1482. Parker, D., Key, A., and Davies, R. S.   Catheter-tip transducer for continuous in-vivo measurement of oxygen tension. *Lancet* 1:952–953, 1971.
1483. Parker, F. B., Jr., Racz, G. B., Wax, S. D., Kusajima, K., Murray, D. G., and Webb, W. R.   The hemodynamics of experimental fat embolism and associated therapy. *Chest* 65(Suppl.): 54S–55S, 1974.
1484. Parker, K. D., Fontan, C. R., and Kirk, P. L.   Rapid gas chromatographic method for screening of toxicological extracts for alkaloids, barbiturates, sympathomimetic amines, and tranquilizers. *Anal. Chem.* 35:356–359, 1963.
1485. Parkes, J. D., Sharpstone, P., and Williams, R.   Levodopa in hepatic coma. *Lancet* 2:1341–1343, 1970.
1486. Parks, C. R., Alden, E. R., Standaert, T. A., Woodrum, D. E., Graham, C. B., and Hodson, W. A.   The effect of water nebulization on cough transport of pulmonary mucus in the mouth-breathing dog. *Am. Rev. Respir. Dis.* 108:513–519, 1973.
1487. Parmley, L. F., Mattingly, T. W., Manion, W. C., and Jahnke, E. J., Jr.   Non-penetrating traumatic injury of the aorta. *Circulation* 17:1086–1101, 1958.
1488. Parmley, W. W., Chatterjee, K., Charuzi, Y., and Swan, H. J. C.   Hemodynamic effects of noninvasive systolic unloading (nitroprusside) and diastolic augmentation (external counterpulsation) in patients with acute myocardial infarction. *Am. J. Cardiol.* 33:819–825, 1974.
1489. Parving, H.-H., Rossing, N., Nielsen, S. L., and Lassen, N. A.   Increased transcapillary escape rate of albumin, IgG, and IgM after plasma volume expansion. *Am. J. Physiol.* 227:245–250, 1974.

1490. Paskin, S., Rodman, T., and Smith, T. C.   The effect of spinal anesthesia on the pulmonary function of patients with chronic obstructive pulmonary disease. *Ann. Surg.* 169:35–41, 1969.

1491. Patton, J. F., and Doolittle, W. H.   Core rewarming by peritoneal dialysis following induced hypothermia in the dog. *J. Appl. Physiol.* 33:800–804, 1972.

1492. Patton, J. F., Doolittle, W. H., and Hamlet, M. P.   Peritoneal clearance of urea and potassium following experimental hypothermia. *J. Appl. Physiol.* 36:403–406, 1974.

1493. Paulson, O. B., Parving, H.-H., Olesen, J., and Skinhoj, E.   Influence of carbon monoxide and of hemodilution on cerebral blood flow and blood gases in man. *J. Appl. Physiol.* 35:111–116, 1973.

1494. Paust, J. C.   Respiratory care in acute botulism: A report of four cases. *Anesth. Analg.* (Cleve.) 50:1003–1009, 1971.

1495. Payne, J. H., and DeWind, L. T.   Surgical treatment of obesity. *Am. J. Surg.* 118:141–146, 1969.

1496. Pazell, J. A., and Peltier, L. F.   Experience with 63 patients with fat embolism. *Surg. Gynecol. Obstet.* 135:77–80, 1972.

1497. Pearce, M. L., Yamashita, J., and Beazell, J.   Measurement of pulmonary edema. *Circ. Res.* 16:482–488, 1965.

1498. Pecora, D. V.   Predictability of effects of abdominal and thoracic surgery upon pulmonary function. *Ann. Surg.* 170:101–108, 1969.

1499. Pedowitz, P., and Bloomfield, R. D.   Ruptured adnexal abscess (tubo-ovarian) with generalized peritonitis. *Am. J. Obstet. Gynecol.* 88:721–729, 1964.

1500. Peirce, E. C., II.   The theory and function of the membrane lung. *Mt. Sinai J. Med. N.Y.* 40:119–134, 1973.

1501. Peirce, E. C., II, Zacharias, A., Alday, J. M., Jr., Hoffman, B. A., Jacobson, J. H., II.   Carbon monoxide poisoning: Experimental hypothermic and hyperbaric studies. *Surgery* 72:229–237, 1972.

1502. Pelled, B., Shechter, Y., Alroy, G., Lichtig, C., Turbati, D., and Ben David, A.   Deleterious effects of oxygen breathing at ambient and hyperbaric pressure in treatment of nitrogen dioxide poisoned mice. *Am. Rev. Respir. Dis.* 108:1152–1157, 1973.

1503. Pelletier, C. L., and Shepherd, J. T.   Venous responses to stimulation of carotid chemoreceptors by hypoxia and hypercapnia. *Am. J. Physiol.* 223:97–103, 1972.

1504. Peltier, L. F.   Fat embolism: A pulmonary disease. *Surgery* 62:756–758, 1967.

1505. Penn, I.   Penetrating injuries of the neck. *Surg. Clin. North Am.* 53:1469–1478, 1973.

1506. Penn, I., and Schwartz, S. I.   Evaluation of low molecular weight dextran in the treatment of frostbite. *J. Trauma* 4:784–790, 1964.

1507. Perchick, J. S., Winkelstein, A., and Shadduck, R. K.   Disseminated intravascular coagulation in heat stroke. Response to heparin therapy. *J.A.M.A.* 231:480–483, 1975.

1508. Perine, P. L., Harris, K. L., and Kirkpatrick, C. H.   Immunologic reaction to duck embryo rabies vaccine. *J.A.M.A.* 205:554–558, 1968.

1509. Perkins, H. A.   Postoperative coagulation defects. *Anesthesiology* 27:456–464, 1966.

1510. Perlo, V. P., Arnason, B., and Castleman, B.   The thymus gland in elderly patients with myasthenia gravis. *Neurology* 25:294–295, 1975.

1511. Perlo, V. P., Poskanzer, D. C., Schwab, R. S., Viets, H. R., Osserman, K. E., and Genkins, G.   Myasthenia gravis: Evaluation of treatment in 1,335 patients. *Neurology* 16:431–439, 1966.

1512. Perry, J. F., Jr., and Galway, C. F.   Factors influencing survival after flail chest injuries. *Arch. Surg.* 91:216–219, 1965.

1513. Perry, J. F., Jr., and Galway, C. F. Chest injury due to blunt trauma. *J. Thorac. Cardiovasc. Surg.* 49:684–693, 1965.

1514. Peskett, W. G. H. Antacids before obstetric anaesthesia. A clinical evaluation of the effectiveness of mist. magnesium trisilicate BPC. *Anaesthesia* 28:509–513, 1973.

1515. Peters, J. M., and Ferris, B. G., Jr. Smoking, pulmonary function, and respiratory symptoms in a college-age group. *Am. Rev. Respir. Dis.* 95:774–782, 1967.

1516. Peters, J. M., Theriault, G. F., Fine, L. J., and Wegman, D. H. Chronic effect of fire fighting on pulmonary function. *N. Engl. J. Med.* 291:1320–1322, 1974.

1517. Peters, R. M. Work of breathing following trauma. *J. Trauma* 8:915–923, 1968.

1518. Peters, R. M., Hilberman, M., Hogan, J. S., and Crawford, D. A. Objective indications for respirator therapy in post-trauma and post-operative patients. *Am. J. Surg.* 124:262–268, 1972.

1519. Peterson, D. I., Lonergan, L. H., and Hardinge, M. G. Smoking and pulmonary function. *Arch. Environ. Health* 16:215–218, 1968.

1520. Petty, T. L., Bigelow, D. B., and Levine, B. E. The simplicity and safety of arterial puncture. *J.A.M.A.* 195:693–695, 1966.

1521. Petty, T. L., Stanford, R. E., and Neff, T. A. Continuous oxygen therapy in chronic airway obstruction. Observations on possible oxygen toxicity and survival. *Ann. Intern. Med.* 75:361–367, 1971.

1522. Peyton, M. D., Hinshaw, L. B., and Elkins, R. C. Effects of coronary vasodilatation on cardiac performance during endotoxin shock. *Crit. Care Med.* 3:48–49, 1975.

1523. Pflug, A. E., Murphy, T. M., Butler, S. H., and Tucker, G. T. The effects of postoperative peridural analgesia on pulmonary therapy and pulmonary complications. *Anesthesiology* 41:8–17, 1974.

1524. Phelps, M. E., Grubb, R. L., Jr., and Ter-Pogossian, M. M. Correlation between Pa_{CO_2} and regional cerebral blood volume by x-ray fluorescence. *J. Appl. Physiol.* 35:274–280, 1973.

1525. Phillips, A. W., and Cope, O. Burn therapy. II. The revelation of respiratory tract damage as a principal killer of the burned patient. *Ann. Surg.* 155:1–12, 1962.

1526. Phillips, A. W., Tanner, J. W., and Cope, O. Burn therapy. IV. Respiratory tract damage (an account of the clinical, x-ray and post-mortem findings) and the meaning of restlessness. *Ann. Surg.* 158:799–811, 1963.

1527. Pierce, A. K., and Sanford, J. P. Bacterial contamination of aerosols. *Arch. Intern. Med.* 131:156–159, 1973.

1528. Pierce, A. K., Sanford, J. P., Thomas, G. D., and Leonard, J. S. Long-term evaluation of decontamination of inhalation-therapy equipment and the occurrence of necrotizing pneumonia. *N. Engl. J. Med.* 282:528–531, 1970.

1529. Pierce, G. E., and Brockenbrough, E. C. The spectrum of mesenteric infarction. *Am. J. Surg.* 119:233–239, 1970.

1530. Pierce, J. A. Age related changes in the fibrous proteins of the lung. *Arch. Environ. Health* 6:50–57, 1963.

1531. Pierce, J. A., and Ebert, R. V. The elastic properties of the lungs in the aged. *J. Lab. Clin. Med.* 51:63–71, 1958.

1532. Plotz, P. H., Berk, P. D., Scharschmidt, B. F., Gordon, J. K., and Vergalla, J. Removing substances from blood by affinity chromatography. I. Removing bilirubin and other albumin-bound substances from plasma and blood with albumin-conjugated agarose beads. *J. Clin. Invest.* 53:778–785, 1974.

1533. Plum, F. Hyperpnea, hyperventilation, and brain dysfunction. *Ann. Intern. Med.* 76:328, 1972.

1534. Plum, F., and Alvord, E. C., Jr. Apneustic breathing in man. *Arch. Neurol.* 10:101–112, 1964.

1535. Plum, F., and Posner, J. B. *The Diagnosis of Stupor and Coma.* Philadelphia: Davis, 1972.

1536. Plum, F., Posner, J. B., and Collins, R. C. Cerebral metabolism during induced seizures in man and animals. *Riv. Patol. Nerv. Ment.* 91:345–356, 1970.

1537. Plum, F., Posner, J. B., and Hain, R. F. Delayed neurological deterioration after anoxia. *Arch. Intern. Med.* 110:18–25, 1962.

1538. Plum, F., and Swanson, A. G. Abnormalities in the central regulation of respiration in acute and convalescent poliomyelitis. *Arch. Neurol. Psychiatry* 80:267–285, 1958.

1539. Plum, F., and Swanson, A. G. Central neurogenic hyperventilation in man. *Arch. Neurol. Psychiatry* 81:535–549, 1959.

1540. Pollak, E. W., Sparks, F. C., and Barker, W. F. Pulmonary embolism. An appraisal of therapy in 516 cases. *Arch. Surg.* 107:66–68, 1973.

1541. Pontoppidan, H. Treatment of respiratory failure in nonthoracic trauma. *J. Trauma* 8:938–945, 1968.

1542. Pontoppidan, H., and Beecher, H. K. Progressive loss of protective reflexes in the airway with the advance of age. *J.A.M.A.* 174:2209–2213, 1960.

1543. Pontoppidan, H., and Bushnell, L. S. Respiratory Therapy for Convalescing Surgical Patients with Chronic Lung Disease. In D. A. Holaday (Ed.), *Clinical Anesthesia: Lung Disease.* Philadelphia: Davis, 1967. Pp. 120–123.

1544. Pontoppidan, H., Geffin, B., and Lowenstein, E. Acute respiratory failure in the adult. *N. Engl. J. Med.* 287:690–698, 743–752, 799–806, 1972.

1545. Pontoppidan, H., Hedley-Whyte, J., Bendixen, H. H., Laver, M. B., and Radford, E. P., Jr. Ventilation and oxygen requirements during prolonged artificial ventilation in patients with respiratory failure. *N. Engl. J. Med.* 273:401–409, 1965.

1546. Pontoppidan, H., Laver, M. B., and Geffin, B. Acute respiratory failure in the surgical patient. *Adv. Surg.* 4:163–254, 1970.

1547. Pool, J. L., Owen, S. E., Meyers, F. K., Coalson, J. J., Holmes, D. D., Guenter, C. A., and Hinshaw, L. B. Response of the subhuman primate in gram-negative septicemia induced by live *Escherichia coli. Surg. Gynecol. Obstet.* 132:469–477, 1971.

1548. Poppers, P. J. Controlled evaluation of ultrasonic measurement of systolic and diastolic blood pressures in pediatric patients. *Anesthesiology* 38:187–191, 1973.

1549. Poppers, P. J., Epstein, R. M., and Donham, R. T. Automatic ultrasound monitoring of blood pressure during induced hypotension. *Anesthesiology* 35:431–435, 1971.

1550. Poppers, P. J., Hochberg, H. M., and Schmalzbach, E. L. A method for ultrasonic measurement of blood pressure in the adult leg. *Anesthesiology* 38:490–494, 1973.

1551. Powell, W. J., Jr., Daggett, W. M., Magro, A. E., Bianco, J. A., Buckley, M. J., Sanders, C. A., Kantrowitz, A. R., and Austen, W. G. Effects of intra-aortic balloon counterpulsation on cardiac performance, oxygen consumption, and coronary blood flow in dogs. *Circ. Res.* 26:753–764, 1970.

1552. Powers, S. R., Jr., Mannal, R., Neclerio, M., English, M., Marr, C., Leather, R., Ueda, H., Williams, G., Custead, W., and Dutton, R. Physiologic consequences of positive end-expiratory pressure (PEEP) ventilation. *Ann. Surg.* 178:265–272, 1973.

1553. Prasertwanitch, Y., Schwartz, J. J. H., and Vandam, L. D.   Arytenoid cartilage dislocation following prolonged endotracheal intubation. *Anesthesiology* 41:516–517, 1974.
1554. Pratt, P. C.   Pulmonary capillary proliferation induced by oxygen inhalation. *Am. J. Pathol.* 34:1033–1042, 1958.
1555. Pratt, P. C.   The reaction of the human lung to enriched oxygen atmosphere. *Ann. N.Y. Acad. Sci.* 121:809–822, 1965.
1556. Pratt, S. A., Smith, M. H., Ladman, A. J., and Finley, T. N.   The ultrastructure of alveolar macrophages from human cigarette smokers and nonsmokers. *Lab. Invest.* 24:331–338, 1971.
1557. Press, E.   Nuclear and fossil-fueled plants generating electricity. Their environmental health hazards. *J.A.M.A.* 222:1281–1283, 1972.
1558. Presscott, L. F., Peard, M. C., and Wallace, I. R.   Accidental hypothermia. A common condition. *Br. Med. J.* 2:1367–1370, 1962.
1559. Preston, F. E., Malia, R. G., Sworn, M. J., and Blackburn, E. K.   Intravascular coagulation and *E. coli* septicaemia. *J. Clin. Pathol.* 26:120–125, 1973.
1560. Priano, L. L., Wilson, R. D., and Traber, D. L.   Lack of significant protection afforded by heparin during endotoxic shock. *Am. J. Physiol.* 220:901–905, 1971.
1561. Price, D. J. E., and Sleigh, J. D.   Control of infection due to *Klebsiella aerogenes* in a neurosurgical unit by withdrawal of all antibiotics. *Lancet* 2:1213–1215, 1970.
1562. Pritchard, J. A., and Stone, S. R.   Clinical and laboratory observations on eclampsia. *Am. J. Obstet. Gynecol.* 99:754–765, 1967.
1563. Proctor, H. J., Ballantine, T. V. N., and Broussard, N. D.   An analysis of pulmonary function following non-thoracic trauma, with recommendations for therapy. *Ann. Surg.* 172:180–189, 1970.
1564. Proctor, H. J., Moss, G. S., Homer, L. D., and Litt, B. D.   Hemorrhagic shock in the baboon. II. Changes in lung compliance associated with hemorrhagic shock and resuscitation. *J. Trauma* 8:842–847, 1968.
1565. Proctor, H. J., and Woolson, R.   Prediction of respiratory muscle fatigue by measurements of the work of breathing. *Surg. Gynecol. Obstet.* 136:367–370, 1973.
1566. Pruitt, B. A., Jr., DiVincenti, F. C., Mason, A. D., Jr., Foley, F. D., and Flemma, R. J.   The occurrence and significance of pneumonia and other pulmonary complications in burned patients: Comparison of conventional and topical treatments. *J. Trauma* 10:519–530, 1970.
1567. Pruitt, B. A., Jr., Flemma, R. J., DiVincenti, F. C., Foley, F. D., and Mason, A. D., Jr.   Pulmonary complications in burn patients. *J. Thorac. Cardiovasc. Surg.* 59:7–18, 1970.
1568. Prys-Roberts, C.   Principles of treatment of poisoning by higher oxides of nitrogen. *Br. J. Anaesth.* 39:432–438, 1967.
1569. Prys-Roberts, C., Corbett, J. L., Kerr, J. H., Crampton Smith, A., and Spalding, J. M. K.   Treatment of sympathetic overactivity in tetanus. *Lancet* 1:542–545, 1969.
1570. Prys-Roberts, C., Kelman, G. R., Greenbaum, R., Kain, M. L., and Bay, J.   Hemodynamics and alveolar arterial P_{O_2} differences at varying Pa_{CO_2} in anesthetized man. *J. Appl. Physiol.* 25:80–87, 1968.
1571. Puglia, C. D., Glauser, E. M., and Glauser, S. C.   Core temperature response of rats during exposure to oxygen at high pressure. *J. Appl. Physiol.* 36:149–153, 1974.
1572. Putnam, C. E., Minagi, H., and Blaisdell, F. W.   The roentgen appearance of disseminated intravascular coagulation (DIC). *Radiology* 109:13–18, 1973.

1573. Puy, R. J. M., Hyde, R. W., Fisher, A. B., Clark, J. M., Dickson, J., and Lambertsen, C. J.   Alterations in the pulmonary capillary bed during early O_2 toxicity in man. *J. Appl. Physiol.* 24:537–543, 1968.

1574. Qvist, J., Pontoppidan, H., Wilson, R. S., Lowenstein, E., and Laver, M. B.   Hemodynamic responses to mechanical ventilation with PEEP: The effect of hypervolemia. *Anesthesiology* 42:45–55, 1975.

1575. Rådegran, K.   Circulatory and respiratory effects of induced platelet aggregation. An experimental study in dogs. *Acta Chir. Scand.* [Suppl.] 420:1–24, 1971.

1576. Raffensperger, J. C., and Ramenofsky, M. L.   A fatal complication of hyperalimentation: A case report. *Surgery* 68:393–394, 1970.

1577. Rahal, J. J., Jr., Meade, R. H., III, Bump, C. M., and Reinauer, A. J.   Upper respiratory tract carriage of gram-negative enteric bacilli by hospital personnel. *J.A.M.A.* 214:754–756, 1970.

1578. Rahimtoola, S. H., Loeb, H. S., Ehsani, A., Sinno, M. Z., Chuquimia, R., Lal, R., Rosen, K. M., and Gunnar, R. M.   Relationship of pulmonary artery to left ventricular diastolic pressures in acute myocardial infarction. *Circulation* 46:283–290, 1972.

1579. Rahn, H., and Fenn, W. O.   *A Graphical Analysis of the Respiratory Gas Exchange. The O_2-CO_2 Diagram.* Washington, D.C.: American Physiological Society, 1955.

1580. Rakower, S. R., and Worth, M. H., Jr.   Autotransfusion: Perspective and critical problems. *J. Trauma* 13:573–574, 1973.

1581. Rakower, S. R., Worth, M. H., Jr., and Lackner, H.   Massive intraoperative autotransfusion of blood. *Surg. Gynecol. Obstet.* 137:633–636, 1973.

1582. Ramachandran, P. R., and Fairley, H. B.   Changes in functional residual capacity during respiratory failure. *Can. Anaesth. Soc. J.* 17:359–369, 1970.

1583. Ramirez-R. J., and O'Neill, E. F.   Endobronchial polymyxin B: Experimental observations in chronic bronchitis. *Chest* 58:352–357, 1970.

1584. Ramirez de Arellano, A. A., Hetzel, P. S., and Wood, E. H.   Measurement of the pulmonary blood flow using the indicator-dilution technic in patients with a central arteriovenous shunt. *Circ. Res.* 4:400–405, 1956.

1585. Ramsey, L. H., Puckett, W., Jose, A., and Lacy, W. W.   Precapillary gas and water distribution volumes of the lung calculated from multiple indicator dilution curves. *Circ. Res.* 15:275–286, 1964.

1586. Rand, P. W., Austin, W. H., Lacombe, E., and Barker, N.   pH and blood viscosity. *J. Appl. Physiol.* 25:550–559, 1968.

1587. Rand, P. W., and Lacombe, E.   Hemodilution, tonicity, and blood viscosity. *J. Clin. Invest.* 43:2214–2226, 1964.

1588. Rand, P. W., Lacombe, E., Hunt, H. E., and Austin, W. H.   Viscosity of normal human blood under normothermic and hypothermic conditions. *J. Appl. Physiol.* 19:117–122, 1964.

1589. Ranson, J. H. C., Roses, D. F., and Fink, S. D.   Early respiratory insufficiency in acute pancreatitis. *Ann. Surg.* 178:75–79, 1973.

1590. Rapaport, E., and Scheinman, M.   Rationale and limitations of hemodynamic measurements in patients with acute myocardial infarction. *Mod. Concepts Cardiovasc. Dis.* 38:55–61, 1969.

1591. Rapaport, F. T., Nemirovsky, M. S., Bachvaroff, R., and Ball, S. K.   Mechanisms of pulmonary damage in severe burns. *Ann. Surg.* 177:472–477, 1973.

1592. Rapaport, S. I., Tatter, D., Coeur-Barron, N., and Hjort, P. F.   *Pseudomonas* septicemia with intravascular clotting leading to the generalized Shwartzman reaction. *N. Engl. J. Med.* 271:80–84, 1964.

1593. Rassaian, N., Marshall, W. E., Greenwald, L., and Omachi, A. Ultrafiltrable ATP and 2,3-DPG in cold-stored human erythrocytes. *Physiologist* 17:318, 1974.

1594. Ratliff, N. B., Wilson, J. W., Hackel, D. B., and Martin, A. M. The lung in hemorrhagic shock. II. Observations on alveolar and vascular ultrastructure. *Am. J. Pathol.* 58:353–373, 1970.

1595. Ratliff, N. B., Wilson, J. W., Mikat, E., Hackel, D. B., and Graham, T. C. The lung in hemorrhagic shock. IV. The role of neutrophilic polymorphonuclear leukocytes. *Am. J. Pathol.* 65:325–334, 1971.

1596. Ratnoff, O. D. Epsilon aminocaproic acid—A dangerous weapon. *N. Engl. J. Med.* 280:1124–1125, 1969.

1597. Ravin, M. B. Comparison of spinal and general anesthesia for lower abdominal surgery in patients with chronic obstructive pulmonary disease. *Anesthesiology* 35:319–322, 1971.

1598. Ravitch, M. M., and Blalock, A. Aspiration of blood from pericardium in treatment of acute cardiac tamponade after injury. *Arch. Surg.* 58:463–477, 1949.

1599. Rea, W. J., Sugg, W. L., Wilson, L. C., Webb, W. R., and Ecker, R. R. Coronary artery lacerations. An analysis of 22 cases. *Ann. Thorac. Surg.* 7:518–528, 1969.

1600. Read, A. E., Emslie-Smith, D., Gough, K. R., and Holmes, R. Pancreatitis and accidental hypothermia. *Lancet* 2:1219–1221, 1961.

1601. Redding, J., Voigt, G. C., and Safar, P. Drowning treated with intermittent positive pressure breathing. *J. Appl. Physiol.* 15:849–854, 1960.

1602. Redding, J. S., Voigt, G. C., and Safar, P. Treatment of sea-water aspiration. *J. Appl. Physiol.* 15:1113–1116, 1960.

1603. Redding, R. A., Arai, T., Douglas, W. H. J., Tsurutani, H., and Overs, J. Early changes in lungs of rats exposed to 70% O_2. *J. Appl. Physiol.* 38:136–142, 1975.

1604. Reeves, J. T., Daoud, F. S., and Estridge, M. Pulmonary hypertension caused by minute amounts of endotoxin in calves. *J. Appl. Physiol.* 33:739–743, 1972.

1605. Rehder, K., Hatch, D. J., Sessler, A. D., and Fowler, W. S. The function of each lung of anesthetized and paralyzed man during mechanical ventilation. *Anesthesiology* 37:16–26, 1972.

1606. Rehder, K., Hatch, D. J., Sessler, A. D., Marsh, H. M., and Fowler, W. S. Effects of general anesthesia, muscle paralysis, and mechanical ventilation on pulmonary nitrogen clearance. *Anesthesiology* 35:591–601, 1971.

1607. Rehder, K., and Sessler, A. D. Effect of Positive Airway Pressure on Pulmonary Blood Flow Distribution in Sitting, Anesthetized, Paralyzed Man. Abstracts of scientific papers, Annual Meeting of the American Society of Anesthesiologists, Washington, D.C., October 12–16, 1974. Pp. 313–314.

1608. Rehder, K., Wenthe, F. M., and Sessler, A. D. Function of each lung during mechanical ventilation with ZEEP and with PEEP in man anesthetized with thiopental-meperidine. *Anesthesiology* 39:597–606, 1973.

1609. Reich, T., Tait, J., Suga, T., Naftchi, N. E., and Demeny, M. Pathogenesis of pulmonary oxygen toxicity: Role of systemic hyperoxia and convulsions. *J. Appl. Physiol.* 32:374–379, 1972.

1610. Reid, D., Bell, E. J., Grist, N. R., and Wilson, T. S. Poliomyelitis: A gap in immunity? *Lancet* 2:899–900, 1973.

1611. Reid, D. J. Intravenous fat therapy. II. Changes in oxygen consumption and respiratory quotient. *Br. J. Surg.* 54:204–207, 1967.

1612. Reinarz, J. A., Pierce, A. K., Mays, B. B., and Sanford, J. P. The potential role of inhalation therapy equipment in nosocomial pulmonary infection. *J. Clin. Invest.* 44:831–839, 1965.

1613. Reintjes, M., Swierenga, J., and Bogaard, J. M.   Effect of smoking one cigarette on airway resistance. *Scand. J. Respir. Dis.* 53:129–134, 1972.

1614. Reitan, J. A., Smith, N. T., Borison, V. S., and Kadis, L. B.   The cardiac pre-ejection period: A correlate of peak ascending aortic blood-flow acceleration. *Anesthesiology* 36:76–80, 1972.

1615. Restall, D. S., Woo, S. W., Hedley-Whyte, J., and Bushnell, L. S.   Recent advances in the prevention and treatment of respiratory failure. *R.I. Med. J.* 57:235–244, 1974.

1616. Reul, G. J., Jr., Greenberg, S. D., Lefrak, E. A., McCollum, W. B., Beall, A. C., Jr., and Jordan, G. L., Jr.   Prevention of post-traumatic pulmonary insufficiency. Fine screen filtration of blood. *Arch. Surg.* 106:386–393, 1973.

1617. Rhoads, J. E.   Supranormal dietary requirements of acutely ill patients. *J. Am. Diet. Assoc.* 29:897–903, 1953.

1618. Ribaudo, C. A., and Grace, W. J.   Pulmonary aspiration. *Am. J. Med.* 50:510–520, 1971.

1619. Richards, J. H., and Marriott, C.   Effect of relative humidity on the rheologic properties of bronchial mucus. *Am. Rev. Respir. Dis.* 109:484–486, 1974.

1620. Ridley, A.   The neuropathy of acute intermittent porphyria. *Q. J. Med.* 38:307–333, 1969.

1621. Rie, M. A., and Wilson, R. S.   Prolonged Morphine Therapy for Control of Sympathetic Hyperactivity and Elevated Peripheral Vascular Resistance During Severe Tetanus. Abstracts of scientific papers, Annual Meeting of the American Society of Anesthesiologists, Washington, D.C., October 12–16, 1974. Pp. 403–404.

1622. Rie, M. W.   Physical therapy in the nursing care of respiratory disease patients. *Nurs. Clin. North Am.* 3:463–478, 1968.

1623. Riordan, J. F., and Walters, G.   Pulmonary oedema in bacterial shock. *Lancet* 1:719–721, 1968.

1624. Rittenhouse, E. A., Dillard, D. H., Winterscheid, L. C., and Merendino, K. A.   Traumatic rupture of the thoracic aorta: A review of the literature and a report of five cases with attention to special problems in early surgical management. *Ann. Surg.* 170:87–100, 1969.

1625. Rivers, J. F., Orr, G., and Lee, H. A.   Drowning. Its clinical sequelae and management. *Br. Med. J.* 2:157–161, 1970.

1626. Robb, J. D. A., and Matthews, J. G. W.   The injuries and management of riot casualties admitted to the Belfast hospital wards, August to October 1969. *Br. J. Surg.* 58:413–419, 1971.

1627. Robboy, S., Colman, R., and Minna, J.   Fibrinolysis *vs* disseminated intravascular coagulation. *N. Engl. J. Med.* 281:222, 1969.

1628. Robboy, S. J., Colman, R. W., and Minna, J. D.   Pathology of disseminated intravascular coagulation (DIC). Analysis of 26 cases. *Hum. Pathol.* 3:327–343, 1972.

1629. Robboy, S. J., Minna, J. D., Colman, R. W., Birndorf, N. I., and Lopas, H.   Pulmonary hemorrhage syndrome as a manifestation of disseminated intravascular coagulation: Analysis of ten cases. *Chest* 63:718–721, 1973.

1630. Roberton, N. R. C., Goddard, P., Rolfe, P., Marcovitch, H., and Scopes, J. W.   The use of an indwelling catheter tip transducer for measurement of arterial Po_2 in the newborn. *Crit. Care Med.* 2:53, 1974.

1631. Roberts, D. V., and Wilson, A.   Electromyography in the diagnosis and treatment of myasthenia gravis. *Br. J. Pharmacol.* 34:229P–230P, 1968.

1632. Roberts, R. B., and Shirley, M.   Reducing the risk of acid aspiration during cesarean section. *Anesth. Analg.* (Cleve.) 53:859–863, 1974.

1633. Roberts, R. B., and Shirley, M.   Aspiration during vaginal delivery. *Anesthesiology* 40:317, 1974.

1634. Robertson, W. G., Hargreaves, J. J., Herlocher, J. E., and Welch, B. E. Physiologic response to increased oxygen partial pressure. II. Respiratory studies. *Aerosp. Med.* 35:618–622, 1964.

1635. Robin, E. D.   The aging lung—Functional aspects. *Arch. Environ. Health* 6:44–50, 1963.

1636. Robin, E. D., Carey, L. C., Grenvik, A., Glauser, F., and Gaudio, R.   Capillary leak syndrome with pulmonary edema. *Arch. Intern. Med.* 130:66–71, 1972.

1637. Robin, E. D., Cross, C. E., and Zelis, R.   Pulmonary edema. *N. Engl. J. Med.* 288:239–246, 292–304, 1973.

1638. Robinson, F. R., and Casey, H. W.   Animal model: Oxygen toxicity in nonhuman primate. *Am. J. Pathol.* 76:175–178, 1974.

1639. Robinson, F. R., Sopher, R. L., Witchett, C. E., and Carter, V. L., Jr.   Pathology of normobaric oxygen toxicity in primates. *Aerosp. Med.* 40:879–884, 1969.

1640. Robinson, N. E., and Gillespie, J. R.   Lung volumes in aging beagle dogs. *J. Appl. Physiol.* 35:317–321, 1973.

1641. Rocchio, M. A., DiCola, V., and Randall, H. T.   Role of electrolyte solutions in treatment of hemorrhagic shock. *Am. J. Surg.* 125:488–495, 1973.

1642. Rockwell, M. A., Shubin, H., Weil, M. H., and Meagher, P. F.   Shock III, a computer system as an aid in the management of critically ill patients. *Comm. Assoc. Computing Mech.* 9:355–357, 1966.

1643. Rodriguez, F., Bierzwinsky, G., and Nassar, M.   Evaluation of noninvasive techniques in acute hemorrhagic shock. *Crit. Care Med.* 1:120–121, 1973.

1644. Rodríguez-Erdmann, F.   Bleeding due to increased intravascular blood coagulation. Hemorrhagic syndromes caused by consumption of blood-clotting factors (consumption-coagulopathies). *N. Engl. J. Med.* 273:1370–1378, 1965.

1645. Roe, B. B.   Prevention and treatment of respiratory complications in surgery. *N. Engl. J. Med.* 263:547–550, 1960.

1646. Roe, B. B.   Physiologic changes occurring after open-heart surgery. *Surg. Annu.* 5:299–314, 1973.

1647. Roe, C. F., and Kinney, J. M.   The caloric equivalent of fever. II. Influence of major trauma. *Ann. Surg.* 161:140–147, 1965.

1648. Roehm, J. N., Haldey, J. G., and Menzel, D. B.   Antioxidants *vs* lung disease. *Arch. Intern. Med.* 128:88–93, 1971.

1649. Rogers, R. M., Braunstein, M. S., and Shuman, J. F.   Role of bronchopulmonary lavage in the treatment of respiratory failure: A review. *Chest* 62(Suppl.):95S–106S, 1972.

1650. Rogers, R. M., Weiler, C., and Ruppenthal, B.   Impact of the respiratory intensive care unit on survival of patients with acute respiratory failure. *Chest* 62:94–97, 1972.

1651. Rolf, L. L., and Travis, D. M.   Pleural fluid-plasma bicarbonate gradients in oxygen-toxic and normal rats. *Am. J. Physiol.* 224:857–861, 1973.

1652. Romhilt, D. W., Bloomfield, S. S., Chou, T.-C., and Fowler, N. O.   Unreliability of conventional electrocardiographic monitoring for arrhythmia detection in coronary care units. *Am. J. Cardiol.* 31:457–461, 1973.

1653. Romney, S. L., Schulman, H., Goldwyn, R. M., Del Guercio, L. R. M., and Siegel, J. H.   Hemodynamic evaluation of patients with puerperal sepsis and shock. *Am. J. Obstet. Gynecol.* 105:797–807, 1969.

1654. Roscher, R., Bittner, R., and Stockman, U.   Pulmonary contusion: Clinical experience. *Arch. Surg.* 109:508–510, 1974.

1655. Rose, H. D., Pendharker, M. B., Snider, G. L., and Kory, R. C.   Evaluation of sodium colistimethate aerosol in gram-negative infections of the respiratory tract. *J. Clin. Pharmacol.* 10:274–281, 1970.

1656. Rosenbaum, R. W., Hayes, M. F., and Matsumoto, T.   Efficacy of steroids in the treatment of septic and cardiogenic shock. *Surg. Gynecol. Obstet.* 136:914–918, 1973.

1657. Rosenberg, R. D.   Heparin action. *Circulation* 49:603–605, 1974.

1658. Rosenberg, R. D.   Actions and interactions of antithrombin and heparin. *N. Engl. J. Med.* 292:146–151, 1975.

1659. Rosenblum, R., and Frieden, J.   Intravenous dopamine in the treatment of myocardial dysfunction after open-heart surgery. *Am. Heart J.* 83:743–748, 1972.

1660. Rosenblum, R., Tai, A. R., and Lawson, D.   Dopamine in man: Cardiorenal hemodynamics in normotensive patients with heart disease. *J. Pharmacol. Exp. Ther.* 183:256–263, 1972.

1661. Rosin, A. J., and Exton-Smith, A. N.   Clinical features of accidental hypothermia, with some observations on thyroid function. *Br. Med. J.* 1:16–19, 1964.

1662. Rosner, F., and Rubenberg, M. L.   Erythrocyte fragmentation in consumption coagulopathy. *N. Engl. J. Med.* 280:219–220, 1969.

1663. Rosoff, L., Weil, M., Bradley, E. C., and Berne, C. J.   Hemodynamic and metabolic changes associated with bacterial peritonitis. *Am. J. Surg.* 114:180–189, 1967.

1664. Ross, E., and Armentrout, S. A.   Myocarditis associated with rabies. Report of a case. *N. Engl. J. Med.* 266:1087, 1962.

1665. Ross, R. S.   Electrical hazards for cardiac patients. *N. Engl. J. Med.* 281:390, 1969.

1666. Ross, S.   Contrast-medium tamponade following insertion of a central venous catheter. *Anesthesiology* 41:518–519, 1974.

1667. Rossen, R., Kabat, H., and Anderson, J. P.   Acute arrest of cerebral circulation in man. *Arch. Neurol. Psychiatry* 50:510–528, 1943.

1668. Rothe, C. F.   Fluid Dynamics. In E. E. Selkurt (Ed.), *Physiology* (3rd ed.). Boston: Little, Brown, 1971. Pp. 239–257.

1669. Roughton, F. J. W., and Darling, R. C.   The effect of carbon monoxide on the oxyhemoglobin dissociation curve. *Am. J. Physiol.* 141:17–31, 1944.

1670. Rovenstein, E. A., and Taylor, I. B.   Postoperative respiratory complications: Occurrence following 7,874 anesthesias. *Am. J. Med. Sci.* 191:807–819, 1936.

1671. Rowe, G. G., and Henderson, R. H.   Systemic and coronary hemodynamic effects of sodium nitroprusside. *Am. Heart J.* 87:83–87, 1974.

1672. Rubin, R. H., Gregg, M. B., and Sikes, R. K.   Rabies in citizens of the United States, 1963–1968: Epidemiology, treatment, and complications of treatment. *J. Infect. Dis.* 120:268–273, 1969.

1673. Rudy, L. W., Jr., Heymann, M. A., and Edmunds, L. H., Jr.   Distribution of systemic blood flow during cardiopulmonary bypass. *J. Appl. Physiol.* 34:194–200, 1973.

1674. Rugberg, R. L., Allen, T. R., Goodman, M. J., Long, J. M., and Dudrick, S. J.   Hypophosphatemia with hypophosphaturia in hyperalimentation. *Surg. Forum* 22:87–88, 1971.

1675. Rushmer, R. F., Baker, D. W., Johnson, W. L., and Strandness, D. E.   Clinical applications of a transcutaneous ultrasonic flow detector. *J.A.M.A.* 199:326–328, 1967.

1676. Russell, M. A. H., Cole, P. V., and Brown, E.   Absorption by non-smokers of carbon monoxide from room air polluted by tobacco smoke. *Lancet* 1:576–579, 1973.

1677. Russell, R. O., Jr., Rackley, C. E., Pombo, J., Hunt, D., Potanin, C., and Dodge, H. T. Effects of increasing left ventricular filling pressure in patients with acute myocardial infarction. *J. Clin. Invest.* 49:1539–1550, 1970.

1678. Rutherford, W. H. Medical consequences of the riots in Belfast in 1969. *Br. J. Hosp. Med.* 4:641–646, 1970.

1679. Ryan, J. A., Jr., Abel, R. M., Abbott, W. M., Hopkins, C. C., McChesney, T., Colley, R., Phillips, K., and Fischer, J. E. Catheter complications of total parenteral nutrition. A prospective study of 200 consecutive patients. *N. Engl. J. Med.* 290:757–761, 1974.

1680. Ryan, J. F., Donlon, J. V., Malt, R. A., Bland, J. H. L., Buckley, M. J., Sreter, F. A., and Lowenstein, E. Cardiopulmonary bypass in the treatment of malignant hyperthermia. *N. Engl. J. Med.* 290:1121–1122, 1974.

1681. Ryan, J. F., Raines, J., Dalton, B. C., and Mathieu, A. Arterial dynamics of radial artery cannulation. *Anesth. Analg.* (Cleve.) 52:1017–1023, 1973.

1682. Rylander, R. Alterations of lung defense mechanisms against airborne bacteria. *Arch. Environ. Health* 18:551–555, 1969.

1683. Sabri, S., Roberts, V. C., and Cotton, L. T. Prevention of early postoperative deep vein thrombosis by passive exercise of leg during surgery. *Br. Med. J.* 3:82–83, 1971.

1684. Sack, R. A. Bilateral internal iliac (hypogastric) artery ligation to control obstetric and gynecologic hemorrhage. *Am. J. Obstet. Gynecol.* 116:493–497, 1973.

1685. Sackner, M. A., Landa, J., Hirsch, J., and Zapata, A. Pulmonary effects of oxygen breathing. A 6-hour study in normal men. *Ann. Intern. Med.* 82:40–43, 1975.

1686. Safar, P., Grenvik, A., and Smith, J. Progressive pulmonary consolidation: Review of cases and pathogenesis. *J. Trauma* 12:955–964, 1972.

1687. Safar, P., Stezoski, W., and Nemoto, E. M. Amelioration of brain damage after cardiac arrest. *Crit. Care Med.* 3:38–39, 1975.

1688. Sahn, S. A., and Lakshminarayan, S. Bedside criteria for discontinuation of mechanical ventilation. *Chest* 63:1002–1005, 1973.

1689. Said, S. I. Abnormalities of pulmonary gas exchange in obesity. *Ann. Intern. Med.* 53:1121–1129, 1960.

1690. Salem, S. N. Neurological complications of heat-stroke in Kuwait. *Ann. Trop. Med. Parasitol.* 60:393–400, 1966.

1691. Saltzman, H. A., and Fridovich, I. Oxygen toxicity. Introduction to a protective enzyme: Superoxide dismutase. *Circulation* 48:921–923, 1973.

1692. Salzman, E. W. Does intravascular coagulation occur in hemorrhagic shock in man? *J. Trauma* 8:867–871, 1968.

1693. Salzman, E. W. Thrombosis in artificial organs. *Transplant. Proc.* 3:1491–1496, 1971.

1694. Salzman, E. W., Deykin, D., Shapiro, R. M., and Rosenberg, R. Management of heparin therapy: Controlled prospective trial. *N. Engl. J. Med.* 292:1046–1050, 1975.

1695. Samaan, H. A. The hazards of radial artery pressure monitoring. *J. Cardiovasc. Surg.* 12:342–347, 1971.

1696. Sanders, C. A., Buckley, M. J., Leinbach, R. C., Mundth, E. D., and Austen, W. G. Mechanical circulatory assistance. Current status and experience with combining circulatory assistance, emergency coronary angiography, and acute myocardial revascularization. *Circulation* 45:1292–1313, 1972.

1697. Sands, J. H., Cypert, C., Armstrong, R., Ching, S., Trainer, D., Quinn, W., and Stewart, D. A controlled study using routine intermittent positive pressure breathing in the post-surgical patient. *Dis. Chest* 40:128–133, 1961.

1698. Sanford, J. P., Barnett, J. A., and Gott, C.   A mechanism of the glycogenolytic action of bacterial endotoxin. *J. Exp. Med.* 112:97–105, 1960.

1699. Sankaran, S., and Wilson, R. F.   Factors affecting prognosis in patients with flail chest. *J. Thorac. Cardiovasc. Surg.* 60:402–409, 1970.

1700. Sarnoff, S. J., Braunwald, E., Welch, G. H., Jr., Case, R. B., Stainsby, W. N., and Macruz, R.   Hemodynamic determinants of oxygen consumption of the heart with special reference to the tension-time index. *Am. J. Physiol.* 192:148–156, 1958.

1701. Sarnquist, F., and Larson, C. P., Jr.   Drug-induced heat stroke. *Anesthesiology* 39:348–350, 1973.

1702. Saunders, S. J., Hickman, R., MacDonald, R., and Terblanche, J.   The Treatment of Acute Liver Failure. In H. Popper and F. Schaffner (Eds.), *Progress in Liver Diseases.* New York: Grune & Stratton, 1972. Vol. IV, pp. 333–344.

1703. Saunders, S. J., Terblanche, J., Bosman, S. C. W., Harrison, G. G., Walls, R., Hickman, R., Biebuyck, J., Dent, D., Pearce, S., and Barnard, C. N.   Acute hepatic coma treated by cross-circulation with a baboon and by repeated exchange transfusions. *Lancet* 2:585–588, 1968.

1704. Savides, E. P., and Hoffbrand, B. I.   Hypothermia, thrombosis and acute pancreatitis. *Br. Med. J.* 1:614, 1974.

1705. Schapira, M., and Stern, W. Z.   Hazards of subclavian vein cannulation for central venous pressure monitoring. *J.A.M.A.* 201:327–329, 1967.

1706. Scharf, S. M., Thames, M. D., and Sargent, R. K.   Transmural myocardial infarction after exposure to carbon monoxide in coronary-artery disease. *N. Engl. J. Med.* 291:85–86, 1974.

1707. Scharschmidt, B. F., Plotz, P. H., Berk, P. D., Waggoner, J. G., and Vergalla, J.   Removing substances from blood by affinity chromatography. II. Removing bilirubin from the blood of jaundiced rats by hemoperfusion over albumin-conjugated agarose beads. *J. Clin. Invest.* 53:786–795, 1974.

1708. Schechter, E., and Parisi, A. F.   Removal of catheter fragments from pulmonary artery using a snare. *Br. Heart J.* 34:699–700, 1972.

1709. Scheidt, S., Wilner, G., Mueller, H., Summers, D., Lesch, M., Wolff, G., Krakauer, J., Rubenfire, M., Fleming, P., Noon, G., Oldham, N., Killip, T., and Kantrowitz, A.   Intra-aortic balloon counterpulsation in cardiogenic shock. Report of a co-operative clinical trial. *N. Engl. J. Med.* 288:979–984, 1973.

1710. Schlenker, J. D., and Hubay, C. A.   The pathogenesis of postoperative atelectasis. A clinical study. *Arch. Surg.* 107:846–850, 1973.

1711. Schloerb, P. R., Hunt, P. T., Plummer, J. A., and Cage, G. K.   Pulmonary edema after replacement of blood loss by electrolyte solutions. *Surg. Gynecol. Obstet.* 135:893–896, 1972.

1712. Schlueter, D. P.   Pulmonary risks. *Clin. Obstet. Gynecol.* 16:91–110, 1973.

1713. Schmid-Schönbein, H., Klose, H. J., Volger, E., and Weiss, J.   Hypothermia and blood flow behavior. *Res. Exp. Med.* (Berl.) 161:58–68, 1973.

1714. Schmidt, G. B., Bennett, E. J., Kotb, K. M., and Hwang, K. K.   Continuous Positive Airway Pressure (CPAP) in the Prophylaxis of the ARDS. Abstracts of scientific papers, Annual Meeting of the American Society of Anesthesiologists, Washington, D.C., October 12–16, 1974. Pp. 251–252.

1715. Schmitz, J. T.   Pregnant patients with burns. *Am. J. Obstet. Gynecol.* 110:57, 1971.

1716. Schneeberger-Keeley, E. E., and Karnovsky, M. J.   The ultrastructural basis of alveolar-capillary membrane permeability to peroxidase used as a tracer. *J. Cell Biol.* 37:781–793, 1968.

1717. Schuler, R., and Kreuzer, F.   Rapid polarographic in vivo oxygen catheter electrodes. *Respir. Physiol.* 3:90–110, 1967.

1718. Schumacher, R. R., Lieberson, A. D., Childress, R. H., and Williams, J. F., Jr. Hemodynamic effects of lidocaine in patients with heart disease. *Circulation* 37:965–972, 1968.

1719. Scott, H. W., Jr., Dean, R., Shull, H. J., Abram, H. S., Webb, W., Younger, R. K., and Brill, A. B. New considerations in use of jejunoileal bypass in patients with morbid obesity. *Ann. Surg.* 177:723–735, 1973.

1720. Scott, H. W., Jr., Law, D. H., IV, Sandstead, H. H., Lanier, V. C., Jr., and Younger, R. K. Jejunoileal shunt in surgical treatment of morbid obesity. *Ann. Surg.* 171:770–782, 1970.

1721. Scott, H. W., Jr., Sandstead, H. H., Brill, A. B., Burko, H., and Younger, R. K. Experience with a new technic of intestinal bypass in the treatment of morbid obesity. *Ann. Surg.* 174:560–571, 1971.

1722. Scott, M. M. Cardiopulmonary considerations in nonfatal amniotic fluid embolism. *J.A.M.A.* 183:989–993, 1963.

1723. Scribner, B. H., Cole, J. J., Christopher, T. G., Vizzo, J. E., Atkins, R. C., and Blagg, C. R. Long-term total parenteral nutrition. The concept of an artificial gut. *J.A.M.A.* 212:457–463, 1970.

1724. Sears, M. R., O'Donoghue, J. M., Fisher, H. K., and Beaty, H. N. Effect of experimental pneumococcal meningitis on respiration and circulation in the rabbit. *J. Clin. Invest.* 54:18–23, 1974.

1725. Selden, R., Lee, S., Wang, W. L. L., Bennett, J. V., and Eickhoff, T. C. Nosocomial *Klebsiella* infections: Intestinal colonization as a reservoir. *Ann. Intern. Med.* 74:657–664, 1971.

1726. Selling, L. S. Clinical study of a new tranquilizing drug. *J.A.M.A.* 157:1594–1596, 1955.

1727. Seltzer, C. C., Siegelaub, A. B., Friedman, G. D., and Collen, M. F. Difference in pulmonary function related to smoking habits and race. *Am. Rev. Respir. Dis.* 110:598–608, 1974.

1728. Senior, R. M., Sherman, L. A., and Yin, E. T. Effects of hyperoxia on fibrinogen metabolism and clotting factors in rabbits. *Am. Rev. Respir. Dis.* 109:156–161, 1974.

1729. Severinghaus, J. W. Respiration and hypothermia. *Ann. N.Y. Acad. Sci.* 80:384–394, 1959.

1730. Severinghaus, J. W. Electrical measurement of pulmonary oedema with a focusing conductivity bridge. *J. Physiol.* (Lond.) 215:53p–55p, 1971.

1731. Severinghaus, J. W., and Bradley, A. F. Electrodes for blood Po_2 and Pco_2 determination. *J. Appl. Physiol.* 13:515–520, 1958.

1732. Severinghaus, J. W., and Mitchell, R. A. Ondine's curse—Failure of respiratory center automaticity while awake. *Clin. Res.* 10:122, 1962.

1733. Sevitt, S. *Fat Embolism.* London: Butterworth, 1962.

1734. Sevitt, S. Reflections on mortality and causes of death after injury and burns. *Injury* 4:151–156, 1972.

1735. Sevitt, S. Diffuse and focal oxygen pneumonitis. A preliminary report on the threshold of pulmonary oxygen toxicity in man. *J. Clin. Pathol.* 27:21–30, 1974.

1736. Sevitt, S., and Gallagher, N. Venous thrombosis and pulmonary embolism. A clinico-pathological study in injured and burned patients. *Br. J. Surg.* 48:475–489, 1961.

1737. Sexton, L. I., Hertig, A. T., Reid, D. E., Kellogg, F. S., and Patterson, W. S. Premature separation of the normally implanted placenta. A clinicopathological study of 476 cases. *Am. J. Obstet. Gynecol.* 59:13–24, 1950.

1738. Shabetai, R., Fowler, N. O., and Guntheroth, W. G. The hemodynamics of cardiac tamponade and constrictive pericarditis. *Am. J. Cardiol.* 26:480–489, 1970.

1739. Shafer, A. W., Tague, L. L., Welch, M. H., and Guenter, C. A. 2, 3-Diphosphoglycerate in red cells stored in acid-citrate-dextrose and citrate-phosphate-dextrose: Implications regarding delivery of oxygen. *J. Lab. Clin. Med.* 77:430–437, 1971.

1740. Shapiro, J. *Radiation Protection. A Guide for Scientists and Physicians.* Cambridge, Mass.: Harvard University Press, 1972. Pp. 250–309.

1741. Sharefkin, J. B., and MacArthur, J. D. Pulmonary artery pressure as a guide to the hemodynamic status of surgical patients. *Arch. Surg.* 105:699–704, 1972.

1742. Sharefkin, J. B., and Silen, W. Diuretic agents: Inciting factor in nonocclusive mesenteric infarction? *J.A.M.A.* 229:1451–1453, 1974.

1743. Sharnoff, J. G., and DeBlasio, G. Prevention of fatal postoperative thromboembolism by heparin prophylaxis. *Lancet* 2:1006–1007, 1970.

1744. Sharp, J. T., Henry, J. P., and Sweany, S. K. Effects of mass loading on the respiratory system in man. *J. Appl. Physiol.* 19:959–966, 1964.

1745. Shay, H., and Sun, D. C. H. Stress and gastric secretion in man. I. A study of the mechanisms involved in insulin hypoglycemia. *Am. J. Med. Sci.* 228:630–642, 1954.

1746. Shear, L., and Brandman, I. S. Hypoxia and hypercapnia caused by respiratory compensation for metabolic alkalosis. *Am. Rev. Respir. Dis.* 107:836–841, 1973.

1747. Sheh, J. M., O'Connor, N. E., and Moore, F. D. In vivo measurement of the extravascular water content of the lungs in pulmonary edema. *Surg. Forum* 19:259–261, 1968.

1748. Shepherd, J. T., Donald, D. E., Linder, E., and Swan, H. J. C. Effect of small doses of 5-hydroxytryptamine (serotonin) on pulmonary circulation in the closed-chest dog. *Am. J. Physiol.* 197:963–967, 1959.

1749. Sheppard, L. C., and Kirklin, J. W. Cardiac surgical intensive care computer system. *Fed. Proc.* 33:2326–2328, 1974.

1750. Sherman, L. A., Wessler, S., and Avioli, L. V. Therapeutic problems of disseminated intravascular coagulation. *Arch. Intern. Med.* 132:446–453, 1973.

1751. Sherry, S. Fibrinolysis and afibrinogenemia. *Anesthesiology* 27:465–474, 1966.

1752. Sherwin, R. P., Dibble, J., and Weiner, J. Alveolar wall cells of the guinea pig. Increase in response to 2 ppm nitrogen dioxide. *Arch. Environ. Health* 24:43–47, 1972.

1753. Shibolet, S., Coll, R., Gilat, T., and Sohar, E. Heatstroke: Its clinical picture and mechanism in 36 cases. *Q. J. Med.* 36:525–548, 1967.

1754. Shils, M. E., Wright, W. L., Turnbull, A., and Brescia, F. Long-term parenteral nutrition through an external arteriovenous shunt. *N. Engl. J. Med.* 283:341–344, 1970.

1755. Shires, G. T. *Care of the Trauma Patient.* New York: McGraw-Hill, 1966.

1756. Shires, G. T. Fluid and electrolyte needs at operation. *S. Afr. Med. J.* 42:867–872, 1968.

1757. Shires, G. T., Cunningham, J. N., Baker, C. R., Reeder, S. F., Illner, H., Wagner, I. Y., and Maher, J. Alterations in cellular membrane function during hemorrhagic shock in primates. *Ann. Surg.* 176:288–295, 1972.

1758. Shires, G. T., Williams, J., and Brown, F. Acute change in extracellular fluids associated with major surgical procedures. *Ann. Surg.* 154:803–810, 1961.

1759. Shizgal, H. M., Goldstein, M., Richard, P. F., and MacLean, L. D. Measurement of cardiac output with radioactive xenon. *Surg. Gynecol. Obstet.* 136:618–622, 1973.

1760. Shnider, S. M., and Moya, F. Amniotic fluid embolism. *Anesthesiology* 22:108–119, 1961.

1761. Shoemaker, W. C.   Cardiorespiratory patterns in complicated and uncomplicated septic shock: Physiologic alterations and their therapeutic implications. *Ann. Surg.* 174:119–125, 1971.

1762. Shoemaker, W. C., Montgomery, E. S., Kaplan, E., and Elwyn, D. H. Physiologic patterns in surviving and nonsurviving shock patients. Use of sequential cardiorespiratory variables in defining criteria for therapeutic goals and early warning of death. *Arch. Surg.* 106:630–636, 1973.

1763. Shoemaker, W. C., Vladeck, B. C., Bassin, R., Printen, K., Brown, R. S., Amato, J. J., Reinhard, J. M., and Kark, A. E.   Burn pathophysiology in man. I. Sequential hemodynamic alterations. *J. Surg. Res.* 14:64–73, 1973.

1764. Shook, C. D., MacMillan, B. G., and Altemeier, W. A.   Pulmonary complications of the burned patient. *Arch. Surg.* 97:215–224, 1968.

1765. Shooter, R. A., Cooke, E. M., Gaya, H., Kumar, P., and Patel, N.   Food and medicaments as possible sources of hospital strains of *Pseudomonas aeruginosa*. *Lancet* 1:1227–1229, 1969.

1766. Shooter, R. A., Faiers, M. D., Cooke, E. M., Breaden, A. C., and O'Farrell, S. M.   Isolation of *Escherichia coli, Pseudomonas aeruginosa,* and *Klebsiella* from food in hospitals, canteens, and schools. *Lancet* 2:390–392, 1971.

1767. Shors, C. M., Kozul, V. J., Christensen, R. C., and Jafri, M. S.   Measurement of stroke volume, cardiac output, ejection fraction, left ventricular mass, and velocity of myocardial contraction by the echocardiogram at the bedside in the ICU. *Crit. Care Med.* 2:46, 1974.

1768. Shubin, H., and Weil, M. H.   The mechanism of shock following suicidal doses of barbiturates, narcotics and tranquilizer drugs, with observations on the effects of treatment. *Am. J. Med.* 38:853–863, 1965.

1769. Shurin, P. A., Permutt, S., and Riley, R. L.   Pulmonary antibacterial defenses with pure oxygen breathing. *Proc. Soc. Exp. Biol. Med.* 137:1202–1208, 1971.

1770. Siegel, D. C., Cochin, A., Geocaris, T., and Moss, G. S.   Effects of saline and colloid resuscitation on renal function. *Ann. Surg.* 177:51–57, 1973.

1771. Siegel, D. C., Moss, G. S., Cochin, A., and Das Gupta, T. K.   Pulmonary changes following treatment for hemorrhagic shock: Saline versus colloid infusion. *Surg. Forum* 21:17–19, 1970.

1772. Siegel, H. W., and Downing, S. E.   Contributions of coronary perfusion pressure, metabolic acidosis and adrenergic factors to the reduction of myocardial contractility during hemorrhagic shock in the cat. *Circ. Res.* 27:875–889, 1970.

1773. Siegel, J. H., Goldwyn, R. M., Farrell, E. J., Gallin, P., and Friedman, H. P.   Hyperdynamic states and the physiologic determinants of survival in patients with cirrhosis and portal hypertension. *Arch. Surg.* 108:282–292, 1974.

1774. Siegel, J. H., Greenspan, M., and Del Guercio, L. R. M.   Abnormal vascular tone, defective oxygen transport and myocardial failure in human septic shock. *Ann. Surg.* 165:504–517, 1967.

1775. Sieker, H. O., Estes, E. H., Jr., Kelser, G. A., and McIntosh, H. D.   A cardiopulmonary syndrome associated with extreme obesity. *J. Clin. Invest.* 34:916, 1955.

1776. Signori, E. E., Penner, J. A., and Kahn, D. R.   Coagulation defects and bleeding in open-heart surgery. *Ann. Thorac. Surg.* 8:521–529, 1969.

1777. Silen, W.   Evaluation of renal-failure treatment. *N. Engl. J. Med.* 288:1303–1304, 1973.

1778. Silen, W.   Potpourri dissected. *N. Engl. J. Med.* 291:974–975, 1974.

1779. Silen, W., and Skillman, J. J.   Stress ulcer, acute erosive gastritis and the gastric mucosal barrier. *Adv. Intern. Med.* 19:195–212, 1974.

512   References

1780. Silverstein, P., and Dressler, D. P.   Effect of current therapy on burn mortality. *Ann. Surg.* 171:124–129, 1970.
1781. Silvis, S. E., and Paragas, P. V., Jr.   Fatal hyperalimentation syndrome. Animal studies. *J. Lab. Clin. Med.* 78:918–930, 1971.
1782. Simmons, R. L., Anderson, R. W., Ducker, T. B., Sleeman, H. K., Collins, J. A., and Boothman, K. P.   The role of the central nervous system in septic shock. II. Hemodynamic, respiratory and metabolic effects of intracisternal or intraventricular endotoxin. *Ann. Surg.* 167:158–167, 1968.
1783. Simmons, R. L., Martin, A. M., Jr., Heisterkamp, C. A., III, and Ducker, T. B.   Respiratory insufficiency in combat casualties. II. Pulmonary edema following head injury. *Ann. Surg.* 170:39–44, 1969.
1784. Simons, J. R., Theodore, J., and Robin, E. D.   Common oxidant lesion of mitochondrial redox state produced by nitrogen dioxide, ozone, and high oxygen in alveolar macrophages. *Chest* 66(Suppl. 2):9S–12S, 1974.
1785. Simpson, B. R., Parkhouse, J., Marshall, R., and Lambrechts, W.   Extradural analgesia and the prevention of postoperative respiratory complications. *Br. J. Anaesth.* 33:628–641, 1961.
1786. Singer, M. M., Wright, F., Stanley, L. K., Roe, B. B., and Hamilton, W. K.   Oxygen toxicity in man. A prospective study in patients after open-heart surgery. *N. Engl. J. Med.* 283:1473–1478, 1970.
1787. Sinha, R. P., Ducker, T. B., and Perot, P. L., Jr.   Arterial oxygenation: Findings and its significance in central nervous system trauma patients. *J.A.M.A.* 224:1258–1260, 1973.
1788. Skillman, J. J.   Ethical dilemmas in the care of the critically ill. *Lancet* 2:634–637, 1974.
1789. Skillman, J. J. (Ed.).   *Intensive Care.* Boston: Little, Brown, 1975.
1790. Skillman, J. J., Bushnell, L. S., Goldman, H., and Silen, W.   Respiratory failure, hypotension, sepsis and jaundice. A clinical syndrome associated with lethal hemorrhage from acute stress ulceration of the stomach. *Am. J. Surg.* 117:523–529, 1969.
1791. Skillman, J. J., Bushnell, L. S., and Hedley-Whyte, J.   Peritonitis and respiratory failure after abdominal operations. *Ann. Surg.* 170:122–127, 1969.
1792. Skillman, J. J., Gould, S. A., Chung, R. S. K., and Silen, W.   The gastric mucosal barrier: Clinical and experimental studies in critically ill and normal man, and in the rabbit. *Ann. Surg.* 172:564–582, 1970.
1793. Skillman, J. J., Hedley-Whyte, J., and Pallotta, J. A.   Cardiorespiratory, metabolic and endocrine changes after hemorrhage in man. *Ann. Surg.* 174:911–922, 1971.
1794. Skillman, J. J., Malhotra, I. V., Pallotta, J. A., and Bushnell, L. S.   Determinants of weaning from controlled ventilation. *Surg. Forum* 22:198–200, 1971.
1795. Skillman, J. J., Parikh, B. M., and Tanenbaum, B. J.   Pulmonary arteriovenous admixture. Improvement with albumin and diuresis. *Am. J. Surg.* 119:440–447, 1970.
1796. Skillman, J. J., Restall, D. S., and Salzman, E. W.   Randomized trial of albumin vs. electrolyte solutions during abdominal aortic operations. *Surgery* 78:291–302, 1975.
1797. Skillman, J. J., and Silen, W.   Acute gastroduodenal "stress" ulceration: Barrier disruption of varied pathogenesis? *Gastroenterology* 59:478–482, 1970.
1798. Skillman, J. J., and Silen, W.   Gastric mucosal barrier. *Surg. Annu.* Pp. 213–237, 1972.
1799. Skinner, J. F., and Pearce, M. L.   Surgical risk in the cardiac patient. *J. Chronic Dis.* 17:57–72, 1964.

1800. Sladen, A., Aldredge, C. F., and Albarran, R.   PEEP vs. ZEEP in the treatment of flail chest injuries. *Crit. Care Med.* 1:187–191, 1973.
1801. Sladen, A., Laver, M. B., and Pontoppidan, H.   Pulmonary complications and water retention in prolonged mechanical ventilation. *N. Engl. J. Med.* 279:448–453, 1968.
1802. Sladen, A., Zanca, P., and Hadnott, W. H.   Aspiration pneumonitis—The sequelae. *Chest* 59:448–450, 1971.
1803. Slovis, T. L., Ott, J. E., Teitelbaum, D. T., and Lipscomb, W.   Physostigmine therapy in acute tricyclic antidepressant poisoning. *Clin. Toxicol.* 4:451–459, 1971.
1804. Small, H. S., Weitzner, S. W., and Nahas, G. G.   Cerebrospinal fluid pressure during hypercapnia and hypoxia in dogs. *Am. J. Physiol.* 198:704–708, 1960.
1805. Smart, R. C.   Measurement of gas pressures and tensions. *Int. Anesthesiol. Clin.* 3:451–472, 1965.
1806. Smith, B. E., Modell, J. H., Gaub, M. L., and Moya, F.   Complications of subclavian vein catheterization. *Arch. Surg.* 90:228–229, 1965.
1807. Smith, B. M., Skillman, J. J., Edwards, B. G., and Silen, W.   Permeability of the human gastric mucosa. Alteration by acetylsalicylic acid and ethanol. *N. Engl. J. Med.* 285:716–721, 1971.
1808. Smith, G., Dewar, K. M. S., and Spence, A. A.   The effect of high inspired partial pressures of oxygen on conscious volunteers. *Br. J. Anaesth.* 43:1199, 1971.
1809. Smith, G., Winter, P. M., and Wheelis, R. F.   Increased normobaric oxygen tolerance of rabbits following oleic-acid induced lung damage. *J. Appl. Physiol.* 35:395–400, 1973.
1810. Smith, G. W.   Use of hemodynamic selection criteria in the management of cirrhotic patients with portal hypertension. *Ann. Surg.* 179:782–790, 1974.
1811. Smith, K., and Fields, H.   The supine hypotensive syndrome—A factor in the etiology of abruptio placentae. *Obstet. Gynecol.* 12:369–372, 1958.
1812. Smith, N. T., and Wesseling, K. H.   An Anesthetic Evaluation of a Beat-to-Beat Cardiac Output Computer. Abstracts of scientific papers, Annual Meeting of the American Society of Anesthesiologists, Washington, D.C., October 12–16, 1974. Pp. 105–106.
1813. Smith, T. W., Butler, V. P., and Haber, E.   Determination of therapeutic and toxic serum digoxin concentrations by radioimmunoassay. *N. Engl. J. Med.* 281:1212–1216, 1969.
1814. Smith, T. W., and Haber, E.   Digitalis. *N. Engl. J. Med.* 289:945–952, 1010–1015, 1063–1072, 1125–1129, 1973.
1815. Smithwick, W., III, Stalheim, A., Keller, G., and Love, J. W.   Removal of foreign bodies from the superior vena cava and right atrium without thoracotomy. *Ann. Thorac. Surg.* 17:197–199, 1974.
1816. Snell, J. D., Jr., and Ramsey, L. H.   Pulmonary edema as a result of endotoxemia. *Am. J. Physiol.* 217:170–175, 1969.
1817. Sochor, F. M., and Mallory, G. K.   Lung lesions in patients dying of burns. *Arch. Pathol.* 75:303–308, 1963.
1818. Sodipo, J. O.   Experience with an intensive care unit in a developing country. *Crit. Care Med.* 3:166–169, 1975.
1819. Solis, R. T., and Gibbs, M. B.   Filtration of microaggregates in stored blood. *Transfusion* 12:245–250, 1972.
1820. Solow, C., Silberfarb, P. M., and Swift, K.   Psychosocial effects of intestinal bypass surgery for severe obesity. *N. Engl. J. Med.* 290:300–304, 1974.

1821. Soloway, H. B., Castillo, Y., and Martin, A. M., Jr.   Adult hyaline membrane disease: Relationship to oxygen therapy. *Ann. Surg.* 168:937–945, 1968.

1822. Sonntag, V. K. H., and Stein, B. M.   Arteriopathic complications during treatment of subarachnoid hemorrhage with epsilon-aminocaproic acid. *J. Neurosurg.* 40:480–485, 1974.

1823. Sorbini, C. A., Grassi, V., Solinas, E., and Muiesan, G.   Arterial oxygen tension in relation to age in healthy subjects. *Respiration* 25:3–13, 1968.

1824. Soroff, H. S., Giron, F., Ruiz, U., Birtwell, W. C., Hirsch, L. J., and Deterling, R. A., Jr.   Physiologic support of heart action. *N. Engl. J. Med.* 280:693–704, 1969.

1825. Spalding, J. M. K., and Crampton Smith, A.   *Clinical Practice and Physiology of Artificial Respiration.* Oxford: Blackwell, 1963.

1826. Sparks, H. V., Kopald, H. H., Carrière, S., Chimoskey, J. E., Kinoshita, M., and Barger, A. C.   Intrarenal distribution of blood flow with chronic congestive heart failure. *Am. J. Physiol.* 223:840–846, 1972.

1827. Spence, A. A., and Alexander, J. I.   Mechanisms of postoperative hypoxaemia. *Proc. R. Soc. Med.* 65:12–14, 1972.

1828. Spence, A. A., and Smith, G.   Postoperative analgesia and lung function: A comparison of morphine with extradural block. *Br. J. Anaesth.* 43:144–148, 1971.

1829. Speroff, L.   Toxemia of pregnancy. Mechanism and therapeutic management. *Am. J. Cardiol.* 32:582–591, 1973.

1830. Spitzer, J. J., Bechtel, A. A., Archer, L. T., Black, M. R., and Hinshaw, L. B.   Myocardial substrate utilization in dogs following endotoxin administration. *Am. J. Physiol.* 227:132–136, 1974.

1831. Spitzer, S. A., Goldschmidt, Z., and Dubrawsky, C.   The bronchodilator effect of salbutamol administered by IPPB to patients with asthma. A controlled study with isoproterenol and placebo. *Chest* 62:273–276, 1972.

1832. Spoerel, W. E., Narayanan, P. S., and Singh, N. P.   Transtracheal ventilation. *Br. J. Anaesth.* 43:932–938, 1971.

1833. Stage, A. H.   Severe burns in the pregnant patient. *Obstet. Gynecol.* 42:259–262, 1973.

1834. Stager, W. R.   Blood conservation by autotransfusion. *Arch. Surg.* 63:78–82, 1951.

1835. Stamm, W. E., Colella, J. J., Anderson, R. L., and Dixon, R. E.   Indwelling arterial catheters as a source of nosocomial bacteremia: An outbreak caused by *Flavobacterium* species. *N. Engl. J. Med.* 292:1099–1102, 1975.

1836. Staples, P. J., and Griner, P. F.   Extracorporeal hemolysis of blood in a microwave warmer. *N. Engl. J. Med.* 285:317–319, 1971.

1837. Starmer, C. F., and Whalen, R. E.   Current density and electrically induced ventricular fibrillation. *Med. Instrum.* 7:158–161, 1973.

1838. Staub, N. C.   The pathophysiology of pulmonary edema. *Hum. Pathol.* 1:419–432, 1970.

1839. Staub, N. C.   Pathogenesis of pulmonary edema. "State of the Art" review. *Am. Rev. Respir. Dis.* 109:358–372, 1974.

1840. Stefadouros, M. A., Dougherty, M. J., Grossman, W., and Craige, E.   Determination of systemic vascular resistance by a noninvasive technic. *Circulation* 47:101–107, 1973.

1841. Stegall, H. F., Kardon, M. B., and Kemmerer, W. T.   Indirect measurement of arterial blood pressure by Doppler ultrasonic sphygmomanometry. *J. Appl. Physiol.* 25:793–798, 1968.

1842. Steiger, E., Allen, T. R., Daly, J. M., Vars, H. M., and Dudrick, S. J.   Beneficial effects of immediate postoperative total parenteral nutrition. *Surg. Forum* 22: 89–90, 1971.

1843. Stein, J. A., and Tschudy, D. P. Acute intermittent porphyria: A clinical and biochemical study of 46 patients. *Medicine* 49: 1–16, 1970.

1844. Stein, J. H., Boonjarern, S., Mauk, R. C., and Ferris, T. F. Mechanism of the redistribution of renal cortical blood flow during hemorrhagic hypotension in the dog. *J. Clin. Invest.* 52: 39–47, 1973.

1845. Stein, M., and Cassara, E. L. Preoperative pulmonary evaluation and therapy for surgery patients. *J.A.M.A.* 211: 787–790, 1970.

1846. Stein, M., Koota, G. M., Simon, M., and Frank, H. A. Pulmonary evaluation of surgical patients. *J.A.M.A.* 181: 765–770, 1962.

1847. Stein, M., and Thomas, D. P. Role of platelets in the acute pulmonary responses to endotoxin. *J. Appl. Physiol.* 23: 47–52, 1967.

1848. Steinberg, A. D., and Karliner, J. S. The clinical spectrum of heroin pulmonary edema. *Arch. Intern. Med.* 122: 122–127, 1968.

1849. Steinberg, D. Disseminated Intravascular Coagulation. In E. A. Stiene (Ed.), *Hematology Laboratory Medicine: Current Aspects.* Miami: Symposia Specialists, 1974.

1850. Stephens, R. V., and Randall, H. T. Use of a concentrated, balanced, liquid elemental diet for nutritional management of catabolic states. *Ann. Surg.* 170: 642–667, 1969.

1851. Stephenson, H. E., Jr. *Cardiac Arrest and Resuscitation.* St. Louis: Mosby, 1969.

1852. Stevens, R. M., Teres, D., Skillman, J. J., and Feingold, D. S. Pneumonia in an intensive care unit. A 30-month experience. *Arch. Intern. Med.* 134: 106–111, 1974.

1853. Stewart, G. N. Researches on the circulation time and on the influences which affect it. IV. The output of the heart. *J. Physiol.* 22: 159–183, 1897.

1854. Stewart, J. D., Williams, J. S., Kluge, D. N., and Drapanas, T. Effect of cross circulation on metabolism following hepatectomy. *Ann. Surg.* 158: 812–819, 1963.

1855. Stiehm, E. R., Kennan, A. L., and Schelble, D. T. Split products of fibrin in maternal serum in the perinatal period. *Am. J. Obstet. Gynecol.* 108: 941–945, 1970.

1856. Stiles, P. J. Tracheal lesions after tracheostomy. *Thorax* 20: 517–522, 1965.

1857. Stock, S. L. Prophylaxis of thromboembolism. *N. Engl. J. Med.* 289: 218, 1973.

1858. Stockard, J. J., Bickford, R. G., and Schauble, J. F. Pressure-dependent cerebral ischemia during cardiopulmonary bypass. *Neurology* (Minneap.) 23: 521–529, 1973.

1859. Stoddart, J. C. Gram-negative infections in the ICU. *Crit. Care Med.* 2: 17–22, 1974.

1860. Stoelting, R. K. Evaluation of external jugular venous pressure as a reflection of right atrial pressure. *Anesthesiology* 38: 291–294, 1973.

1861. Stone, H. H., and Martin, J. D., Jr. Pulmonary injury associated with thermal burns. *Surg. Gynecol. Obstet.* 129: 1242–1246, 1969.

1862. Stone, H. H., Rhame, D. W., Corbitt, J. D., Given, K. S., and Martin, J. D., Jr. Respiratory burns: A correlation of clinical and laboratory results. *Ann. Surg.* 165: 157–168, 1967.

1863. Stone, H. L. Change in atrial function with cardiac pacing. *Fed. Proc.* 33: 397, 1974.

1864. Stott, R. B., Cameron, J. S., Ogg, C. S., and Bewick, M. Why the persistently high mortality in acute renal failure? *Lancet* 2: 75–79, 1972.

1865. Strauss, J., Beran, A. V., and Baker, R.   Continuous O_2 monitoring of new-born and older infants and of children. *J. Appl. Physiol.* 33:238–243, 1972.

1866. Strauss, M. B., Lee, W. S., and Cantrell, R. W.   Serous otitis media in divers breathing 100% oxygen. *Aerosp. Med.* 45:434–437, 1974.

1867. Strieder, D. J., Murphy, R., and Kazemi, H.   Mechanism of postural hypoxemia in asymptomatic smokers. *Am. Rev. Respir. Dis.* 99:760–766, 1969.

1868. String, T., Robinson, A. J., and Blaisdell, F. W.   Massive trauma. Effect of intravascular coagulation on prognosis. *Arch. Surg.* 102:406–410, 1971.

1869. Stromme, W. B., and Wagner, R. M.   Bleeding from other than major obstetric causes. *Clin. Obstet. Gynecol.* 3:616–636, 1960.

1870. Strunin, L., Ward, M. E., Weston, M. J., Smith, M. G. M., and Williams, R.   Development of a New Liver Failure Unit and the Particular Problem of Cardio-respiratory Emergencies. Scientific abstracts, First World Congress on Intensive Care, London, England, June 24–27, 1974. P. 7.

1871. Struxness, D. F.   Cardiac Output by Non-invasive Technique. Abstracts of scientific papers, Annual Meeting of American Society of Anesthesiologists, Washington, D.C., October 12–16, 1974. Pp. 111–112.

1872. Sturm, J. T., Strate, R. G., Mowlem, A., Quattlebaum, F. W., and Perry, J. F., Jr.   Blunt trauma to the subclavian artery. *Surg. Gynecol. Obstet.* 138:915–918, 1974.

1873. Sugerman, H. J., Berkowitz, H. D., Davidson, D. T., and Miller, L. D.   Treatment of the hepatorenal syndrome with metaraminol. *Surg. Forum* 21:359–361, 1970.

1874. Sugerman, H. J., Davidson, D. T., Vibul, S., Delivoria-Papadopoulos, M., Miller, L. D., and Oski, F. A.   The basis of defective oxygen delivery from stored blood. *Surg. Gynecol. Obstet.* 131:733–741, 1970.

1875. Sugerman, H. J., Miller, L. D., Oski, F. A., Diaco, J., Delivoria-Papadopoulos, M., and Davidson, D.   Decreased 2,3-diphosphoglycerate (DPG) and reduced oxygen (O_2) consumption in septic shock. *Clin. Res.* 18:418, 1970.

1876. Sugg, W. L., Craver, W. D., Webb, W. R., and Ecker, R. R.   Pressure changes in the dog lung secondary to hemorrhagic shock: Protective effect of reimplantation. *Ann. Surg.* 169:592–598, 1969.

1877. Sugg, W. L., Rea, W. J., Ecker, R. R., Webb, W. R., Rose, E. F., and Shaw, R. R.   Penetrating wounds of the heart. An analysis of 459 cases. *J. Thorac. Cardiovasc. Surg.* 56:531–543, 1968.

1878. Sugg, W. L., Webb, W. R., and Ecker, R. R.   Prevention of lesions of the lung secondary to hemorrhagic shock. *Surg. Gynecol. Obstet.* 127:1005–1010, 1968.

1879. Sullivan, R. D.   Continuous arterial infusion cancer chemotherapy. *Surg. Clin. North Am.* 42:365–388, 1962.

1880. Suter, P. M., Fairley, H. B., and Isenberg, M. D.   Optimum end-expiratory airway pressure in patients with acute pulmonary failure. *N. Engl. J. Med.* 292:284–289, 1975.

1881. Suter, P. M., Fairley, H. B., and Schlobohm, R. M.   The response of lung volume and pulmonary perfusion to short periods of 100% oxygen ventilation in acute respiratory failure. *Crit. Care Med.* 2:43–44, 1974.

1882. Suter, P. M., Lindauer, J. M., Fairley, H. B., and Schlobohm, R. M.   The Swan-Ganz catheter: Criteria for wedging. *Crit. Care Med.* 1:119, 1973.

1883. Suwa, K., Hedley-Whyte, J., and Bendixen, H. H.   Circulation and physiologic dead space changes on controlling the ventilation of dogs. *J. Appl. Physiol.* 21:1855–1859, 1966.

1884. Swan, H.   Clinical hypothermia: A lady with a past and some promise for the future. *Surgery* 73:736–758, 1973.

1885. Swan, H. J. C., Ganz, W., Forrester, J., Marcus, H., Diamond, G., and

Chonette, D.   Catheterization of the heart in man with use of a flow-directed balloon-tipped catheter. *N. Engl. J. Med.* 283:447–451, 1970.

1886. Swank, R. L.   Alteration of blood on storage: Measurement of adhesiveness of "aging" platelets and leukocytes and their removal by filtration. *N. Engl. J. Med.* 265:728–733, 1961.
1887. Swank, R. L.   Adhesiveness of platelets and leukocytes during acute exsanguination. *Am. J. Physiol.* 202:261–264, 1962.
1888. Swank, R. L.   Platelet aggregation: Its role and cause in surgical shock. *J. Trauma* 8:872–879, 1968.
1889. Swank, R. L., and Edwards, M. J.   Microvascular occlusion by platelet emboli after transfusion and shock. *Microvasc. Res.* 1:15–22, 1968.
1890. Swank, R. L., Hissen, W., and Bergentz, S. E.   5-Hydroxytryptamine and aggregation of blood elements after trauma. *Surg. Gynecol. Obstet.* 119:779–784, 1964.
1891. Swank, R. L., Roth, J. G., and Jansen, J.   Screen filtration pressure method and adhesiveness and aggregation of blood cells. *J. Appl. Physiol.* 19:340–346, 1964.
1892. Swann, H. G., Brucer, M., Moore, C., and Vezien, B. L.   Fresh water and sea water drowning: A study of the terminal cardiac and biochemical events. *Tex. Rep. Biol. Med.* 5:423–437, 1947.
1893. Swann, H. G., and Spafford, N. R.   Body salt and water changes during fresh and sea water drowning. *Tex. Rep. Biol. Med.* 9:356–382, 1951.
1894. Sykes, M. K., Young, W. E., and Robinson, B. E.   Oxygenation during anaesthesia with controlled ventilation. *Br. J. Anaesth.* 37:314–325, 1965.
1895. Szidon, J. P., Pietra, G. G., and Fishman, A. P.   The alveolar-capillary membrane and pulmonary edema. *N. Engl. J. Med.* 286:1200–1204, 1972.
1896. Takala, I., and Niinikoski, J.   Role of lysosomal damage in the development of pulmonary oxygen poisoning. *Acta Chir. Scand.* 140:167–170, 1974.
1897. Talley, R. C., and Beller, B. M.   Dopamine in low resistance human shock. *Circulation* 43, 44(Suppl. II):232, 1971.
1898. Talley, R. C., Goldberg, L. I., Johnson, C. E., and McNay, J. L.   A hemodynamic comparison of dopamine and isoproterenol in patients in shock. *Circulation* 39:361–378, 1969.
1899. Taplin, D., and Mertz, P. M.   Flower vases in hospitals as reservoirs of pathogens. *Lancet* 2:1279–1281, 1973.
1900. Tarhan, S., Moffitt, E. A., Taylor, W. F., and Giuliani, E. R.   Myocardial infarction after general anesthesia. *J.A.M.A.* 220:1451–1454, 1972.
1901. Tatelman, M., and Sheehan, S.   Total vertebral-basilar arteriography via transbrachial catheterization. *Radiology* 78:919–929, 1962.
1902. Taylor, A. E., and Gaar, K. A., Jr.   Estimation of equivalent pore radii of pulmonary capillary and alveolar membranes. *Am. J. Physiol.* 218:1133–1140, 1970.
1903. Taylor, G., and Pryse-Davies, J.   The prophylactic use of antacids in the prevention of the acid-pulmonary-aspiration syndrome (Mendelson's syndrome). *Lancet* 1:288–291, 1966.
1904. Taylor, G., and Pryse-Davies, J.   Evaluation of endotracheal steroid therapy in acid pulmonary aspiration syndrome (Mendelson's syndrome). *Anesthesiology* 29:17–21, 1968.
1905. Taylor, S. H., Sutherland, G. R., MacKenzie, G. J., Staunton, H. P., and Donald, K. W.   The circulatory effects of intravenous phentolamine in man. *Circulation* 31:741–754, 1965.
1906. Teabeaut, J. R., II.   Aspiration of gastric contents. An experimental study. *Am. J. Pathol.* 28:51–68, 1952.

1907. Tector, A. J., Reuben, C. F., Hoffman, J. F., Gelfand, E. T., Keelan, M., and Worman, L. Coronary artery wounds treated with saphenous vein bypass grafts. *J.A.M.A.* 225:282–284, 1973.

1908. Teichholz, L. E., Cohen, M. V., Sonnenblick, E. H., and Gorlin, R. Study of left ventricular geometry and function by B-scan ultrasonography in patients with and without asynergy. *N. Engl. J. Med.* 291:1220–1226, 1974.

1909. Teplitz, C., Davis, D., Mason, A. D., and Moncrief, J. A. *Pseudomonas* burn wound sepsis. I. Pathogenesis of experimental *Pseudomonas* burn wound sepsis. *J. Surg. Res.* 4:200–222, 1964.

1910. Teplitz, C., Epstein, B. S., Rose, L. R., and Moncrief, J. A. Necrotizing tracheitis induced by tracheostomy tube. *Arch. Pathol.* 77:6–19, 1964.

1911. Teplitz, C., Epstein, B. S., Rose, L. R., Switzer, W. E., and Moncrief, J. A. Pathology of low tracheostomy in children. *Am. J. Clin. Pathol.* 42:58–63, 1964.

1912. Teres, D. ICU-acquired pneumonia due to *Flavobacterium meningosepticum*. *J.A.M.A.* 228:732, 1974.

1913. Teres, D., Roizen, M. F., and Bushnell, L. S. Successful weaning from controlled ventilation despite high deadspace-to-tidal volume ratio. *Anesthesiology* 39:656–659, 1973.

1914. Teres, D., Schweers, P., Bushnell, L. S., Hedley-Whyte, J., and Feingold, D. S. Sources of *Pseudomonas aeruginosa* infection in a respiratory/surgical intensive-therapy unit. *Lancet* 1:415–417, 1973.

1915. Terman, J. W., and Newton, J. L. Changes in alveolar and arterial gas tensions as related to altitude and age. *J. Appl. Physiol.* 19:21–24, 1964.

1916. Thaning, N. O., and Hinder, R. A. Penetrating stab wounds of the heart—Experience with 23 cases. *S. Afr. J. Surg.* 11:209–212, 1973.

1917. Thomas, A. N., and Hall, A. D. Mechanism of pulmonary injury after oxygen therapy. *Am. J. Surg.* 120:255–262, 1970.

1918. Thompson, H. L., and Decker, W. J. Analysis of blood. A simplified gas chromatographic approach for toxicologic purposes. *Am. J. Clin. Pathol.* 49:103–107, 1968.

1919. Thoren, L. Post-operative pulmonary complications. Observations on their prevention by means of physiotherapy. *Acta Chir. Scand.* 107:193–205, 1954.

1920. Thornton, D., Ponhold, H., Butler, J., Morgan, T., and Cheney, F. W. Effects of pattern of ventilation on pulmonary metabolism and mechanics. *Anesthesiology* 42:4–10, 1975.

1921. Tierney, D. F. Lung metabolism and biochemistry. *Annu. Rev. Physiol.* 36:209–231, 1974.

1922. Tierney, D. F. Intermediary metabolism of the lung. *Fed. Proc.* 33:2232–2237, 1974.

1923. Tierney, D. F., Ayers, L., Herzog, S., and Yang, J. Pentose pathway and production of reduced nicotinamide adenine dinucleotide phosphate. A mechanism that may protect lungs from oxidants. *Am. Rev. Respir. Dis.* 108:1348–1351, 1973.

1924. Tillotson, J. R., and Finland, M. Bacterial colonization and clinical superinfection of the respiratory tract complicating antibiotic treatment of pneumonia. *J. Infect. Dis.* 119:597–624, 1969.

1925. Tilney, N. L., Bailey, G. L., and Morgan, A. P. Sequential system failure after rupture of abdominal aortic aneurysms: An unsolved problem in postoperative care. *Ann. Surg.* 178:117–122, 1973.

1926. Tinstman, T. C., Dines, D. E., and Arms, R. A. Postoperative aspiration pneumonia. *Surg. Clin. North Am.* 53:859–862, 1973.

1927. Todres, I. D., Ryan, J. F., and Rogers, M. C. Percutaneous Radial Artery

Cannulation in the Newborn Infant. Abstracts of scientific papers, Annual Meeting of the American Society of Anesthesiologists, Washington, D.C., October 12–16, 1974. P. 299.

1928. Tolman, K. G., and Cohen, A.   Accidental hypothermia. *Can. Med. Assoc. J.* 103:1357–1361, 1970.

1929. Toothill, C.   The chemistry of the in vivo reaction between haemoglobin and various oxides of nitrogen. *Br. J. Anaesth.* 39:405–412, 1967.

1930. Topkins, M. J., and Artusio, J. F., Jr.   Myocardial infarction and surgery. A five year study. *Anesth. Analg.* (Cleve.) 43:716–720, 1964.

1931. Toren, M., Goffinet, J. A., and Kaplow, L. S.   Pulmonary bed sequestration of neutrophils during hemodialysis. *Blood* 36:337–340, 1970.

1932. Tovell, R. M., and D'Ambruoso, D. C.   Humidity in inhalation therapy. *Anesthesiology* 23:452–459, 1962.

1933. Towne, W. D., Geiss, W. P., Yanes, H. O., and Rahimtoola, S. H.   Intractable ventricular fibrillation associated with profound accidental hypothermia— Successful treatment with partial cardiopulmonary bypass. *N. Engl. J. Med.* 287:1135–1136, 1972.

1934. Travis, K. W., Carson, H. S., III, Uhl, R. R., and Bendixen, H. H.   Report on the first year's activities of a multidisciplinary respiratory intensive care unit. *Crit. Care Med.* 1:235–238, 1973.

1935. Travis, S. F., Sugerman, H. J., Rugberg, R. L., Dudrick, S. J., Delivoria-Papadopoulos, M., Miller, L. D., and Oski, F. A.   Alterations of red-cell glycolytic intermediates and oxygen transport as a consequence of hypophosphatemia in patients receiving intravenous hyperalimentation. *N. Engl. J. Med.* 285:763–768, 1971.

1936. Trey, C., Burns, D. G., and Saunders, S. J.   Treatment of hepatic coma by exchange blood transfusion. *N. Engl. J. Med.* 274:473–481, 1966.

1937. Trey, C., and Davidson, C. S.   The Management of Fulminant Hepatic Failure. In H. Popper and F. Schaffner (Eds.), *Progress in Liver Diseases.* New York: Grune & Stratton, 1970. Vol. III, pp. 282–298.

1938. Trichet, B., Falke, K., Togut, A., and Laver, M. B.   The effect of pre-existing pulmonary vascular disease on the response to mechanical ventilation with PEEP following open-heart surgery. *Anesthesiology* 42:56–67, 1975.

1939. Tristani, F. E., and Cohn, J. N.   Studies in clinical shock and hypotension. VII. Renal hemodynamics before and during treatment. *Circulation* 42:839–851, 1970.

1940. Troupp, H.   Intraventricular pressure in patients with severe brain injuries. *J. Trauma* 7:875–883, 1967.

1941. Trubuhovich, R. V., and Spence, M.   Treatment of Acute Brain Swelling. Scientific abstracts, First World Congress on Intensive Care, London, England, June 24–27, 1974. Pp. 85–86.

1942. Truscott, D. G., Firor, W. B., and Clein, L. J.   Accidental profound hypothermia. Successful resuscitation by core rewarming and assisted circulation. *Arch. Surg.* 106:216–218, 1973.

1943. Tschudy, D. P.   Porphyrin Metabolism and the Porphyrias. In P. K. Bondy and L. E. Rosenberg (Eds.), *Duncan's Diseases of Metabolism.* Vol. 1, *Genetics and Metabolism* (7th ed.). Philadelphia: Saunders, 1974. Pp. 775–824a.

1944. Tucker, A. D., Wyatt, J. H., and Undery, D.   Clearance of inhaled particles from alveoli by normal interstitial drainage pathways. *J. Appl. Physiol.* 35:719–732, 1973.

1945. Tucker, D. H., and Sieker, H. O.   The effect of change in body position on lung volumes and intrapulmonary gas mixing in patients with obesity, heart failure and emphysema. *Am. Rev. Respir. Dis.* 82:787–791, 1960.

1946. Tullis, J. L., and Lionetti, F. J.   Preservation of blood by freezing. *Anesthesiology* 27:483–493, 1966.

1947. Turell, D. J., Austin, R. C., and Alexander, J. K.   Cardiorespiratory response of very obese subjects to treadmill exercise. *J. Lab. Clin. Med.* 64:107–116, 1964.

1948. Turner, J. M., Mead, J., and Wohl, M. E.   Elasticity of human lungs in relation to age. *J. Appl. Physiol.* 25:664–671, 1968.

1949. Turney, S. Z., Labrosse, E., Paul, R., McAslan, T. C., Dunn, J., and Cowley, R. A.   The sympathetic response in head trauma: Catecholamine and cardiopulmonary changes upon altering Pco_2. *Ann. Surg.* 177:86–92, 1973.

1950. Turnier, E., Hill, J. D., Kerth, W. J., and Gerbode, F.   Massive pulmonary embolism. *Am. J. Surg.* 125:611–622, 1973.

1951. Tyberg, J. V., Keon, W. J., Sonnenblick, E. H., and Urschel, C. W.   Effectiveness of intra-aortic balloon counterpulsation in the experimental low output state. *Am. Heart J.* 80:89–95, 1970.

1952. Tyler, W. S., and Pearse, A. G. E.   Oxidative enzymes of the interalveolar septum of the rat. *Thorax* 20:149–152, 1965.

1953. Tysinger, D. S., Jr.   Common misconceptions in inhalation therapy. I. Humidity. II. Particulate water. *J. Med. Assoc. State Ala.* 40:439–445, 503–510, 1971.

1954. Udhoji, V. N., and Weil, M. H.   Hemodynamic and metabolic studies on shock associated with bacteremia. Observations on 16 patients. *Ann. Intern. Med.* 62:966–978, 1965.

1955. U. S. Department of Health, Education, and Welfare, Public Health Service.   Smoking and Health: Report of the Advisory Committee to the Surgeon General of the Public Health Service. Publication no. 1103. Washington, D.C., 1964.

1956. U.S. Department of Health, Education, and Welfare, Public Health Service.   The Health Consequences of Smoking: A Public Health Service Review. Publication no. 1696. Washington, D.C., 1967.

1957. U.S. Department of Health, Education, and Welfare, Public Health Service, National Communicable Disease Center. Botulism in the United States: Review of Cases 1899–1967 and Handbook for Epidemiologists, Clinicians, and Laboratory Workers. Atlanta, 1968.

1958. U.S. Department of Health, Education, and Welfare, Public Health Service, Center for Disease Control.   National Nosocomial Infections Study. DHEW Publication No. (HSM) 73–8226. Washington, D.C., 1973. Pp. 2–26.

1959. U.S. Department of Health, Education, and Welfare, Public Health Service.   Vital Statistics of the United States, 1969. Vol. II. Mortality, Part A. Rockville, Md.: National Center for Health Statistics, 1974. Pp. 122–123.

1960. U.S. Department of Health, Education, and Welfare, Public Health Service.   Vital Statistics of the United States, 1971. Vol. II. Mortality, Part A. Rockville, Md.: National Center for Health Statistics, 1974.

1961. U.S. Government, National Heart and Lung Institute, Division of Lung Disease, National Institutes of Health.   Protocol for Extracorporeal Support for Respiratory Insufficiency. Collaborative Program. Washington, D.C., February 10, 1974.

1962. Urabe, M., Segawa, Y., Tsubokawa, T., Yamamoto, K., Araki, K., and Izumi, K.   Pathogenesis of the acute pulmonary edema occurring after brain operations and brain trauma. *Jpn. Heart J.* 2:147–169, 1961.

1963. Urban, B. J., and Weitzner, S. W.   Avoidance of hypoxemia during endotracheal suction. *Anesthesiology* 31:473–475, 1969.

1964. Urschel, C. W., Eber, L., Forrester, J., Matloff, J., Carpenter, R., and Sonnenblick, E.   Alteration of mechanical performance of the ventricle by intraaortic balloon counterpulsation. *Am. J. Cardiol.* 25:546–551, 1970.

1965. Uzawa, T., and Ashbaugh, D. G. Continuous positive-pressure breathing in acute hemorrhagic pulmonary edema. *J. Appl. Physiol.* 26:427–432, 1969.

1966. Vago, T., and Jhirad, A. Mechanism of rupture of the unscarred uterus. *Am. J. Obstet. Gynecol.* 113:848–849, 1972.

1967. Valeri, C. R., and Collins, F. B. Physiologic effects of 2,3-DPG-depleted red cells with high affinity for oxygen. *J. Appl. Physiol.* 31:823–827, 1971.

1968. Valeri, C. R., and Collins, F. B. The physiologic effect of transfusing preserved red cells with low 2,3-diphosphoglycerate and high affinity for oxygen. *Vox Sang.* 20:397–403, 1971.

1969. Valeri, C. R., and Hirsch, N. M. Restoration in vivo of erythrocyte adenosine triphosphate, 2,3-diphosphoglycerate, potassium ion, and sodium ion concentrations following the transfusion of acid-citrate-dextrose-stored human red blood cells. *J. Lab. Clin. Med.* 73:722–733, 1969.

1970. Valeri, C. R., and Zaroulis, C. G. Rejuvenation and freezing of outdated stored human red cells. *N. Engl. J. Med.* 287:1307–1313, 1972.

1971. Välimäki, M., Kivisaari, J., and Niinikoski, J. Permeability of alveolar-capillary membrane in oxygen poisoning. *Aerosp. Med.* 45:370–374, 1974.

1972. Välimäki, M., and Niinikoski, J. Development and reversibility of pulmonary oxygen poisoning in the rat. *Aerosp. Med.* 44:533–538, 1973.

1973. Valtis, D. J., and Kennedy, A. C. The causes and prevention of defective function of stored red blood cells after transfusion. *Glasgow Med. J.* 34:521–543, 1953.

1974. Valtis, D. J., and Kennedy, A. C. Defective gas-transport function of stored red blood cells. *Lancet* 1:119–124, 1954.

1975. Van Bergen, F. H., and Buckley, J. J. Management of severe systemic tetanus. *Anesthesiology* 13:599–604, 1952.

1976. Vandam, L. D. Aspiration of gastric contents in the operative period. *N. Engl. J. Med.* 273:1206–1208, 1965.

1977. Vandam, L. D., and Moore, F. D. Adrenocortical mechanisms related to anesthesia. *Anesthesiology* 21:531–552, 1960.

1978. Van De Water, J. M., Kagey, K. S., Miller, I. T., Parker, D. A., O'Connor, N. E., Sheh, J.-M., MacArthur, J. D., Zollinger, R. M., Jr., and Moore, F. D. Response of the lung to six to 12 hours of 100 per cent oxygen inhalation in normal man. *N. Engl. J. Med.* 283:621–626, 1970.

1979. Van De Water, J. M., Miller, I. T., Milne, E. N. C., Hanson, E. L., Sheldon, G. F., and Kagey, K. S. Impedance plethysmography. A noninvasive means of monitoring the thoracic surgery patient. *J. Thorac. Cardiovasc. Surg.* 60:641–647, 1970.

1980. Van De Water, J. M., Watring, W. G., Linton, L. A., Murphy, M., and Byron, R. L. Prevention of postoperative pulmonary complications. *Surg. Gynecol. Obstet.* 135:229–233, 1972.

1981. Van Hemert, P., Kilburn, D. G., Righelato, R. C., and Van Wezel, A. L. A steam-sterilizable electrode of the galvanic type for the measurement of dissolved oxygen. *Biotechnol. Bioeng.* 11:549–560, 1969.

1982. Vapalahti, M., and Troupp, H. Prognosis for patients with severe brain injuries. *Br. Med. J.* 3:404–407, 1971.

1983. Vatner, S. F., Higgins, C. B., and Braunwald, E. Effects of norepinephrine on coronary circulation and left ventricular dynamics in the conscious dog. *Circ. Res.* 34:812–823, 1974.

1984. Vatner, S. F., McRitchie, R. J., and Braunwald, E. Effects of dobutamine on left ventricular performance, coronary dynamics, and distribution of cardiac output in conscious dogs. *J. Clin. Invest.* 53:1265–1273, 1974.

1985. Vatner, S. F., McRitchie, R. J., Maroko, P. R., Patrick, T. A., and Braunwald, E. Effects of catecholamines, exercise, and nitroglycerin on the normal and ischemic myocardium in conscious dogs. *J. Clin. Invest.* 54:563–575, 1974.

1986. Vaughan, R. W., and Weygandt, G. R. Reliable percutaneous central venous pressure measurement. *Anesth. Analg.* (Cleve.) 52:709–716, 1973.

1987. Vaughn, D. L., Gunter, C. A., and Stookey, J. L. Endotoxin shock in primates. *Surg. Gynecol. Obstet.* 126:1309–1317, 1968.

1988. Veasy, L. G., Clark, J. S., Jung, A. L., and Jenkins, J. L. A system for computerized automated blood gas analysis: Its use in newborn infants with respiratory distress. *Pediatrics* 48:5–17, 1971.

1989. Verstraete, M., Vermylen, J., and Collen, D. Intravascular coagulation in liver disease. *Annu. Rev. Med.* 25:447–455, 1974.

1990. Victor, M. The role of hypomagnesemia and respiratory alkalosis in the genesis of alcohol-withdrawal symptoms. *Ann. N.Y. Acad. Sci.* 215:235–248, 1973.

1991. Victor, M., and Adams, R. D. Delirium Tremens. In M. M. Wintrobe et al. (Eds.), *Harrison's Principles of Internal Medicine* (7th ed.). New York: McGraw-Hill, 1974. Pp. 676–678.

1992. Vilinskas, J., Schweizer, R. T., and Foster, J. H. Experimental studies on aspiration of contents of obstructed intestine. *Surg. Gynecol. Obstet.* 135:568–570, 1972.

1993. Vinnars, E. Recent advances in parenteral nutrition. *Crit. Care Med.* 2:143–151, 1974.

1994. Vinnars, E., Fürst, P., Hermansson, I. L., Josephson, B., and Lindholmer, B. Protein catabolism in the postoperative state and its treatment with amino acid solution. *Acta Chir. Scand.* 136:95–109, 1970.

1995. Visick, W. D., Fairley, H. B., and Hickey, R. F. The effects of tidal volume and end-expiratory pressure on pulmonary gas exchange during anesthesia. *Anesthesiology* 39:285–290, 1973.

1996. Vito, L., Dennis, R. C., Weisel, R. D., and Hechtman, H. B. Sepsis presenting as acute respiratory insufficiency. *Surg. Gynecol. Obstet.* 138:896–900, 1974.

1997. Vladeck, B. C., Bassin, R., Kim, S. I., and Shoemaker, W. C. Burn pathophysiology in man. II. Sequential oxygen transport and acid base alterations. *J. Surg. Res.* 14:74–79, 1973.

1998. Vogel, C. M., Kingsbury, R. J., and Baue, A. E. Intravenous hyperalimentation. A review of two and one-half years' experience. *Arch. Surg.* 105:414–419, 1972.

1999. Vogel, J. M., and Vogel, P. Transfusion of blood components. *Anesthesiology* 27:363–373, 1966.

2000. Voss, H. J., Macnicol, M. F., Saravis, C. A., Altug, K., and Clowes, G. H. A., Jr. The pathogenesis of pneumonitis in sepsis. *Surg. Forum* 22:27–29, 1971.

2001. Voukydis, P. C., and Cohen, S. I. Catheter induced arrhythmias. *Am. Heart J.* 88:588–592, 1974.

2002. Waddell, W. G., Fairley, H. B., and Bigelow, W. G. Improved management of clinical hypothermia based upon related biochemical studies. *Ann. Surg.* 146:542–559, 1957.

2003. Wagner, P. D., Laravuso, R. B., Uhl, R. R., and West, J. B. Continuous distributions of ventilation-perfusion ratios in normal subjects breathing air and 100% O_2. *J. Clin. Invest.* 54:54–68, 1974.

2004. Wahrenbrock, E. A., Carrico, C. J., Amundsen, D. A., Trummer, M. J., and Severinghaus, J. W. Increased atelectatic pulmonary shunt during hemorrhagic shock in dogs. *J. Appl. Physiol.* 29:615–621, 1970.

2005. Waisbren, B. A.   Gram-negative shock and endotoxin shock. *Am. J. Med.* 36: 819–824, 1964.

2006. Wald, A., Hass, W. K., Siew, F. P., and Wood, D. H.   Continuous measurement of blood gases in vivo by mass spectrography. *Med. Biol. Eng.* 8: 111–128, 1970.

2007. Wald, A., Jason, D., Murphy, T. W., and Mazzia, V. D. B.   A computer system for respiratory parameters. *Comput. Biomed. Res.* 2: 411–429, 1969.

2008. Waldenström, J., and Haeger-Aronsen, B.   Different patterns of human porphyria. *Br. Med. J.* 2: 272–276, 1963.

2009. Walder, A. I., Summerlin, W. T., Mason, A. D., Foley, F. D., and Moncreif, J. A.   Respiratory complications in the acutely burned patient. *Milit. Med.* 132: 379–384, 1967.

2010. Walinsky, P., Chatterjee, K., Forrester, J. S., Parmley, W. W., and Swan, H. J. C.   Enhanced left ventricular performance with phentolamine in acute myocardial infarction. *Am. J. Cardiol.* 33: 37–41, 1974.

2011. Walker, W. J.   Treatment of heart failure. *J.A.M.A.* 228: 1276–1278, 1974.

2012. Wallace, C. T., Marks, W. E., Jr., Adkins, W. Y., and Mahaffey, J. E.   Perforation of the tympanic membrane, a complication of tympanic thermometry during anesthesia. *Anesthesiology* 41: 290–291, 1974.

2013. Wallace, J. E., and Dahl, E. V.   The determination of amitriptyline by ultraviolet spectrophotometry. *J. Forensic Sci.* 12: 484–496, 1967.

2014. Walley, R. V.   Control of artificial respiration in poliomyelitis patients with paralysis of swallowing. *Lancet* 2: 1143–1145, 1957.

2015. Walston, A., II, and Kendall, M. E.   Comparison of pulmonary wedge and left atrial pressure in man. *Am. Heart J.* 86: 159–164, 1973.

2016. Waltemath, C. L., and Bergman, N. A.   Increased respiratory resistance provoked by endotracheal administration of aerosols. *Am. Rev. Respir. Dis.* 108: 520–525, 1973.

2017. Waltemath, C. L., and Bergman, N. A.   Respiratory compliance in obese patients. *Anesthesiology* 41: 84–85, 1974.

2018. Waltemath, C. L., Erbguth, P. H., and Sunderland, W. A.   Increased respiratory resistance after ultrasonic humidification of anesthesia gas. *Anesthesiology* 39: 547–549, 1973.

2019. Waltemath, C. L., and Preuss, D. D.   Determination of blood pressure in low-flow states by the Doppler technique. *Anesthesiology* 34: 77–79, 1971.

2020. Walters, M. B., Stranger, H. A. D., and Rotem, C. E.   Complications with percutaneous central venous catheters. *J.A.M.A.* 220: 1455–1457, 1972.

2021. Wangensteen, S. L., Geissinger, W. T., Lovett, W. L., Glenn, T. M., and Lefer, A. M.   Relationship between splanchnic blood flow and a myocardial depressant factor in endotoxin shock. *Surgery* 69: 410–418, 1971.

2022. Wanner, A., Landa, J. F., Nieman, R. E., Jr., Vevaina, J., and Delgado, I.   Bedside bronchofiberscopy for atelectasis and lung abscess. *J.A.M.A.* 224: 1281–1283, 1973.

2023. Ward, B. D., and Hood, A. G.   Annual Report: Membrane Oxygenator Comparison. Salt Lake City: Utah Biomedical Test Laboratory, 1973.

2024. Ward, R. J., Danziger, F., Bonica, J. J., Allen, G. D., and Bowes, J.   An evaluation of postoperative respiratory maneuvers. *Surg. Gynecol. Obstet.* 123: 51–54, 1966.

2025. Ward, R. J., and Green, H. D.   Arterial puncture as a safe diagnostic aid. *Surgery* 57: 672–675, 1965.

2026. Ware, H. H., Jr.   Bleeding and hemorrhage in late pregnancy. Rupture of the uterus. *Clin. Obstet. Gynecol.* 3: 637–645, 1960.

2027. Ware, H. H., Jr., Jarrett, A. Q., and Reda, F. A. Rupture of the gravid uterus. Report of 40 cases. *Am. J. Obstet. Gynecol.* 76:181–187, 1958.

2028. Ware, R. W., Laenger, C. J., Sr., Heath, C. A., and Crosby, R. J. Development of an ultrasonic indirect blood pressure sensing technique for aerospace application. AMRL-TR-67-201, Vol. 1. Aerospace Medical Research Laboratories, Aerospace Medical Division, Air Force Systems Command, Wright-Patterson Air Force Base, Ohio, July 1968.

2029. Warmolts, J. R., and Engel, W. K. Benefit from alternate-day prednisone in myasthenia gravis. *N. Engl. J. Med.* 286:17–20, 1972.

2030. Warner, H. R. Experiences with computer-based patient monitoring. *Anesth. Analg.* (Cleve.) 47:453–462, 1968.

2031. Warner, H. R., Gardner, R. M., and Toronto, A. F. Computer-based monitoring of cardiovascular functions in postoperative patients. *Circulation* 37(Suppl. 2):68–74, 1968.

2032. Warner, H. R., Swan, H. J. C., Connolly, D. C., Tompkins, R. G., and Wood, E. H. Quantitation of beat-to-beat changes in stroke volume from the aortic pulse contour in man. *J. Appl. Physiol.* 5:495–507, 1953.

2033. Warner, H. R., and Wood, E. H. Simplified calculation of cardiac output from dye dilution curves recorded by oximeter. *J. Appl. Physiol.* 5:111–116, 1952.

2034. Watanabe, T., Covell, J. W., Maroko, P. R., Braunwald, E., and Ross, J., Jr. Effects of increased arterial pressure and positive inotropic agents on the severity of myocardial ischemia in the acutely depressed heart. *Am. J. Cardiol.* 30:371–377, 1972.

2035. Waterhouse, K., and Gross, M. Trauma to the genitourinary tract: A 5-year experience with 251 cases. *J. Urol.* 101:241–246, 1969.

2036. Waters, E. G., and Hall, W. M. Rupture of the uterus in late pregnancy. Changing concepts based upon studies of 50 cases. *Obstet. Gynecol.* 20:585–593, 1962.

2037. Watson, W. E. Some circulatory responses to Valsalva's manoeuvre in patients with polyneuritis and spinal cord disease. *J. Neurol. Neurosurg. Psychiatry* 24:19–23, 1962.

2038. Webb, G. E. Comparison of esophageal and tympanic temperature monitoring during cardiopulmonary bypass. *Anesth. Analg.* (Cleve.) 52:729–733, 1973.

2039. Webre, D. R., and Arens, J. F. Use of cephalic and basilic veins for introduction of central venous catheters. *Anesthesiology* 38:389–392, 1973.

2040. Weenig, C. S., Pietak, S., Hickey, R. F., and Fairley, H. B. Relationship of preoperative closing volume to functional residual capacity and alveolar-arterial oxygen difference during anesthesia with controlled ventilation. *Anesthesiology* 41:3–7, 1974.

2041. Weil, M. H., Shubin, H., and Biddle, M. Shock caused by gram-negative micro-organisms. Analysis of 169 cases. *Ann. Intern. Med.* 60:384–400, 1964.

2042. Weinberger, L. M., Gibbon, M. H., and Gibbon, J. H., Jr. Temporary arrest of the circulation to the central nervous system. I. Physiologic effects. *Arch. Neurol. Psychiatry* 43:615–634, 1940.

2043. Weinberger, L. M., Gibbon, M. H., and Gibbon, J. H., Jr. Temporary arrest of the circulation to the central nervous system. II. Pathologic effects. *Arch. Neurol. Psychiatry* 43:961–986, 1940.

2044. Weiner, A. E., and Reid, D. E. The pathogenesis of amniotic-fluid embolism. III. Coagulant activity of amniotic fluid. *N. Engl. J. Med.* 243:597–598, 1950.

2045. Weinstein, L., Goldfield, M., and Ching, T.-W. Infections occurring during chemotherapy. A study of their frequency, type, and predisposing factors. *N. Engl. J. Med.* 251:247–255, 1954.

2046. Weinstein, L., and Klainer, A. S. Management of emergencies. IV. Septic shock—Pathogenesis and treatment. *N. Engl. J. Med.* 274:950–953, 1966.

2047. Weintraub, R. M., Voukydis, P. C., Aroesty, J. M., Cohen, S. I., Ford, P., Kurland, G. S., LaRaia, P. J., Morkin, E., and Paulin, S. Treatment of preinfarction angina with intraaortic balloon counterpulsation and surgery. *Am. J. Cardiol.* 34:809–814, 1974.

2048. Weir, F. W., Bath, D. W., Yevich, P., and Oberst, F. W. Study of effects of continuous inhalation of high concentrations of oxygen at ambient pressure and temperature. *Aerosp. Med.* 36:117–120, 1965.

2049. Weiskopf, R. B., and Gabel, R. A. Doxapram in Awake Man: Comparison with Hypoxia in Stimulation of Ventilation. Abstracts of scientific papers, Annual Meeting of the American Society of Anesthesiologists, Washington D.C., October 12–16, 1974. Pp. 195–196.

2050. Weisz, G. M., and Barzilai, A. Nonfulminant fat embolism: Review of concepts on its genesis and physiopathology. *Anesth. Analg.* (Cleve.) 52:303–309, 1973.

2051. Welch, B. E., Morgan, T. E., Jr., and Clamann, H. G. Time-concentration effects in relation to oxygen toxicity in man. *Fed. Proc.* 22:1053–1056, 1963.

2052. Wessel, H. U., Paul, M. H., James, G. W., and Grahn, A. R. Limitations of thermal dilution curves for cardiac output determinations. *J. Appl. Physiol.* 30:643–652, 1971.

2053. West, J. B. Causes of carbon dioxide retention in lung disease. *N. Engl. J. Med.* 284:1232–1236, 1971.

2054. West, J. B. Blood flow to the lung and gas exchange. *Anesthesiology* 41:124–138, 1974.

2055. West, J. B. Pulmonary gas exchange in the critically ill patient. *Crit. Care Med.* 2:171–180, 1974.

2056. Wexler, L., and Silverman, J. Traumatic rupture of the innominate artery—A seat belt injury. *N. Engl. J. Med.* 282:1186–1187, 1970.

2057. Whalen, R. E., Starmer, C. F., and McIntosh, H. D. Electrical hazards associated with cardiac pacemaking. *Ann. N.Y. Acad. Sci.* 111:922–931, 1964.

2058. Whaun, J. M., and Oski, F. A. Experience with disseminated intravascular coagulation in a children's hospital. *Can. Med. Assoc. J.* 107:963–967, 1972.

2059. Whelton, A., Snyder, D. S., and Walker, W. G. Acute toxic drug ingestions at the Johns Hopkins Hospital, 1963 through 1970. *Johns Hopkins Med. J.* 132:157–167, 1973.

2060. White, D. C., and Nowell, N. W. The effect of alcohol on the cardiac arrest temperature in hypothermic rats. *Clin. Sci.* 28:395–399, 1965.

2061. White, M. G., and Asch, M. J. Acid base effects of topical mafenide acetate in the burned patient. *N. Engl. J. Med.* 284:1281–1286, 1971.

2062. White, M. K., Shepro, D., and Hechtman, H. B. Pulmonary function and platelet-lung interaction. *J. Appl. Physiol.* 34:697–703, 1973.

2063. Wightman, J. A. K. A prospective survey of the incidence of postoperative pulmonary complications. *Br. J. Surg.* 55:85–91, 1968.

2064. Wilhelmsen, L. Effects on bronchopulmonary symptoms, ventilation, and lung mechanics of abstinence from tobacco smoking. *Scand. J. Respir. Dis.* 48:407–414, 1967.

2065. Wilks, S. S., and Clark, R. T., Jr. Carbon monoxide determinations in postmortem tissues as an aid in determining physiologic status prior to death. *J. Appl. Physiol.* 14:313–320, 1959.

2066. Williams, B. T., Sancho-Fornos, S., Clarke, D. B., Abrams, L. D., and Schenk,

W. G., Jr. Continuous, long-term measurement of cardiac output after open-heart surgery. *Ann. Surg.* 174:357–363, 1971.

2067. Williams, I. M. Central nervous system dysfunction with open heart operations. *Proc. Aust. Assoc. Neurol.* 10:1–6, 1973.

2068. Williams, J. R., and Bonte, F. J. Pulmonary damage in nonpenetrating chest injuries. *Radiol. Clin. North Am.* 1:439–448, 1963.

2069. Williams, M., and Crawford, J. S. Titration of magnesium trisilicate mixture against gastric acid secretion. *Br. J. Anaesth.* 43:783–784, 1971.

2070. Willson, R. A., Hofmann, A. F., and Kuster, G. G. R. Toward an artificial liver. II. Removal of cholephilic anions from dogs with biliary obstruction, by hemoperfusion through charged and uncharged resins. *Gastroenterology* 66:95–107, 1974.

2071. Willson, R. A., Webster, K. H., Hofmann, A. F., and Summerskill, W. H. J. Toward an artificial liver: In vitro removal of unbound and protein-bound plasma compounds related to hepatic failure. *Gastroenterology* 62:1191–1199, 1972.

2072. Willson, R. A., Winch, J., Thompson, R. P. H., and Williams, R. Rapid removal of paracetamol by haemoperfusion through coated charcoal. In-vivo and in-vitro studies in the pig. *Lancet* 1:77–79, 1973.

2073. Wilmore, D. W., and Dudrick, S. J. Growth and development of an infant receiving all nutrients exclusively by vein. *J.A.M.A.* 203:860–864, 1968.

2074. Wilmore, D. W., Moylan, J. A., Bristou, B. F., Mason, A. D., Jr., and Pruitt, B. A., Jr. Anabolic effects of human growth hormone and high caloric feedings following thermal injury. *Surg. Gynecol. Obstet.* 138:875–884, 1974.

2075. Wilmore, D. W., Moylan, J. A., Helmkamp, G. M., and Pruitt, B. A., Jr. Clinical evaluation of a 10% intravenous fat emulsion for parenteral nutrition in thermally injured patients. *Ann. Surg.* 178:503–511, 1973.

2076. Wilson, J. D., and Taswell, H. F. Autotransfusions: Historical review and preliminary report on a new method. *Mayo Clin. Proc.* 43:26–35, 1968.

2077. Wilson, J. W. Treatment or prevention of pulmonary cellular damage with pharmacologic doses of corticosteroid. *Surg. Gynecol. Obstet.* 134:675–681, 1972.

2078. Wilson, J. W. Pulmonary microcirculation. *Crit. Care Med.* 2:186–199, 1974.

2079. Wilson, J. W., Ratliff, N. B., and Hackel, D. B. The lung in hemorrhagic shock. I. In vivo observations of pulmonary microcirculation in cats. *Am. J. Pathol.* 58:337–351, 1970.

2080. Wilson, R. F., Chiscano, A. D., Quadros, E., and Tarver, M. Some observations on 132 patients with septic shock. *Anesth. Analg.* (Cleve.) 46:751–763, 1967.

2081. Wilson, R. F., McCarthy, B., LeBlanc, L. P., and Mammen, E. Respiratory and coagulation changes after uncomplicated fractures. *Arch. Surg.* 106:395–399, 1973.

2082. Wilson, R. F., Sarver, E., and Birks, R. Central venous pressure and blood volume determinations in clinical shock. *Surg. Gynecol. Obstet.* 132:631–636, 1971.

2083. Wilson, R. F., Thal, A. P., Kindling, P. H., Grifka, T., and Ackerman, E. Hemodynamic measurement in septic shock. *Arch. Surg.* 91:121–129, 1965.

2084. Wilson, R. S., and Laver, M. B. Oxygen analysis: Advances in methodology. *Anesthesiology* 37:112–126, 1972.

2085. Wilson, R. S., and Pontoppidan, H. Acute respiratory failure: Diagnostic and therapeutic criteria. *Crit. Care Med.* 2:293–304, 1974.

2086. Wilson, W. R., Martin, W. J., Wilkowske, C. J., and Washington, J. A., II. Anaerobic bacteremia. *Mayo Clin. Proc.* 47:639–646, 1972.

2087. Wingate, M. B.   Fatal pulmonary embolism in pregnancy. *Br. Med. J.* 2:685, 1957.

2088. Winnie, A. P., Gladish, J. T., Angel, J. J., Ramamurthy, S., and Collins, V. J. Chemical respirogenesis. II. Reversal of postoperative hypoxemia with the "pharmacologic sigh." *Anesth. Analg.* (Cleve.) 50:1043–1052, 1971.

2089. Winslow, E. J., Loeb, H. S., Rahimtoola, S. H., Kamath, S., and Gunnar, R. M.   Hemodynamic studies and results of therapy in 50 patients with bacteremic shock. *Am. J. Med.* 54:421–432, 1973.

2090. Winter, P. M., Gupta, R. K., Michalski, A. H., and Lanphier, E. H. Modification of hyperbaric oxygen toxicity by experimental venous admixture. *J. Appl. Physiol.* 23:954–963, 1967.

2091. Winter, P. M., Henry, R. F., Wheelis, R. F., and Pflug, A. E.   The Effect of Corticosteroids on the Rate of Development of Oxygen Toxicity in the Injured and Uninjured Lung. Abstracts of scientific papers, Annual Meeting of the American Society of Anesthesiologists, Washington, D.C., October 12–16, 1974. Pp. 417–418.

2092. Winter, P. M., and Smith, G.   The toxicity of oxygen. *Anesthesiology* 37:210–241, 1972.

2093. Winter, P. M., Smith, G., and Wheelis, R. F.   The effect of prior pulmonary injury on the rate of development of fatal oxygen toxicity. *Chest* 66(Suppl., Pt. 2):1S–4S, 1974.

2094. Winternitz, M. C., Smith, G. H., and McNamara, F. P.   Effect of intrabronchial insufflation of acid. *J. Exp. Med.* 32:199–204, 1920.

2095. Winters, W. D., Mori, K., Spooner, C. E., and Bauer, R. O.   The neurophysiology of anesthesia. *Anesthesiology* 28:65–79, 1967.

2096. Wiot, J. F.   The radiologic manifestations of blunt chest trauma. *J.A.M.A.* 231:500–503, 1975.

2097. Wisch, N., Litwak, R. S., Luckban, S. B., and Glass, J. L.   Hematologic complications of open heart surgery. *Am. J. Cardiol.* 31:282–285, 1973.

2098. Witoszka, M. M., Tamura, H., Indeglia, R., Hopkins, R. W., and Simeone, F. A.   Electroencephalographic changes and cerebral complications in open-heart surgery. *J. Thorac. Cardiovasc. Surg.* 66:855–864, 1973.

2099. Woldring, S., Owens, G., and Woolford, D. C.   Blood gases: Continuous in vivo recording of partial pressures by mass spectrography. *Science* 153:885–887, 1966.

2100. Wolfe, S. M., Mendelson, J., Ogata, M., Victor, M., Marshall, W., and Mello, N.   Respiratory alkalosis and alcohol withdrawal. *Trans. Assoc. Am. Physicians* 82:344–350, 1969.

2101. Wolfe, S. M., and Victor, M.   The relationship of hypomagnesemia and alkalosis to alcohol withdrawal symptoms. *Ann. N.Y. Acad. Sci.* 162:973–984, 1969.

2102. Wolfe, W. G., DeVries, W. C., Anderson, R. W., and Sabiston, D.C., Jr.   Changes in pulmonary capillary filtration and ventilatory dead space during exposure to 95% oxygen. *J. Surg. Res.* 16:312–317, 1974.

2103. Wolfe, W. G., and Ebert, P. A.   Relationship of ventilation and inspired oxygen concentration to mucociliary clearance. *Surg. Forum* 21:217–219, 1970.

2104. Wolfe, W. G., Ebert, P. A., and Sabiston, D.C., Jr.   Effect of high oxygen tension on mucociliary function. *Surgery* 72:246–252, 1972.

2105. Wolfe, W. G., and Sabiston, D. C., Jr.   Lung function in spontaneously breathing and mechanically ventilated dogs exposed to 95% oxygen. *Surg. Gynecol. Obstet.* 137:763–768, 1973.

2106. Wollman, H., Smith, T. C., Stephen, G. W., Colton, E. T., III, Gleaton, H. E., and Alexander, S. C.   Effects of extremes of respiratory and metabolic alkalosis on cerebral blood flow in man. *J. Appl. Physiol.* 24:60–65, 1968.

2107. Woo, S. W., Berlin, D., Büch, U., and Hedley-Whyte, J. Altered perfusion, ventilation, anesthesia and lung-surface forces in dogs. *Anesthesiology* 33:411–418, 1970.

2108. Woo, S. W., and Hedley-Whyte, J. Macrophage accumulation and pulmonary edema due to thoracotomy and lung overinflation. *J. Appl. Physiol.* 33:14–21, 1972.

2109. Woo, S. W., and Hedley-Whyte, J. Oxygen therapy. The titration of a potentially dangerous drug. *Br. J. Hosp. Med.* 9:487–490, 1973.

2110. Worman, L. W., Hurley, J. D., Pemberton, A. H., and Narodick, B. G. Rupture of the esophagus from external blunt trauma. *Arch. Surg.* 85:333–338, 1962.

2111. Wren, H. B., Texada, P. J., and Krementz, E. T. Traumatic rupture of the diaphragm. *J. Trauma* 2:117–125, 1962.

2112. Wright, C. B., and Solis, R. T. Microaggregation in canine autotransfusion. *Am. J. Surg.* 126:25–29, 1973.

2113. Wright, G. P. The use of ATS in the treatment and prophylaxis of tetanus. *Proc. R. Soc. Med.* 51:997–1000, 1958.

2114. Wyche, M. Q., Jr., and Marshall, B. E. Lung function, pulmonary extravascular water volume and hemodynamics in early hemorrhagic shock in anesthetized dogs. *Ann. Surg.* 174:296–303, 1971.

2115. Wyche, M. Q., Jr., Teichner, R. L., Kallos, T., Marshall, B. E., and Smith, T. C. Effects of continuous positive-pressure breathing on functional residual capacity and arterial oxygenation during intra-abdominal operations: Studies in man during nitrous oxide and d-tubocurarine anesthesia. *Anesthesiology* 38:68–74, 1973.

2116. Wyler, F., Forsyth, R. P., Nies, A. S., Neutze, J. M., and Melmon, K. L. Endotoxin-induced regional circulatory changes in the unanesthetized monkey. *Circ. Res.* 24:777–786, 1969.

2117. Yawata, Y., Craddock, R., Hebbel, R., Hone, R., Silvis, S., and Jacob, H. Hyperalimentation hypophosphatemia: Hematologic-neurologic dysfunction due to ATP depletion. *Clin. Res.* 21:729, 1973.

2118. Yeager, H., Jr., Zimmet, S. M., and Schwartz, S. L. Pinocytosis by human alveolar macrophages: Comparison of smokers and nonsmokers. *J. Clin. Invest.* 54:247–251, 1974.

2119. Yeo, M. T., Gazzaniga, A. B., Bartlett, R. H., and Shobe, J. B. Total intravenous nutrition. Experience with fat emulsion and hypertonic glucose. *Arch. Surg.* 106:792–796, 1973.

2120. Yin, E. T., Wessler, S., and Stoll, P. J. Identity of plasma-activated factor X inhibitor with antithrombin III and heparin cofactor. *J. Biol. Chem.* 246:3712–3719, 1971.

2121. Yoshikawa, T., Tanaka, K. R., and Guze, L. B. Infection and disseminated intravascular coagulation. *Medicine* 50:237–258, 1971.

2122. Young, D. S. "Normal laboratory values" (case records of the Massachusetts General Hospital) in SI units. *N. Engl. J. Med.* 292:795–802, 1975.

2123. Yuen, T. G. H., and Sherwin, R. P. Hyperplasia of type 2 pneumocytes and nitrogen dioxide (10 ppm) exposure. A quantitation based on electron photomicrographs. *Arch. Environ. Health* 22:178–188, 1971.

2124. Zapol, W. M., Bloom, S., Carvalho, A., Wonders, T., Skoskiewicz, M., Schneider, R., and Snider, M. Improved platelet economy using filter free silicone rubber in long term membrane perfusion. *Trans. Am. Soc. Artif. Intern. Organs* 21:587–591, 1975.

2125. Zapol, W. M., and Kitz, R. J. Buying time with artificial lungs. *N. Engl. J. Med.* 286:657–658, 1972.

2126. Zapol, W. M., Pontoppidan, H., McCullough, N., Schmidt, V., Bland, J., and Kitz, R. J. Clinical membrane lung support for acute respiratory insufficiency. *Trans. Am. Soc. Artif. Intern. Organs* 18:553–560, 1972.

2127. Zapol, W. M., Schneider, R., Snider, M., and Rie, M. Partial bypass with membrane lungs for acute respiratory failure. *Int. Anesthesiol. Clin.* 14(1):119–133, 1976.

2128. Zarem, H. A., Rattenborg, C. C., and Harmel, M. H. Carbon monoxide toxicity in human fire victims. *Arch. Surg.* 107:851–853, 1973.

2129. Zeidifard, E., Silverman, M., and Godfrey, S. Reproducibility of indirect (CO_2) Fick method for calculation of cardiac output. *J. Appl. Physiol.* 33:141–143, 1972.

2130. Zervas, N. T., and Hedley-Whyte, J. Successful treatment of cerebral herniation in five patients. *N. Engl. J. Med.* 286:1075–1077, 1972.

2131. Zervas, N. T., Hori, H., and Rosoff, C. B. Experimental inhibition of serotonin by antibiotic: Prevention of cerebral vasospasm. *J. Neurosurg.* 41:59–62, 1974.

2132. Zervas, N. T., Kuwayama, A., Rosoff, C. B., and Salzman, E. W. Cerebral arterial spasm: Modification by inhibition of platelet function. *Arch. Neurol.* 28:400–404, 1973.

2133. Zieve, L., and Vogel, W. C. Measurement of lecithinase A in serum and other body fluids. *J. Lab. Clin. Med.* 57:586–599, 1961.

2134. Zikria, B. A., Sturner, W. Q., Astarjian, N. K., Fox, C. L., and Ferrer, J. M., Jr. Respiratory tract damage in burns: Pathophysiology and therapy. *Ann. N.Y. Acad. Sci.* 150:618–626, 1968.

2135. Ziment, I. Why are they saying bad things about IPPB? *Respir. Care* 18:677–689, 1973.

2136. Zimmerman, J. E. Respiratory failure complicating post-traumatic acute renal failure. Etiology, clinical features and management. *Ann. Surg.* 174:12–18, 1971.

2137. Zimmerman, J. E., Dunbar, S. K., and Klingenmaier, C. Management of Patients Developing Subcutaneous Emphysema, Pneumomediastinum and Pneumothorax During Respirator Therapy. Scientific abstracts, First World Congress on Intensive Care, London, England, June 24–27, 1974. P. 73.

2138. Zinner, S. H., and McCabe, W. R. Specific IgG and IgM antibody in gram-negative bacteremia. *J. Clin. Invest.* 53:88a, 1974.

2139. Zivin, I., and Shalowitz, M. Acute toxic reaction to prolonged glutethimide administration. *N. Engl. J. Med.* 266:496–498, 1962.

2140. Zoll, P. M. Countershock and pacemaking in cardiac arrhythmias. *Hosp. Practice* 10(3):125–132, 1975.

2141. Zorab, J. S. M. Continuous display of the arterial pressure. A simple manometric technique. *Anaesthesia* 24:431–437, 1969.

2142. Zucker, M. B., and Lundberg, A. Platelet transfusions. *Anesthesiology* 27:385–398, 1966.

2143. Zumbro, G. L., Jr., Mullin, M. J., and Nelson, T. G. Central venous catheter placement utilizing common facial vein. A technique useful in hyperalimentation and venous pressure monitoring. *Am. J. Surg.* 125:654–656, 1973.

2144. Zuskin, E., Mitchell, C. A., and Bouhuys, A. Interaction between effects of beta blockade and cigarette smoke on airways. *J. Appl. Physiol.* 36:449–452, 1974.

2145. Zweig, R. M. CO levels and auto accidents. *N. Engl. J. Med.* 291:1258, 1974.

Index